Nevirapine and the Quest
to End Pediatric AIDS

Nevirapine and the Quest to End Pediatric AIDS

REBECCA J. ANDERSON

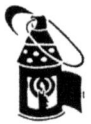

McFarland & Company, Inc., Publishers
Jefferson, North Carolina

LIBRARY OF CONGRESS CATALOGUING-IN-PUBLICATION DATA

Anderson, Rebecca J. (Rebecca Jane), 1949–
Nevirapine and the quest to end pediatric AIDS / Rebecca J. Anderson.
          p.   cm.
Includes bibliographical references and index.

ISBN 978-0-7864-7780-7
softcover : acid free paper ∞

1. HIV infections—Transmission—Prevention.   2. AIDS (Disease) in pregnancy—Transmission—Prevention.   3. AIDS (Disease) in infants—Chemoprevention.   4. Antiretroviral agents.   5. Breastfeeding—Health aspects.   I. Title.
RA643.8.A592 2014
614.5'99392—dc23   2013043757

BRITISH LIBRARY CATALOGUING DATA ARE AVAILABLE

© 2014 Rebecca J. Anderson. All rights reserved

No part of this book may be reproduced or transmitted in any form or by any means, electronic or mechanical, including photocopying or recording, or by any information storage and retrieval system, without permission in writing from the publisher.

On the cover: Child and physicians in the Call to Action program (photographer, Mia Collis, for Elizabeth Glaser Pediatric AIDS Foundation)

Manufactured in the United States of America

*McFarland & Company, Inc., Publishers
Box 611, Jefferson, North Carolina 28640
www.mcfarlandpub.com*

For the children who are still waiting.

Acknowledgments

I have many people to thank for helping me write this book. At the top of that list are Peter Farina and Susan Aiello, who have encouraged my efforts throughout. Peter has been an unfailing champion. At Boehringer Ingelheim, he was closely associated with nevirapine from its initial discovery to the most recent product line extensions, and he assured me that this was a book worth writing. He provided a wealth of institutional knowledge, connecting me to the right people, steering me to the most important literature citations, and reminding me of key events when my own knowledge was insufficient, misguided, or lacking. In an ongoing series of discussions, from my first fragmentary concept to the book's final printed page, he has been an invaluable sounding board.

Likewise, Susan has been a longstanding champion of my writing and her knowledge of the publishing industry guided me as I navigated the very challenging process of attracting a publisher. Her early editorial critiques and suggestions strengthened my writing and helped me focus my efforts, which turned a mediocre early draft into a much better manuscript. Writers need encouragement to sustain and reassure them through months of frustration and the years of hard work that it takes to produce a book. I am indeed fortunate that Peter and Susan were solidly in my corner throughout this arduous process. I simply cannot thank them enough.

From the beginning, I wanted to relate this narrative through the eyes of those who did the work and those whose lives were transformed, directly or indirectly, by nevirapine. I was therefore largely dependent on obtaining the cooperation and winning the confidence of dozens of people, some of whom were former coworkers at Boehringer Ingelheim but most of whom I had never met. I am very grateful to them for generously setting aside time from their busy schedules to answer my long lists of questions and provide me with so many personal insights. They freely explained the hurdles they faced, the choices they made, and the things that inspired and frustrated them. Our conversations frequently revived clear memories of distant events long forgotten. They shared humorous anecdotes as well as details of the tragic situations they sought to overcome. And often, I found, the circumstances surrounding their extraordinary contributions were just as interesting as the contributions themselves. I am deeply indebted to each of them for sharing their personal experiences and allowing me to put them in print.

Hundreds of people were involved with developing nevirapine, AZT, and the other AIDS drugs described herein. Thousands of others at clinics, non-profit organizations, government agencies, advocacy organizations, and in the HIV/AIDS community were also involved with pediatric AIDS in significant ways. I wish I could have included all of them by name and elaborated on each of their contributions. Faced with this multitude of interesting perspectives, I inevitably had to make choices. My choices reflect a desire to highlight the people and events that defined the path of pediatric AIDS. Certainly, many others were involved in these events as well. I take responsibility for the choices I made.

I was fortunate that many contemporary authors chronicled AIDS not only in the scientific and medical literature but also in the lay press and in social, cultural, political, and economic commentaries. These print and online publications were valuable sources of first-hand information about pediatric AIDS and, as it evolved, its impact on individuals, communities, and various organizations. I especially want to thank Carol Kaliff at the *Danbury News-Times*, Cindy Lachlin and Richard Klein at the Food and Drug Administration, Susan Malsbury at the New York Public Library, and Charles Huber at the Davidson Library for responding to my requests for information, as well as Stewart Memorial Library, Reeves Medical Library, and the National Library of Medicine, whose archive collections I consulted repeatedly. The administrative staffs at the FDA and the National Institutes of Health were especially responsive to my requests for reports and transcripts from their archives. In addition to those publicly available sources, I am also indebted to Art Ammann, Maureen Myers, Jay Merluzzi, Bob Eckner, John Sullivan, and Brooks Jackson, who generously provided source documents from their personal files. Most importantly, I want to thank David Townson for his creative investigative work, which helped me track down some of the most elusive but essential bits of information. This book is much richer for his hard work, advice, and encouragement.

Boehringer Ingelheim kindly provided press releases and citations for abstracts, conference presentations, and publications related to nevirapine. I am especially grateful to Amy Shortlidge-Cox and Len Sierra for their literature searches and to Kate O'Connor and others at Boehringer Ingelheim who responded to my many requests and assisted with fact checking key events.

Special thanks goes to the Elizabeth Glaser Pediatric AIDS Foundation for the important work they do. Elizabeth Glaser and her Foundation's initiatives to address pediatric AIDS predate almost everyone else, and I am grateful to the Foundation's leaders, especially Trish Karlin, Nick Hellmann, and Susan DeLaurentis, for sharing their collective institutional knowledge with me. I also want to thank Jane Coaston, Taylor Moore, Haley Donovan, John Sheeran, Bob Yule, and Evan Von Leer, who were helpful in so many ways: arranging interviews, providing archived documents and photos, fact checking, and always cheerfully responding to my questions and requests.

To balance my natural temptation, as a scientist, to emphasize the scientific and technical aspects, I am grateful to those who helped me understand the social, political, and human impact of AIDS on individuals and whole communities. My conversations with David Selberg (Pacific Pride), Doug Nelson (AIDS Resource Center of Wisconsin), and Mark Harrington (Treatment Action Group), in particular, gave me invaluable insights regarding the issues facing the HIV/AIDS community in the 1980s and 1990s. Likewise, Kimberly Lanegran and Justice Edwin Cameron patiently explained the nuances of the political ideology prevailing in South Africa in the 1990s and 2000s and provided their personal insights of the factors at play during those troubling times.

Mike Benge, Lori Hahn, Peter Jaynes, Doug Nelson, and Arlene Townson graciously took the time to read the early drafts of the manuscript, and I am extremely grateful for their efforts. Each of them reviewed the text from a different perspective, and their comments, critiques, and suggestions have helped to make the manuscript much stronger than it otherwise would have been. However, as is customary, despite all the proofing, fact checking, and editing by all of those who have reviewed this manuscript along the way, any remaining flaws are my own.

Table of Contents

Acknowledgments vii
Preface 1
Introduction 3

1. Eureka! 13
2. The Second Time Around 24
3. A Star Is Born 37
4. A Cast of Thousands 48
5. In the Spotlight 60
6. The Christmas Tree 66
7. The Journey Begins, Finally 73
8. Patient Pressure Points 83
9. Resistance Is Futile — Or Not 94
10. A Rash Decision 106
11. The Road to Prevention 110
12. The Trifecta 122
13. Supply and Demand: Getting to PICNIC 132
14. Surrogates and Accelerated Approval 139
15. To Peds or Not to Peds 147
16. And the Winner Is... 159
17. Oh, Canada! 165
18. Into Africa 185
19. I Remember Montreal 199
20. The Kids' Turn 206
21. Justice Delayed 215
22. Am-Bushed 231
23. If Nothing Else... 246

Epilogue 259
Chapter Notes 265
List of Author Interviews 293
Bibliography 295
Index 311

Preface

The grueling quest to conquer AIDS was one of the great medical dramas of the twentieth century. Triggered by a deadly virus that struck indiscriminately, the rapid downward spiral of AIDS symptoms propagated anxiety, fear, and grief throughout entire communities, countries, and continents. People who faced certain death demanded action and scientists responded. During the first decade of AIDS research, while investigators made steady progress in adult therapeutics, pediatric AIDS received less attention, with only isolated pockets of success. It was an era in which the difference between life and death from pediatric AIDS was determined only by when and where a child was born. For many people, living through that era was a very personal struggle filled with frustrations and setbacks.

This book takes a historical journey from the emergence of pediatric AIDS in the early 1980s to the present state of AIDS therapeutics, and at each step along the way highlights the people who helped shape that path, set its direction, or benefitted from traveling on it. The narrative extends from the United States (where most of the AIDS therapies were developed) to Canada, Germany, the Netherlands, Nigeria, Uganda, South Africa, and other parts of the world, where investigators, parents, and activists all played pivotal roles in tackling pediatric AIDS. In addition, I have included the firsthand accounts of pharmaceutical scientists and clinicians, who raced against the clock, overcame enormous obstacles, and pushed the bounds of scientific knowledge and technical know-how to deliver the lifesaving drugs that eventually conquered pediatric AIDS.

Unifying all of these events is nevirapine, a drug that emerged from goal-oriented efforts to find a novel treatment for adults with AIDS. The discovery of nevirapine's unique ability to combat pediatric AIDS led to unanticipated, emotionally charged social crusades, and those events drive the narrative. Nevirapine became a target of suspicious AIDS dissidents, a rallying point for AIDS activists, the subject of landmark court decisions, and the centerpiece of early international AIDS prevention campaigns. Advocates praised its virtues while critics reminded everyone of its faults. Scientifically and medically, nevirapine's discovery represented a breakthrough in the treatment of AIDS. It was the first drug in a new class of AIDS agents, and its ability to prevent mother-to-child HIV transmission marked a turning point in the feasibility and economics of AIDS healthcare. It is by no means a perfect drug, but despite its faults nevirapine remains one of the most widely used AIDS drugs in the world. Now, more than twenty years after nevirapine's discovery, the narrative arc has reached the point where it makes sense to review—the evolution of pediatric AIDS from a vicious killer to inevitable extinction and the intertwined evolution of nevirapine and the other treatment regimens responsible for eradicating HIV infections.

This book is not a scientific treatise. Medical textbooks cover all aspects of the causes, symptoms, and treatment of AIDS in both adults and children. Similarly, all of the data on nevirapine have been published in medical and scientific journals. Rather, this book focuses on the people who were touched by pediatric AIDS: the children infected with HIV and their families, the physicians who treated them, and the scientists who sought to understand the virus. Overlying their experiences are the personal accounts of the people who created nevirapine, discovered its unique properties, and worked tirelessly to get it to the patients who needed it. At a time when these researchers were doing their best work, many of them were also raising young children at home. They nevertheless gave up their children's little league games, band concerts, parent-teacher conferences, and quality time to save the lives of children — and adults — whom they had never met.

I have interviewed pediatric AIDS patients, their HIV-infected mothers, and pediatric AIDS researchers. I have also considered the experiences of AIDS patients who did not survive. To relate these personal recollections to the social, political, and cultural setting in which they took place, I have drawn on a wide variety of archival material including published research reports, monographs, government records, meeting transcripts, newsletters, position papers, conference proceedings, commission reports, memoirs, press releases, and archived news articles. The result is an account of unprecedented scientific achievement, unprecedented influence of multi-national patient advocacy groups to change government healthcare policies, unprecedented industry humanitarianism that put patient welfare above intellectual property rights and corporate profits, and unprecedented international cooperation to eliminate trade barriers to drug access. And at the center of it all is a drug that saved children from AIDS.

Nevirapine proved that simple, inexpensive, and effective remedies can prevent HIV infection and, according to one researcher, it "changed the face of AIDS globally." Yet, despite the success of nevirapine and other antiviral drugs, the World Health Organization estimates that 300,000 babies are born each year with HIV, and only one-quarter of HIV-infected children in the world receive adequate drug treatment. The problem now is not poor quality drugs but limitations in service delivery. Complacency, diminished financial commitment, and redirected political priorities threaten to roll back the medical gains of the past two decades in the United States and slow the momentum in the developing world. AIDS no longer makes the headlines, but HIV infection remains a threat and still contributes to rising healthcare costs both in the United States and in developing countries. More than ever, public awareness is needed to prevent recurrence of pediatric AIDS in the United States and to invigorate efforts to eliminate pediatric AIDS in impoverished countries. I hope this book will encourage expansion of healthcare services and wider use of those treatments to eradicate, once and for all, one of the world's most tenacious health problems.

Introduction

Hauwa, a resident of Bakin Kogi, deep in the interior of Nigeria, was a woman on a mission. It was March 2004, and the AIDS epidemic had been escalating unchecked for twenty years, affecting more people in Nigeria than in any other country in the world, except South Africa. Although Nigeria had been among the first African nations to take steps to curb the disease, those efforts could not keep pace with the expanding epidemic. Hundreds of thousands of Nigerians were dying, and in impoverished rural areas like Bakin Kogi, which had no medical facilities or healthcare professionals, villagers accepted their fate as inevitable. But not Hauwa.

Hauwa was a traditional birth attendant, responsible for assisting mothers in Bakin Kogi and the surrounding community during childbirth.[1] Most of those pregnant women did not realize that they were infected with the AIDS virus, although many were clearly sick. They passed the virus to their babies, who were often born frail or became infected through breast milk and died before the age of two. Each year, Hauwa watched in frustration as more and more women and babies developed the all-too-familiar symptoms. She knew they could be treated, but they died because, despite all her birthing skills, they needed drugs she did not have. Then, one day, Hauwa learned that doctors at the Faith Alive Foundation Clinic in Jos were offering an AIDS training workshop for traditional birth attendants.[2] Nothing was going to stop her from attending.

Filled with expectation, Hauwa ventured from her home, leaving behind Bakin Kogi's tropical rainforests and lush green soybean fields. For three hours, she jostled over bumpy dirt roads that led up a temperate plateau to Jos, a thriving metropolis of nearly one million people in the exact center of Nigeria. At the Faith Alive facility, a neighborhood clinic in the heart of Jos, Arthur Ammann, a physician representing a private foundation in the United States, along with the director of the Faith Alive clinic, conducted the AIDS workshop. They explained how the AIDS virus spread from mothers to their babies and taught Hauwa and her fellow birth attendants how to use a simple drug treatment to prevent babies from becoming infected. Armed with supplies from the workshop, Hauwa returned to Bakin Kogi and set up a tiny clinic, anxious to apply her new skills.

The technique she had learned was simple and inexpensive—just a single dose of a drug called nevirapine—but the impact of her work was immediately evident to everyone, not only the expectant mothers she assisted in her clinic, but also other residents of the village and their tribal leaders. Starting with the very first baby who received nevirapine under her care, babies were more frequently born healthy, and they were more likely to stay that way.

In September 2004, a group of visitors from an American philanthropic group came to meet Hauwa and see her clinic. She enthusiastically greeted them at the outskirts of the

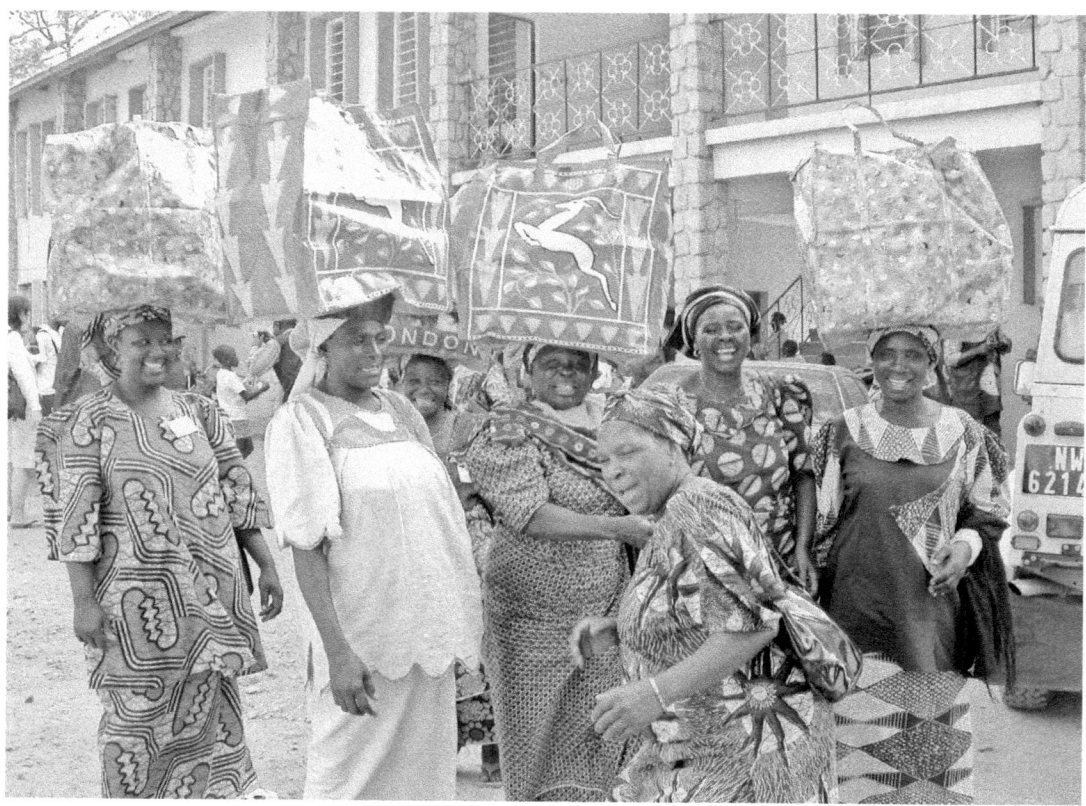

Traditional birth attendants leaving their single-dose nevirapine training session at the Faith Alive Foundation clinic in Jos, Nigeria, in March 2004. They are carrying their training materials and medical supplies on their heads (courtesy Global Strategies for HIV Prevention).

village and personally escorted them to the first stop on their tour. As they walked down the dusty road to the village chief's "palace," women and children fell in behind them in an impromptu parade, singing and dancing in an ever-growing display of gratitude and celebration. At the palace, the chief and village elders graciously received the visitors and gave them a photograph, insisting that they accept it on behalf of Dr. Ammann, who had trained Hauwa. It was a small but heartfelt token of their appreciation for what Hauwa and her newfound skills meant to them: a photograph of the first Bakin Kogi baby who had been saved by nevirapine. Here, in a village where two-thirds of the people were infected with the AIDS virus, was a child that the entire village celebrated. A child with a future.[3]

Hauwa's return trip down the Jos plateau, over the rough country roads that cut through wild, emerald lowlands to Bakin Kogi, was the final leg of a fifteen-year journey — a journey of medical discoveries frequently stalled by twists and turns, detours and dead ends. And it was a journey that might very well have been aborted — a closed and unfulfilled chapter of medicine — had it not been for a sequence of events that aligned by chance in 1990.

In April 1990, a rather ordinary Indiana teenager, who had become a cause célèbre, died. In June, scientists gathered in San Francisco and called the world's attention to a disturbing trend: the rising number of children with AIDS. And in July, federal regulators met with representatives of a drug company in Washington, DC, to discuss the firm's experimental AIDS drug — a drug so new that it had not yet been given a name. The federal regulators' unexpected and unusual recommendations at that otherwise ordinary meeting became the starting point for an extraordinary journey.

*　*　*

For as long as he could remember, Ryan White had been coping with doctors, hospitals, and an incurable disease. Boys have a one in 10,000 chance of inheriting hemophilia, and Ryan was one of them. When most people get a cut, their blood starts to clot. In less than twelve minutes a scab forms and the cut begins to heal. Ryan's blood took thirty to forty minutes to clot, which meant he could bleed to death from even a minor cut or scrape.[4] Equally dangerous were bumps and bruises, which caused internal bleeding and painful swelling that often lasted for days or weeks. Repeated internal bleeding episodes damaged his muscles and joints, making Ryan skinny with knobby knees and elbows.[5]

Ryan's blood lacked Factor VIII, a protein necessary for normal blood clotting. Fortunately, scientists had discovered a way to extract Factor VIII from blood donated by volunteers. In a concentrated form, this Factor VIII product is an effective treatment for hemophilia.

Ryan played during school recess, rode his bike on his newspaper delivery route, and was as active as most boys. The difference, of course, was that each of his injuries meant a quick trip to the hospital, where the medical staff injected Factor VIII. After he turned five, Ryan started taking Factor VIII regularly at home as a precaution. His doctors taught his mother the intravenous procedure, and she gave him injections two to three times a week. If he had a bleeding episode, she injected Factor VIII more frequently, sometimes every day.[6]

When Ryan was twelve, he began to feel sluggish and was less active than he had usually been during summer vacations. By September, he was having night sweats, stomach cramps, and diarrhea. His pediatrician attributed those symptoms and his swollen lymph glands to the flu. During his regular hemophilia checkup in November, blood tests showed that he had recently had hepatitis.[7] As he approached his thirteenth birthday in December, Ryan began having coughing spells, had difficulty breathing, and generally felt rundown. He developed a high fever and was admitted to the hospital, where an x-ray revealed that he had pneumonia in both lungs. When his condition did not improve, the doctors performed a lung biopsy to determine the cause of his illness.[8]

The tests confirmed that Ryan had pneumocystis pneumonia. PCP is a rare form of pneumonia that typically does not bother people with a healthy immune system.[9] But in 1984, PCP was the hallmark of a newly recognized disease, acquired immune deficiency syndrome. Ryan had AIDS.[10]

Only a few months earlier, scientists had discovered AIDS was caused by a virus. Mandatory testing to determine if donated blood was infected with the virus, which was eventually called the human immunodeficiency virus, was not started until the spring of 1985. Consequently, many blood donors up to that time did not know whether they were infected with HIV, and much of the Factor VIII supplied to hemophilia patients was contaminated. Nine out of ten people who received contaminated blood products became infected with HIV. The initial HIV infection causes mild, flu-like symptoms that quickly disappear, and many hemophilia patients, like Ryan, only realized they were infected when they began experiencing AIDS symptoms such as pneumocystis pneumonia.

Ryan's classmates and neighbors had not been concerned that he had hemophilia, but

AIDS frightened them. No one knew much about the disease, except that it was contagious and people infected with the virus died. After Ryan recovered from pneumonia, he wanted to return to school, but school officials advised against it. For eight months, Ryan's family fought a legal battle in the county and state courts, and eventually Ryan won the right to attend school. But apprehension and misperceptions in the community persisted. Parents incorrectly thought that Ryan posed an unacceptable risk to their children. In an uneasy compromise, Ryan agreed to eat lunch with disposable utensils, use a private toilet, and drink from a separate water fountain.[11] Parents and the teaching staff wanted the entire school disinfected every night. Many people along Ryan's newspaper delivery route canceled their subscriptions. After an unhappy year, Ryan and his family moved to the nearby community of Cicero, Indiana, where school officials and student leaders had made a concerted effort to educate the faculty, students, and parents about AIDS.

The publicity surrounding Ryan's determination to attend school attracted the attention of numerous public officials and celebrities. He was interviewed by television and newspaper reporters, appeared at AIDS fundraisers, campaigned for better AIDS education, testified before the President's Commission on AIDS, and addressed the National Education Association's annual meeting in the New Orleans Superdome. Articulate, sincere, and determined to lead a normal life, Ryan gave pediatric AIDS a face, raised the public's awareness of the impact of AIDS on children and their families, and highlighted the need for effective and safer treatments for HIV-infected children.

In parallel with the publicity surrounding his battle to go to school, Ryan also battled his accumulating AIDS symptoms. HIV attacks the immune system, making it more difficult to fight all sorts of infections. In AIDS patients, these are called opportunistic infections, because they take advantage of the person's weakened immune system. Ryan's pneumonia infection cleared, but he contracted thrush, an unpleasant yeast infection that produced funny-tasting white patches inside his mouth and throat. The thrush, along with a herpes infection, made Ryan's throat sore, and swallowing was painful. AIDS also affected his sense of taste and smell, and not surprisingly, he lost his appetite.[12] When he was discharged from the hospital in February 1985, he had lost twenty pounds and still had thrush, diarrhea, and a persistent cough.[13]

In September, he was again hospitalized because of a high fever and continuous coughing and vomiting. While in the hospital, Ryan had two seizures. His vomiting and lack of eating had created low blood sugar and an imbalance in other blood nutrients.[14] This type of imbalance sometimes causes seizures in normal children, but the HIV infection made his brain more vulnerable. In Ryan's case, improved nutrition prevented further seizures. Over the next few years, he had recurring nausea, vomiting, diarrhea, and night sweats, but he also experienced periods — especially during warm weather — when his symptoms eased. Unfortunately, the cough and thrush persisted, and AIDS-related muscle wasting reduced his arms and legs to little more than a skin-covered skeleton.

In January 1988, he was hospitalized to treat a second flare-up of pneumocystis pneumonia.[15] Later that year, his HIV infection induced shingles: itchy, painful blisters that left scars on his back.[16] A year later, he developed a hernia, his liver became inflamed, and he had a bloated belly.[17] His fevers continued to come and go, but his cough was a constant, if unwelcome, companion. By October 1989, Ryan only had enough energy to attend school for a few days at a time. By December, he also had laryngitis, bloody noses that persisted despite Factor VIII treatment, and at times difficulty hearing.[18]

For the next few months, Ryan continued to struggle with his sore throat and coughing, which made it difficult to breathe and sleep. The shingles cleared, but he developed open sores on his legs. His hernia, swollen belly, and liver problems were painful, and he had difficulty walking upright.[19] A few months after his eighteenth birthday, Ryan's liver, spleen, and kidneys began to fail, and he was again admitted to the hospital. AIDS was wearing him down, and this time his body was too weak to fight it.[20] The doctors could treat his opportunistic infections with drugs, but they were unable to boost his failing immune system and stop the spiral of his accumulating AIDS symptoms. On April 8, 1990, Ryan White died. But Ryan's passing, instead of marking the end of a boy's stubborn struggle to simply go to school and lead a normal life, accelerated the pace, deepened the intensity, and redoubled everyone's efforts to conquer pediatric AIDS.

* * *

Around the time that Ryan learned he had AIDS, 2000 researchers from around the world gathered in Atlanta, Georgia, concerned about the growing AIDS epidemic and the lack of early-stage tests to diagnose it. Subsequently, the annual International AIDS Conferences grew in size, scope, and prestige. Within a few years, it became the largest venue for discussing AIDS, attracting researchers, representatives from governmental and non-governmental organizations, and AIDS advocates. For all of those who had a stake in the AIDS issue, it was the place to be and be seen. Scientists presented their latest research findings. Clinicians described how AIDS symptoms developed and their progress in finding treatments. Policy makers proposed public health programs to control the spread of the virus. Government regulators discussed their initiatives to facilitate approval of effective new drugs. Advocacy groups ensured that their voices were heard. And the news media covered it all, communicating the highlights and lowlights to their worldwide audience.

The 6th International AIDS Conference was held in San Francisco in June 1990. Today, it is remembered mostly for the people who did not attend. For the first time, and unlike the previous Conferences held in France, Sweden, and Canada, the leader of the host country's government did not address the Conference. President George H. W. Bush had initially rejected the organizers' invitation to speak and then asked to be re-invited. The program committee extended a second invitation but included a strong statement criticizing the president's executive order banning HIV-infected individuals from traveling to the United States. Bush declined again, choosing instead to attend a fund-raiser for Senator Jesse Helms (R-NC), who coincidently had authored the initial travel ban legislation.[21] Although the United States State Department temporarily eased travel restrictions to allow delegates to attend the Conference, 100 groups chose to boycott it, four plenary speakers declined to appear, and thirty invited scientific presenters withdrew their papers.[22]

The 12,000 participants who attended the International AIDS Conference came from 121 countries and included 2000 media representatives.[23] Among them was a delegation from Boehringer Ingelheim Pharmaceuticals, Inc., who had traveled to San Francisco from their offices in Ridgefield, Connecticut. BI marketed drugs to treat heart and lung diseases, and the delegation's presence in San Francisco was hardly noticed. Like many attendees, they sought out and huddled around the "big names" in AIDS and HIV research, but no one sought out or huddled around them. They asked many questions but answered few. Mostly, they just listened, learned, and took lots of notes.

In methodical, measured, and deliberate steps, the unassuming BI team had been conducting HIV research for two years. Their experimental drug only had a company-assigned code number, and they were not ready to present their results publicly. But they had made steady progress and were now poised to begin testing their drug in people. With no internal experience in conducting AIDS clinical trials, the BI team had been seeking and consulting AIDS clinicians and the leading experts in HIV research. The San Francisco conference was just one of the many scientific gatherings where the BI team was doing its homework.

They were aware of the intense public pressure to get new AIDS drugs on the market. AIDS deaths were mounting, and the fear of AIDS among those at risk was intense. AIDS patients and advocates organized effectively, were aggressively exerting pressure, and would be a significant influence on expediting new AIDS drugs. Recognizing the urgency, the BI team wanted to obtain market approval for its drug as quickly as possible. But because BI had entered the field of HIV research much later than other companies and its internal resources to mount a "fast track" drug development program were limited, BI's clinical trials needed to be bare-bones, focused, and executed perfectly. In 1990, the fastest way to complete a drug development program was to conduct all of the clinical trials in adults, and all of BI's plans were aimed at testing its new drug in HIV-infected adults.

When Ryan White was first diagnosed, only 148 pediatric AIDS cases had been reported in the United States.[24] But by the time of the San Francisco AIDS Conference only a few years later, more than 2500 children had been diagnosed, AIDS was among the leading causes of death in children, and the number of new pediatric AIDS cases was increasing at an alarming rate.[25] Every AIDS clinic in the United States was admitting children who were severely ill and dying.[26] Although some, like Ryan, became infected through infusion of contaminated blood or blood products, most pediatric AIDS cases were infants who acquired the disease from their HIV-infected mothers.[27] AIDS symptoms progressed more rapidly in children than in adults. In infants and young children, the disease also stunted physical growth and brain development, often causing significant brain damage.[28] Ryan stopped growing at age twelve and reached a height of only five feet.[29] Fortunately, Ryan's brain had matured before he began experiencing AIDS symptoms. But when HIV attacks infants and young children whose brains are still developing, AIDS impairs their ability to concentrate, remember, and perform complex mental tasks.

The need for drugs to treat pediatric AIDS had become a pressing concern, but conducting pediatric clinical trials is complicated. Children (especially infants) have limited ability to describe their reactions to drugs, making it more difficult to assess both the drug's therapeutic value and its side effects. To enroll minors in an experimental drug trial, investigators must obtain permission from parents or guardians, who are often reluctant to consent. Investigators also must address ethical issues. Can they justify exposing children to an untested new drug whose side effects might cause permanent damage and a lifetime of suffering? How do they avoid coercing children to participate? Because of these difficulties, many drugs had never been systematically studied in children. And without data from pediatric clinical trials, drug companies could not obtain approval to label or market the drug for pediatric use.

Physicians are allowed to prescribe marketed drugs for unapproved uses as part of the "practice of medicine," and approximately three-fourths of the drugs prescribed by pediatricians were not approved for pediatric use.[30] But in AIDS therapeutics in 1990, this prescribing practice was unwise and insufficient. Children handle and react to drugs differently than adults, raising sobering concerns about causing more harm than good in children who were already very sick. And pediatricians were limited to only one commercially available AIDS drug: zidovudine—originally called azidothymidine and commonly abbreviated to AZT.

The Food and Drug Administration approved AZT in March 1987 for HIV-infected adults who had pneumocystis pneumonia and who had too few white blood cells to fight infections. Unfortunately, the high doses of AZT used during those early years caused a number of unpleasant side effects, which could not be tolerated by half of the AIDS population.[31] Bone marrow suppression was the most serious AZT side effect, and it made patients anemic. The anemia could be corrected by blood transfusions or lowering the AZT dose.[32] But clinicians worried that the lower AZT dose might not adequately treat pediatric AIDS, especially the HIV-induced loss of brain function.

By 1990, investigators were conducting clinical trials with a number of experimental drugs chemically similar to AZT, but none of them had yet been approved. Although these drugs did not appear to suppress bone marrow, they caused other serious side effects such as peripheral nerve damage, which is painful, and inflammation of the pancreas, which in some cases is fatal. These side effects posed very serious concerns when treating infants and children.

So, in 1990, pediatric AIDS was an urgent issue. Ryan White's funeral, the most publicized in Indiana history, was still fresh in everyone's mind.[33] The number of HIV-infected women and the number of their HIV-infected babies were increasing rapidly. And patient advocates were pressing for more pediatric testing of AIDS drugs.[34] Any discussion of HIV research and AIDS treatment required consideration of the pediatric population. Those attending the International AIDS Conference in San Francisco knew it. Clinicians desperately wanting to treat sick children knew it. And so did the FDA.

On July 17, 1990, scientists and clinicians from BI traveled to the FDA's headquarters in Rockville, Maryland. It was the first of many meetings, either in person or by teleconference, that BI would hold with federal regulators regarding their experimental AIDS drug. But the presence of several distinguished participants underscored the importance of this first meeting. Prominent external clinicians involved with AIDS clinical trials asked to join the BI delegation and lend their support. On the FDA side, the group of reviewers who had been assigned to evaluate BI's data and plans were joined by their Division Director, Ellen Cooper.

* * *

In a few short years, Ellen Cooper had risen from a bench scientist to one of the most influential federal regulators in the country. After completing a clinical fellowship in pediatrics and infectious diseases at Children's Hospital Medical Center in Washington, DC, Cooper joined the FDA in 1982 as a researcher in the Division of Virology.[35] Although she enjoyed biologics research, she was soon drawn into the regulatory side of the agency, a fortuitous convergence of opportunity and work style preference. In 1984, she officially transferred to the FDA's Drug Division as a medical reviewer and reviewed the New Drug Application for the oral formulation of acyclovir. Initial approval of the intravenous formulation of acyclovir two years earlier for treating serious herpes infections had marked a major milestone, the first antiviral drug approved by the FDA, and the new oral formulation marked another medical achievement, quickly becoming the treatment of choice for preventing herpes recurrences. With the discovery (also in 1984) that AIDS was caused by a virus, the search for new antiviral drugs escalated, and the FDA reorganized to meet the challenge.

From the time Burroughs Wellcome notified FDA of its intension to initiate clinical trials with AZT in March 1985, Cooper fostered ongoing communications with the company.[36] She and her FDA colleagues knew people were dying, the situation was increasingly desperate, and "there was a lot of urgency to do what we could" to get AZT to patients as quickly as possible.[37] When Burroughs Wellcome submitted its application for AZT approval in December 1986, Cooper was already familiar with the drug, worked around the clock to review the data, and approved the drug in record time.[38]

In February 1988, FDA created the Antiviral Drug Products Division to consolidate regulatory oversight for all types of drugs used in patients with AIDS: the drugs that attacked the virus directly and those designed to treat AIDS-related opportunistic infections.[39] Cooper was the obvious choice to head the new division—the person in charge of regulating all AIDS drugs in the United States. The job also put her in the crosshairs of every critic, investigator, activist, politician, editorialist, bureaucrat, stockholder, and manufacturer who had a stake in AIDS.

Over the next three years, Cooper met frequently with representatives from the AIDS community and listened to their concerns. Among them was a determined mother from Los Angeles who had lost a child to AIDS. Although Cooper explained that they were doing everything they could, this mother came armed with her own plan for moving pediatric AIDS trials "forward like a race car at Le Mans."[40] Pediatric trials gave children early access to experimental AIDS drugs and shortened the time for approving those drugs specifically for use in children. She urged Cooper to grease the bureaucratic wheels so that new AIDS drugs could be approved for pediatric use right after they were approved for adults. Ryan White, at the age of fifteen, was one of the first pediatric AIDS patients to receive AZT, but the drug had not been approved specifically for use in children until a month after his death.[41] This determined mother told the FDA to "turn up the juice."[42] And they did.

* * *

At their meeting with the FDA, the BI delegation sought confirmation that they had accumulated enough data from laboratory and animal studies to justify starting trials of their experimental drug in people. They were also eager to hear the FDA reviewers' reaction to their clinical plans, which proposed testing the drug in adults. The discussion on that sultry day in July was wide-ranging, but the documents presented by BI clearly showed that the researchers had found an interesting new drug. The presence and active participation of Cooper at the meeting elevated BI's hope that its drug might represent not just an alternative to AZT but an actual breakthrough for treating AIDS.

The FDA reviewers found no gaps that would delay testing the drug in people. In fact, in a number of ways, they made suggestions that would speed up BI's timetable. And they wanted BI to incorporate children in the clinical trials. Mindful of the growing need for pediatric AIDS drugs, Cooper and her colleagues were encouraging all developers of AIDS drugs to conduct pediatric trials as an integral part of their clinical trial strategy. "We were committed to getting a drug in kids as soon as possible."[43]

When FDA officials make suggestions, it is usually prudent to heed their advice. Despite no previous experience in conducting pediatric clinical trials, the BI team revamped the development strategy that they had been so carefully planning for the previous two years. They promised to start the first pediatric trial within six months from the start of the first adult AIDS trial, and after that, they would enroll both children and adults.

* * *

The events of those few months in 1990 were the culmination of many forces that had been building momentum for years. The unbridled spread of pediatric AIDS, the passionate protests of advocacy groups, the determined lobbying of desperate parents, and the highly publicized death of an Indiana teenager compelled Boehringer Ingelheim to change course and conduct pediatric AIDS trials as a priority. Because of that major shift, a drug that might otherwise have fallen by the wayside made an extraordinary journey, from a laboratory in Ridgefield, Connecticut, to villages — like Hauwa's — in the most remote corners of the world. Along the way, BI's drug would have its ups and downs. It would not live up to all of its inventors' early expectations, and in fact researchers would eventually expose serious flaws in it.

But on that humid summer day in 1990, the BI researchers returned to their laboratories in Connecticut with a new plan, eager to begin their clinical trials. They would rally hundreds of determined researchers and solicit the cooperation of thousands of patients. They would also make many contributions to our understanding of the virus and AIDS. But even they could not anticipate that their drug would eventually claim a unique place in AIDS therapeutics: a method of drug use as yet unknown and untested, but one that in the coming years would save the lives of millions of children.

1

Eureka!

In the fall of 1985, four-year-old Ariel Glaser began complaining of stomach aches and cramps, unusual for the little girl who liked to take long nature walks and romp on the beach.[1] Ariel had recently returned with her family from a trip to Puerto Rico, and her pediatrician thought she had just picked up a bug. He was not concerned that her hematocrit, the number of red blood cells in her blood, was in the lower part of the normal range. Her other tests were normal, and he recommended a diet to ease her diarrhea, thinking she would recover in a few weeks.

But the painful stomach cramps persisted, and her lips turned a chalky white. She also tired easily, often falling asleep on the drive home from her half-day nursery school. A specialist in pediatric gastroenterology examined Ariel and came to the same conclusion as her pediatrician. It was probably just that "Puerto Rican bug." But he admitted Ariel to the hospital for three days of laboratory tests, intending to examine a series of stool samples and make a definitive diagnosis. Instead, Ariel's doctors quickly shifted their attention to another problem when they received the results of her first hospital blood test. They were alarmed that her hematocrit had dropped to a dangerously low level and gave her an immediate blood transfusion.[2] Ariel stayed in the hospital until her blood count improved, and when she was discharged, she was stronger, and color had returned to her face and lips. But she was still not well. The bouts of diarrhea persisted, and she often woke up in pain. The doctors' extensive tests revealed no bugs — Puerto Rican or otherwise — to explain her symptoms, and they concluded that she probably had hemolytic uremic syndrome, a blood disorder that can lead to kidney failure but usually clears spontaneously in children.[3]

Ariel's condition stabilized. An active child with bright blue eyes, Ariel attended nursery school and went on play dates. She brought home precious treasures from her nature walks — unusual plants, feathers, and flowers — and spent hours painting and drawing the beautiful things she had seen.[4] But the recurring bouts of diarrhea and painful cramps weakened her delicate frame and drained her energy. For four months, her doctors conducted test after test, trying to find the cause of Ariel's symptoms.[5] In addition to the pain and diarrhea, Ariel's white blood cell count was low. Those cells help an individual's immune system fight infections, but the doctors ruled out the two most likely explanations: lupus and leukemia.[6] Finally, in the spring of 1986, her doctors were left with only one remaining diagnosis. It was a long-shot, because Ariel's family history did not put her in a high risk group, but follow up tests soon confirmed their suspicions.[7] Ariel had AIDS.

She began taking gamma globulin, the only treatment then available to treat children with AIDS, to boost her weakened immune system. Every three weeks, she traveled to nearby UCLA Medical Center and sat for her four-hour intravenous infusion of gamma globulin.[8] Unfortunately, Ariel's diagnosis, while solving one mystery, created other prob-

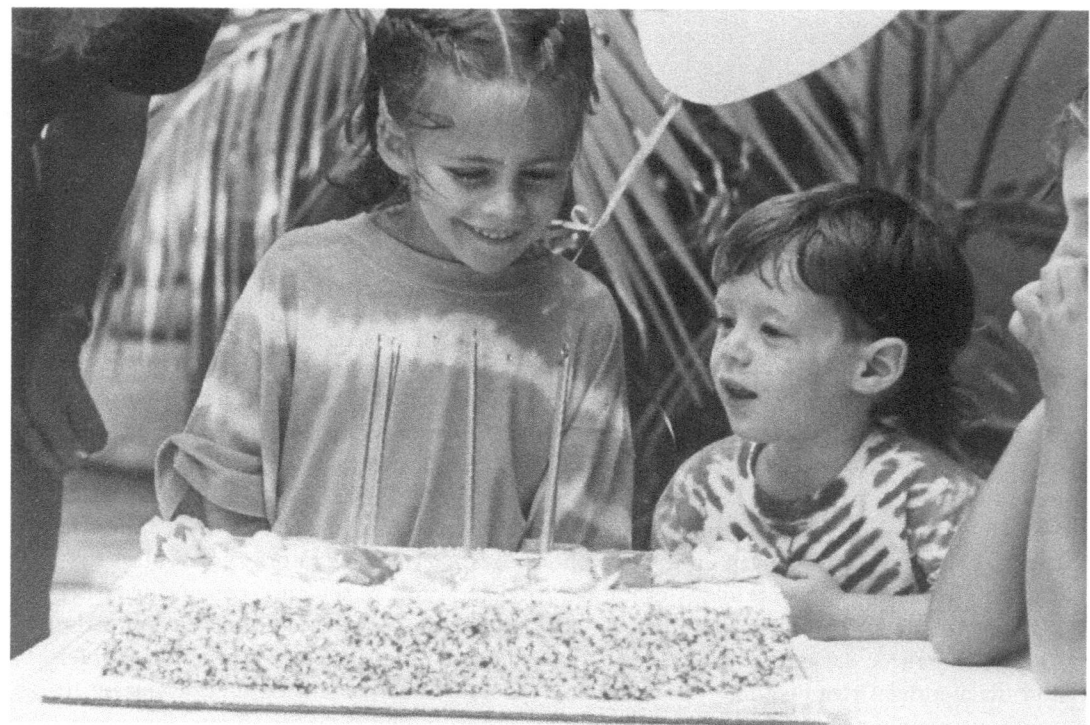

Ariel Glaser on her sixth birthday, with her brother Jake (courtesy Elizabeth Glaser Pediatric AIDS Foundation).

lems. To comply with guidelines issued by the Centers for Disease Control, her parents faced an agonizing choice: either inform Ariel's nursery school that she had AIDS or take her out of school. They took her out. Summer was approaching and Ariel had enrolled in day camp, but the camp would not accept children with AIDS.[9] Ariel spent the summer at home.

* * *

In September 1986, Burroughs Wellcome was wrapping up its historic clinical trial of AZT in adults. The investigators had stopped the trial early, because the AIDS patients who received AZT showed a dramatic improvement compared to those who received a placebo.[10] Investigators at Duke University, located near the Burroughs Wellcome headquarters in North Carolina, had participated in the clinical trial, and news of the AZT results quickly spread throughout the medical center. Catherine Wilfert, a pediatrician at Duke, immediately recognized the potential of AZT for treating children suffering with AIDS. She had seen her first pediatric AIDS cases three years earlier, and the number of HIV-infected children was rapidly growing in the Southeast.[11]

Through her contacts with the AZT investigators at Duke and officials at Burroughs Wellcome, Wilfert persuaded the drug company to conduct a pediatric trial with AZT.[12] Children respond differently to drugs than adults, and the goal of this trial was to establish the safety and optimal dosing conditions for treating children with AZT. In October, Wilfert's team at Duke treated the first child in the world with AZT. The trial, under Wilfert's leadership, ultimately enrolled thirty-five children at Duke, the University of Miami, and the National Cancer Institute in Bethesda, Maryland.[13]

* * *

Because Ariel and her family lived in California, she could only participate in the AZT clinical trial if her family moved across country with her or she was separated from her family for months at a time. Neither option seemed acceptable. Instead, she attended a public-school kindergarten throughout the school year and continued taking her gamma globulin shots, which seemed to keep her strong.[14] But by the summer of 1987, she had again lost her usual energy. The severe stomach pains returned, and she had no appetite.[15] In the fall, Ariel started first grade, still plagued by stomach pains. She cried and screamed when she went to the bathroom, which frightened her classmates and teachers.[16] Unfortunately, the doctors had nothing to treat her pain. After just two weeks at school and to make her more comfortable — along with her classmates and teachers — the school arranged to tutor Ariel at home.[17]

Just before Thanksgiving, Ariel's pain escalated and her parents rushed her to the UCLA emergency room. After so many months of uncertainty and guesswork, the doctors finally determined Ariel's pain was caused by acute pancreatitis, which had been caused by her weakened immune system. Because her pancreas was inflamed, Ariel could not digest food, making it impossible for her to eat. Not eating further inflamed her pancreas, which intensified the pain — a vicious, endless cycle. Consequently, Ariel had lost weight and grew weaker.[18] Now, her only nutrition came from intravenous feeding, a procedure that kept her in the hospital.

An alternative feeding method, though complicated, could be used at home, and Ariel's parents readily agreed to perform it. The doctors surgically implanted an intravenous tube, and her parents learned how to infuse a liquid diet of calories and nutrients through it.[19] After one month in the hospital, Ariel was discharged and her parents began performing the nightly ten-hour infusion. The intricate, sixteen-step sterile procedure took forty minutes to prepare each night and twenty minutes to dismantle each morning.[20] Ariel also began taking AZT. The drug had been approved in March for use in adults, but Ariel's doctors could prescribe it "off-label," confident that they were giving her the right dose, thanks to Wilfert's efforts. Everyone hoped that the AZT capsules, which Ariel took by mouth, and the nightly intravenous infusions would ease her symptoms so that she could start eating normally again.

Instead, the infusions made Ariel uncomfortable and bloated, and the doctors sent a nurse to administer a diuretic and flush excess fluid out of her system several times a week.[21] Still, Ariel slowly deteriorated. In January 1988, she stopped walking and by February she was unable to speak.[22] After three months of treatment, Ariel stopped taking AZT, because it appeared to be having no effect. She began a continuous infusion of morphine to blunt her excruciating pain.[23] In March, Ariel developed pneumonia and was again admitted to the hospital. Among other tests, the doctors did a brain scan, which showed that Ariel's brain had severely shrunk. Everyone was certain that the damage, which accounted for Ariel's inability to walk and talk, was irreversible.[24]

Then, as Ariel slipped deeper and deeper into her unconscious world, her parents learned about a new experimental procedure, a constant infusion of AZT, which seemed to work better than the capsules. The intravenous formulation was not commercially available, but Ariel's doctors, after some political string-pulling, obtained a sample and began infusing it through her implanted intravenous tube.[25] Day and night for three weeks, the AZT solution flowed into her bloodstream, one drop at a time with no apparent affect. Then, Ariel suddenly looked up and spoke for the first time in three months. Every day for the next six weeks, she steadily improved, eventually able to sit up, hold a marking pen, read, walk by herself, and go swimming.[26] She resumed her nature walks, picking wildflowers that served as models for her drawings. One day while drawing with her father in his office behind the Glasers' house, Ariel painted a very special picture, capturing the beauty of the world as only a child can — a garden of colorful flowers bathed in sunlight and surrounded by love.[27]

Taken by mouth, the AZT capsules had not been absorbed through her damaged stomach and intestines, but the direct intravenous infusion allowed AZT to reach her vital organs, including her brain.[28] Although Ariel still needed to be fed intravenously, she was able to eat a few things on her own.[29] By early July, the AZT infusion had markedly improved her brain function, but it had not cured her AIDS nor eased her stomach pain. Two weeks later, Ariel was again admitted to UCLA hospital with a high fever. The doctors found that her white blood cell count had fallen dangerously low (a side effect of AZT) and they stopped the intravenous AZT infusion.[30] The doctors tried to bring down her fever and restore her white blood cells by giving another experimental drug, GM-CSF.[31]

In August, Ariel celebrated her seventh birthday while in the hospital. In a few short weeks, she lost most of her recent improvements, and the doctors again started the intravenous AZT infusions. But this time without success. Ariel grew weaker and her fever would not break. One day, she asked her cousin to bring her paints and drawing paper.[32] Although her eyesight was fading, she still wanted to make pictures. Then, a week after her birthday, she began coughing, gasping, and struggling to breathe. The hospital staff administered oxygen, but despite their efforts, on Friday, August 12, 1988, Ariel Glaser died.[33]

* * *

Around the time that Ariel was first diagnosed with AIDS, Alan Rosenthal made a personal decision that would have far-reaching implications. He left Merck, considered by many the gold standard among pharmaceutical firms, to assume his new position as vice president of the Boehringer Ingelheim Pharmaceuticals, Inc., research and development facility in Connecticut. A prominent immunologist, Rosenthal had spent twelve years at the National Institute of Allergy and Infectious Diseases before joining Merck in 1978, where he led the company's immunology and inflammation research efforts. At BI, Rosenthal seized the opportunity to turn a fledgling set of laboratories into a first-class R&D center.

In 1971, the Boehringer Ingelheim name and the rights to distribute BI products in the United States were licensed from the German company, Boehringer Ingelheim International GmbH. In 1977, BI obtained use of a 193-acre Connecticut estate straddling the border between Ridgefield and Danbury, a site on which the new occupants cleverly blended environmental friendliness with business efficiency. The resident population of wild turkeys and miniature deer roamed freely through the thickets and densely wooded hills, laden with an earthy musk on damp, cool mornings, just as in colonial times. The biannual invasion of Canada geese was less welcome.

The first building BI constructed on the Ridgefield estate, in 1979, was an R&D laboratory building. Mindful of BI's desire to preserve the campus's bucolic charm, the architects chose a site adjacent to the estate's historic Manor House, which they restored and repurposed as a guest house for visiting dignitaries. Schotze, the German housekeeper, maintained the Manor House with an old-world elegance befitting a four star hotel. Returning visitors were drawn as much by her attentive service as by the comfortable rooms. But Schotze ran a tight ship. Even the most distinguished guests quickly learned to eat all their breakfast and not throw their towels on the floor. In return for their good manners, she pampered them, remembering each one's favorite wine and children's names. The proximity of the Manor House to the R&D building offered guests the irresistible combination of Schotze's mothering, pastoral tranquility, and business convenience.[34] Visiting executives jockeyed for the privilege of staying there.

BI's established R&D centers in Europe focused on drugs to treat heart and lung diseases. To avoid duplication with those research efforts, the new Ridgefield laboratories initially concentrated on finding new ways to treat allergies, asthma, and lung inflammation conditions, research that would complement and expand BI's worldwide product line. But Rosenthal was determined to broaden the company's American research efforts. Shortly after his arrival, he engaged his small staff of scientists in developing a new strategic plan.

As part of this broader strategy, Rosenthal assigned Vincent "Jay" Merluzzi to outline some virology research projects.[35] Merluzzi, an unabashed Madonna fan, had arrived at BI a year earlier from Memorial Sloan-Kettering Cancer Center, where he had directed a well-funded research laboratory. Like many talented academic scientists at the time, he was attracted to pharmaceutical research by the stable research funding, modern laboratory facilities, and administrative support that industry offered.[36] And like Rosenthal, Merluzzi was an immunologist. He was not an expert in virology, but he tackled the assignment. After considering a variety of research options, Merluzzi produced a convincing proposal for two virology projects, one of which focused on AIDS. Of all the diseases caused by a virus, AIDS offered the greatest scientific opportunities and represented the greatest unmet medical need. At that time, AZT was the only drug on the market to treat AIDS. Merluzzi knew that several other drug companies were investigating experimental drugs that were chemically related to AZT, and they all worked by inhibiting an HIV-specific enzyme called reverse transcriptase. Clearly, a drug that disabled this enzyme would be beneficial in treating AIDS. But the AZT-like drugs caused a number of unpleasant side effects. Merluzzi proposed a

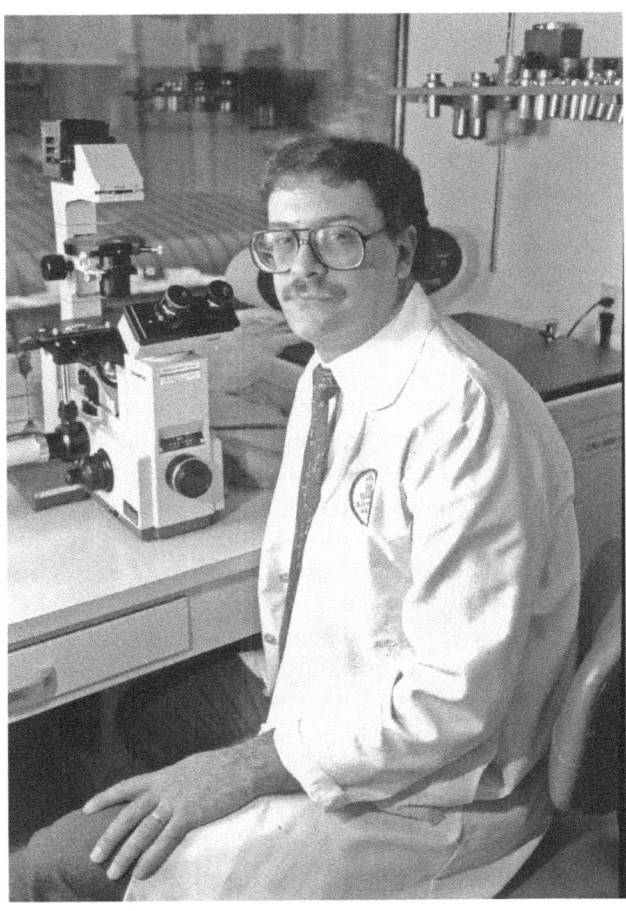

Vincent J. Merluzzi in his laboratory at Boehringer Ingelheim (courtesy *Danbury News-Times*, photographer Wendy Carlson).

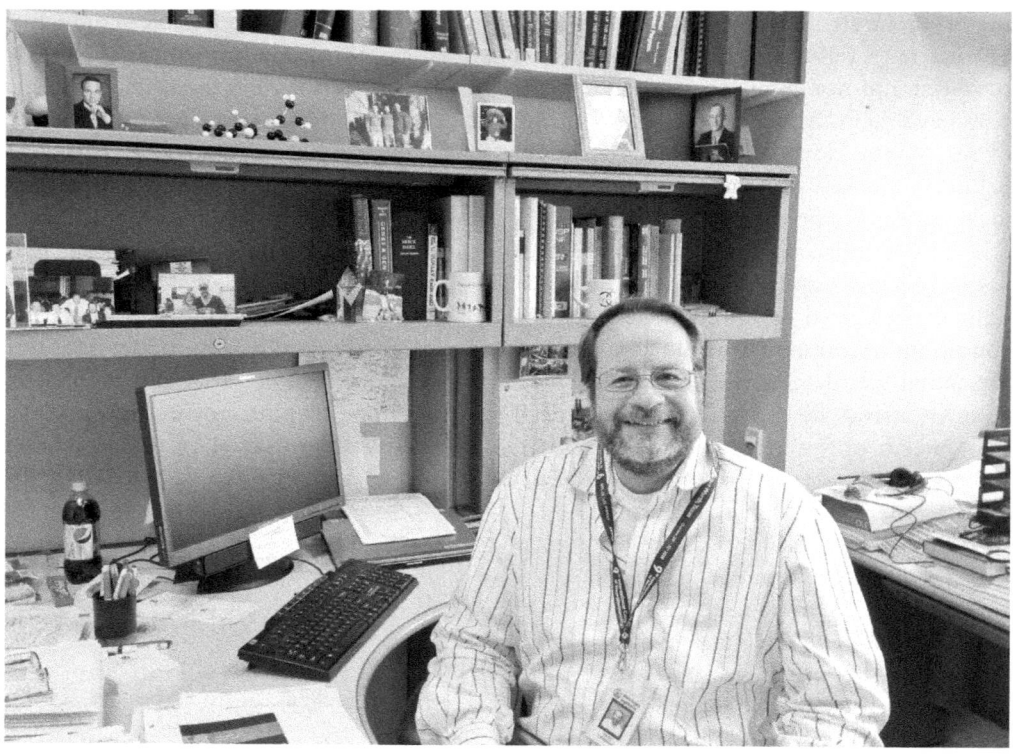

Mark Labadia in his office at Boehringer Ingelheim.

research program to look for a drug that was chemically different, was more potent, and caused fewer side effects than the AZT-like drugs. Rosenthal agreed.

For enzymes that are well understood, chemists use the enzyme's molecular structure as a guide in designing new drugs to inhibit it. Unfortunately, HIV reverse transcriptase had only recently been isolated and little was known about it. Instead, Merluzzi decided to set up a simple laboratory test (known as an assay) that measured the ability of drugs to inhibit the enzyme. BI had an extensive collection of drug samples, the cumulative output of hundreds of BI chemists over many decades. He proposed testing randomly selected compounds from the company's chemical archives, knowing that most of them would fail in the assay. Some companies tested random compounds for years in such screening assays without any success, but if he was lucky, he might find one that worked.

Merluzzi handed his research proposal to Mark Labadia, who was working in his laboratory. Labadia had joined BI a year before Merluzzi as a laboratory scientist and under Merluzzi's direction had been conducting various immunology and cell biology assays in support of BI's other research projects. Now, Merluzzi asked Labadia to set up the enzyme assay referenced in his HIV proposal. Despite his lack of virology experience and no existing standard assays for this HIV enzyme, Labadia embraced the challenge and the opportunity to learn new techniques. He read Merluzzi's proposal, consulted other scientists at BI, and searched the scientific literature for guidance on how to set up his new assay.[37] No commercial suppliers sold the human enzyme. To get things started, Merluzzi purchased supplies of a similar mouse enzyme, and Labadia used it to work out the methods for a screening assay.

Over the next few months, he refined the optimal conditions for rapidly screening the randomly selected compounds and identifying those that inhibited the enzyme.[38]

* * *

Rosenthal and Merluzzi soon realized that they needed to add a virology expert to their research project, preferably someone who understood viruses like HIV, which belongs to a subclass of viruses called retroviruses.[39] As part of this talent search, Merluzzi contacted a colleague at the University of Massachusetts, who passed the inquiry to Robert Eckner, a professor in the Microbiology and Radiation Oncology Department.[40] Merluzzi and Eckner had previously met at Boston University, when Merluzzi was a graduate student and Eckner was on the university faculty, but they had worked in different departments. Eckner had subsequently held several faculty positions and was an accomplished researcher, familiar with a variety of viruses including retroviruses. Although he had not studied HIV, Eckner understood — like everyone else — the urgency in finding ways to curb the raging epidemic caused by this virus and welcomed the opportunity to join the BI team.[41]

Eckner and his wife, Kristine, moved to BI in December 1987. The two had met when he was a post-doctoral fellow at Roswell Park Cancer Research Institute and she was hired as a laboratory assistant in the same laboratory. They developed a close working and personal relationship, coauthoring a number of scientific publications, and eventually they married. Along with his faculty positions at Boston University School of Medicine and the University of Massachusetts Medical School, Bob headed his own research laboratory, where Kris managed the day-to-day laboratory activities, conducting much of the work herself, and handled

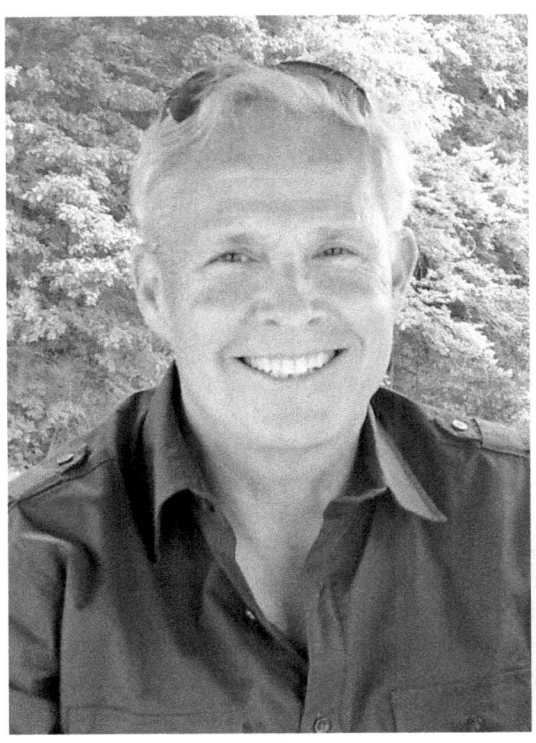
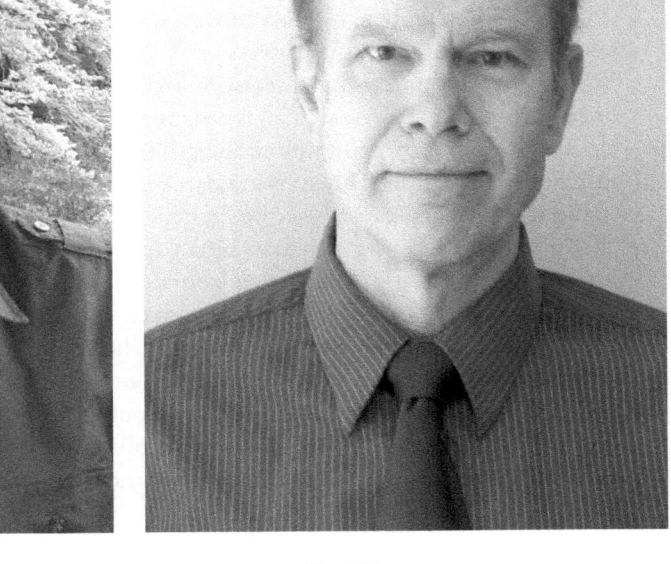

Robert Eckner. **Karl Hargrave.**

the administrative details of his research grants. At BI, Rosenthal immediately assigned Bob to the HIV research project, and Kris took a temporary position in an adjoining laboratory, substituting for a technician who was on maternity leave.[42]

By January 1988, Labadia had refined his mouse enzyme assay sufficiently to begin testing compounds. As a first step, he used his assay to test a broad collection of standards, compounds with known biological properties, to confirm that his assay was running smoothly and producing accurate, reliable results. After testing only a few hundred standards and much to his surprise, he found one that appeared to inhibit the enzyme. He quickly repeated his tests to make sure.[43] Having confirmed the result, Merluzzi and Labadia took their data, along with the compound's chemical structure, to Karl Hargrave and discussed what they should do next.

Hargrave was a mild-mannered and skillful chemist who spoke with a soft, Southern accent. He had joined BI in August 1979, directly after completing his graduate and post-doctoral studies in North Carolina and only two months after the R&D building opened in Ridgefield.[44] Over the following ten years, he had directed one of the Ridgefield unit's five chemistry laboratories and gained considerable experience making new compounds, primarily for an allergy research program. Like the rest of the BI group, he had no previous research experience with HIV, but he selected a few chemically-related compounds for Labadia to test. Those compounds also showed some promise in Labadia's mouse-enzyme assay.[45]

But the mouse enzyme was not the same as the HIV enzyme. To confirm Labadia's findings, Eckner obtained a sample of HIV reverse transcriptase from Ron Swanstrom at the University of North Carolina, who had developed a way to manufacture the human enzyme genetically in a strain of bacteria.[46] Unfortunately, the compounds that Labadia had identified in his mouse assay did not inhibit this human enzyme.[47] This cast doubt that these compounds would be useful AIDS drugs. To make sure, they wanted to test the compounds under more relevant laboratory conditions, an assay that would determine whether the compounds could prevent HIV from infecting and multiplying in living human cells. Unfortunately, the BI laboratories were not equipped to conduct assays using the live human virus.

Eckner remembered John Sullivan, whose laboratory was just down the hall from Eckner's when he worked at the University of Massachusetts in Worcester.[48] During his residency in pediatrics and infectious disease, Sullivan had spent two years at the National Institutes of Health conducting research on the viruses responsible for measles, influenza, and mononucleosis, as well as studying immunology. He joined the new Medical School in Worcester in 1978 and established an active research program, developing cell lines to understand the immune deficiency caused by the Epstein Barr virus, a virus in the herpes family. When children with immune deficiencies began appearing at the University of Massachusetts Medical Center in the early 1980s, he collaborated with his clinical colleagues to study the origins of the children's disease. Sullivan developed an early, indirect method for detecting HIV and, in addition to his laboratory research, he set up a community testing site, where gay and bisexual men, injection drug users, and others at risk for HIV infection could get tested for HIV anonymously. It was an important public service and "something I thought I should do."[49] By the late 1980s, Sullivan ran an established, well-funded research laboratory studying HIV, and the Worcester campus's AIDS clinic served all of central and western Massachusetts.

Sullivan had developed methods to safely isolate HIV from infected patients and use it to observe the virus's ability to infect and proliferate in human cells under controlled lab-

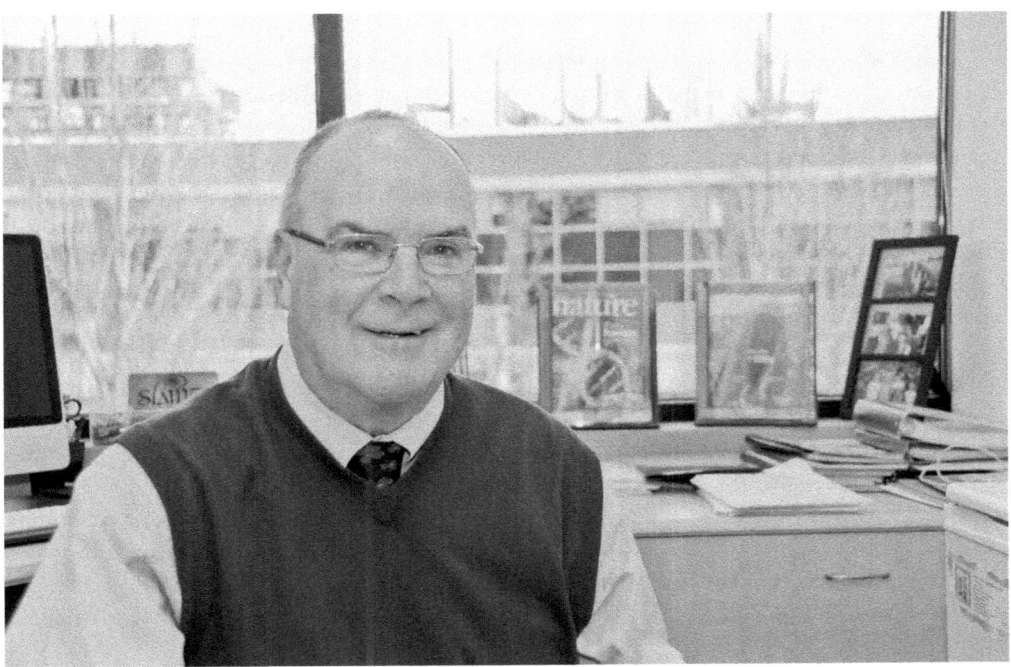

John Sullivan in his office at the University of Massachusetts.

oratory conditions. Sullivan had not screened AIDS drugs for other companies, but he saw the BI drugs as an opportunity to enhance his HIV research activities.[50] At Eckner's request, Sullivan agreed to test the compounds that had shown activity in Labadia's mouse enzyme assay. Unfortunately, the BI compounds were inactive in Sullivan's cell-based assays, the second clue that these compounds would probably not be useful as AIDS drugs.[51]

Because the mouse enzyme was sufficiently different from the human enzyme, Labadia proceeded to develop a new and more relevant screening assay with enzyme derived from HIV, the human virus. By now, Kristine Eckner had been offered a full-time, permanent position, and the two Eckners were again working as a professional team in his laboratory. Using the clone they had received from Swanstrom's laboratory, the Eckners grew colonies of bacteria that had been tricked into producing the human enzyme, spitting out large quantities of HIV reverse transcriptase like a miniature factory.[52] Because the bacteria produced only one enzyme and no other components of the virus, it did not cause HIV infection and was safe to handle in the laboratory. Kris harvested batches of the bacteria's output, isolated the enzyme, and gave it to Labadia for use in his new assay.[53]

For the next few months, Labadia reworked the assay using the HIV enzyme, refined the assay conditions, and confirmed that the new HIV assay was robust and produced reliable, reproducible results.[54] In September 1988, he was ready to begin screening randomly selected compounds from BI's archives, at the rate of 200 compounds per week.[55] Merluzzi, Labadia, and Eckner knew they might go through many thousands of compounds before they found one that showed promising results. Indeed, they might never find one. After all, other drug companies had been studying HIV much longer than BI, and none of them (so far as the BI researchers knew) had found a novel inhibitor of HIV reverse transcriptase.

* * *

Contrary to popular belief, scientists never announce new discoveries by running down the hall gripping a test tube and shouting, "Eureka!" In practice, scientific discoveries do not occur at a moment in time but rather by the accumulation and convergence of ideas, data, and insight. Merluzzi had a bright idea, but most bright ideas dim when put to the test. Labadia accumulated the data, knowing that most of his work would lead only to dead ends. Merluzzi, Labadia, Eckner, and Hargrave's insight would come, both from using the multitude of dead ends to redirect their attention to a few promising paths and from knowing what to do when a surprising result defied conventional wisdom. Their task was daunting, with no North Star to guide them and no promise of success. In addition, they were novices who had jumped on a bandwagon full of scientists who were experts in the field and had already gained years of experience.

Week after week for three months, Labadia tested compounds by the hundreds, and as expected, none gave the slightest hint of activity in his HIV assay. Then, one day as he looked at the dismal columns of numbers, the results for one compound stuck out, screaming for attention. Thinking it was a fluke, he retested it but got the same result. This compound was a robust inhibitor of the HIV enzyme.[56] He obtained a copy of the compound's chemical structure from the company's database, and with the data and chemical structure in hand, he proceeded to inform his colleagues.[57]

It was late in the afternoon, and Eckner was packing his briefcase, anxious to head home after another long day in the laboratory.[58] He looked up to see Labadia, who showed him the results. Tired and with other things on his mind, Eckner at first did not comprehend what Labadia said. It was a good result, the exact result they hoped to find and wanted. But it had come too easily and too quickly. Remembering the earlier active compound, which failed the specific HIV tests, they knew that they had much more work to do.

Labadia's next stop was Hargrave's office. Sitting at his desk, tenting his fingertips, and staring at the chemical structure, Hargrave realized that this compound had lots of potential.[59] Its chemical structure was much different than the AZT-like drugs being pursued by other investigators, and he knew that the molecule could easily be modified to make a whole series of novel compounds. Also, because this active compound had originally been made by a BI chemist, the company's chemical archives probably contained a series of compounds with related chemical structures.

Hargrave combed through BI's chemical database looking for them. It was a laborious, mostly manual process. The database cataloged the compounds, but there was no way to conduct an automatic search by structural class.[60] From his initial search, Hargrave identified and requested 75 compounds for testing. In addition, a BI chemist from the German R&D laboratories who was familiar with this series of chemicals gathered another fifty compounds and sent them to Ridgefield.

A few days after obtaining his original assay results, Labadia and his colleagues sat at the big, round table in Rosenthal's plush corner office, briefing the vice president on their observations and discussing what to do next.[61] Rosenthal energized the research efforts in Ridgefield from the day he arrived, engaging everyone from department heads to entry-level technicians, setting the bar higher than anyone could reach, cheering them on, and praising every accomplishment. Perpetually in motion, he darted through the Ridgefield laboratories like a hummingbird collecting nectar. He loved fine wine and frozen yogurt. But most of all, he loved the quest, probing the edge of scientific knowledge and pushing his scientists beyond it. They were unaccustomed to sitting in a vice president's office, but he encouraged them to come, and they remembered every moment of those invigorating meetings. Rosenthal immediately recognized the chemical structure of Labadia's active compound, recalling that similar compounds were being tested in another research program in Ridgefield.[62] Labadia obtained samples of them to test in his assay, while waiting for the compounds that Hargrave had requested from the archives.

2

The Second Time Around

In 1928, Albert Boehringer, the company's founder, acquired another German pharmaceutical company, Dr. Karl Thomae — a savvy business move to increase Boehringer Ingelheim's market share in opiates. Located near the enchanting Black Forest in southern Germany, Thomae enhanced BI's research, development, and manufacturing capabilities in a setting that seamlessly combined the nineteenth century charms of the rural German grand-duchy with modern industrial knowhow. BI allowed Thomae to continue marketing products under its own label — among them, Thomapyrin, a best-selling headache medication containing aspirin, acetaminophen, and caffeine. In the 1960s and long before anyone knew about AIDS, Thomae scientists began investigations to find a drug that reduced gastric acid and could be used to treat peptic ulcers. They synthesized hundreds of chemically related compounds before settling on pirenzepine as the best drug in its class, and BI subsequently marketed pirenzepine (Gastrozepin) as an anti-ulcer drug in Europe.[1] Instead of discarding the inactive and low-performing drugs in this chemical series, the scientists kept the samples in a storage facility — a sort of chemical graveyard. And there the chemical failures sat for twenty years on a dusty shelf in Germany, until Mark Labadia tested one of them at random in his HIV enzyme assay and found that it was remarkably active.

Labadia continued screening random compounds, but he gave priority to the pirenzepine-related compounds that Karl Hargrave had selected. Some were active, but none were as good as the compound he initially discovered. Then, in February 1989, another compound from the pirenzepine series caught his attention. Its BI code number was L-S 1170, and it was about twenty times more potent than the first active compound.[2] Labadia repeated his tests and verified his results. Bob Eckner quickly arranged for John Sullivan to test L-S 1170 in the cell-based HIV assays at the University of Massachusetts. Unlike the earlier compounds that proved to be "false positives," L-S 1170 prevented HIV replication in Sullivan's laboratory assays, an indication that this compound really might work as an AIDS drug.

For Rosenthal, the timing could not have been better. He had been looking for impressive research findings that he could use to justify his ambitious plans for expanding Ridgefield's research and development operations. L-S 1170, a potential breakthrough in the treatment of AIDS, was just the kind of research progress he sought. The compound's structure was in a completely different chemical class than AZT or any of the AZT-like drugs — Jay Merluzzi's first research objective — and it represented a brand new approach to treating AIDS. Now, with Hargrave's guidance, they hoped to find a more potent drug in the series and one with fewer side effects than AZT — Merluzzi's other two objectives.

Although L-S 1170 presented an opportunity, it also forced Rosenthal to address several critical issues. No one on Rosenthal's team had ever developed an antiviral drug, and Boehringer Ingelheim had never conducted a development program like this.[3] The special sensitivities surrounding treatment of AIDS patients were very much on his mind. In addition to the usual pressures associated with new drug development, drug companies with AIDS programs were working under the watchful eye of news media, which reported every advance and setback. Rosenthal knew that, with the whole world watching, his scientists needed to do things right and do them fast — faster than BI had ever developed a new drug.

The first issue was whether to proceed with developing L-S 1170 as a drug to treat AIDS or let Labadia and Hargrave continue their evaluation of compounds in the L-S 1170 series. Drug development requires extensive preliminary testing, and the sooner they collected these data on L-S 1170, the sooner they could begin testing it in people. Everyone knew the urgent need for new drugs to treat AIDS, and if they had one, they were morally obligated to develop it as fast as possible. On the other hand, if one of the compounds on Labadia and Hargrave's long list of untested compounds was significantly more potent, it would be a better development candidate than L-S 1170. But, there

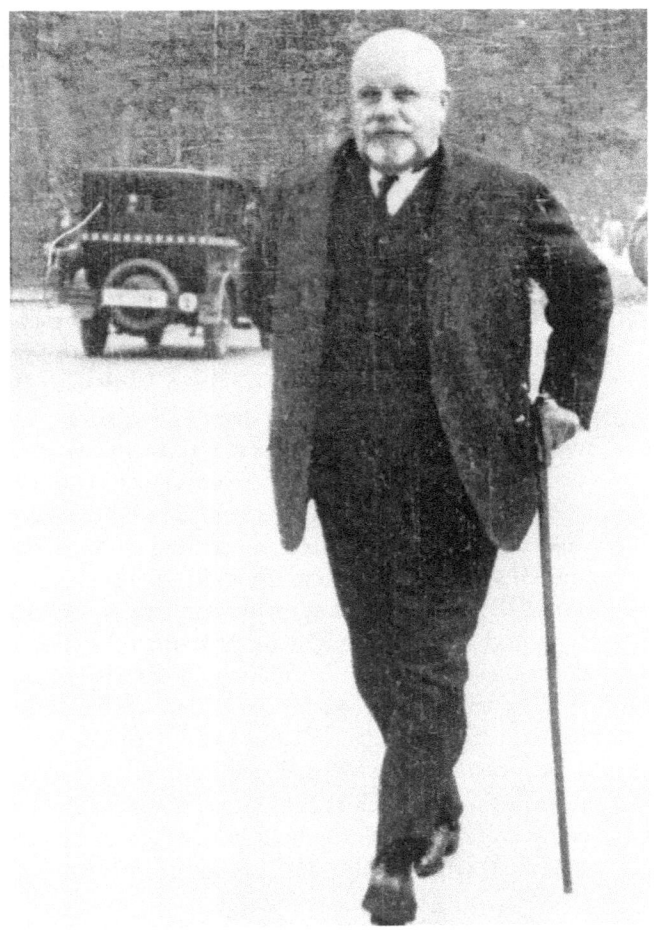

Albert Boehringer, the founder of Boehringer Ingelheim (courtesy Boehringer Ingelheim).

were no guarantees. Labadia might test compounds for years and still not find anything better, and all the while, BI would lose valuable time that could have been spent developing L-S 1170. Faced with this choice, Rosenthal decided to do both: they would move forward with L-S 1170 as a development candidate and Labadia would continue screening compounds in his HIV assay. Rosenthal was determined that, one way or the other, BI would produce a drug to treat AIDS.

The second issue facing Rosenthal was the patent status of L-S 1170. Drug companies have different philosophies on obtaining patents, but they usually file a chemical patent application that covers several related chemical structures in the series, not just the drug that is approved for market. If L-S 1170 had been included in Thomae's original pirenzepine patent, that patent would soon expire, making the drug unattractive from a business perspective. Fortunately, because L-S 1170 had been a failure as an anti-ulcer drug, it had not been covered in Thomae's patent, and consequently, the molecule represented a fertile, new area for chemical research — one that BI was now eager to exploit. Rosenthal directed Hargrave to work with BI's patent attorneys in Ridgefield and at Thomae on a patent application covering L-S 1170. He wanted the application filed within two weeks.

Writing the patent application turned out to be more complicated than Rosenthal anticipated. One key issue concerned who would be named as co-inventors. Chemists at both R&D centers deserved co-inventor recognition, but the status of inventor carried different meanings in the two countries.[4] In the United States, industry scientists typically assign their patent rights to their employer. The scientist may be the designated inventor but his or her employer retains ownership of invented products and the right to profit from them. Some companies may compensate the scientist-inventor through stock, a cash bonus, or other awards, but these incentives are only meant to acknowledge the scientist's contributions and are not related to the value of the commercial product. By contrast, German companies and chemists who are listed on patents as inventors receive payments from the product's sales, based on their share of the patent rights. Therefore, the designation of co-inventors on the L-S 1170 patent was an important issue for Thomae. Determining who was entitled to be listed as a co-inventor would not be sorted out in two weeks. The internal negotiations, Rosenthal was informed, would take time to resolve, and the patent filing could not proceed without first reaching an understanding on inventorship.[5] In the meantime, BI's rights to make and use L-S 1170 were vulnerable. With so much aggressive research to find AIDS drugs and so many companies with similar compounds in their cupboards, other bright scientists might stumble upon the same discovery as Labadia. And they might take the lead by filing a competing patent application.

The third challenge for Rosenthal was finding a way to support and harmonize the research teams in Ridgefield and Laval, Canada. Six months earlier, in the summer of 1988, BI had acquired Bio-Méga, a small Canadian research laboratory. BI designated Rosenthal to oversee the research at Bio-Méga, as well as the R&D center in Ridgefield. In the intervening months, he had frequently traveled to the industrial park near Montreal to become acquainted with the Bio-Méga staff and smooth their transition into the BI organization. Bio-Méga only conducted research to discover new drugs. When the Bio-Méga scientists identified a promising drug candidate, it would be transferred to Ridgefield, where other scientists had the R&D resources to develop the compound into a commercial product. As head of both units, Rosenthal was responsible for coordinating those activities.

Prior to the acquisition, Bio-Méga's research projects included one centered on HIV. The Bio-Méga researchers wanted to find a drug that inhibited another important viral enzyme, HIV protease. Scientists at Bio-Méga and elsewhere were motivated to find HIV protease inhibitors because they knew a lot about the enzyme.[6] They knew how to make significant amounts of HIV protease by standard chemical synthesis or cloning techniques. They knew the enzyme's molecular structure in detail and how it worked. And they had developed efficient laboratory assays for testing and identifying compounds that inhibited it.

Not surprisingly, several major drug companies had large research programs aimed at finding a drug that inhibited HIV protease. Even so, the Bio-Méga chemists felt they were among the leaders in this effort. At that time, the only compounds known to inhibit HIV protease were difficult to make, decomposed easily, and probably would not work when taken by mouth.[7] But the Bio-Méga chemists had succeeded in solving some of those problems and were confident that they could make a compound that was good enough to develop as an AIDS drug.

To prevent the Laval and Ridgefield scientists from working at cross-purposes, Rosenthal had encouraged the Bio-Méga team to continue its HIV protease research and advised the

Ridgefield scientists to limit their efforts to HIV reverse transcriptase.[8] The two research groups worked independently on their respective research projects, an internal competition that Rosenthal knew would spawn two high-performing teams, each motivated to outdo the other.[9] With L-S 1170, the Ridgefield team scored first.

* * *

Initially, the HIV research in Ridgefield was conducted by a small team, including Bob Eckner, the resident virologist, Hargrave, who handled the chemistry activities, Labadia, who screened the compounds in his HIV enzyme assay, Kris Eckner, who provided technical support, and Merluzzi, who continued to play an active role in guiding their efforts. As a graduate student, Hargrave had studied x-ray crystallography, a field of chemistry that gave him a three-dimensional understanding of chemical molecules and their interactions with biological tissues.[10] Now, he applied that knowledge to refine his search for the most promising compounds in BI's sample collection. He also obtained several hundred commercially available compounds with similar chemical structures.

As Labadia reported the results from testing those compounds, Hargrave noted the chemical features that were optimal for inhibiting the HIV reverse transcriptase enzyme. With each new test result, Hargrave gained a better understanding of those features and could predict more accurately the types of compounds that would work best. Unfortunately, most of those compounds had never been synthesized. So, he devised a plan for making these new compounds in his laboratory. At the end of March 1989, he was directing two of the laboratories in his group (four chemists) to make the new compounds. A month later, three of his laboratories (six chemists) were working full time to synthesize the new compounds on his list.[11]

With Rosenthal's mandate to continue the search for better compounds, Eckner's research team steadily grew, adding biochemists who were experts at purifying and characterizing enzymes and other scientists who profiled the biologic properties and side effects of the active compounds. In addition, Eckner continued his efforts to acquire better sources of the HIV enzyme, eventually obtaining several versions of it.[12] Rosenthal repeatedly pressed the research team to verify their results. He wanted assurance that the BI compounds were true inhibitors of HIV and not the result of an error in laboratory technique or impurities in the assay. With each new source of enzyme and each improvement in the assay methods, the active compounds were retested, and the assay was "recertified over and over again."[13]

When they found new compounds that were active in the HIV enzyme assay, Eckner and Labadia would pack them up and drive the

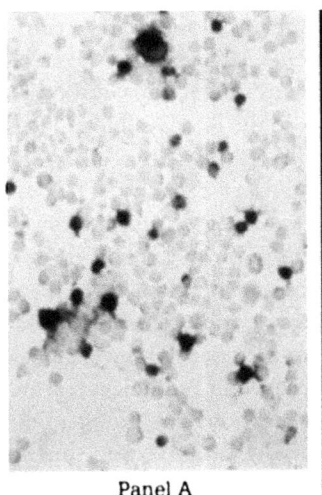 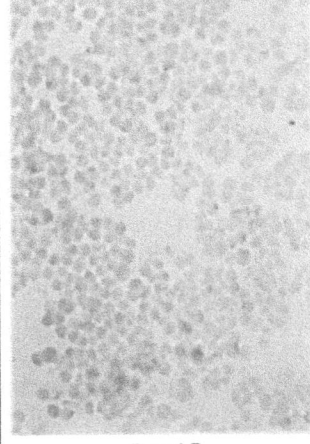

Panel A | Panel B

Replication of the virus (HIV-1) as detected by non-isotopic in situ hybridization. The black splotches in Panel A are human cells infected with HIV. In Panel B, after treatment with BIRG-587, no HIV is detected in any of the cells (courtesy John Sullivan).

130-mile stretch of Interstate 84 from Danbury to Worcester to hand-deliver the compounds to Sullivan's laboratory.[14] While there, they could peer through the microscope and look at living cells infected with HIV, marveling at what they saw. The BI compounds "shut down the virus."[15]

* * *

In addition to Eckner's research team, Rosenthal established a new team specifically focused on L-S 1170 and charged the team with characterizing the compound's pharmaceutical properties and potential side effects.[16] He wanted to start clinical trials with L-S 1170 as soon as possible. To lead this development team, Rosenthal chose Jay Merluzzi — an inspired, if not obvious, choice. In his first three years at BI, Merluzzi had established himself as a productive industrial scientist, playing a key role in the discovery of a biological compound that the researchers thought might prevent the common cold. His research contributions and leadership impressed Rosenthal, but Merluzzi had no experience in drug development and certainly had never led a drug development team.[17]

Even-tempered, unpretentious, and a quick study, Merluzzi let his "naïveté help," seeking out experienced people and asking them to explain the details of drug development that he did not know.[18] Unlike many research scientists, he was also a pragmatic, velvet-gloved taskmaster and diligent about meeting deadlines. After his move to Connecticut, he maintained his academic ties by teaching evening classes at CUNY/Queens College, experience that put him at ease in front of an audience, answering tricky questions and thinking on his feet.[19] His knowledge of HIV, ability to communicate effectively, and easygoing rapport with everyone from vice presidents to laboratory technicians all contributed to his success in leading his team through the frenzied months that lay ahead.

Mindful of the progress at Bio-Méga, Rosenthal asked Merluzzi to prepare plans that would accommodate developing an HIV protease inhibitor — yet to emerge from the researchers at Bio-Méga — as well as L-S 1170, and he assigned two Bio-Méga chemists as members of Merluzzi's team. In addition, the team included representatives from each of BI's development departments, all located in the R&D laboratory building. Their proximity to each other fostered frequent interactions, not only during the team's weekly meetings but also impromptu discussions in the R&D cafeteria, hallways, and even the parking lot. Rounding out the team were the clinical, regulatory affairs, and project management representatives, who served mostly in an advisory capacity. Their offices were located in a rented wing of Union Carbide's corporate building, one mile from the BI campus, and the distance limited their day-to-day interactions with Merluzzi and the other laboratory-based team members. They would switch from advisors to active participants when L-S 1170 entered clinical trials, which would not start — even under the most favorable conditions — for more than a year.

The development team members who were located in BI's R&D building were responsible for profiling the chemical and biological features of L-S 1170 by collecting data under various laboratory testing conditions, including animal studies. Some of those studies would help them understand how the drug worked, but most of the data was needed to satisfy federal regulatory requirements, primarily establishing the drug's safety, prior to giving the drug to people. And all of these preclinical studies required significant amounts of L-S 1170.

Labadia and Sullivan only needed a few specks of the compound for their laboratory assays, and only a small amount of L-S 1170 had been shipped from the chemical archives for this purpose. Because the development team now required much larger quantities, Hargrave and his assistants set out to make an additional sample, but the size of their laboratory equipment limited the amount they could produce. Their first batch was less than half an ounce, which was enough for the first biochemical and biological assays. For the planned series of animal studies, the team needed around seven kilograms (about fifteen pounds) of L-S 1170. The clinical trials, of course, would require even more. To make those kilogram quantities efficiently, the chemists needed larger facilities and equipment, which the Ridgefield campus currently did not have.

* * *

BI's plans for the Ridgefield campus had always included a pilot plant capable of making drug batches up to ten kilograms.[20] This facility would allow the chemists to test various methods for improving production of an experimental drug in bulk quantities, larger than was possible in the small chemistry laboratories. For quantities greater than ten kilograms, they would transfer production to one of BI's large-scale manufacturing plants. Rosenthal supported construction of a pilot plant and saw L-S 1170 as an opportunity to justify approving the long-delayed plans to build it. But even if he obtained approval, the pilot plant would take time to build. Merluzzi's team could not afford to wait. They needed an alternative plan, and the mastermind who solved their immediate drug supply problem was Karl Grozinger.

Born in Germany, Grozinger earned his undergraduate and Ph.D. degrees in chemistry while working full time at Pharma Research Ltd., a small Montreal-based research institute that contributed to BI's international research efforts. In 1979, BI consolidated its North American research facilities, and sixteen of the Pharma Research scientists, including Grozinger, moved to Ridgefield, the first occupants of the new R&D laboratories. Grozinger, an expert in scale up chemistry, had been lured to Ridgefield by an offer to design the new pilot plant and oversee drug production there. But the construction plans were repeatedly delayed in favor of BI's other building expansion priorities in Ridgefield. While waiting for the pilot plant to become a reality, Grozinger maintained a chemistry laboratory in the R&D building, like Hargrave's and the other chemists', but his laboratory equipment was larger, and he could

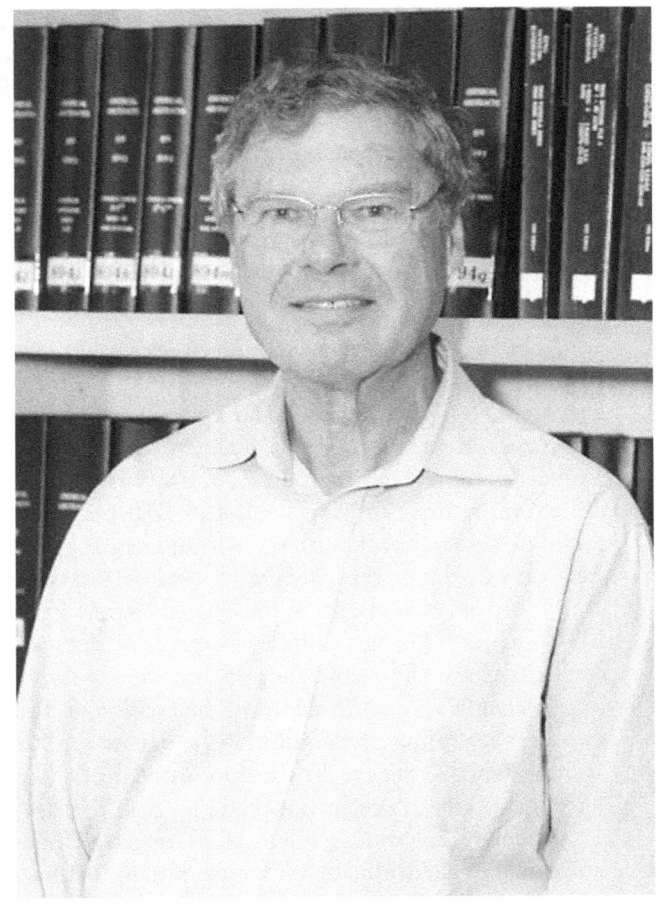

Karl Grozinger.

make drug batches up to one kilogram. Because his colleagues rarely needed kilo-sized batches, he supported the ongoing research teams by making small samples of novel compounds alongside his chemistry colleagues. Grozinger spoke rapidly and enthusiastically about each compound he made — whether it was a small amount of a novel compound or a kilo-batch — and never let his disappointment about the construction delays hinder the quality or efficiency of his work.

Grozinger was as productive and hardworking as the other chemists, but the difference in his work habits was strikingly apparent to anyone who visited his laboratory. Although the R&D building was only ten years old, most of the chemistry laboratories bore the scars of many harsh chemical campaigns. But not Grozinger's. In his spit-polished laboratory, the cabinets were pristine, the bench tops shined, the glassware gleamed, and the floor sparkled. Reagent and solvent bottles stood in regimental order on the shelves, each neatly labeled. The strict standards for cleanliness and equipment maintenance that are required for large-scale pharmaceutical production came naturally to Grozinger, and he applied them to all his work.

To meet the needs of Merluzzi's team for testing L-S 1170 in their various preclinical studies, Grozinger began making batches in his kilo-laboratory. He was still making his first test batch of 50 grams when Merluzzi asked him to start production of a second 50 gram batch. When he delivered those two batches, the team asked for 500 grams (about one pound). Even with Grozinger's skill, the kilo-laboratory was just not suitable to meet the team's increasing drug supply needs. If L-S 1170 performed well in the team's preclinical studies, and everyone hoped it would, Rosenthal wanted to proceed with clinical trials without a delay caused by a shortage of drug supply. So, in addition to making small batches of L-S 1170 in his kilo-laboratory, Grozinger held initial discussions with contract laboratories capable of making larger scale batches. In parallel, Hargrave explored options with his European chemistry colleagues for producing large batches of L-S 1170 at their BI facilities.

* * *

The early test results encouraged Merluzzi's team, who soon discovered that L-S 1170 was well suited to development as an AIDS drug. Except for its ability to inhibit the HIV enzyme, L-S 1170 appeared to have no other biological actions that might cause side effects in patients. It had no effect on the heart, lungs, brain, or other organs, except making some animals sleepy at very high doses, and it was not toxic to living cells that had been grown under laboratory conditions.[21] If L-S 1170 performed the same way in people, the drug might be able to knock out HIV without causing the unpleasant side effects associated with AZT and the other experimental drugs being developed.

In April 1989, Hargrave traveled to Germany to continue detailed discussions with his BI colleagues.[22] He met with the German chemists who had made compounds for the pirenzepine research effort, and they offered valuable advice on how to make novel compounds in this chemical class. In addition, he continued discussions with the chemists and patent attorneys regarding preparation of the patent application for L-S 1170. Finally, he pursued arrangements to engage BI's European facilities to produce the scaled up batches of L-S 1170 that Merluzzi's team was requesting, in preparation for the first clinical trials.

One evening during this visit, Hargrave's dinner with colleagues was interrupted by a waiter who called him to the house phone.[23] Amazed that anyone could track him to a restaurant in Germany, Hargrave listened as the Ridgefield caller informed him of some breaking news about L-S 1170. Along with the encouraging test results, Merluzzi's team was also uncovering some unattractive features of the compound. The most discouraging property, just reported by the scientists in Ridgefield, was that L-S 1170 was metabolized quickly. When given orally to animals, only a small fraction of the compound was absorbed into the bloodstream, and the animals efficiently eliminated it in a couple of hours. Patients took the short-acting AZT three or four times a day, making it a rather inconvenient drug for long-term use. The new L-S 1170 findings meant that it would need to be taken even more frequently, too frequently to be useful as an AIDS drug. Consequently, Hargrave was told, large-scale batches of L-S 1170 were no longer needed. The compound was not good enough for clinical trials.

* * *

Hargrave and his colleagues had found or synthesized a number of compounds that were active in Labadia's HIV assay, and Rosenthal wanted the BI patent to cover them all, hopeful that one would prove to be better than L-S 1170. When Hargrave returned to Ridgefield, he ramped up his efforts on the patent application. For weeks, three secretaries typed draft after draft, incorporating revisions as Hargrave and the lawyers wrote, proofread, and rewrote this complicated document, section by section. The BI group in Ridgefield took responsibility for writing the patent application, but the question of inventorship was still unresolved. BI's attorneys interviewed Hargrave and the other chemists on both sides of the Atlantic to determine the contributions each had made to the discovery of L-S 1170 as a reverse transcriptase inhibitor. Finally, on April 20, 1989, two months after Labadia reported the initial L-S 1170 results, BI filed the patent application. That evening, a long row of plastic bags stuffed full of shredded drafts stretched down the hallway in the R&D building.

The filing date secured BI's claim to the L-S 1170 series of HIV-active compounds, but the patent's claims were already insufficient by the time the application reached the U.S. Patent Office. Labadia had found another compound from BI's chemical archives that was as potent as L-S 1170. Within a few weeks, Hargrave used this compound's chemical structure as a guide to synthesize an equally potent but novel compound. Hargrave and his colleagues now seemed to be on the right track, refining chemical features that led to even more potent compounds.

By May, Labadia reported that three of those newly synthesized compounds were, indeed, more potent than L-S 1170. Hargrave's progress in making better compounds put Merluzzi's team at a crossroad. Should they continue to follow their original directive, which was to collect a comprehensive preclinical dataset on L-S 1170, knowing that it was an inferior compound and would not be given to people? Or, should they discontinue work on L-S 1170 and begin development of a new and more potent compound? But if so, which one? Each week, Labadia's assay results confirmed that the chemists were creating better compounds than the week before — a process that could go on forever. The number of possible variations in this chemical series was astronomical.

For the past three months, Merluzzi had held weekly team meetings, communicated almost daily with his team members, met regularly with Eckner, Labadia, and Hargrave, issued formal reports, and sent countless email updates. He also frequently consulted privately with Rosenthal and the R&D department directors, updating them on the status of L-S 1170 and asking their advice.[24] But contradictory, inconsistent, and rapidly changing opinions left the development team without clear guidance. They were running, enthusiastically, in all directions. Merluzzi, the traffic cop at the crossroad, wanted "to just get on with it."[25] But the push-pull continued. Merluzzi's team continued to evaluate L-S 1170 in various preclinical studies to learn as much as they could about the compound's properties, while Eckner's team continued the search for a better compound to replace it.[26] Not knowing which compound would be selected or when that would happen, Merluzzi took a long weekend at the end of May and headed to Vermont. He was scouting real estate to build a house for his retirement.[27]

The hallway chatter during the summer of 1989 mostly concerned the new and more potent compounds. Merluzzi's team shifted priorities from studies of L-S 1170 to preparing a generic plan to develop one or more of the new compounds, yet to be chosen. They cancelled new preclinical studies of L-S 1170, but they still needed drug supplies to continue the studies they had already started.[28] Grozinger got lots of practice making batches of the chemical, but in the end, his laboratory produced only one kilogram of L-S 1170.[29]

* * *

In parallel with Hargrave's efforts to make better inhibitors of reverse transcriptase in Ridgefield, the chemists at Bio-Méga had been making steady progress in finding HIV protease inhibitors, generating dozens of new compounds per month. Because the Bio-Méga team had limited capability for evaluating these new compounds in their Laval laboratories, they shipped the compounds to Ridgefield. When Eckner sent Hargrave's compounds to Sullivan and other external investigators for further evaluation in various HIV replication assays, he sent Bio-Méga's compounds, too.[30] So far, the Bio-Méga team had not found an HIV protease inhibitor that was good enough to develop as an AIDS drug. But with their rapid progress and the setback imposed by L-S 1170's limitations, the Bio-Méga team now had a chance of finding an AIDS drug candidate before Eckner's team in Ridgefield.

One link between the research efforts at Laval and Ridgefield was Julian Adams. Adams had joined Bio-Méga in 1987 after five years as a medicinal chemist at Merck Frosst Canada in Montreal. At Merck, Rosenthal's responsibilities as vice president of immunology research included overseeing the company's Montreal unit, and the two scientists forged a close working relationship. Subsequently, Rosenthal moved to BI,

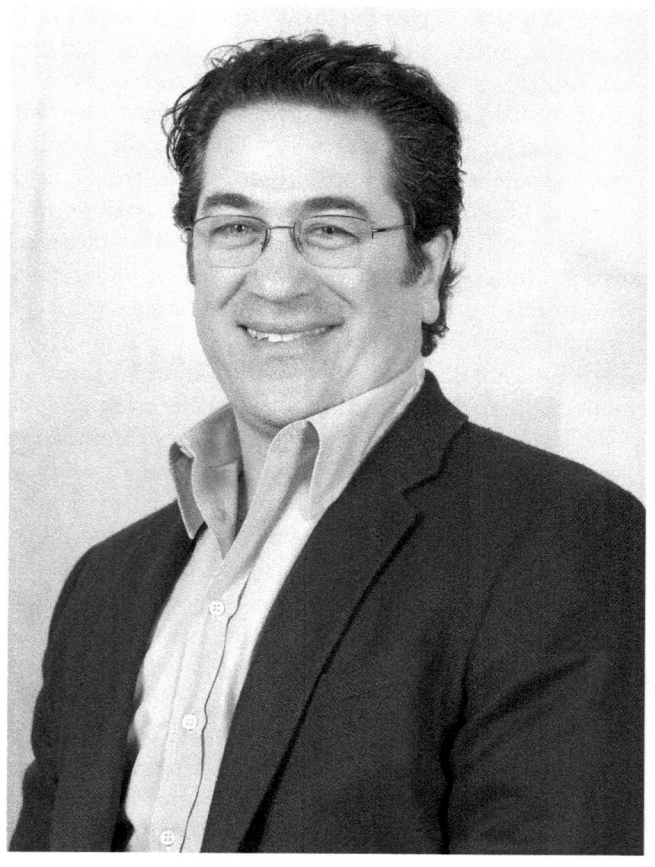

Julian Adams.

Adams moved to Bio-Méga, BI acquired Bio-Méga, and, in 1989, the head of medicinal chemistry at BI's Ridgefield R&D center retired. As Rosenthal crafted the rapidly growing Ridgefield unit, he took advantage of the chemistry vacancy to redefine and restructure BI's medicinal chemistry resources. In parallel with the search for a new department head, Rosenthal asked Adams, whom he trusted and respected, to move to Ridgefield for a year, evaluate the department, and assist with the restructuring effort.[31] Although younger than Grozinger and Hargrave, Adams had apprenticed under senior drug development experts at Merck, and he now applied that insight and experience to the fledgling unit in Ridgefield. He had already been serving as one of the two Bio-Méga chemists on Merluzzi's development team. Once in Ridgefield, Adams accelerated the chemistry department's HIV research efforts, reassigning chemists to supplement Hargrave's laboratory. Soon, fourteen chemists were making novel compounds for the HIV research program.[32] Like everyone else, Adams felt the huge public pressure and the urgent need for new AIDS drugs, but he also knew the importance of finding the best possible drug candidate. He asked Rosenthal for six months, enough time for the chemists to optimize their series of compounds but still a short time that ensured they would work fast.[33]

Adams soon demonstrated not only his command of medicinal chemistry but also his broad understanding of virology and his leadership skills. Rosenthal ended his recruiting efforts for the new head of the chemistry department and officially appointed Adams to the post. Adams organized weekly brainstorming sessions where Hargrave led the chemists in discussing which compounds to make, who would make them, and in what order.[34] With each passing week and guided by the test results from Labadia's and Sullivan's laboratory assays, the best compounds had chemical structures that looked less and less like L-S 1170.

Unfortunately, many of those newer compounds were not claimed in BI's original patent application. Rosenthal once again asked Adams and Hargrave to amend the patent. Over the summer, this was a moving target. Each week, new test results directed them to explore further modifications to the chemical structure, make the new compounds, and test them. Incorporating this evolving knowledge into the patent claims meant multiple revisions to the patent documents. One of BI's patent attorneys moved from his office in the off-campus Union Carbide building to a vacant office in the R&D building to work side-by-side with Hargrave. Four secretaries typed the drafts, as Hargrave wrote, proofread, updated, and rewrote the text. Throughout that "intense" summer, Hargrave often arrived at his office before dawn, and he and his coworkers continued hammering away at the patent documents long after everyone else had gone home each evening—even convincing the computer room staff to delay their routine maintenance shutdowns until the patent drafts were saved.[35] On June 18, 1989, BI's patent attorneys filed the first of the patent application's Continuation-in-Part, which amended and broadened BI's original patent claims. On August 29, 1989, they filed another update covering more chemical structures, ones that were even more distantly related to L-S 1170.[36]

* * *

If the summer of 1989 was intense for Hargrave, it energized Labadia. He "couldn't wait to get out of bed and get to work" each morning.[37] His colleagues in BI's other research programs churned through endless racks of randomly chosen compounds, hoping to find just one that gave a hint of activity. But for Labadia, it was not a question of finding an active compound. He wondered how much the chemists could improve the activity of this chemical series.

Meanwhile, Merluzzi's team was growing increasingly impatient. Nearly a year had passed since the first active compounds had surfaced in Labadia's HIV assay, and they still had not selected the drug destined for clinical trials. About sixty experimental AIDS drugs from other drug companies were in or nearing clinical testing, and BI's clinicians worried that by the time their drug was ready for clinical trials they would have difficulty finding interested clinical investigators and patients.

They were also monitoring a new problem that put greater urgency in finding alternative drugs to treat AIDS, but it was a problem that might also hamper the success of their AIDS drug. The day after Merluzzi held his first team meeting in March, *Science*, a premier scientific journal, published data showing that the AIDS virus developed resistance to AZT.[38] HIV could outsmart AZT by morphing into a mutant form that could proliferate in patients despite continued treatment with the drug. The data suggested that the usefulness of AZT, the only drug so far approved to treat AIDS, might be severely limited, because the virus was able to resist AZT's effects. This raised many questions. Would people who developed AZT resistance respond to other AIDS drugs? Would other AIDS drugs also induce resistant HIV strains? Most importantly for BI, would L-S 1170 and its newer cousins be effective in people who were resistant to AZT, and would the BI compounds induce resistant HIV strains?

Two of the *Science* article's authors were scientists at Wellcome Research Laboratories, the manufacturer of AZT. The third author was Douglas Richman, Professor of Pathology and Medicine at the University of California, San Diego, and a physician at the San Diego Veterans Affairs Medical Center. Richman conducted clinical trials of AIDS drugs and, like Sullivan, headed an active HIV research laboratory. The AZT-resistant virus reported in the *Science* article had been extracted from blood samples of Richman's patients and analyzed in his laboratory.

After the article appeared, Bob Eckner approached Richman at a scientific meeting and proposed a research collaboration.[39] Richman's laboratory had developed cell culture assays for characterizing the effects of AIDS drugs, complementing those that Sullivan

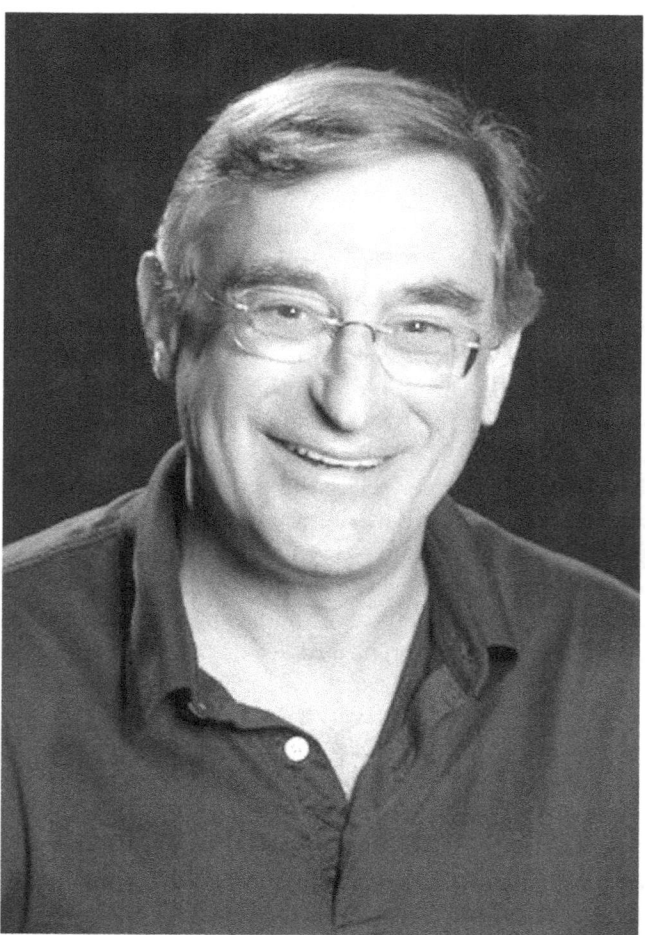

Douglas Richman.

2. The Second Time Around

was conducting at the University of Massachusetts. Most importantly, Eckner and Merluzzi wanted to know whether the BI compounds would inhibit the strains of HIV that had become resistant to AZT. Richman readily agreed to test them.[40] By the summer of 1989, arrangements for the collaboration were in place, and Eckner shipped samples of L-S 1170 and other selected BI compounds to Richman's laboratory in San Diego.[41] The BI compounds knocked out HIV in Richman's assays, just as they had in Sullivan's laboratory assays. Even better, Richman found that the BI compounds also knocked out the mutant HIV strains that were resistant to AZT.[42] Those results suggested not only that the BI compounds might work in patients but also that the BI compounds might be an effective alternative for patients who had become resistant to AZT.

Richman's laboratory also ran assays that could determine the effect of AIDS drugs on various subtypes of the human immunodeficiency virus. HIV-1 is the deadly virus that causes AIDS, and it was spreading rapidly around the world. HIV-2 is a less infectious virus, does not seem to cause as much damage to a person's immune system, and is confined mostly to western Africa. In their efforts to learn as much as possible about the strengths and weaknesses of L-S 1170, Merluzzi's team wanted Richman to test their compound in these selective assays. L-S 1170 inhibited the reverse transcriptase found in HIV-1 but not that associated with HIV-2.[43] AZT, on the other hand, inhibited the enzyme in both HIV-1 and HIV-2. No one knew whether this difference was important in treating AIDS. But some argued that, given a choice, it might be better for an AIDS drug to attack both viruses, rather than just one. This posed another challenge for Adams and Hargrave: Could they modify their active compounds and create one that inhibited both the HIV-1 and HIV-2 enzymes?

Having seen how well the initial BI compounds performed in their laboratory assays, Sullivan and Richman broadened and strengthened their collaborations with the BI researchers. Eckner sent a steady stream of BI's best compounds to Worcester and San Diego, and Sullivan and Richman immediately tested them. Because Sullivan and Richman were both physicians, BI also benefited from their clinical insight and connections in the AIDS community. Their guidance, advocacy, and influence would be indispensable when the yet-to-be-selected BI drug approached testing in the increasingly crowded field of AIDS clinical trials.

* * *

The main topic at the 4th AIDS Advisory Committee meeting, held at the National Institutes of Health on June 18–19, 1989, was pediatric AIDS. Children represented only about two percent of AIDS cases in the United States, but the recent trends were disturbing. In nearly four out of every five pediatric AIDS cases, infants became infected by their HIV-infected mothers before, during, or shortly after birth. The National Institutes of Health was conducting and planning pediatric clinical trials with AZT in an effort to find the best way to treat AIDS in children. At the June meeting, the AIDS Advisory Committee discussed at length various designs for these pediatric AIDS trials: single drug treatment versus drug combinations, whether to use placebos or not, and whether pediatric trials should start only after knowing the results from adult trials or start much earlier when less was known about the drug. The Committee could identify all the critical issues, but it offered no solutions. To design pediatric AIDS trials appropriately, clinicians really needed an experimental AIDS drug that was safe enough to give to children — one that was much safer than AZT.

Among his studies at the University of Massachusetts, Sullivan, a pediatrician, had collected viral samples from 136 hemophilia patients who, like Ryan White, had become infected with HIV through tainted Factor VIII injections. At the time, about one-tenth of all hemophilia patients in the United States had developed AIDS symptoms. But AIDS symptoms developed slowly, usually appearing eight to ten years after the initial HIV infection. Many clinicians, including Sullivan, assumed that most hemophilia patients were infected with HIV and predicted that they would all eventually develop AIDS. As part of the profiling studies requested by Merluzzi's team, Sullivan exposed samples of virus taken from these HIV-infected pediatric patients to L-S 1170. He found that the drug prevented the virus in these samples from proliferating—just as it had in his other cell-based assays. This observation was the first green light in a long and convoluted journey suggesting that the BI compounds might be good enough to give to children. But would they be safe enough?

By the end of September 1989, Mark Labadia and his colleagues had screened 2600 compounds in the HIV enzyme assay. Of those compounds, most of which were structurally related to L-S 1170, he identified several hundred that—more or less—suppressed the enzyme, and at least a dozen of them were more potent than L-S 1170.[44] Although the chemists were still making new compounds in an effort to find one that was even better, two compounds had already emerged as leading contenders to replace L-S 1170: BIRH-414 and BIRG-587.

3

A Star Is Born

When Ariel Glaser was first diagnosed with AIDS, her parents were also tested. Her father, Paul Michael Glaser, who had starred in the television series *Starsky and Hutch*, was not infected, but her mother, Elizabeth, was HIV-positive. Elizabeth's first pregnancy had been difficult. At six months, she was diagnosed with placenta previa, a condition in which the placenta grows across the cervix and causes bleeding, which can be severe.[1] She was confined to bed rest for the last trimester, and Ariel was delivered by Cesarean section in August 1981. There were no complications with Ariel's birth except that Elizabeth began bleeding again, and this time the doctors had difficulty in stopping it. Eventually, they succeeded but not before transfusing her with seven pints of blood.[2]

Only two months before, Michael Gottlieb, who would become Elizabeth's personal physician, had published the first report of an unusual and still unnamed immune deficiency syndrome.[3] Unaware of this syndrome or the virus that caused it, blood banks collected donations from individuals who appeared healthy but were unknowingly contaminating the country's blood supply. One of the pints given to Elizabeth contained HIV, a stealthy invader determined to conquer new territory, not only her body but also Ariel's through breastfeeding. For years, Elizabeth led a normal, active life, unaware of the stubborn microbe colonizing in her and Ariel's blood. At the time of Ariel's diagnosis, Elizabeth's white blood cell count was lower than normal, a telltale sign of HIV infection, but she had no AIDS symptoms.[4]

Shortly after her diagnosis, Elizabeth had a dream.[5] Not an ordinary dream. The kind that wakes you up. The kind you

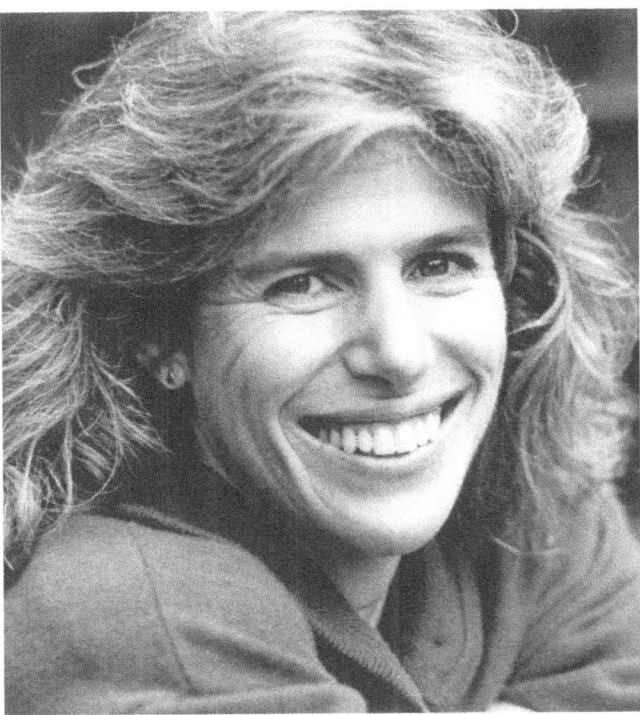

Elizabeth Glaser (courtesy Elizabeth Glaser Pediatric AIDS Foundation).

remember and replay over and over in your mind. She was standing on a cliff overlooking a peaceful bay on a sunny day. Suddenly, a gigantic dragon emerged overhead, its ice-blue and white markings at first camouflaged against the sky and clouds. Cold and menacing, it plummeted from the heights and plunged into the water, creating a huge wave. Then it shot up from the ocean's depths, so large that it blocked the sun. Although the dragon did not attack, it frightened Elizabeth, and she ran to escape its powerful presence.

The memory of the swooping dragon haunted Elizabeth for weeks. It was unlike any dream she had ever had, and it crept back into her thoughts. She tried to suppress it, purge it from her mind, but it persisted. To Elizabeth, the dragon symbolized the AIDS virus, and she was afraid that it would kill her. But, eventually, as she thought more about it, she mustered her courage and strengthened her resolve. She wanted to have that dream again. Next time, she would not fear the dragon. Next time, instead of running away, she would defy it, feet firmly planted on the ground, and battle the demon with all her strength.[6]

* * *

In the early 1960s, Jerome Horwitz, a chemist at the Michigan Cancer Foundation in Detroit, thought he could design a compound that would inhibit the growth of cancer cells.[7] Among more than one hundred compounds, he synthesized azidothymidine, commonly called AZT, and dideoxycitidine, commonly called ddC. AZT and ddC were chemically classified as nucleosides, molecules that were nearly identical to key building blocks of DNA but sufficiently different, hopefully, to damage the DNA in cancer cells and kill

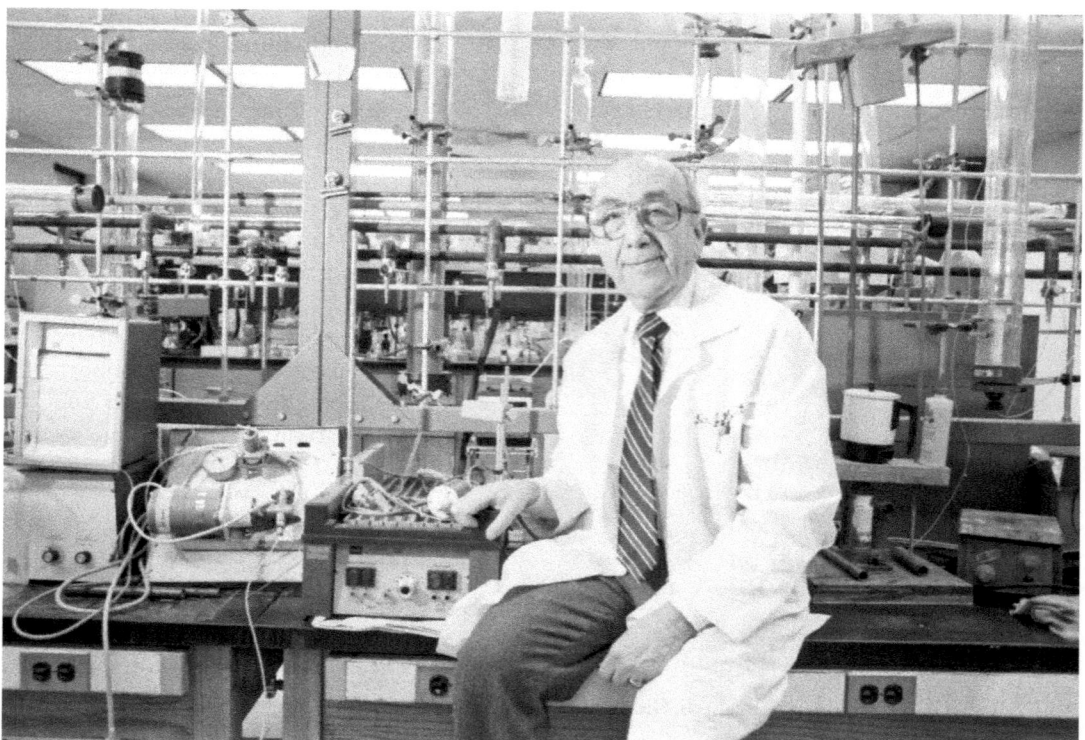

Jerome Horwitz in his laboratory at Wayne State University (courtesy Walter P. Reuther Library, Wayne State University).

them.[8] Unfortunately, when Horwitz tested the compounds in mice with leukemia, they had no activity. Like all scientists, Horwitz was accustomed to "more valleys than peaks and you learn to cope with failure."[9] In 1964, he published the dismal results, shelved the drugs, and turned to more promising approaches for treating cancer.[10]

Twenty years later, with the announcement that the human immunodeficiency virus caused AIDS, scientists at Burroughs Wellcome brainstormed ideas for a new research program. They had considerable experience developing drugs for herpes and other viruses, and they now applied those skills to find an AIDS drug. One of the first compounds supplied by the company's chemists, which they coded 509U81 but in fact was AZT, showed potent activity in their laboratory assay.[11] Like Mark Labadia's original assay at Boehringer Ingelheim, the investigators at Burroughs Wellcome used a mouse-derived assay, and their results, although promising, did not prove that their compound truly inhibited HIV, a human virus.[12] To confirm the activity of 509U81, they sent the compound to several researchers who had developed HIV assays, including Samuel Broder at the National Cancer Institute, a division of the National Institutes of Health in Bethesda, Maryland. When Broder and the other laboratories reported that 509U81 inhibited HIV in their assays, Burroughs Wellcome mounted the most aggressive drug development campaign in its history.[13] The company collaborated with the National Cancer Institute and Duke University to conduct a small safety study, and on July 3, 1985, the first HIV-infected patient was treated with AZT. In February 1986, Burroughs Wellcome launched a larger and definitive clinical trial at twelve medical centers.[14] AZT proved to be an effective treatment for AIDS, and it received approval from the Food and Drug Administration on March 19, 1987.[15]

AZT caused a long list of side effects including headache, insomnia, nausea, vomiting, diarrhea, malaise, muscle pain, rash, and fever. For most patients, these symptoms decreased over time, enabling them to continue taking the drug. AZT's most serious side effect was bone marrow toxicity, which reduced the ability of patients to make new red blood cells. About one-third of AIDS patients with advanced disease required blood transfusions to correct AZT-induced anemia. By 1989, clinicians had gained considerable experience in treating AIDS patients with AZT. They found that by reducing the dose they could minimize AZT's side effects, but bone marrow toxicity remained a serious problem. Viral resistance was another concern. As Doug Richman and the team at Burroughs Wellcome had shown, the virus mutated into strains that were resistant to AZT's antiviral effect, typically occurring after patients had taken the drug for about six months.[16] Although the researchers had not proven the clinical significance of these findings, many investigators assumed that AZT would be less effective and AIDS symptoms would worsen when patients developed AZT-resistant strains of HIV. Scientists therefore intensified their search for alternative drugs.

Broder and his team at the National Cancer Institute evaluated other AZT-like nucleosides as potential AIDS treatments, including ddI.[17] Like AZT, ddI proved to be a potent inhibitor of HIV in their laboratory assay and was effective in treating AIDS patients. Broder's team received patents for their discovery of ddI's effects. But because these investigators worked at a government laboratory and were not in the business of marketing drugs, the National Institutes of Health awarded Bristol-Myers Squibb an exclusive license to continue development of ddI.[18] More than fifty medical centers in the United States were participating in Bristol-Myers Squibb's clinical trials with ddI.[19] By 1989, data from these early clinical trials confirmed the observations of Broder's group, but the investigators at Bristol-Myers Squibb were still experimenting to find the best dose level and dosing schedule. The most common side effects of ddI were headache, insomnia, rash, diarrhea, and mental symptoms such as confusion. Unlike AZT, ddI did not appear to be toxic to bone marrow, but high doses caused inflammation of the pancreas, which could be fatal, and painful nerve damage, especially in the feet.[20]

Researchers were encouraged that ddI suppressed strains of HIV that had become resistant to AZT. But not everyone who wanted to take the drug qualified for the ddI clinical trials, and some patients lived too far away from the medical centers where the ddI clinical trials were being conducted. Consequently, Bristol-Myers Squibb developed a program under FDA's existing guidelines to provide ddI free of charge to needy patients in parallel with the ongoing clinical trials. This expanded access program began in the fall of 1989.[21]

Broder's group at the National Cancer Institute also explored Horwitz's nucleoside compound, ddC, as an AIDS treatment. Similar to the deal that it struck with Bristol-Myers Squibb for ddI, the National Institutes of Health licensed ddC to Hoffmann-La Roche. Although ddC was more potent than ddI in Broder's laboratory assays, clinicians quickly noted serious side effects, which they felt might limit its usefulness as an AIDS drug. Up to one-third of AIDS patients developed peripheral nerve damage after taking ddC. As of 1989, Hoffmann-La Roche had only recently begun its clinical trials and had not yet established ddC's therapeutic value.[22] Clinicians were trying various dosing schemes, including the use of lower ddC doses and alternating treatment between ddC and AZT, to reduce its side effects, particularly the nerve damage problem. But most investigators felt that the best way to avoid the side effects produced by AZT, ddI, and ddC was to find better drugs.

Because AZT, ddI, and ddC were nucleosides with chemical structures similar to the natural components of DNA, scientists thought the drugs' toxic side effects were the result of damage to DNA in normal human cells. If they could find a drug with a "non-nucleoside" chemical structure to inhibit HIV, it might not damage the DNA in normal human cells as the nucleoside drugs did. The scientists at Boehringer Ingelheim thought they had found such a drug. In fact, they had found quite a few. Their challenge in the latter part of 1989 was to decide which one was the best to use in their clinical trials.

* * *

When Mark Labadia and Bob Eckner began reporting the results of BI compounds that were more potent than L-S 1170, Alan Rosenthal — optimistic as always — thought the team would be able to quickly choose one for clinical trials. In June, Eckner's team set August 22 as the target date for selecting the new compound. But throughout the summer of 1989, Julian Adams's chemists continued to crank out new compounds, many of which were active in Labadia's HIV enzyme assay.

At this point, Jay Merluzzi's development team had gathered a substantial amount of information about the strengths and weaknesses of L-S 1170. The compound that would replace it needed to be better than L-S 1170 in all categories, not just a potent inhibitor in Labadia's assay.[23] Although such tough selection criteria meant simultaneously testing compounds under many laboratory conditions, an arduous undertaking, they knew that prematurely selecting an inferior compound would set back their efforts in the long run.[24]

One of the major limitations of L-S 1170 was its rapid metabolism, making it too short-acting to be useful as an AIDS drug. The drug that would replace L-S 1170 needed to be absorbed better and last longer. Scientists call the ability of a drug to be absorbed from the gut into the bloodstream "bioavailability," and they measure it as a percentage of the total drug dose. A high percent bioavailability means the drug is well absorbed. Scientists also measure how long the drug remains in the bloodstream and compare drugs by calculating a number called half-life, which is the time it takes for half of the drug to be eliminated from the blood. A longer half-life means the drug stays longer in the bloodstream, and patients can take the drug less frequently. Eckner's team was looking for a compound that had a bioavailability much higher than the fifteen percent bioavailability of L-S 1170 and a half-life much longer than its 2.5 hours. To do the assessments of bioavailability and half-life of the new compounds, they turned to the scientists in BI's drug metabolism and pharmacokinetics department, headed by James Keirns.

An introspective, meticulous, and articulate scientist, Keirns applied those same skills at the piano in his limited leisure time. Parts of BI's R&D building were still under construction when he arrived in Ridgefield in 1979 to head the newly created biochemistry department. By the time that Rosenthal arrived with his ideas for expansion, Keirns had assembled a staff of thirty biochemists and assistants.[25] In 1988, Rosenthal accelerated the growth of Ridgefield's drug development resources, and he appointed Keirns director of the new drug metabolism and pharmacokinetics department. Keirns had gained experience in drug development at American Cyanamid's Lederle Laboratories before joining BI, and he recruited scientists to expand the department's capabilities for assessing new drug candidates.

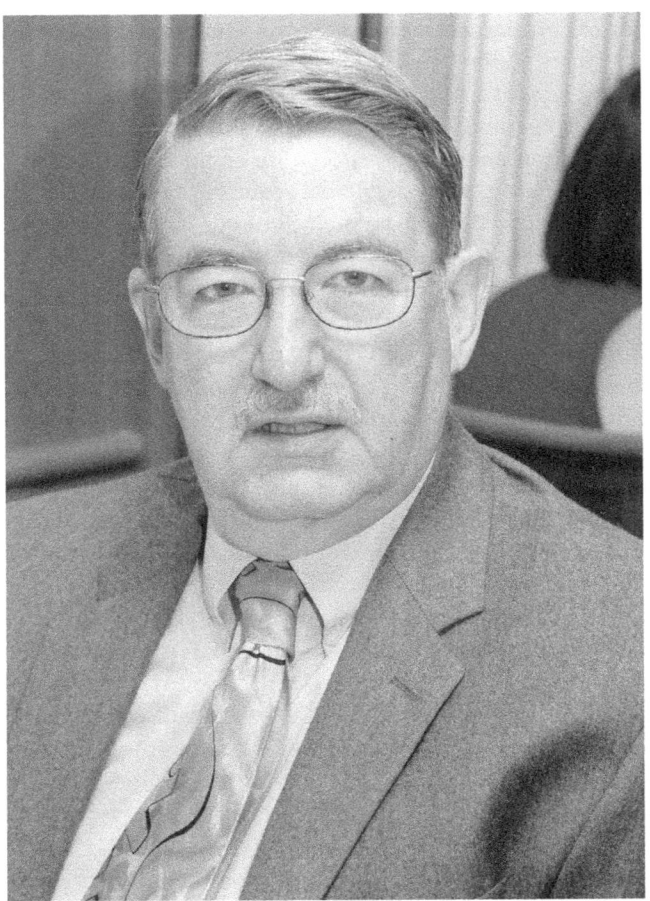

James Keirns.

With the discovery of L-S 1170 a few months later, Keirns assigned members of his staff to serve on Merluzzi's development team, but he continued his active involvement and closely supervised their work. Keirns's staff had collected the influential data showing that L-S 1170 had poor bioavailability and a short half-life in animals — the news that had cut short Karl Hargrave's German trip and that redirected the chemists' efforts to find a replacement for L-S 1170.

When Labadia found a compound that was potent in his HIV assay, Keirns's scientists dosed animals to determine its bioavailability and half-life. Each new compound required a new assay to measure the amount of that compound in the animals' blood. For months, Keirns's scientists worked nonstop to develop, validate, and conduct the compound-specific assays, but they managed to keep pace with the chemists who were systematically making newer and more potent compounds. Many of these compounds, like L-S 1170, had poor bioavailability, a short half-life, or both, and Eckner's team quickly ruled them out. But the data that Keirns generated — even on the poor compounds — gave the chemists important clues about how to optimize the chemical structure. The scientists frequently visited each other's laboratories, discussing the latest results and prioritizing which compounds the chemists should make next.[26] One by one, Labadia and Keirns queued the newly synthesized compounds for testing, looking for ones that were potent in Labadia's HIV assay and had good bioavailability and half-life characteristics in Keirns's assays.

In July, the chemists produced BIRH-414.[27] It was a potent inhibitor in the HIV assay, and Keirns's scientists found that it had about twice the bioavailability of L-S 1170 and a reasonable half-life in rats.[28] Consequently, BIRH-414 became a leading contender, and Eckner's research team scheduled the compound for more detailed testing. Because Eckner and his team wanted to include the results of these follow-up studies in their deliberations, they moved the target date for compound selection to September 1, 1989.

In September, Eckner's research team discussed the results of another new compound, BIRG-587, which appeared to be as potent as BIRH-414 in the HIV assay. Encouraged by this result and thinking his colleagues could make an even better compound, Hargrave added new compounds to his list for chemical synthesis. And the team again delayed the date for compound selection. The cycle of chemical synthesis and testing could go on forever. To prevent that from happening, Adams set Halloween as the deadline for his chemists to finish making the new compounds on Hargrave's list. At that time, Eckner's and Merluzzi's teams would collaborate in putting the best compounds through an extensive battery of tests to characterize their biologic properties and potential side effects. By comparing the data side-by-side, they hoped one compound would emerge as the best drug for development.

As had been the case with L-S 1170, Merluzzi's team would require a substantial amount of each of the compounds on the short list to do their follow up testing. So, Adams promised to redirect the chemists' efforts after October 31 to concentrate on making adequate supplies of the short-list compounds. If necessary, he would assign the entire chemistry department to do the scale-up work so that the detailed studies could proceed as fast as possible. The target date for compound selection, which now would be based on the extensive data collected from the yet-to-be chosen compounds on the short list, was postponed until January 1990.

On October 30, 1989, Eckner's team gathered in the R&D building's Main Conference Room to review the data they had collected. The chemists had completed their eight-month campaign making novel compounds, and Eckner's team had tested most of them in the HIV enzyme assay. About a dozen of the compounds were potent inhibitors of reverse transcriptase. The research team had submitted the best compounds to their colleagues at BI and to several outside investigators to gather additional data on each compound's properties. They had accumulated more data on the earlier compounds, including BIRH-414, than on those that had been discovered more recently, such as BIRG-587. Although the profiling studies were still ongoing, everyone felt the pressure to get on with compound selection as quickly as possible. "Everyone realized what was at stake."[29] They were all anxious to slay Elizabeth Glaser's dragon.

But so far, all of the potent compounds performed equally well in their laboratory assays. Like L-S 1170, they all showed "exquisite specificity," eliciting no biologic activity besides the HIV effect and no side effects.[30] Little distinguished one compound from the others, except their bioavailabilities and half-lives. Based on the data they had collected so far, Keirns's scientists ranked BIRH-414 and BIRG-587 as the best compounds in the series.

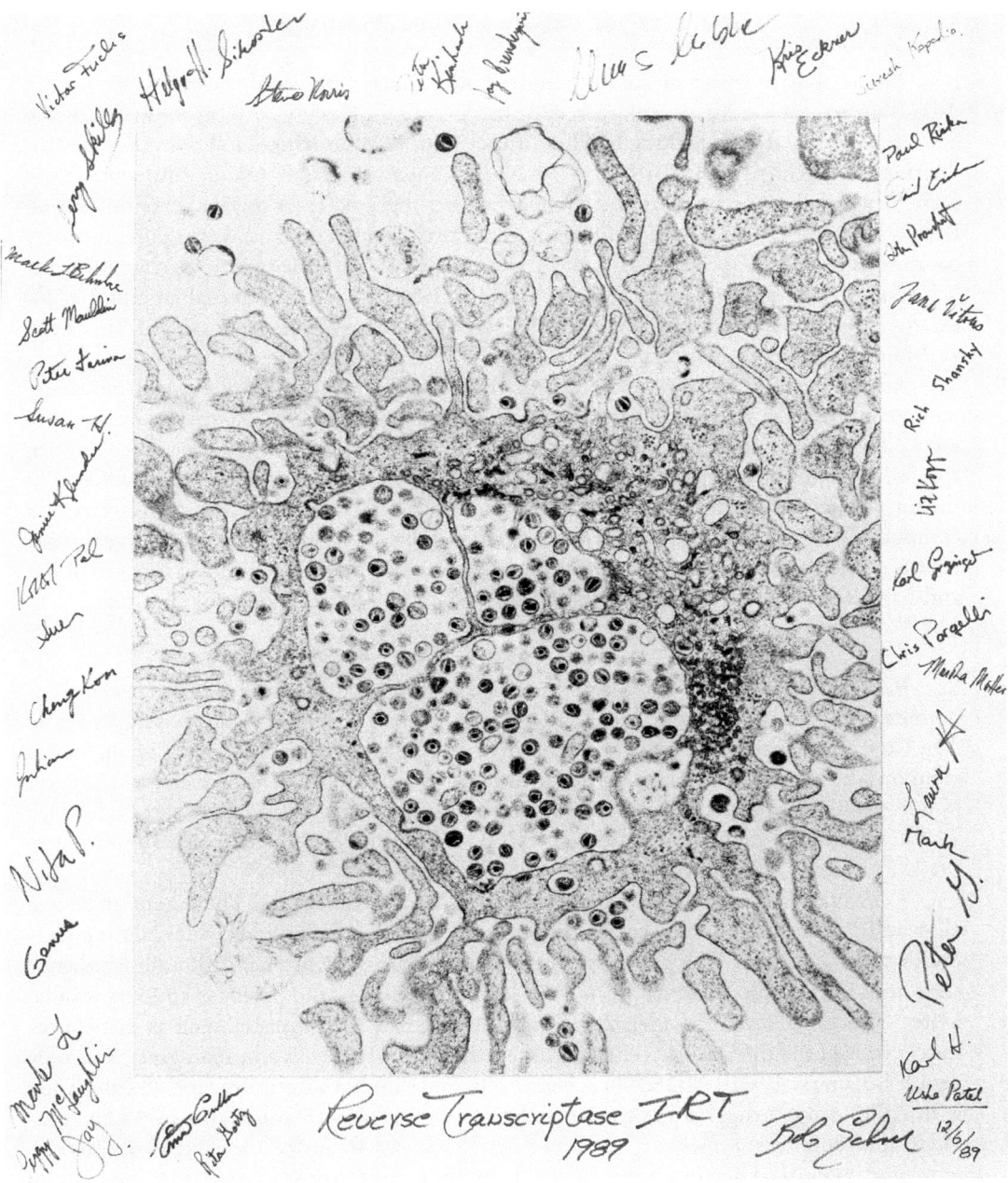

An electron micrograph of human cells teeming with HIV (the small circular particles). This photograph was signed by members of the HIV research team at Boehringer Ingelheim and presented to Alan Rosenthal in December 1989 (courtesy Julian Adams).

Rosenthal encouraged the scientists to continue their evaluation of the newly synthesized compounds, but clearly BIRH-414 and BIRG-587 were the leading contenders. Eckner's team and members of Merluzzi's development team moved forward with their detailed studies of BIRH-414 and BIRG-587, a head-to-head comparison that would hopefully determine the better compound.[31] The list of planned studies was long, and consequently the target date for compound selection was delayed from January to February 1990.

This extensive roster of studies required additional supplies of the compounds, and Adams shifted his chemistry resources, as he had promised. Having by this time accumulated considerable practice in making batches of L-S 1170, Karl Grozinger led the scale-up production of BIRH-414 and BIRG-587, making about 100 grams (about four ounces) of each.[32] In parallel, the Eckners and the biochemists repeated their original experiments on BIRH-414 and BIRG-587 to certify, again, that the enzyme in their assay was pure, the assay conditions were appropriate, and their initial results were not due to an experimental error or anomaly. Eckner also sent BIRH-414 and BIRG-587 to several external laboratories for extensive testing in various cell-based HIV assays, including Doug Richman's in San Diego and John Sullivan's in Worcester.

Among the most influential studies were the follow-up bioavailability and half-life assessments conducted in Keirns's department. Like most drug companies, Keirns's scientists used rats in their initial studies. Because the bioavailability and half-life of drugs often differ between species, they routinely repeated the studies in a second species, usually dogs or monkeys. At the time of Eckner's October meeting, Keirns had collected data from BIRG-587 (a very new compound) in rats, and only slightly more data with BIRH-414. With so much at stake, Keirns needed to be thorough. Over the next two months, his staff conducted bioavailability and half-life studies of BIRH-414 and BIRG-587 in rats, mice, monkeys, and dogs.

* * *

Because Eckner's and Merluzzi's teams were now concentrating on the newer compounds, the chemists realized that the BI patent application needed to be revised yet again. The Continuation-in-Part that they submitted in August incorporated some of the newer compounds, including BIRH-414, but it did not cover BIRG-587. Once again, Hargrave huddled with BI's patent attorneys to expand the list of compounds in their patent claims.[33] The new claims, which included the chemical structure of BIRG-587, were submitted to the U.S. Patent Office on November 17, 1989.[34]

As 1989 drew to a close, key elements of the patent were secure. The patent office had allowed BI's claims for the invention of this novel series of compounds. But claiming their use to treat or prevent HIV infection proved to be more contentious. Although Merluzzi's team provided ample evidence from their laboratory assays, the patent examiners wanted more "clinically relevant" evidence.[35] Data from animals with diseases such as diabetes or cancer proved the therapeutic claims of other drugs. But HIV was a human virus, and only people became sick with AIDS. There were no suitable animal substitutes, and all companies with AIDS drugs struggled to provide proof that the examiners would accept.[36] The arguments and counterarguments in BI's case flew back and forth for the next two years. As more and more data accumulated, BI would submit three more Continuations-in-Part to extend its claims, and BI's patent finally became official on November 22, 1994.[37] Karl Hargrave, who led the chemical synthesis work, was named first in the list of inventors, followed by Grozinger, Adams, and John Proudfoot from Ridgefield. In addition, four chemists from BI's R&D center at Thomae were listed as co-inventors.[38]

* * *

Before choosing either BIRH-414 or BIRG-587, Merluzzi's team wanted evidence that the drugs were free of toxic side effects. Keirns's staff had exposed animals to a single dose of each drug in their bioavailability and half-life experiments, and the animals showed no obvious signs of toxicity. But the team wanted to assess drug safety systematically. Because rigorous safety assessment in animals is time-consuming, the team instead opted to perform a "mini-safety" experiment.[39] This preliminary toxicology assessment involved dosing rats and dogs daily for two weeks. The toxicologists had a sufficient amount of each compound to conduct the preliminary 14-day toxicology studies in rats, but the 14-day toxicology studies in dogs required much larger quantities, about 1.5 kilograms (about 3 pounds) of each compound. Despite Grozinger's skill and experience, producing kilogram quantities with his existing equipment was a major challenge. The days and weeks rolled by, and discussion of the 14-day dog studies—and the chemists' scale up progress—became a regular agenda item at Merluzzi's team meetings.[40]

When the New Year began, members of Eckner's and Merluzzi's teams were making rapid progress with their experiments to profile both BIRH-414 and BIRG-587, and they were able to set a more specific date for compound selection. Although both teams were contributing data, Eckner's research team was officially responsible, under BI's R&D rules, for selecting the compound. In January, they set February 14, 1990, as the date for making this important decision.

Eckner's team was compiling a long table of data, comparing their extensive test results of BIRH-414 versus BIRG-587, but choosing between them would not be easy.[41] Both compounds were potent inhibitors of HIV reverse transcriptase. In ranking all of the compounds in the HIV enzyme assay, BIRH-414 was the second-most potent and BIRG-587 ranked sixth, overall. In the cell-based assays at the University of Massachusetts and University of California, San Diego, both compounds were equally potent in preventing HIV proliferation. Sullivan and Richman also reported that both BIRH-414 and BIRG-587 inhibited mutant HIV strains that were resistant to AZT. Like L-S 1170, both compounds were selective in inhibiting the HIV-1 virus. Neither compound affected HIV-2.

Unlike AZT, ddI, and ddC, neither BIRH-414 nor BIRG-587 harmed the DNA of normal, healthy cells.[42] In addition, neither compound appeared to have the unacceptable side effects associated with AZT, ddI, and ddC. Merluzzi asked Malcolm Moore, a former colleague at Memorial Sloan-Kettering Cancer Center, to assess the compounds in his assays and found that neither BI compound suppressed bone marrow.[43]

Neither compound caused any significant toxicity when given to rats in the 14-day "mini-safety" study. Likewise, in dogs, the toxicologists saw no notable side effects with either compound after a single dose, even in the dogs that received a very high dose. The toxicologists moved forward with plans for the 14-day dog studies, but they could not start those studies until Grozinger completed production of the scale-up batches. Eckner's team decided not to wait for those results.

Among the most important data that Eckner's team considered was Keirns's comprehensive studies of the bioavailability and half-life of BIRH-414 and BIRG-587. In all of the species that Keirns's staff studied, BIRH-414 and BIRG-587 each remained in the animals' bloodstream more than twice as long as L-S 1170—a significant improvement. Both drugs also had much better bioavailability than L-S 1170, but BIRG-587 had slightly better absorption in all species, especially in monkeys.[44] The difference meant that at a given dose, much more BIRG-587 would reach the bloodstream than BIRH-414, a significant advantage.

* * *

On February 1, 1990, Eckner's team was on the verge of officially selecting between BIRH-414 and BIRG-587 when they received some surprising news. Belgian researchers from the Rega Institute and Janssen Research Foundation, an affiliate of Johnson & Johnson, published a report in the prestigious scientific journal, *Nature*, announcing their discovery of a new class of potent AIDS drugs.[45] The chemical name for this class of compounds was tetrahydro-imidazo-benzodiazepin-ones, which the researchers abbreviated to TIBO. The similarities between Janssen's and BI's compounds were striking. Like BI, Janssen had discovered its first active compounds by testing randomly selected compounds in its HIV assays. Like BI's compounds, the TIBO compounds had been systematically improved by making specific changes to the chemical structure of the molecule. Like BI's compounds, the TIBO compounds were non-nucleosides — they were not chemically related to AZT, ddI, or ddC. Like BI's compounds, the TIBO compounds inhibited the reverse transcriptase enzyme associated with HIV-1 but not HIV-2. And like BI's compounds, the TIBO compounds did not affect the function of DNA in normal cells.

The news, although unexpected, was reassuring to the BI scientists. The pharmaceutical profile that the Janssen scientists had compiled on the TIBO compounds was virtually identical to the data they had assembled on the BI compounds. Remarkably, the two companies, working independently, had discovered non-nucleoside compounds that were chemically different from each other but which worked essentially the same.[46] In essence, the Janssen scientists had validated BI's results using a different class of chemicals.

Because the BI and Janssen compounds produced identical biological effects despite very different chemical structures, many more types of chemical structures might also inhibit HIV reverse transcriptase. Perhaps other companies, all of whom had large sample collections sitting on their shelves, were developing their own HIV drugs, just like BI. And perhaps some of them, like Janssen, were further along in developing their compounds than the BI team. The BI scientists had been diligently working for a full year and were close to beginning clinical trials, but the *Nature* paper reported that Janssen had already started clinical trials and had given one of the TIBO compounds to six people.[47]

Despite Janssen's success in discovering a new class of AIDS drugs, the TIBO compounds were difficult and time-consuming to make. Janssen chemists had only made small amounts of the compounds, and scaling up supplies for extended clinical trials might be difficult.[48] By contrast, BI's compounds were simpler to make, and Grozinger had gained considerable scale-up experience, which would aid the chemists in making larger and larger batches of BI's drug. Still, the BI scientists knew that, going forward, they would be required to compare their results to the performance of the TIBO compounds under the same testing conditions. They could not justify developing either BIRH-414 or BIRG-587 if the TIBO compounds proved to be better. The chemists studied the European patent, which described the methods for preparing the TIBO compounds and listed Janssen's claims for using the compounds to treat HIV infections.[49] The BI scientists would need reference samples to compare with their compounds.

* * *

When Eckner's team met to review the accumulated data on BIRH-414 and BIRG-587, each scientist pointed to a favorite study, trying to justify selecting one compound over the other. But the choice was not obvious to anyone. In most of the tests, the two compounds were indistinguishable. The decisive data came from Keirns's studies. BIRG-587 had a better bioavailability profile, a property that could be an advantage clinically.[50] Although no one knew how well their compounds would perform in HIV-infected people, the team wanted a drug that got into the bloodstream and stayed there a long time — at least until the patient could conveniently take the next dose. And so, from the beginning, they had worked hard to create a compound with the highest bioavailability and longest half-life.[51]

Karl Hargrave made most of the novel BI compounds on the short list, including BIRH-414. But a large number of chemists participated in this ambitious chemistry campaign, many of them made insightful contributions, and all of them could honestly claim a share of the bragging rights. On February 7, 1990, Eckner formally notified Merluzzi that the research team had selected BIRG-587 as the development candidate. According to the scheme that BI used to distinguish its novel experimental compounds, the "BI" stood for Boehringer Ingelheim, the "R" identified the location of the BI R&D center where the compound had been made (in this case, Ridgefield), and the "G" designated the chemist who had first synthesized the compound (in this case, Karl Grozinger). Therefore, BIRG-587 was the 587th compound that Karl Grozinger had made in his long career at Boehringer Ingelheim.

Thanks to the TIBO compounds, BIRG-587 would not be viewed as a scientific breakthrough. Instead, the international scientific community hailed the TIBO compounds as the first non-nucleoside reverse transcriptase inhibitors and hoped that the TIBOs would offer advantages over the AZT-like drugs in treating AIDS. But the BI scientists had set the bar very high when they systematically engineered their compounds. They had moved quickly, but they had insisted on not rushing into development with an inferior compound. Ultimately, they found several compounds that met their tough standards, and they settled on one that they hoped would be good enough to survive the even tougher road ahead.

The year, from the initiation of his HIV enzyme screening assay in September 1988 to the discovery of BIRG-587 in September 1989, had been the most fun in Labadia's four years at BI. It "stoked" his interest in becoming an independent researcher, and he headed back to graduate school to earn a Ph.D. in immunology.[52] For Merluzzi, whose development team now took charge, the fun and challenges were just beginning. His objective was to start clinical trials as soon as possible. Clinical results were the only way to prove that BIRG-587 was a useful AIDS drug and that it did not have the same limitations as the AZT-like drugs. Merluzzi's team had been discussing their clinical plans for almost a year, and they had already set the target date for starting those clinical trials.

4

A Cast of Thousands

On the day that BIRG-587 was selected for development, James Wright walked into Julian Adams's office and asked for a sample.[1] Wright had joined Boehringer Ingelheim six months earlier, in the summer of 1989, as Associate Director of Pharmaceutics, and the AIDS project had not been one of his assignments. But BI's active HIV compounds fascinated him. With a solid grounding in academic research, Wright approached all of his work with a university professor's curiosity. In his downhome, aw-shucks manner, he shrugged off the constraints of job descriptions and organizational pigeonholes and dove into the AIDS project, reading everything he could find about HIV, antiviral drugs, and reverse transcriptase.[2] He tagged along, participated at the team meetings, and soon became an official member of the team. Wright quickly earned Jay Merluzzi's respect, and the two became a powerful tag team professionally. In their rare moments of leisure time, they shared a passion for outer space. The two would set up their telescopes (Wright's deep reflector and Merluzzi's smaller refractor) in Wright's backyard and gaze at the stars.[3]

Of all the people on Merluzzi's team, Wright was always the first one to predict the rough spots and apply the grease before the hinges squeaked and the gears jammed. Whenever anything needed to get done, Wright stepped up to do it.[4] Now, in Adams's office, he was pushing to start work immediately on a drug formulation for use in the clinical trials. Unfortunately, Adams had only a precious, small amount of BIRG-587, and the team had already earmarked all of it for use in high-priority studies. They both knew that the clinical trials could start sooner if they used unformulated drug, dissolving the pure powder in water or juice or putting it in capsules. But Wright argued that those trials would need to be repeated with the formulated drug. He wanted to use formulated tablets from the start, eliminating the need for this equivalence testing. And the sooner he started his formulation work, the more likely he would have the tablets ready for the first clinical trial.

Through persistent and persuasive negotiations, Wright managed to get a small amount of BIRG-587. Over the following months, he partnered with the most experienced scientists in his department and inspired them to do their best formulation work.[5] They thoroughly studied the physical and chemical properties of BIRG-587, and Wright, with his training in physical chemistry and pharmacy, set high standards for the tablet formulation. He would have preferred a compound that dissolved better in water, but otherwise the formulation "process was reasonably simple."[6] The first time they put their formulation mixture through their test equipment, they pressed tablets that were suitable for use in the clinical trials. They would make small adjustments to their ingredients and procedures, but this first formulation changed very little throughout the clinical trials.[7]

Wright's role on Merluzzi's team put him at the interface between the chemists who were producing batches of BIRG-587, the scientists who analyzed each batch to confirm

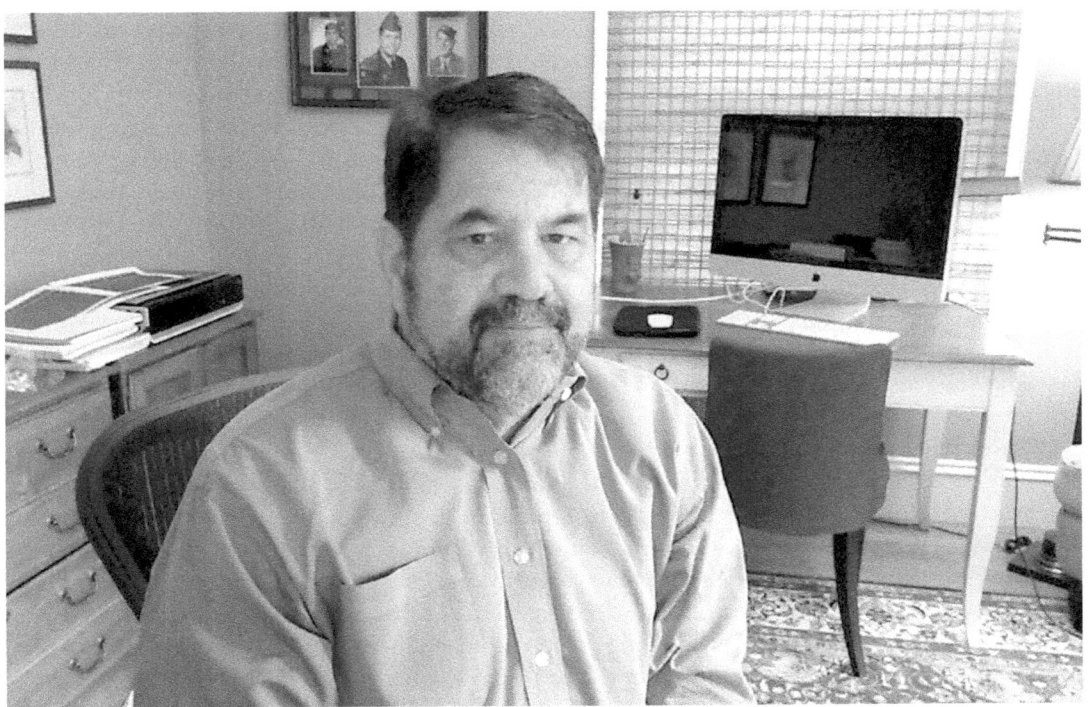

James Wright.

the drug's purity, the scientists in his department who were formulating the drug, other scientists who needed liquid formulations for their animal studies, and the clinicians who relied on him for the tablets they gave to patients. Anything that involved handling BIRG-587 involved Jim Wright, and everyone on the team, in one way or another, needed supplies of BIRG-587. Wright knew and meticulously complied with all of the rules and restrictions for handling experimental drugs, ensuring that BIRG-587 was produced, formulated, packaged, stored, and dispensed safely and securely. But rather than using those rules and restrictions as an excuse, he took personal pride in finding the fastest and most efficient way to get the job done.

One day, Merluzzi's team was discussing how to overcome a delay in laboratory testing because no one had written an official procedure for transferring samples of BIRG-587 from the room where it was being stored to the laboratory where it was needed — a distance separated by only one flight of stairs. Merluzzi and Wright listened for a while, as the others described the problem and brainstormed various ways of solving it, each procedure more elaborate than the last. Increasingly exasperated, Merluzzi turned to Wright and silently gave him a quick nod of encouragement.[8] That signal was all Wright needed, because he had heard enough, too. "Just take the fucking thing, put it in a beaker, and walk it downstairs."[9]

* * *

Starting in April 1989, Merluzzi scheduled team meetings every Tuesday afternoon in the windowless Pharmacology Conference Room of BI's Research and Development building, pushing and prodding, pulling and praising, doing anything and everything to get their AIDS drug into clinical trials. The team's initial discussions and work revolved around

L-S 1170, now long abandoned. But it was time not wasted.[10] During those early months, the core members of Merluzzi's team learned to work together and evolved into a harmonious, high performing team — due in no small measure to Merluzzi's leadership skills. In the course of profiling L-S 1170, they had identified its weaknesses, information that guided their evaluation of the newer compounds and confirmed that BIRG-587 was the right compound to replace it. Now, much of the team's discussions, considerations, plans, and procedures for developing L-S 1170 would be directly applied to BIRG 587.[11] In January 1990, Merluzzi cut back the scheduled team meetings to once every two weeks, partly because their meetings had become more efficient and partly because they now spent more time doing work than talking about it.

At the center of all discussions at Merluzzi's team meetings were the toxicology studies. The Food and Drug Administration set detailed and specific requirements for the design of toxicology studies and the types of toxicology data needed prior to starting clinical trials. These regulatory standards were spelled out in the FDA's Good Laboratory Practices, and only data from toxicology studies that precisely followed those regulatory requirements were acceptable proof that the drug was safe enough to give to people. The length of animal exposure to an experimental drug determined how long it could be given to people — the longer animals had been dosed without harmful side effects, the longer patients could be treated. When Eckner's research team selected BIRG-587 for development in February 1990, they had only evaluated the drug in a preliminary 14-day toxicology study in rats and a single-dose toxicology study in dogs. The 14-day study in dogs had been delayed until a sufficient amount of drug could be produced. And, although the data from these "mini-safety" studies were sufficient for compound selection, the toxicology studies in both species needed to be repeated under Good Laboratory Practices conditions to satisfy the regulatory authorities.

Those toxicology studies and the ones that followed were under the supervision of Laura Andrews, a veterinary pathologist who had joined BI in 1988, part of Alan Rosenthal's initiative to add talented drug development expertise in Ridgefield. After completing her veterinary intern and residency programs, Andrews worked at Parke, Davis & Company for seven years, gaining considerable toxicology experience and serving on a number of clinical project teams.[12] A native Texan who had consciously suppressed all traces of a southern accent, Andrews quickly earned the respect of her BI colleagues through her reserved, thoughtful professionalism and her firm grasp of regulatory requirements, toxicology study design, and animal pathology. On Merluzzi's team, she understood the need to go fast, but she also insisted on doing things right.[13]

Andrews's ability to conduct toxicology studies was limited by the small toxicology staff, shortage of laboratory space, and lack of animal rooms for dogs in Ridgefield.[14] State-of-the-art toxicology laboratories were another part of Rosenthal's R&D expansion plans. While she was conducting the preliminary toxicology studies with BIRG-587, Andrews was simultaneously planning for that expansion. Andrews and her toxicology colleagues met regularly with contractors and BI's engineers to design the animal rooms, set the requirements for environmental controls, and select laboratory equipment. They wanted to conduct the BIRG-587 toxicology studies in Ridgefield, but the new toxicology facilities would not be ready for at least another year. In the meantime, Andrews made arrangements to conduct the regulatory-required toxicology studies at a commercial laboratory in Canada.[15]

Andrews's progress depended upon having a sufficient supply of BIRG-587, and the dog toxicology studies needed the greatest amount, 7.5 kilograms (about 16 pounds). Instead of beagle dogs, which are commonly used for toxicology studies, the team proposed cynomolgus monkeys as an alternative, because they are smaller and would therefore consume less drug. Some team members also argued that monkeys might be a better choice, anyway, because they are genetically closer to humans — a factor worth considering for drugs that attacked HIV, a human virus. But Andrews explained that monkeys offered no advantages over dogs for toxicology studies and actually had several drawbacks. Monkeys did not necessarily handle drugs the same as humans, and because they are caught in the wild and vary in age, they responded less consistently in experimental studies than beagles, which are bred uniformly for research. While Karl Grozinger continued his campaign through the winter months to produce a 1.5 kilogram batch of BIRG-587, Merluzzi's team debated the pros and cons of dogs versus monkeys, favoring monkeys to stretch their limited drug supplies.

At the end of March 1990, the plans for the monkey toxicology studies took an unexpected turn. Andrews informed the team that the Centers for Disease Control had imposed a ban on importing cynomolgus monkeys because of a concern over Ebola virus, a virus more deadly to humans than either herpes or HIV.[16] Because of the ban, the monkeys that Andrews had ordered had not been shipped. Not knowing when the ban would be lifted, she recommended that they return to their original plan and use dogs for the toxicology studies, which would allow her to start immediately but would require about twice as much drug. Grozinger had just delivered the first 200 grams (about a half pound) of BIRG-587, and Merluzzi's team assigned most of it to Andrews so she could begin preparations for the dog toxicology studies.

* * *

While Grozinger was busily making scale up batches, he finally received news that he had waited ten years to hear. He had worked with the architects, engineers, and BI's decision makers, preparing and revising the blueprints for the Ridgefield pilot plant too many times to count, and now those plans had been approved.[17] Ignoring the chill on a wintry Connecticut afternoon, Grozinger led a small group of BI dignitaries and elected officials on the short walk from the front door of the R&D building to the spot where the new pilot plant was to be constructed. As if on cue, big fluffy snowflakes began falling just as the ceremonial shovels jabbed the frozen soil, a picture-perfect moment that Currier and Ives would envy. The dignitaries hastened through their official duties and as they scurried back to the R&D building for warmth and refreshments, the snowy confetti stopped as quickly as it had started.

Throughout the following year, Grozinger — always a dynamo — had an extra spring in his step as he shuttled between construction meetings and his old laboratory, where he continued making batches of BIRG-587. When he walked down the hall, he carried rolls of blueprints under his arm, and in his office he bent over his desk and credenza, both overflowing with building plans. The pilot plant's design, equipment configuration, and utility installations changed constantly, but Grozinger stayed on top of it all, working to satisfy Connecticut's strict standards for environmental protection and regulatory requirements for worker safety, equipment monitoring, and plant cleanliness. He set the requirements for the pilot plant's efficiency, quality, and performance, suggested every design feature, and approved every change. When the building was completed in May 1990, he knew every beam, bolt, and pipe in it.[18] And the pilot plant's opening could not have been more timely.

Now, Grozinger could draw on his thirty years of experience to produce drug batches on an appropriate scale. He soon delivered the first kilogram of BIRG-587 and proceeded with an aggressive schedule, turning out an additional kilogram every month for six months. In addition, he saved the reaction solutions from each of his batches and reprocessed them to extract nearly one additional kilogram of drug.[19]

With a steady and predictable supply of "Grozinger's Finest" now streaming out of the pilot plant, Merluzzi and Andrews could proceed with plans for the next series of toxicology studies. A flurry of discussions took place during April and May to sort out the details. Andrews had made considerable progress in establishing standard procedures for animal handling, record keeping, and equipment calibration, and she was on the verge of scheduling the regulatory-required rat toxicology studies in the Ridgefield laboratories. Then, the team was notified that construction for a new parking structure (another of Rosenthal's planned expansion projects at the R&D center) might cause occasional noise, vibration, and unplanned power outages over the next six months. The parking deck was being erected next to the wing of the R&D building that housed the laboratory animals. Andrews worried that the uncontrolled, erratic environmental disturbances would spook the animals, making it difficult to interpret the results of the toxicology studies. Several rounds of discussions led to some carefully orchestrated and creative scheduling, but finally both the toxicology studies and the parking deck construction moved forward with only minor delays. Having settled on dogs because of the ban on monkey imports, Andrews began the 14-day dog toxicology study at BI in June 1990. The 28-day rat toxicology study, also conducted at BI, followed soon after. Starting the 28-day dog toxicology study would be more challenging.

* * *

Merluzzi's team was acutely aware that advocacy by AIDS activists was growing in numbers and intensity and that there was an urgent need for more rapid development of new AIDS drugs. They put themselves under intense pressure to start clinical trials with BIRG-587 as quickly as possible.[20] To achieve that goal, they realized that they needed to engage a broader group of experts for clinical advice and guidance. Going forward, their discussions about development of BIRG-587 would extend far beyond the team's meetings in the Pharmacology Conference Room.

BI's clinical department added John Sullivan and Doug Richman as clinical consultants. Both of them had done yeoman's service in testing BI's compounds in their cell culture assays, and they now played an equally active role as clinicians, offering suggestions, serving as BI advocates in discussions with other influential groups, and facilitating the arrangements for starting the clinical trials. They also introduced Merluzzi's team to a wide range of other external experts who knew much more about conducting AIDS clinical trials than BI did. Before beginning clinical trials with BIRG-587, the team also needed to notify the FDA of their intentions. And Rosenthal wanted that notification backed up by data that was as impressive as they could make it.

The date for starting clinical testing of BIRG-587 would depend on Merluzzi's ability to steer the team not only to collect the required supporting data efficiently but also to orchestrate a complicated series of presentations and discussions with consultants, key investigators, and federal regulators. The sequence and interdependence of these interactions required careful planning, constant communication, frequent scheduling adjustments, and infinite patience.

* * *

In the early 1980s, the AIDS research activities sponsored by various institutes of the National Institutes of Health in Bethesda, Maryland, were uncoordinated and hampered by a lack of government funding.[21] But after scientists determined that AIDS was caused by a viral infection, the National Institute of Allergy and Infectious Diseases became the lead institute, and Anthony Fauci, the institute's director, became the coordinator for AIDS research across all of the National Institutes of Health.[22] Fauci successfully negotiated a large increase in the institutes' budget for AIDS research and was then faced with building an administrative staff to oversee it. One day, he called Maureen Myers and John LaMontagne, two of his most capable administrators, into his office and asked them to "set something up."[23]

Myers joined the Clinical Center at the National Institutes of Health in 1965 as a technician in a newly established viral diagnostic laboratory. Several years later, a supervisor in the National Cancer Institute encouraged her to enter graduate school. She earned her Ph.D. in three years and returned to NCI to work on interferon as a postdoc. In 1980, following a year's training to become a "scientist-administrator" in the extramural program, Myers joined NIAID as Director of the Antiviral Substances Program.[24] LaMontagne came to NIAID in 1976 as the program officer for influenza research, and his first challenge was the swine flu crisis. Over the next eight years, his responsibilities expanded to include overseeing the funding for viral vaccine and viral respiratory disease programs.

Although Myers and LaMontagne had not previously been involved with AIDS research, both held doctoral degrees in virology, understood the nuances of government-funded research, and were highly skilled program managers. If anyone could navigate the bureaucracy and build an AIDS Division from scratch, they could.

Sitting at Myers's dining room table, the two began sketching out the various sections of the new division. AIDS had more facets than the Hope diamond, and to be of any use, the AIDS Division needed to fund all of them, all at once: epidemiology, vaccines, drug discovery, preclinical research, and clinical drug development, among others.[25] Myers was particularly interested in drug development and treatment and chose to focus on those areas, while LaMontagne assumed leadership for the Division overall. For most of the new Division's research areas, they could draw on the institute's existing programs and basic know-how. But NIAID had limited experience with large multi-center clinical trials, so Myers began by visiting sister institutes to learn about their established clinical trial networks for heart, neurology, and cancer research. Although the lessons from those networks were helpful, AIDS clearly posed challenges for which there was no simple blueprint.

Undeterred, Myers solicited proposals from investigators across the country.[26] In a matter of months, the submitted proposals were reviewed, and contracts were awarded to the first fourteen clinical units in the new AIDS clinical network. The network was still taking shape when LaMontagne transferred from the AIDS program to become director of the institute's Division of Microbiology and Infectious Diseases. Myers stayed with the AIDS Division. In addition to the clinical unit grants, she managed contract awards for the infrastructure services that supported the network's clinical trials: statistics and data management, clinical monitoring, and pharmaceutical and operational support.[27]

In June 1986, Myers gathered the group of clinical network investigators for an organizational meeting on the National Institutes of Health campus in Bethesda. They sat around a conference table on the seventh floor of Building 31, "trying to figure out exactly what we were, where we were going, and how we might get there."[28] AIDS was the only common denominator. The experts around the table did not know each other and represented disciplines that had not worked together before, but they quickly forged alliances. This group evolved into the clinical network's Executive Committee, and at this first meeting they selected Martin Hirsch, an investigator from Harvard Medical School, as the committee's first chairman.[29]

Hirsch had been studying viral diseases since the 1960s and shifted his attention to AIDS when the new disease was first reported in the early 1980s. But the AIDS clinical network was a bold new venture with no roadmap.[30] The evening before their second meeting with the investigators, Myers and Hirsch sat in her home brainstorming the agenda for the next day. "We were flying by the seat of our pants."[31] Driven by a common purpose, guided only by their professional discipline, and fueled by generous funding, they forged ahead. Myers and Hirsch facilitated the Executive Committee's ongoing discussions between the National Institutes of Health, FDA, drug companies, and clinical investigators to plan and conduct AIDS clinical trials on a large scale. Some thought their progress was frustratingly slow, but by historical standards, their accomplishments were unprecedented. Within two years, the AIDS Division grew from two people (Myers and LaMontagne) to a staff of sixty people, and the clinical trials network — now officially called the AIDS Clinical Trials Group — expanded to 36 clinical centers headed by prominent investigators throughout the United States.[32] By 1990, the ACTG was the largest and most influential network of HIV clinical trial sites in the world.[33]

* * *

Sullivan and Richman urged BI to consider conducting its clinical trials, at least in part, within the ACTG. The National Institute of Allergy and Infectious Diseases provided funding, operational support, and a center for processing the data collected from AIDS clinical trials. The hierarchy of ACTG's multiple committees served as a focal point and clearinghouse for scientists, clinical investigators, drug makers, regulatory officials, and advocacy groups who were all interested in one thing: finding a solution to the AIDS epidemic. Sullivan and Richman both served as clinical investigators in ACTG-sponsored trials and had seen firsthand how quickly the ACTG network could martial its resources to evaluate new AIDS drugs.

Rosenthal also had strong ties to the National Institutes of Health. Prior to joining Merck as Vice President of Immunology and Infectious Diseases in 1978, he had spent twelve years at the National Institute of Allergy and Infectious Diseases as a clinical investigator. He knew the inner workings of the government's clinical research operations and although he had been away for more than a decade, he maintained professional relationships with many investigators there. News of BI's AIDS drug began circulating in whispers through the corridors of the institute, and the ACTG officials were anxious to see the data.[34] When they contacted BI, Rosenthal personally made the arrangements to add BIRG-587 to the agenda of ACTG's meeting on May 4, 1990.

Aside from individual consultants such as Sullivan and Richman, this would be the first disclosure of the BIRG-587 results to people outside the company. In planning the presentation, Rosenthal limited the amount of data that the team would disclose, but he wanted the presentation sufficiently compelling to convince the ACTG to put BIRG-587 on its priority list. Rosenthal and the BI clinicians had not yet decided whether to conduct the BIRG-587 clinical trials within the ACTG network, but he wanted to reserve BI's place in the clinical queue.

On May 4, 1990, Rosenthal led a contingent that included Merluzzi, Adams, and Sullivan to Washington, DC, for their presentation to a small committee representing the ACTG.[35] In addition to the BI presenters, Sullivan shared his laboratory results and, as a member of the ACTG network, spoke in support of BI's clinical plans. The committee was impressed with the data, and they urged BI to speed up its timetable for starting clinical trials, offering suggestions for streamlining the preclinical toxicology studies. They were eager to sponsor BI's clinical trials within the ACTG network and gave BIRG-587 their highest priority rating. In addition, a couple of the committee members offered to accompany the BI team and lend their support during the company's discussions with the FDA.[36]

* * *

Throughout the spring and summer of 1990, individual BI scientists and small BI delegations traveled to a series of scientific conferences, gathering the latest information on HIV, the design of AIDS clinical trials, and the performance of other AIDS drugs under development. Prominent among these meetings was the 6th International AIDS Conference, held in San Francisco in June — a rare opportunity for the team to absorb information and insights from the world's leaders in AIDS clinical trials. They learned that clinicians were able to reduce the serious side effects of AZT without losing its therapeutic benefits by cutting the daily dose in half. Investigators were also exploring ways to enhance AZT therapy and overcome AZT-induced resistance by giving the drug at earlier stages of HIV infection and giving AZT in combination with one of the other AZT-like drugs such as ddI or ddC. The BI team noted with interest how investigators had structured clinical trials with the newer experimental drugs, including the TIBO compounds and HIV protease inhibitors. Those investigators were under pressure to report their clinical results promptly and to provide their drugs to people who did not qualify for the clinical trials. BI would likely face the same pressures.

In addition, AIDS in women and children had reached a tipping point and became an integral part of the conversation in San Francisco. Although pediatric AIDS only represented two percent of the total cases reported in the United States, one in every five AIDS cases in developing countries occurred in children.[37] In 1990, an estimated 150,000 children worldwide became infected with HIV, most of whom would eventually develop AIDS symptoms and die.[38] And investigators expected the number of pediatric cases would continue to grow. As more and more women of childbearing age became infected, so would their babies. Public health officials and AIDS advocates at the Conference urged investigators to include women and children in clinical trials of new AIDS drugs.

* * *

Elizabeth Glaser was among the voices demanding greater and faster access to these new AIDS drugs, particularly to treat children. In March 1988, she had watched helplessly as Ariel struggled with pneumonia in her hospital bed, the sickest the little girl had ever been. Ariel's doctors thought she would not make it through the weekend.[39] Although Elizabeth wanted to maintain her privacy, she resolved that weekend "to do something about AIDS" and make a difference.[40] In the spring of 1988, while Ariel stubbornly clung to life, Elizabeth left the safety of her Santa Monica neighborhood and made her first trip to Washington, DC, intending to join the team that was fighting for children with AIDS. But she discovered that very few clinical trials were being conducted in children, and much to her surprise, there was no pediatric AIDS team. Despite 1346 reported cases of pediatric AIDS in the United States, "no one was paying any attention to the children."[41] Doctors and policy makers had few answers for her questions. She knew firsthand what most of them did not: AIDS affects children differently than adults. She had watched HIV debilitate Ariel's brain, leading to her inability to walk, talk, and write—problems that rarely occurred in HIV-infected adults.[42] Elizabeth also knew that drugs worked differently in children than adults. The intravenous infusion of AZT had reversed Ariel's brain damage, something the drug did not do in adults.[43]

Elizabeth realized that if she wanted things to change, she would have to do it herself. Along with two of her friends, Susan DeLaurentis and Susie Zeegen, she took on the overwhelming challenge and responsibility of creating a pediatric AIDS team. They called it the Pediatric AIDS Foundation.[44] Working from a cramped one-room office with one phone, a computer, and three desks in Los Angeles, they began building their team, which soon included a stellar panel of scientific and medical advisors. Elizabeth and her friends would make many trips to Washington, DC, to mobilize what she perceived as government inaction, lobbying government officials and scientists, advocating more pediatric AIDS research, and urging faster approval of AIDS drugs for pediatric use.[45]

At the FDA, Elizabeth went straight to the top, requesting a meeting with Commissioner Frank Young. Ellen Cooper, the FDA's most knowledgeable expert on AIDS drugs, facilitated the arrangements for the meeting.[46] In March 1989, Elizabeth walked into Young's office with a long list of topics, but the main question she wanted Young and Cooper to answer was: Why can't drug testing start in children simultaneously with adults?[47] Doctors at the National Institutes of Health and the medical advisors to her Pediatric AIDS Foundation believed that investigators could begin testing most experimental drugs in children two months after they started clinical trials in adults.[48] Simultaneous clinical trials would make new AIDS drugs available to both children and adults.

* * *

The issue that Merluzzi's team debated most frequently in the spring of 1990 was the plan for the regulatory-required toxicology studies. Andrews had started the 14-day toxicology studies in both rats and dogs, but FDA's minimum requirement for starting clinical trials with a new AIDS drug was data from 28-day toxicology studies.[49] Those studies were on Andrews's schedule, but despite Grozinger's best efforts, the rollout of additional drug supplies and the length of the 28-day toxicology studies pushed the date for starting clinical trials into mid–1991. Everyone was anxious to start testing BIRG-587 in AIDS patients sooner than that. Every day, Merluzzi coordinated discussions between Andrews, Grozinger, and other key team members, searching for ways to speed up the work and shorten the timetable. They discussed a number of options without reaching a satisfactory solution.[50]

Before a drug company can begin clinical trials with an experimental drug in the United States, it must notify the FDA by submitting an Investigational New Drug application. If the FDA reviewers are not satisfied with the application's data describing the drug's safety and other pharmaceutical properties, they can prevent the trials from starting. For drugs intended to treat most medical conditions, the process of regulatory review was formal, methodical, and often slow. The AIDS Coalition to Unleash Power (known as ACT UP), AIDS service organizations (such as Gay Men's Health Crisis in New York City and AIDS Project Los Angeles), national AIDS policy agencies (such as the AIDS Action Council and the National Minority AIDS Council in Washington, DC), and people living with HIV, like Elizabeth Glaser, criticized the FDA's bureaucratic procedures and demanded faster and broader access to new AIDS drugs.

To expedite FDA oversight and help drug developers avoid costly pitfalls and unproductive trials, Cooper fostered a cooperative and flexible relationship with industry, patient advocates, and her colleagues in the government's research institutes. She sat on the ACTG's steering committee, regularly attended its meetings, and used her position to share information back and forth between the FDA and the National Institutes of Health. She also frequently consulted investigators and other AIDS experts.[51] Being part of the process — from both a clinical trial and regulatory perspective — helped Cooper understand her critics' issues and make informed decisions aimed at streamlining FDA's procedures.[52] Regulators could protect the public health and still be responsive to the needs of dying patients.

Merluzzi's team welcomed the opportunity to meet with the FDA in a "pre-IND meeting," where they could exchange ideas, float their various scenarios, and negotiate an acceptable plan prior to submitting their formal Investigational New Drug application. Encouraged by the reaction of the ACTG officials, who were enthusiastic about BIRG-587 and had urged the team to accelerate the pace of the development program, the team pulled together all of their data and outlined their clinical plans in a package for the pre-IND meeting discussion. They hoped that Cooper's reviewers would work with them to streamline the toxicology data requirements and allow them to start clinical testing sooner.

On Monday, July 16, 1990, the BI delegation, led by Rosenthal, arrived in Bethesda, Maryland. Adams and Merluzzi flew separately from the rest of the group, the only passengers in a small commuter plane. Merluzzi checked his luggage, which unfortunately was not waiting for him when they landed.[53] That afternoon, the team held one final rehearsal at the Crowne Plaza Hotel, discussing the data they would present, the questions they wanted to ask, and the key points they wished to make at the pre-IND meeting. Jim Keirns sketched some last minute data with a felt-tipped marker on three blank transparencies for his part of the presentation. "It was not the first time or last time" he had incorporated last-minute data for discussions with the FDA.[54]

At 9:00 A.M. on Tuesday morning, the BI delegation, including a rather scruffy looking Merluzzi, was ushered into a conference room at FDA's Parklawn Building in Rockville, Maryland.[55] Typical of the FDA's meeting rooms, the furnishings were simple, 1980s government-issue. The BI team arranged themselves in the molded-plastic chairs and rested their notes and briefing books on the modular, Formica-topped tables. Joining Rosenthal, Merluzzi, Andrews, Keirns, Adams, and several others from BI were John Sullivan from the University of Massachusetts and two representatives from the National Institutes of Health, who

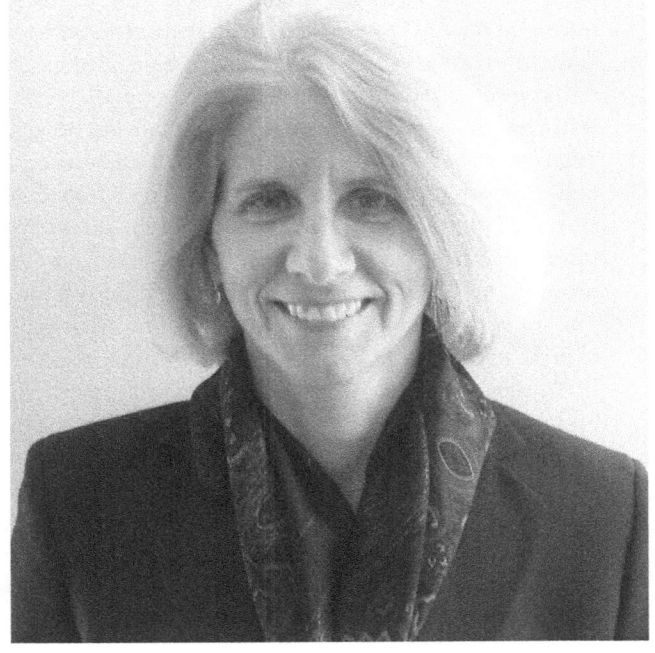

Ellen C. Cooper.

had participated in BI's meeting with the ACTG in May.[56] The conference room was equipped with a slide projector, but they would primarily use the overhead projector during their presentation. Ordinarily, Eileen Leonard, a medical reviewer and pre-IND team coordinator, would have led the FDA reviewers' discussions, but on this day, they were joined by Ellen Cooper, the Director of the Antiviral Drug Products Division. The young division had not held many pre-IND meetings, and as its most experienced medical reviewer, Cooper wanted to make sure the meeting ran smoothly.[57]

In the first thirty minutes, the BI team summarized two years of work and their development plans for BIRG-587. Merluzzi, Keirns, and Andrews presented the preclinical data, showing that BIRG-587 was a potent inhibitor of HIV, had good bioavailability and a long half-life, and, so far, had produced no toxic effects in animals.[58] BI's clinicians, with the backing of Rosenthal and the support of BI's clinical consultants, explained their proposed clinical trials — a solid, thoughtful, and conventional clinical plan centered on treating HIV-infected adults.

For the remaining hour, the FDA reviewers, led by Cooper and Leonard, made a number of comments on BI's development plans, framed within the context of the FDA's requirements for Investigational New Drug applications and mindful of the overwhelming urgency to get new AIDS drugs to the people who desperately needed them. It was an interactive discussion, with the BI representatives clarifying their data, justifying their proposals, offering alternative strategies, and restating key discussion points to ensure they understood the reviewers' comments, intent, and rationale. Cooper and Leonard intentionally avoided telling the BI team what to do or not do, but in their characteristically well-chosen comments, their intent and rationale were unmistakable. "They told us to hurry up."[59]

And, they said, BI should conduct robust pediatric trials, along the same lines as the adult trials. Cooper was a pediatrician and understood both the challenges and value of pediatric drug testing.[60] The growing number of pediatric AIDS cases demanded early testing of new AIDS drugs in children, and those pediatric trials needed to be designed well enough to "stand alone," without the benefit of extensive data from adult trials.[61] Pediatric trials of ddI and ddC were proceeding in parallel with the adult clinical trials of those drugs, setting a precedent that Cooper encouraged other drug companies to follow.[62] That advice reflected what Elizabeth Glaser had been advocating for over a year in her crusade for early and aggressive pediatric clinical trials of AIDS drugs. And Glaser's advocacy had been amplified by the emotionally charged discussions about the pediatric AIDS epidemic at the International AIDS Conference in San Francisco, held just a month before the BI-FDA meeting, and by Ryan White's highly publicized funeral a few months before that.

But the emphasis on pediatric clinical trials represented a major shift in the BI team's clinical trial strategy and caught them by surprise.[63] At the end of this muggy July day in 1990, they returned to Ridgefield, delighted by the FDA reviewers' clear message to hurry up but also burdened with reworking a large part of their clinical plans. BI had never conducted pediatric clinical trials.

* * *

Throughout 1990, Merluzzi's team had expanded the number of individuals and groups they included in discussions of their data and clinical trial plans. But they were not yet ready to publicly disclose BIRG-587 or acknowledge their efforts in HIV research. The ACTG and FDA officials were bound by governmental policies to respect proprietary information. The consulting agreements that BI established with Sullivan, Richman, and other investigators included terms that ensured the confidentiality of those discussions. And, when BI employees represented the company at scientific and professional meetings, they were reminded not to discuss BIRG-587. There would be a time and place to announce the results that BI had obtained on BIRG-587, but that time had not yet come.

Patient advocacy groups probed every obscure corner and followed every rumor, seeking hints about new AIDS drugs and grasping every glimmer of hope that better treatments for this dreaded disease were on the horizon. In conjunction with the International AIDS Conference in San Francisco, ACT UP, a high-profile advocacy group, issued a background document, which included a table of experimental drugs thought to be entering clinical trials in the coming year.[64] Some of those drugs, such as Janssen's TIBO compounds, had already been publicly disclosed and were no surprise. But the alphabetically organized list also included a number of unfamiliar compounds, without any explanation of the compounds' biological or chemical characteristics and no mention of which drug companies had made them. One compound on that list was "BIRG 6587."[65]

Somewhere along the way, as the ACT UP document's author compiled the table from various sources, a typographical error had been made in the BI compound's designation. This error, coupled with a lack of published data and the fact that BI's compound was buried in a list of sixty, mostly unfamiliar compounds, lessened the possibility that anyone would notice — or care about — the drug. Still, this unforeseen and unplanned listing represented the first public disclosure of BIRG-587 and confirmed that BI was, indeed, conducting AIDS research. The date of BI's planned, authorized, and high-profile public disclosure of BIRG-587 was still months away.

5

In the Spotlight

Nestled in the hilly woodlands of western Connecticut, Boehringer Ingelheim was about to reach a turning point. The reserved, unassuming, and inconspicuous company was privately owned and managed by the Boehringer family, and the company's executives relied on superior products rather than publicity campaigns to maintain its reputation. They took a long-term view and never made decisions based "on what's going to be written in the *Wall Street Journal* tomorrow."[1] But that was about to change.

Jay Merluzzi and his team had conducted discussions with government officials, such as the AIDS Clinical Trials Group (within the National Institutes of Health) and the Food and Drug Administration, without media coverage. But those discussions and the ongoing interactions with a lengthening list of external researchers increased the chance that news reporters, hungry for any advances in AIDS research, would become aware of BIRG-587 and begin asking about it.

To Alan Rosenthal, this concern was all too real. One of his first successes as BI's Vice President of Research and Development in Ridgefield was the discovery of a possible breakthrough in treating, and perhaps preventing, the common cold. Disclosure of this finding unleashed a brief but intense burst of publicity. Rosenthal granted interviews with television network reporters, but he had been caught off-guard. His efforts to limit speculation about the significance of BI's work were lost in the media's coverage that asserted a possible cure for the common cold.

Rosenthal knew the media's interest in the common cold discovery was just a taste of what the researchers could expect when they published the BIRG-587 data. He was determined that this time he would be prepared. Public relations needed to be factored into the BIRG-587 development plans. BI's Ridgefield unit was accustomed to responding to questions about the company's marketed products, but media inquiries about research projects was something new and different. So in August 1989, when Merluzzi's team was still focused on L-S 1170 and Karl Grozinger had not yet synthesized the first speck of BIRG-587, Rosenthal announced plans to engage Fleishman Hillard, a public relations firm in New York City, to help BI manage the expected publicity surrounding its AIDS drug development program.

* * *

Like BI, Elizabeth Glaser and her family had fiercely protected their privacy. From the moment that Ariel had been diagnosed with AIDS, her parents wanted to ensure that she did not suffer the social isolation that Ryan White and so many other HIV-infected children had endured. Despite legislation and court decisions that affirmed their civil rights, people known to have HIV disease received death threats, were terminated from their jobs, were discharged from the military, were dismissed from their schools, churches, and even their own families, and were refused admission to apartments and restaurants. In some cases, their homes were burned to the ground.[2] Ariel's parents might not be able to ease her AIDS symptoms but they were determined to protect her from that onslaught of publicity, prejudice, and abuse.

For the sake of Ariel's younger brother, who was also HIV-positive, Elizabeth continued to guard the family's privacy, sharing his HIV status with only close friends and family, and remaining in the background of the Pediatric AIDS Foundation. But as she lobbied government officials, orchestrated fundraisers, and pushed researchers for more pediatric clinical trials, the chances grew that her secret would be exposed. When tabloid reporters began making widespread inquiries, the Glasers decided that if their story was to be made public, they would at least tell it on their terms. Elizabeth cooperated with a *Los Angeles Times* reporter, who published a feature story on the family's three-year AIDS struggle in August 1989.[3] For the next few months, a television production crew from CBS's *60 Minutes* followed Elizabeth as she worked at the Foundation, attended fundraisers, walked the halls of Congress, and consulted AIDS experts at the National Institutes of Health, the FDA, and pharmaceutical companies.[4] The fifteen-minute segment aired on February 4, 1990, a story that reached fifty million Americans.[5] Elizabeth was "flabbergasted by the positive and enthusiastic reaction."[6] Strangers responded, encouraged her efforts, and offered to help. All of a sudden, she was the center of attention. Although she felt conflicted, knowing that her mission and the fame had come only because of her daughter's death, Elizabeth became, from that moment, the most passionate, eloquent, and influential spokesperson for children with AIDS and their families.

* * *

Four hundred miles north of the Glasers' home in Santa Monica, David Feigal was facing other public disclosure issues. After medical training at Stanford and the University of California, Davis, Feigal's interests drifted toward public health. He earned a master's degree in epidemiology and biostatistics from UC-Berkeley and then spent several years learning how to conduct clinical trials by serving as the data coordinator for cardiovascular research programs. One day, he wandered into a journal club presentation at San Francisco General Hospital, where his wife was a fellow in oncology.[7] The journal club topic was bowel diseases among gay men, and Feigal was intrigued by the unusual types of infectious diseases that physicians were observing in gay men, especially the lung infection, pneumocystis pneumonia. No one understood what was happening, but the number of cases kept increasing, and the death rate was high. When the funding for his cardiovascular projects ended, both Feigals decided to make career changes: she was interested in AIDS-related cancers, especially Kaposi's sarcoma, and he wanted to study pneumocystis pneumonia. AIDS "was *the* public health problem of our age," and San Francisco General Hospital was seeing one out of every ten AIDS cases in the country.[8]

Many of Feigal's patients on the crowded AIDS ward at San Francisco General died alone, rejected by their families, abandoned by their former friends, and fired from their jobs. Attending funerals became a part of the Feigals' routine. "I buried so many of my patients."[9] In a few fortunate cases, families accepted and supported a loved one who was suffering from AIDS. But like the Glasers, they feared the backlash of their friends and neighbors. The family of one patient asked Feigal to report cancer as the cause of death on their son's death certificate. His sister was a school teacher, and they feared that she would lose her job if people knew her brother had died from AIDS.[10]

* * *

To handle the media relations aspects of the BIRG-587 project, Rosenthal created an ad hoc public relations task force. From the beginning, their strategy for BIRG-587 was coordinated between Rosenthal's R&D division and the Product Public Relations unit in BI's marketing department.[11] A product PR manager was hired specifically to coordinate the planned communications within BI, manage public disclosures of the scientific findings, and serve as a liaison with Fleishman Hillard. Rosenthal, Merluzzi, and others in R&D generated the information about BI's AIDS research efforts and determined when and where the data were presented. In conjunction with those disclosures to scientific audiences, the public relations unit organized and packaged information for use by the media and other general audiences.[12]

Throughout the spring of 1990, Merluzzi and the other members of the task force met regularly to discuss the strategy for disclosing the BIRG-587 data. They decided that the first data presentation would be at the Interscience Conference on Antimicrobial Agents and Chemotherapy meeting in Atlanta, Georgia, in October 1990. In addition, Merluzzi proposed a series of eight scientific papers, each to highlight a certain aspect of the accumulated data, authored by those who had collected the corresponding data, and published in appropriately chosen scientific journals. The first of those manuscripts, which described the discovery of BIRG-587, would be the most widely quoted, and Rosenthal wanted it published in the prestigious scientific journal, *Science*. *Science* was reporting new HIV research findings in virtually every issue and was the place where the BIRG-587 data would get the broadest visibility within the scientific community.[13]

But Merluzzi's team was uncertain whether the editors of *Science* would accept the manuscript. Only high caliber, cutting edge, scientific reports survived the editors' critical eyes, and those manuscripts usually came from academic scientists, not commercial laboratories. In June, BI representatives contacted Steven Benkovic, who was serving as a research consultant to the BI teams and was on the editorial board of *Science*, and asked him to give the manuscript a "pre-read."[14]

Rosenthal wanted the paper published before the end of the year. Ordinarily, the process of publishing scientific results, from manuscript submission to a published article, took considerably longer than six months, especially in top-tier scientific journals. But AIDS advocacy groups and the general public, impatient with the long delays in publishing data that might help desperately ill patients, had been pressing editors to accelerate their review procedures and publication timetables. Journal editors responded by shifting from their traditional practices to expedited publication of breakthrough research findings on serious diseases such as AIDS.[15] Encouraged by Benkovic's assessment that BI's data might qualify for expedited publication, Merluzzi formally submitted the manuscript to *Science* in mid-June.

* * *

As they prepared their manuscripts for publication, Merluzzi's team and the public relations task force realized that they needed to address one other issue. The press, public, and research community would view BI's results more favorably if the compound had a name rather than a serial number. All drug companies routinely assign a unique number to each of their newly created compounds. When promising experimental drugs are destined to be widely referenced in scientific papers, discussed at scientific meetings, and reported in the media, drug companies take steps to give the compound a name.

BI's Nomenclature Committee asked Merluzzi's team to make recommendations for a non-proprietary name, and the team assigned the task to Karl Hargrave. Incorporating factors such as the drug's chemical structure, biologic properties, and intended clinical use, Hargrave generated a list of possible names and distributed it to the team for review. Their top five choices were tricyclovir, virazepine, tricyclovirin, dipyridovir, and diazevir. Rosenthal, in consultation with his management team, revised the choices to include tricyclidine and diciclovir. The Nomenclature Committee reviewed Rosenthal's list and recommended virazepene, diazevir, and provirazone to BI's executives for their consideration. After additional internal discussions, the group settled on provirazone, virazepine, and divirone. BI's attorneys submitted these three names to the United States Adopted Names Council, a clearing house for assigning unique generic drug names for use in the United States. They hoped that one of their recommended names for BIRG-587 would be approved in time to use at the ICAAC meeting and in the *Science* paper.

* * *

Also in June 1990, a BI delegation traveled to San Francisco to attend the 6th International Conference on AIDS. They monitored the scientific sessions, walked through the exhibit hall, listened to the attendees' informal discussions, and noted the media's involvement. From those observations, they gleaned valuable insight on how BI should prepare for the BIRG-587 presentation at ICAAC. Although clinicians were making some progress with existing drug treatments and researchers were following up on new discoveries, no one reported any scientific breakthroughs in San Francisco. Consequently, the political and social aspects of AIDS dominated the meeting. They learned that instead of being called patients, victims of AIDS, or AIDS sufferers, advocacy groups preferred the term, "people living with AIDS." Drug companies received harsh criticism, especially those firms that charged a high price for their AIDS drugs or that appeared to be unsympathetic to patient needs. The ICAAC meeting would be much smaller than the San Francisco AIDS conference, but BI would be prepared to respond to those issues.

In August, the editors of *Science* informed Merluzzi that the BIRG-587 manuscript had been accepted for publication with minor revisions. He responded to the editors' suggestions and submitted the revised manuscript within a week. It would be close, but Rosenthal was still optimistic that the *Science* article would be published before the end of the year.

Merluzzi's team and the public relations task force now knew that their public relations strategy must consider the impact of both the presentation at the ICAAC meeting in October and the *Science* paper which, hopefully, would appear shortly afterward. Consistent with BI's corporate philosophy, they would not seek press attention or issue a press release. But they would be prepared to address any question or issue that was raised by the media, scientific community, or general public. Among those preparations, BI's public relations advisors asked Merluzzi to consider what failure looked like.[16] In all of the team's discussions over the preceding two years, "that was something we had not considered."[17] But in the high stakes industry where only one drug reaches the market for every two hundred entering development, failure was not only possible but likely.[18] Their plans for BIRG-587 needed to include criteria for stopping development as well as proceeding with clinical trials, and they soberly prepared a risk management strategy.

Some of the media relations plans depended on whether BI's research at the ICAAC meeting would be presented as a platform talk, in which Merluzzi would present the data to an assembled audience of attendees, or assigned to a poster session, in which attendees had a few hours to stroll around the convention hall and view a poster-sized display of the data. A platform talk would likely attract more attention by both the scientific and media attendees. In either case, the BI delegation would follow a disciplined, reactive strategy. They would answer questions about BIRG-587 if asked, but they would limit their comments to a discussion of the scientific data. Over sixty compounds were known to be in development to treat AIDS, and none of them had received much attention at the San Francisco meeting, except the few drugs that were already in clinical trials. They did not expect that BIRG-587 would be singled out by the ICAAC attendees or generate much media attention, but they would be prepared.

Prior to the ICAAC meeting, Rosenthal, Merluzzi, and Julian Adams traveled to Fleishman Hillard's New York City offices and received a full day of media training.[19] They practiced answering questions, sat for mock-interviews, reviewed their videotaped performance, and were given basic tips for their media interactions. A similar media training session was arranged for John Sullivan, who was a coauthor on the BIRG-587 paper and would also be attending the meeting.[20]

On October 21, 1990, the contingent of BI scientists, including Merluzzi, Hargrave, and Adams, traveled to Atlanta, Georgia, to attend the ICAAC meeting. Two days later, they presented their data on BIRG-587. The ICAAC organizers had decided to schedule BI's disclosure in one of the poster sessions, rather than as a platform presentation. In a convention hall filled with posters, scientists crowded around BI's poster display, including at least one Nobel laureate. Gertrude Elion, who had made legendary discoveries of new cancer drugs and was part of the Burroughs Wellcome team that developed AZT, congratulated the BI scientists on their work.[21] For the entire three hours of the session, visitors to the BIRG-587 poster peppered the BI team with questions and took extensive notes. Many of them grabbed one of the letter-sized copies of the poster display and tucked it away for future reference. Often, the authors were asked, "Is BIRG-587 active in humans?" and "Is this a TIBO-like compound?" The answer to the first question, of course, was that the clinical trials had not yet begun. The BI authors bristled at the suggestion that BIRG-587 was a TIBO look-alike — they tactfully explained the differences. Academic scientists were impressed with the quality of the research. Industry scientists from competing firms had a more pragmatic interest, one of whom was overheard saying, "Why couldn't we have done this?"[22]

An article about Sullivan's involvement with the BIRG-587 research at the University of Massachusetts appeared in the Worcester newspaper the same day the poster was on display in Atlanta.[23] Two days later, as inquiries from local reporters flowed into Ridgefield, BI's director of public affairs issued a press release confirming BI's research program and the data that had been disclosed in Atlanta.[24] For the next few days, news about BI's new AIDS drug appeared in the local newspapers and on radio and television broadcasts. Some of these stories featured interviews with Rosenthal or Merluzzi, but the drug had only been tested in laboratory assays, and public interest soon faded. Everyone was waiting to know how BIRG-587 would perform when it was given to people with AIDS.

Around Thanksgiving, the editors of *Science* notified Merluzzi that the BIRG-587 article would appear in the December 7, 1990, issue. The media would receive advance copies of the issue's abstracts on November 30, and BI anticipated that media inquiries would begin arriving on December 3 or 4. *Science* embargoed media reports of its stories until the date of publication, but reporters would likely seek information and perhaps request interviews to incorporate into their stories, which they would publish when the embargo was lifted on December 7. Not knowing how extensive that reaction might be, Merluzzi's team and the public relations task force planned for three possible scenarios: no media interest, mild-to-moderate interest, and excessive interest. They prepared press packets, alerted key BI personnel, and waited.[25] By December 6, it was clear that the *Science* article was generating significant media interest. BI's public relations office supplied press packets when asked and arranged for interviews at the request of the *New York Times, Wall Street Journal,* and *Newsday,* as well as the Associated Press, United Press International, and Dow Jones wire services.

On December 7, 1990, BI's first published report, which included the chemical structure of BIRG-587 and the team's accumulated laboratory data, appeared in *Science.*[26] Merluzzi led the long list of authors, which also included chemists Karl Hargrave, Karl Grozinger, and Julian Adams, the original virologists Kristine and Robert Eckner, several other scientists from the BI team, Alan Rosenthal, and Richard Koup and John Sullivan from the University of Massachusetts.[27] Acknowledging the significance of BI's research, the journal's editors featured the BI article on its editorial page, which fueled the interest of not only the scientific community but also the media.[28]

Over the next month, articles about BIRG-587 continued to appear in national and local newspapers, trade publications, and specialty newsletters from coast to coast. Network and local radio and television reporters mentioned BIRG-587 in their news reports. Altogether, the news of BIRG-587 reached over 200 million people in the United States and Europe.

The media keyed on Jay Merluzzi, the lead author on the *Science* paper. Drawing on his media training and with the approval of BI's management, Merluzzi granted interviews to top science reporters at major newspapers and wire services.[29] He was gratified that all of the team's hard work, after years of silent labor, was finally receiving public acclaim.[30] It swelled his ego — behavior not lost on his wife. One evening, when his sustained excitement again dominated their dinner conversation, she turned to him and said, "Brigitte Gerney."[31]

Five years earlier, when the Merluzzis were living in a New York City suburb, a huge crane collapsed at a Manhattan construction project, trapping a woman in the rubble. The rescue effort, as often happens in cases of trapped victims, attracted local media, and the human interest story dominated several news cycles. Hour after hour, the city collectively held its breath, the Merluzzis among them, as rescue workers inched their way toward her. But unlike the rest of New York City, Merluzzi and his wife realized that this woman — suddenly the most well-known person in town — would be forgotten as soon as the media left the scene. They resolved not to let that happen. Unlike everyone else, they would always remember her name, Brigitte Gerney. So, in December 1990, while the media's spotlight still shone brightly on Jay Merluzzi, his wife reminded him of Brigitte Gerney. His fame, too, would be fleeting. People would soon forget, and he should keep things in perspective.[32]

News of BI's drug soon reached the scientists at Janssen Pharmaceuticals. They formally requested a sample of BIRG-587 in exchange for a sample of their TIBO compound. The BI scientists readily agreed to the exchange, confident that their drug would out-perform the TIBO drugs. Similarly, Merck reacted to the news of BIRG-587 by issuing a press release and announcing that its scientists had produced two compounds, L-697,639 and L-697,661, which were also potent HIV-1 reverse transcriptase inhibitors.[33] Although the chemical structures of these "L" compounds were markedly different from BIRG-587, they seemed to produce remarkably similar effects on the virus in laboratory assays. And, like Janssen's TIBO compounds but unlike BI's BIRG-587, Merck also reported that its "L" drugs had already been given to a small number of people. Two major pharmaceutical companies had indeed stumbled upon potent compounds that seemed to perform as well as BIRG-587, and both of those firms were further ahead in the race to develop better AIDS drugs.

6

The Christmas Tree

From the time that BIRG-587 was selected for development in February 1990, Jay Merluzzi included clinical planning on the agenda of every team meeting, and it was always the most hotly debated topic. At that time, there was no standard, no rule book, and little reliable experience for designing AIDS clinical trials. Everyone brought ideas and suggestions to the table. Jim Keirns, who had compiled an impressive profile of the drug's half-life and bioavailability in animals, translated that knowledge into what he hoped would be a safe dosing schedule for people.[1] Jim Wright, who led the effort to formulate the drug into tablets, continued his scholarly quest to understand HIV infections and became fascinated with the logistics of handling drug supplies and assaying the patients' blood samples.[2] Julian Adams, who headed the chemistry department, sought clinicians and other key opinion leaders, engaged them in detailed discussions, and from those interactions contributed his own ideas about how to design the clinical trials.[3] And Alan Rosenthal, himself a physician, invigorated BI's clinicians and pushed them to set aggressive clinical target dates. Merluzzi's team meetings resembled a jazz improvisation — discordant, independent voices somehow meshing into a like-minded track with a single beat, rhythm, and direction.[4] They energized each other. And out of those discussions, week by week, a plan for the BIRG-587 clinical trials began to take shape.

Merluzzi's team also incorporated the suggestions of their clinical consultants, John Sullivan at the University of Massachusetts in Worcester and Doug Richman at the University of California in San Diego. Both physicians were caring for AIDS patients who desperately needed new and better drugs, and BIRG-587 represented an attractive alternative to AZT.[5] They "wanted to move things along quickly."[6] Periodically, Sullivan and his colleagues would make the 130-mile drive to Ridgefield and sit in a conference room with the Boehringer Ingelheim scientists — Rosenthal, the laboratory scientists, chemists, and clinicians — all sharing data, reporting progress, and planning the next studies, an industry-academic collaboration without barriers.[7] And a very productive one.

The first clinical trial with any investigational drug must establish its safety, and for that reason, early clinical trials typically test the drug in disease-free, healthy people. Merluzzi's team, in conjunction with the clinical consultants, weighed the risks and decided to enroll HIV-infected people instead. Each person would receive only a single dose of BIRG-587, a very small dose, to assess the drug's safety. But they hoped, as they gingerly increased the dose level in the next subjects, that they might see some evidence that BIRG-587 inhibited the virus in the patients' blood. Sarah Cheeseman, a clinical colleague of Sullivan's at the University of Massachusetts and an investigator in the AIDS Clinical Trials Group network, agreed to serve as the physician in charge of conducting this first BIRG-587 clinical trial.

But Sullivan and Richman were more interested in conducting the second clinical trial, the one that Merluzzi's team spent the most time discussing, debating, and designing. This trial would be their first opportunity to determine whether BIRG-587 actually worked in people, and they packed all of their ideas into the study's protocol. They would give BIRG-587 to HIV-infected adults for twelve weeks, which was the minimum time necessary to show that an AIDS drug worked. From each patient throughout the twelve week dosing schedule, the investigators would draw a series of blood samples and perform a battery of laboratory tests, in addition to constantly monitoring the patients' health and noting side effects. If the patients showed signs of improvement, they would continue taking BIRG-587 for another twelve weeks. Not knowing the optimal dose, the team decided to treat several groups of HIV-infected people, each at a different dose level.

Based on the impressive data from the cell-based assays in Sullivan and Richman's laboratories, Merluzzi's team hoped that the higher doses of BIRG-587 would be sufficient to inhibit HIV in the patients' blood. But because Richman had observed that patients developed resistance to AZT, clinicians needed alternative treatment regimens. Among the ideas being explored by investigators was an attempt to boost the antiviral effect of AZT by combining it with one of the new experimental AIDS drugs. Richman used his cell culture assays to show that AZT in combination with BIRG-587 suppressed HIV proliferation much better than either drug alone, a synergistic effect.[8] The BI team therefore embellished the clinical study protocol to include groups that would receive AZT in addition to various dose levels of BIRG-587.

For BI's entry into the world of AIDS clinical trials, this was an ambitious and complex way to start. Drawing a schematic diagram of this complicated clinical trial — a graph showing the dosing groups and sequence of events — proved to be a particular challenge, given the limitations of graphics software available at the time. Someone thought the resulting diagram, which had multiple branches with every conceivable thing hanging off of it, looked like a Christmas tree, and the name stuck.[9]

* * *

Following the meetings with the AIDS Clinical Trials Group in May 1990 and the FDA reviewers in July, Merluzzi's team maintained an ongoing dialog with each government agency as they revised and refined the BIRG-587 clinical plans. The FDA reviewers had suggested design changes that would make it easier for patients to qualify for the clinical trials, reduce the complexity of the Christmas tree study, and incorporate testing BIRG-587 in children as well as adults. Those suggestions streamlined the clinical trials, but the FDA reviewers also insisted on certain minimum requirements to protect patients from being harmed by an experimental, largely unknown new drug. They were concerned about one gap in particular. The accumulated toxicology data on BIRG-587 was insufficient to support the ambitious clinical trials that the team — and everyone else — wanted to conduct.

Prior to starting the initial, single-dose safety study in people, the FDA guidelines required data from 28-day toxicology studies in animals.[10] So far, Laura Andrews had only completed the 14-day toxicology studies, and the 28-day toxicology studies were ongoing. For the Christmas tree study, in which patients would be treated for twelve weeks, BI needed to provide data from 3-month toxicology studies — studies that were still on the drawing boards at BI. In addition, BI proposed treating some patients in the Christmas tree study with a combination of BIRG-587 and AZT. The FDA reviewers wanted evidence from animal tests that those two drugs given together were safe and did not interfere with each other. But doing toxicology studies with the combined drugs was daunting—a complicated matrix of treatment groups, each dosed with various amounts of the drugs alone and in combination for various lengths of time. That type of testing would set back the team's timetable by many months.

During the fall of 1990, Merluzzi's team pondered how to close the gap, and three issues dominated their discussions: Could they demonstrate sufficient safety from the 14-day toxicology data to justify giving BIRG-587 to the HIV-infected patients who would be enrolled in the first clinical study? How quickly could they generate acceptable laboratory data showing that the combination of BIRG-587 and AZT was safe? And what could they do to start the crucial Christmas tree study earlier?

According to the team's calculations, the timing to deliver the crucial toxicology data was tight. Andrews would be able to finish the reports for both the rat and dog 14-day toxicology studies by December, but the reports of the 28-day toxicology studies would not be completed until January 1991. The 3-month rat toxicology study was slated to start in December, but unfortunately, the dog 3-month toxicology study would not start until March 1991. The FDA reviewers had assisted BI in streamlining the clinical plans in a number of ways, but would they be willing to compromise on the toxicology requirements?

The second issue was how to determine whether AZT and BIRG-587 were safe when given together. Merluzzi's team already had some data on the drug combination from Richman's laboratory assays. They knew that the two drugs given in combination had a powerful effect on suppressing HIV and were not toxic to the living cells in the assay. To elaborate on this observation, Keirns's staff gave the drug combination to animals, measured the bioavailability and half-life of each drug, and showed that neither drug affected the blood levels of the other drug.[11] These results, although less extensive than a toxicology study, indicated that AZT and BIRG-587 did not interact in a harmful manner. But would this be sufficient evidence to convince the FDA reviewers?

To address the third issue, the complexity of the Christmas tree study, Merluzzi's team decided to split it down the middle, creating two smaller and simpler studies. In the first of these, essentially the first branch of the Christmas tree, patients would receive only BIRG-587. If all went well, they would then begin the next study, essentially the second branch of the Christmas tree, treating patients with both BIRG-587 and AZT.[12]

As Merluzzi's team worked through these issues, they shared their ideas and plans with the FDA reviewers. This ongoing dialog reassured the team and increased their confidence that they were doing the right studies in the right way and that their plans for the clinical trials would be productive. Likewise, the FDA reviewers were pleased with the quality of BI's work.[13] They acknowledged the company's cooperation in making adjustments to the development plan and in general agreed with BI's new proposals. They accepted Keirns's data, showing that BIRG-587 and AZT did not cause any worrisome interactions. They were especially pleased at BI's new plans for the pediatric clinical trials, which had been beefed up to resemble the adult trials and would start within six months of the start of the first adult study. But the toxicology studies remained a sticking point.

Merluzzi's team had become accustomed to the FDA reviewers' cooperation, knowing that everyone was working to speed up clinical trials with new AIDS drugs. But the team had finally pushed their plans to the limit of what the regulators would accept. At the end of the day, the FDA behaves like the FDA, bound by its mandate to protect the public health. The reviewers compromised little on the requirements for toxicology data prior to treating people. They would allow BI to start the single-dose safety study with supporting data from the 14-day toxicology studies, but BI could not start the first Christmas tree study, in which patients would be dosed for twelve weeks, until Andrews had completed the 28-day toxicology studies and had at least started the 3-month toxicology studies. The team adjusted its plans accordingly.

* * *

Impressed with the clinical capabilities and resources that the ACTG network could offer, Rosenthal wanted to keep the ACTG involved in BI's clinical discussions. In November 1990, a BI delegation, along with Sullivan, Richman, and Cheeseman, traveled to Washington, DC, to attend the tenth AIDS Clinical Trial Group meeting, where the ACTG investigators were scheduled to discuss their latest advances in sessions open to the public. Richman was co-chair of ACTG's Primary Infection Committee, and Sullivan and Cheeseman were investigators in the ACTG network. Cheeseman presented the concept sheets for the first BIRG-587 clinical safety study and the newly split branches of the Christmas tree study to the ACTG Working Group and to the ACTG's Core Committee. In addition, BI shared its concept for the pediatric trials, which, with significant input from Sullivan, had been reconfigured along the same lines as the Christmas tree study. Among the ACTG members in attendance were Joep Lange and Martin Hirsch, who would become key investigators in later clinical trials of BIRG-587.

The ACTG Working Group and Core Committee, which represented a large circle of AIDS experts, enthusiastically supported BI's proposals. BIRG-587 was the first drug in its class to reach the ACTG, and the ACTG members, desperate for good drugs, wanted to do "whatever they could to facilitate and expedite the trials."[14] Martin Delaney, who represented the patient advocacy group Project Inform, was pleased that BI was "forward thinking" in submitting study designs for both the adult and pediatric trials to the ACTG.[15] Like his ACTG colleagues, he fully endorsed the first adult trial, but he also strongly urged BI to follow through with the pediatric trial and the BIRG-587/AZT combination trials.

* * *

Before BI could start giving BIRG-587 to people, it needed to submit an Investigational New Drug application to the FDA, containing all of the team's accumulated data on BIRG-587 and its plans for the first clinical trials. The faster that Merluzzi's team submitted the Investigational New Drug application, the sooner they could start giving the drug to people. At the time BIRG-587 was selected for development, Merluzzi's team had set October 1991 as the target date for submitting the Investigational New Drug application. Rosenthal pressed the team to speed things up so that the clinical trials could begin much sooner. So, they repeatedly reworked their plans, moving the target date up to July 1991, then to May 1991, and then to March 1991. The suggestions offered by the ACTG officials and FDA reviewers at their meetings in the summer of 1990, and the ongoing discussions that followed, encouraged the team to squeeze several more months out of the schedule. After Andrews completed her analysis of the 14-day toxicology studies in rats and dogs in August, the team settled on a target date of December 1990—a mere four months away.

Merluzzi knew the scientists had not kept up with writing and filing the research reports that were needed for the Investigational New Drug application. The results of each experiment were exciting, and new AIDS drugs were desperately needed, fueling the supercharged scientists to stay in their laboratories and collect more data to move the project forward. Consequently, a mountain of raw data and unfinished reports had accumulated.

Merluzzi compiled a list of the backlogged reports, set deadlines for completing each one, and then closely monitored the authors' progress.

Every week, Merluzzi met with John Tiso, a project manager assigned to the team, to review and coordinate the activities for preparing the Investigational New Drug application. The process of compiling it was anything but efficient. Merluzzi continually pushed the laboratory scientists to write reports. But some of them, including Andrews and Keirns's staff, faced the difficult choice of conducting studies versus writing reports, both of which were critical for the Investigational New Drug application. They worked weekends and did both.[16]

Another challenge was that Merluzzi's team members used different software and hardware systems. The laboratory scientists preferred software that could produce graphs and tables of their data as well as text. The clinical department, on the other hand, used a Wang word processing platform, a popular and leading system at the time. But the Wang system had limitations for producing graphics and tables. In addition, some of the critical data had been generated by external collaborators and contract laboratories, which submitted hardcopy reports rather than electronic documents. A technical writer in the toxicology department compiled the reports written by the laboratory scientists and the other documents from various sources, organizing the information on 5¼-inch magnetic floppy disks. Proofreading and editing these documents for inclusion in the Investigational New Drug application required printing hard copies of the text and literally cutting, rearranging, and taping together small slips of paper with new handwritten text in between. The reordered text was then retyped by a team of word-processing technicians in the clinical department.[17]

For Merluzzi, in particular, it was a stressful time. He was juggling trips to the hospital to visit his gravely ill mother with his team leader responsibilities, prodding the team to finish reports for the Investigational New Drug application, making arrangements for the ICAAC presentation in Atlanta, and finalizing the *Science* paper. Rosenthal wanted the presentation at the ICAAC meeting, publication of the *Science* paper, and the submission of the Investigational New Drug application to follow one another in rapid succession, systematically announcing BIRG-587 to an anxious public, and it was Merluzzi's job to orchestrate it all. One evening, he was driving his pickup truck along the narrow winding roads of Putnam County, New York, with his young son strapped into the front seat. An oncoming car crossed the center line and collided with them head-on. They were rushed to the hospital and treated for minor cuts and bruises. And through it all Merluzzi kept thinking, "I wish my mother wasn't sick."[18]

By Thanksgiving, the word processing group had compiled everything in the Investigational New Drug application except the results from the 28-day toxicology studies. Because these results were needed to support BI's proposed clinical plans, the Christmas tree studies in particular, the team had no choice but to wait until the data were available. That data arrived in mid–December and was quickly incorporated. The completed Investigational New Drug application circulated through the company, receiving the necessary reviews and internal approvals with lightning speed, and Alan Rosenthal, now promoted to Senior Vice President of Scientific Affairs in Ridgefield, signed it on behalf of BI.

On December 26, 1990, BI officially submitted the Investigational New Drug application for BIRG-587.[19] Merluzzi's team had already shared and discussed virtually everything in it with the FDA officials, and they had every reason to expect that the review would be expedited. The team had even asked Cheeseman to start scheduling beds in the clinic at the University of Massachusetts. But unfortunately, an expedited review was far from certain.

One week before BI's application arrived at the FDA, Ellen Cooper asked to be transferred from her position as Director of the Antiviral Drug Products Division.[20] For years, the tenacious, open-minded, and resilient regulator had withstood withering criticism from AIDS advocacy groups, drug company officials, and clinical investigators, all of whom wanted the FDA to go faster.[21] While upholding the agency's legal mandate to base new drug licenses on scientifically rigorous data, she worked tirelessly to streamline regulatory procedures. Her efforts had resulted in AZT's lightning-speed development and approval, shortened the clinical development path for Bristol-Myers Squibb's ddI and Hoffmann-La Roche's ddC, and hastened clinical trials of emerging AIDS drugs such as BIRG-587. She was the most influential person involved in regulating and licensing new AIDS drugs in the country, and she would be hard to replace.[22] Her departure and the loss of her leadership heightened the uncertainty among drug companies about how to proceed with their new AIDS drugs. The Investigational New Drug application of BIRG-587 was a significant milestone for BI. But without Cooper in charge, how would the FDA view BI's request to start clinical testing?

* * *

For Merluzzi, reaching this regulatory milestone was bittersweet. His mother lost her battle with leukemia in November, not living to read the news articles displaying her son's photograph or to share his pride in successfully guiding the team to the threshold of clinical trials with a potentially life-saving drug, achievements that are rare for scientists at any company and were a first for BI's Ridgefield facility.[23]

Submitting the Investigational New Drug application also marked the transition of Merluzzi's leadership. For the past two years, the development team had consumed nearly all of his time and energy. He had led the team through the chaotic early days of the L-S 1170 studies, the fits and starts of uncertainty while BI settled on a new development compound, and the frenzy and flurry of activity to get BIRG-587 into clinical trials. From this point forward, the laboratory scientists would take a backseat to the clinicians. The chemists would continue to make batches of the drug, and other laboratory scientists would continue to collect toxicology and bioavailability data from animals. But from now on, their main job was to support the clinicians' efforts and the all-important clinical trials. BI now referred to the group as a project team, rather than a development team. And Merluzzi officially turned over leadership of the project team to John Tiso, a highly experienced project manager in Ridgefield's project management group.

As Tiso shouldered the burden of leading the team, Merluzzi settled into a new role. He would represent the laboratory scientists on the project team and coordinate their efforts in support of the BIRG-587 clinical trials.[24] But the bulk of his time and energy would now be devoted to new research initiatives in his laboratory, experiments that needed more of his attention and guidance.

Tiso had previously served as the project manager for several of BI's pulmonary and cardiovascular products, which had been discovered and largely developed at BI's other R&D centers. When his department learned that the Ridgefield R&D laboratories were making progress with a newly discovered AIDS drug, the project management unit took steps to support the team, knowing that eventually a full-time project manager would be needed.[25] Tiso initially joined Merluzzi's team in an auxiliary capacity. For a year, he regularly attended team meetings, familiarizing himself with the team members and their roles and learning about the compound and the team's plans. When asked, he offered his advice.

During preparation of the Investigational New Drug application, Tiso assisted Merluzzi and began forming an administrative structure for managing the project during clinical development. At the same time, Rosenthal approached the head of Tiso's department, and they vetted candidates to lead the BIRG-587 project team, quickly settling on Tiso.[26] Well informed and well equipped to take charge, Tiso seamlessly assumed responsibilities for coordinating the project team's cross-functional activities, chairing the team meetings, assembling the project plans, obtaining the team's consensus on project issues, overseeing the team's progress, and reporting the project's status. It would take all of Tiso's talent and experience to manage this project, which had greatly expanded in scope and visibility and would face demanding internal and external audiences in the years ahead.

* * *

As of December 1990, the Centers for Disease Control had accumulated 161,073 reports of AIDS in the United States.[27] Of the reported cases, 100,813 people had died, leaving 60,260 AIDS patients alive and available for treatment beginning in 1991. More than a dozen AIDS drugs were already in clinical trials, and more than sixty drugs were being readied for testing in people.[28] With so many choices, would patients be interested in taking BIRG-587?

On January 16, 1991, the project team received the news they had been waiting for — expedited by the FDA reviewers, despite the holidays and the loss of their Director.[29] Having reviewed the data and reports in the Investigational New Drug application, the FDA officials said that BI could proceed with the first clinical trial of BIRG-587. Sarah Cheeseman had already identified patients for the study, and Jim Wright had already shipped BIRG-587 tablets to the University of Massachusetts.

7

The Journey Begins, Finally

On January 21, 1991, Phil sat in the clinic at the University of Massachusetts in Worcester, uncertain how the day would end.[1] He and two other volunteers were waiting to become the first humans to take an investigational drug called BIRG-587. Beginning with this first clinical trial, Boehringer Ingelheim welcomed both men and women, but most of the participants, like Phil, were gay men in their mid–30s.[2] They had been vibrant, active men who went for a daily run and regularly worked out at the gym. When their HIV infections progressed to the first stages of AIDS, their only treatment option was AZT. Initially, they responded to treatment, and their renewed energy allowed them to resume their normal daily activities. Phil and his fellow trial participants were spared the nasty and dangerous side effects that plagued patients who had taken AZT in earlier years, because physicians realized that they could lower the dose and still get a good response. AZT's side effects at the lowered dose, although unpleasant, usually cleared within a few months.

The men tackled their illness aggressively and holistically. In addition to AZT and their fitness routines, they took pentamidine aerosol to prevent pneumocystis pneumonia and embraced acupuncture, meditation, herbal treatments, and macrobiotic diets. Unfortunately, after a year or two, and despite all their efforts to preserve their health, AZT could no longer hold back the onslaught of this persistent virus. Their weakened immune systems struggled to fight even mild infections, serious side effects of AZT loomed as a possibility, and AZT-induced anemia was a constant threat. They became impatient with AZT and with medicine in general. But instead of complaining and accepting their fate, they resolved to do something, to be active participants in the fight to find answers.

Phil and the other volunteers saw the BIRG-587 clinical trial as an opportunity to help find some of those answers. It was a way of taking control of their situation and doing something constructive. They willingly agreed to be poked and punctured dozens of times, donating their blood to science so that the investigators could learn how this drug performed in people. They knew that the dose of BIRG-587 they would be taking was too small and probably came too late to help them. They also knew that the drug might cause some unanticipated and dangerous side effects — effects the investigators had not seen in the preceding animal studies. But they were willing to take those risks. This drug might turn out to be more effective and less toxic than anything else that was currently available, and somebody had to take the first step. It was a very empowering feeling.

The tiny 2.5 milligram tablet that Phil and the other two volunteers swallowed on that cold January morning marked the beginning of BI's clinical trials with BIRG-587. Sarah Cheeseman closely monitored the men for side effects and drew a series of blood samples. Jim Keirns and his staff took turns waiting to process the samples in a nearby laboratory at the University of Massachusetts. Then, they packed the tubes in ice and drove the 130 miles from Worcester to Boehringer Ingelheim's laboratories in Ridgefield, where the scientists immediately assayed the amount of BIRG-587 in each blood sample.[3] Over the next few weeks, Cheeseman gave additional patients, in groups of three, successively larger doses of BIRG-587, and Keirns's staff quickly analyzed their blood. Cheeseman observed no drug-related side effects in any of the patients. And Keirns's staff soon discovered that the bioavailability of BIRG-587 in people is very high and the half-life is long, significant advantages over AZT.[4] BIRG-587 reached levels in the patients' blood that exceeded the amount needed to stop HIV proliferation (at least, as predicted by their original cell culture results), and those findings increased the project team's confidence that BIRG-587 might actually stop HIV proliferation in patients. This first, small clinical trial had achieved its goals. BIRG-587 could be given safely to people, and the drug had much more attractive pharmaceutical properties than AZT. So far, BIRG-587 was performing exactly as the team wanted.

* * *

While Phil and his fellow volunteers were taking their dose of BIRG-587, the BI project team in Ridgefield concentrated on the plans for the next clinical trials, especially the critical Christmas tree studies. They had reached an agreement defining the relationship between BI and the AIDS Clinical Trials Group at the National Institutes of Health. For clinical trials of BIRG-587 conducted in the United States, investigators in the ACTG network would recruit and treat the patients. BI would retain responsibility for managing the clinical data, monitoring the sites, and communicating with the Food and Drug Administration. The project team was also planning clinical trials in other countries. BI would conduct those international trials without support from the ACTG.

As soon as these agreements were reached, BI's clinicians scheduled a clinical investigator meeting, to be held in Dana Point, a resort town in southern California. It was the first time that BI's American and international clinical consultants would meet to discuss BIRG-587. To ensure that BI's clinical plans incorporated the latest views about how to conduct AIDS clinical trials, representatives from the AIDS divisions at the National Institutes of Health and the FDA had also been invited.[5] Then, three days before the meeting, the United States and coalition forces began bombing Baghdad in the First Gulf War. Fearing retaliation by Saddam Hussein, many businesses curtailed non-essential business travel to destinations in the United States, a situation that threatened to derail the Dana Point meeting. Airports remained open, but in many terminals, airport workers outnumbered passengers.[6] For all of those invited to the Dana Point meeting, the prospect that BIRG-587 might represent a major advance in the treatment of AIDS outweighed any reluctance to travel. They bravely boarded their planes and arrived safely in California.

For the Ridgefield contingent and most of the other travelers, the Dana Point meeting was an opportunity to escape the dreary doldrums of mid-winter. In between the long sessions debating the best ways to stage the BIRG-587 clinical trials, they strolled along the beach, breathed the salty air, and watched carefree Californians surf and play beach volleyball in brilliant sunshine.[7] Far from a distraction, these blissful surroundings invigorated them, and they returned to the conference table eager to tackle their deadly serious work. They mapped the clinical strategy like general staff officers conducting war games, outlining the sequence of studies, setting each study's objectives and design, and deciding where each study would be conducted. In the course of four days, they established their battle plan and forged a close collaboration that would last for many years, spanning a wide range of clinical trials with BI's new drug. Prominent among those plans were the pediatric clinical trials and the first international clinical trials, both of which were based on the design of the first Christmas tree study.

Shortly after the Dana Point meeting, the project team continued discussing plans for the Christmas tree studies with the ACTG officials. The study team for these trials consisted of representatives from both BI and ACTG, and they met for the first time in Washington, DC, in March 1991. In those days, before the internet, BI and the ACTG maintained separate email platforms. ACTG made arrangements to establish a special account on its email system so that the BI and ACTG team members could rapidly exchange critical trial information such as laboratory results and treatment side effects.

Representatives from the FDA also attended the March ACTG meeting. Although the Christmas tree studies would be conducted within the ACTG network, the protocols needed to be reviewed by the FDA. This close collaboration between BI, ACTG, and FDA expedited completion of the plans for the Christmas tree trials and ensured that the necessary regulatory review step would not cause delays. Cheeseman at the University of Massachusetts and Doug Richman at the University of California in San Diego, were already compiling a list of patients who expressed interest in the Christmas tree studies.

* * *

The Christmas tree studies represented a quantum leap in complexity compared to the first, single-dose safety study, and transitioning smoothly from one to the other required meticulous planning and disciplined coordination. Because patients would be treated for a minimum of twelve weeks and, hopefully, for another twelve weeks, the project team needed to show that BIRG-587 was safe in animals that had been dosed at least that long. So far, Laura Andrews had completed the 28-day toxicology studies in rats and dogs. She had also started dosing rats and dogs in the 3-month toxicology studies. The FDA reviewers would permit BI to start the first Christmas tree study, based on the 28-day toxicology data, but BI needed to finish the 3-month toxicology studies before the patients had been dosed longer than 28 days. The scheduling was extremely tight.

Equally critical for Andrews was scheduling the 52-week toxicology studies in rats and dogs. These studies also needed to start in a timely manner, to support continued dosing in the Christmas tree patients beyond the first twelve weeks. The 52-week rat toxicology study required a relatively small batch of drug, which Karl Grozinger could produce in his new pilot plant, and Andrews moved forward with the study. But the 52-week dog toxicology study would require 75 kilograms (about 165 pounds) of BIRG-587, and the toxicologists wanted all of it to come from a single batch. This was far beyond the capabilities of Grozinger's kilogram-scale facility. Andrews continued making plans for the 52-week dog study and conducted several preliminary tests to sort out the experimental details. But the start date of the definitive 52-week dog toxicology study would be delayed multiple times, mainly awaiting delivery of the large batch of BIRG-587. To meet this need for bulk drug supplies, Grozinger, in conjunction with his own production schedule, held ongoing discussions with his colleagues in BI's large-scale chemical plant.[8] Together, they planned production of BIRG-587 batches ten times larger than those Grozinger was producing in his pilot plant.

Clinical planning for the Christmas tree studies was also complex. On paper, the two branches of the original Christmas tree had been split into two separate clinical trials. The first of these trials would test BIRG-587 in HIV-infected adults for twelve weeks, and if all went well, for an additional twelve weeks.[9] The second branch of the Christmas tree followed the same design—daily doses of BIRG-587 for the same length of time at each of the same dose levels — but each patient also received AZT daily. In practice, the two branches of the Christmas tree were intertwined.[10] The University of Massachusetts in Worcester and the University of California in San Diego enrolled patients into both clinical trials, which ran simultaneously.[11]

In early April 1991, BI submitted the 28-day rat and dog toxicology reports and the results of Cheeseman's clinical safety study to the FDA. Those results confirmed the safety of BIRG-587 both in animals and people. BI also confirmed that Andrews had started the 3-month rat and dog toxicology studies, a prerequisite for starting the first Christmas tree study. One week later, the FDA officials allowed BI to begin enrolling patients in the Christmas tree study, the first real test of whether BIRG-587 would suppress HIV in people.

* * *

Following the Dana Point meeting, the project team continued discussions with BI's international clinical investigators. Premier AIDS treatment centers headed by Joep Lange in the Netherlands, David Cooper in Australia, and Stefano Vella in Italy were the most desirable locations for conducting clinical trials with BIRG-587. The project team eagerly sought these investigators, and the investigators were equally eager to access BI's new experimental AIDS drug.[12] Together, they finalized plans for an international clinical trial using HIV-infected patients. Because the country-specific regulatory reviews were lengthy and complex, the international investigators wanted to submit the applications to their respective regulatory authorities as soon as possible. Even under the best circumstances, they would not be able to start the international trial for many months. The logistics for coordinating this international effort was complicated not only by the assortment of regulatory requirements and the wide span of time zones but also by the limited communication technologies available at the time. BI's internal email system connected the Ridgefield unit with the BI R&D centers in Europe. But the Ridgefield team did not have an email connection with the BI office in Australia. Computer technicians at the two locations worked diligently to install the necessary software and hardware on the Australian office's local area network, but the email link to Ridgefield took several weeks to complete.

The project team was also mindful of the special relationship between the R&D units in Ridgefield and Canada. Jay Merluzzi had routinely included Bio-Méga and BI's Canadian business unit when he distributed his status reports of the team's progress. The Bio-Méga laboratories continued to search for an HIV protease inhibitor that would be a suitable AIDS drug, and Merluzzi as well as the clinical team made frequent trips to Montreal to brief the Bio-Méga scientists on the BIRG-587 clinical development plans.[13] Now that the first clinical trials had begun and plans were being made to start the international trials, Merluzzi and other members of the team traveled to Ottawa for meetings with the Health Protection Branch, Canada's drug regulatory agency.[14] The Health Protection Branch officials welcomed the opportunity to have an early discussion about BIRG-587. Although the Canadian regulatory review of new clinical programs took up to sixty days (compared with the thirty-day turnaround time of the FDA), the regulatory officials had expedited their procedures to accommodate clinical trials of other AIDS drugs that used sites in both the United States and Canada.[15] The BI project team viewed Canada as an attractive country in which to expand the BIRG-587 clinical program, but they were currently focused on launching their first international clinical trial in Australia, Italy, and the Netherlands, countries with larger populations of HIV-infected adults and with experienced AIDS clinical centers.[16] In the meantime, they maintained a rapport with the Canadian authorities and fostered relationships with key Canadian investigators.

One key investigator was Julio Montaner, a young clinician at St. Paul's Hospital and the University of British Columbia in Vancouver. Born and raised in Buenos Aires, Argentina, Montaner intended to follow in the footsteps of his father, a prominent respiratory specialist well known for his work on tuberculosis.[17] To establish his own professional credentials, the younger Montaner trained at St. Paul's as a resident in respiratory medicine in 1981, fully intending to return to Argentina and practice on an equal footing with his father. Instead, he met his future wife, an X-ray technician at the hospital, and "found a reason to stay" in Canada.[18] Physicians were increasingly referring cases of AIDS-related pneumocystis pneumonia to Montaner, the hospital's respiratory specialist, and he drew on his background in tuberculosis to tackle the infection with innovative drug regimens. When AZT came along, St. Paul's had the opportunity to test the new AIDS drug. The head of the hospital's department of medicine asked Montaner, because of his success in treating opportunistic infections, to set up an AIDS research program. For Montaner, who by default had become the hospital's most experienced AIDS physician, it was a diversion from his respiratory interests, but he agreed to do HIV/AIDS clinical research for a year. As new AIDS drugs emerged, though, Montaner was drawn more deeply into antiviral research. Step by step, his work shifted, until eventually he was treating AIDS patients exclusively.

Those early AIDS drugs, such as AZT, ddI, and ddC, gave short-term relief, but they were insufficient. For Montaner and his patients, "it was a dark time."[19] He was searching for the next scientific advance — the next drug that would hopefully provide incremental improvement — when the BI team contacted him in 1991 to discuss BIRG-587. Montaner and the BI team instantly meshed, Montaner intrigued by BIRG-587's potential and BI impressed with the Vancouver research unit — the largest HIV/AIDS facility in Canada. But the BI project team had already engaged some of the world's best AIDS experts to test BIRG-587 in the first international clinical trial. The outcome of that trial, along with the ongoing clinical program through the ACTG network in the United States, would determine the course of BIRG-587's continued development. For the time being, the BI team put Montaner, a young and less-known investigator, on hold.[20] But he closely followed the progress of BIRG-587, anxiously awaiting his opportunity to join the international team.

* * *

Because the results from Cheeseman's clinical safety study in adults were encouraging, BI moved forward with its commitment to the FDA to begin the pediatric trials within six months. That meant starting the first pediatric study by the end of July, and there was still much to do. In addition to Cheeseman's safety data and the pediatric study protocol, they needed to develop a suitable liquid formulation of the drug to give to the children.

Amale Hawi, a scientist in BI's formulations group, led the efforts to develop the liquid formulation. Following the same philosophy as Jim Wright who wasted no time in beginning his work on the tablets, Hawi and her colleagues began exploring liquid formulations soon after BIRG-587 had been selected for development. At that time, the project team planned to conduct only adult clinical trials, and the only formulation they needed was tablets. Consequently, Hawi approached her early experiments as an academic exercise, learning about the compound's properties without pressure from the team to produce a certain type of liquid formulation by a fixed date.[21]

As Wright had already discovered, the only property of BIRG-587 that posed a formulation challenge was that the compound did not easily dissolve in water. To obtain a clear liquid, Hawi needed a large volume of water to dissolve a small amount of the compound.

Children would have to drink several quarts of this very dilute liquid each day to get an adequate dose of BIRG-587. Looking for a better option, Hawi explored a different kind of formulation, suspending particles of the powdered BIRG-587 in a thickened liquid, like raisins in a cake batter. She tinkered with the ingredients and soon found a way to prepare a concentrated suspension that contained enough BIRG-587 to reduce the volume to about one tablespoon of liquid.

Then, one day in 1990, the team asked Hawi to accelerate her formulation work. They had made a commitment to the FDA to incorporate the pediatric clinical trials as an integral part of the development plan, and those trials would start soon after the first adult study. With a new sense of urgency and the target date for starting the pediatric clinical trials fast approaching, Hawi applied her accumulated knowledge and ramped up her efforts to make a clinically acceptable formulation — one that children would be willing take.[22]

When embarking on a pediatric clinical trial with a new investigational drug, the first thing pediatricians do is taste the drug.[23] If it tastes bad, they know that children will refuse to take it. For some of the early pediatric AIDS trials, no pediatric formulation of the experimental drugs existed. Pediatricians resorted to purchasing syrups from the supermarket and concocted drug-containing liquids that they hoped would be more palatable than the hard-to-swallow pills.[24] Many of the AIDS drugs tasted bad, and drug company scientists struggled to prepare pleasant-tasting liquid formulations. Some were chalky or gritty, and one tasted like peppermint flavored gasoline.[25] Hawi experimented with grape and cherry, the usual children's flavoring agents, but ultimately decided not to use them.[26] BIRG-587 did not have an objectionable taste, and she settled on a simple formulation containing only a mild sweetener to offset the suspension's otherwise bland taste. The resulting white liquid looked and tasted like runny icing.[27]

Hawi's biggest challenge was the formulation's stability. Her early liquid suspensions were acceptable in many ways, but unfortunately they required storage in a refrigerator. If the liquid formulation sat on the shelf at room temperature, the suspended particles of BIRG-587 began to form larger and larger crystals, like rock candy growing in a sugar solution.[28] After only one month, the crystals of BIRG-587 grew too large and ruined the suspension.[29] If this formulation were given to patients, the large crystals would simply pass through the gut without being absorbed, and none of the BIRG-587 would reach the virus in the blood and other tissues.

For those early experiments, Hawi had used the same, highly purified BIRG-587 that her colleagues were using to prepare tablets. But she discovered that when she used a different crystal form of BIRG-587 (called a hemihydrate) in her recipe, the finished suspension was stable at room temperature and did not coalesce into large crystals.[30] This requirement for two different types of BIRG-587 — the original dry powder for tablets and the hemihydrate for the suspension — would pose another challenge for Karl Grozinger and his colleagues. As the clinical trials proceeded, they needed to produce bulk drug supplies using two different chemical procedures, one for supplies that would be used to make tablets and the other for the liquid formulation.

* * *

Meanwhile, the BI team and ACTG officials continued planning the first pediatric trial using BIRG-587. In January 1991, the ACTG Operations Office appointed an ACTG staff specialist to the study.[31] John Sullivan worked with the BI project team and the ACTG's Pediatric Core Committee to finalize the study protocol. Hawi's suspension formulation was suitable for this first study, which would enroll only a small number of children. But the project team realized that the following pediatric trials would be larger and enroll children with a wide range of ages and weights.[32] The drug dose would be adjusted for the child's age and size, and the project team wanted to avoid giving large volumes of the suspension to the larger, older children. They decided to use both formulations in the pediatric trials. The suspension would be easier for small children to take, and the older children would be given tablets. In March and April, the project team compiled the BIRG-587 data and updated other documents that were needed to support the first pediatric clinical trial. Like Cheeseman's first adult trial, this first pediatric trial of BIRG-587 would be conducted at the University of Massachusetts.

In June 1991, Katherine Luzuriaga, a pediatrician and Sullivan's colleague, gave the first dose of BIRG-587 to children, one month sooner than the BI project team had promised to the FDA. This pediatric safety study was similar to Cheeseman's safety study in adults, and the results were similar. The children achieved blood levels of BIRG-587 that were comparable to those seen in the adults, and Luzuriaga detected no drug-related side effects. Encouraged by these results, the project team began making plans to conduct additional pediatric trials, comparable to the adult Christmas tree studies. At this point, the future of BIRG-587 as a pediatric AIDS drug seemed bright.

* * *

BIRG-587 still did not have a name. In February 1991, the United States Adopted Name Council rejected all three names that BI had proposed. They were all too similar to the names used for other classes of drugs. Instead, USAN had consulted the World Health Organization's International Nonproprietary Name Expert Committee and the two organizations had devised a name that they found acceptable for use both in the United States and worldwide: azevirpine. Because their deliberations had taken a long time, USAN and WHO-INN offered to expedite the paperwork, and if BI agreed, they could authorize official use of the new name in a matter of weeks.

Alan Rosenthal and the project team disliked USAN's choice. After discussions between BI's Nomenclature Committee and the project team, they countered with hivirapine as their primary choice and proposed rovirapine and alvirapine as backups. Unfortunately, the USAN rejected those names and instead proposed two alternatives: davirapine and nevirapine. The project team was not particularly enthused with either name. Rosenthal preferred nevirapine. In March, BI formally submitted its application to USAN for the non-proprietary name of BIRG-587, indicating nevirapine as the primary choice and proposed lovirapine as a backup. USAN and WHO then vetted the names through their organizations. Having received no challenges to BI's application, the USAN Council voted in May 1991 to adopt nevirapine. BIRG-587 now had a name.

The project team next turned its attention to brainstorming a brand name for BIRG-587, the unique trademarked name that BI would use to market the product. Unlike the generic name, nevirapine, which corresponded to BIRG-587's unique chemical composition and would be used by everyone to identify the chemical substance, the brand name would be owned by BI and would be used to identify the drug product that was solely made and sold by BI.[33] The brand name for nevirapine needed to be easy to remember, easy to pronounce in multiple languages, and not associated with negative meanings in any language. From a list of about thirty choices, the project team prioritized their favorites: Notran, Replix, Virune, Alvir, and Viramun. The team knew that whittling down this list to a final name would be a long, complicated, and tedious process.

* * *

Assigning nevirapine as the name for BIRG-587 had come in time to be incorporated into BI's presentations at the 7th International AIDS Conference in Florence, Italy. A year earlier, the BI delegation had traveled to the 6th International Conference in San Francisco primarily to gather information from other investigators. At the Florence Conference, they would showcase their data on nevirapine. Hargrave, Grozinger, and the other chemists submitted a paper describing the chemical synthesis campaign that led to the discovery of nevirapine.[34] Joe Wu, a BI biochemist, represented the team of scientists who had investigated how nevirapine bound to the viral enzyme, HIV reverse transcriptase, and prevented it from functioning.[35]

To conduct his experiments, Wu used a chemical probe, and his approach was as clever as it was unconventional. Julian Adams had first suggested the concept of a chemical probe, a molecule that not only mimicked nevirapine's ability to inhibit the HIV enzyme but also could be triggered to fuse with the enzyme, gluing it permanently in place. The molecule that John Proudfoot, a chemist in Adams's department, designed was triggered by ultraviolet light, and for that reason they called it a photoaffinity probe.[36] In their initial attempts, the BI scientists had been unsuccessful in getting the probe to stick, and when Wu joined the company, they asked him to give it a try — his first project after completing graduate school.

The secret of Wu's success was finding an appropriate light source to activate the chemical probe. Lights designed for scientific experiments produce pure and specific wavelengths of light, but Wu knew that pure ultraviolet light would fry the delicate proteins in his assay. He needed a milder, more diffuse light source. Eschewing scientific supply catalogs, he went to a local hardware store and bought a sunlamp, a light source designed to mimic sunlight and generate milder ultraviolet light. Making meticulous calculations and numerous adjustments, Wu shone the sunlamp on his assay solution in experiment after experiment, month after month. His colleagues would walk by his laboratory, shake their heads, and kid him about his suntan lamp experiments. But Wu's persistence paid off. He finally achieved the desired fusion between the probe and enzyme, and his results earned him a trip to Florence.

Just like the ICAAC meeting eight months earlier, BI did not seek any media attention at the Florence AIDS Conference. But the company ensured everyone was prepared to respond to any inquiry. Rosenthal informed the R&D staff about BI's planned scientific presentations, BI's public relations task force drafted responses to anticipated media inquiries, and the departmental secretaries were briefed on how to handle incoming calls from the general public. But Wu brushed aside media training, which the public relations task force offered to all of the scientist-presenters. He had attended other scientific meetings and knew how to present laboratory data.[37] Why should this Conference be any different?

The lay press coverage in Florence made no mention of nevirapine, but Wu's presentation generated considerable interest among the research scientists, especially those representing competitor companies. Throughout the rest of the Conference, they hounded Wu everywhere he went. Faced with the constant barrage of questions, he now understood the importance of media training. Without it, but remembering Rosenthal's philosophy of sharing data, Wu struck his own balance, describing his data in detail but declining to speculate about its significance. "It was an interesting and awkward status" for the newly minted industrial scientist.[38] One evening after another long day of hide-and-seek, Wu ducked into the hotel bar, only to be cornered again by a couple of scientists from other drug companies and once again trapping him in a discussion of his work. The conversation dragged on, collegial but probing, through round after round of drinks, as a fidgety Wu searched in vain for an opportunity to make a graceful retreat. He finally sauntered back to his room in the wee hours of the morning wearing a broad smile. Wu is allergic to alcohol, and the sunlamp guru had just made another discovery. Florentine coffee is the best in the world.[39]

* * *

The International AIDS Conference in Florence drew the attention of research scientists to Boehringer Ingelheim as a company conducting HIV research and to nevirapine. But by 1991, the media, clinicians, and the AIDS community had seen many compounds that never matured beyond the research laboratory. To them, nevirapine was just another interesting research tool. They were waiting for data from clinical trials.

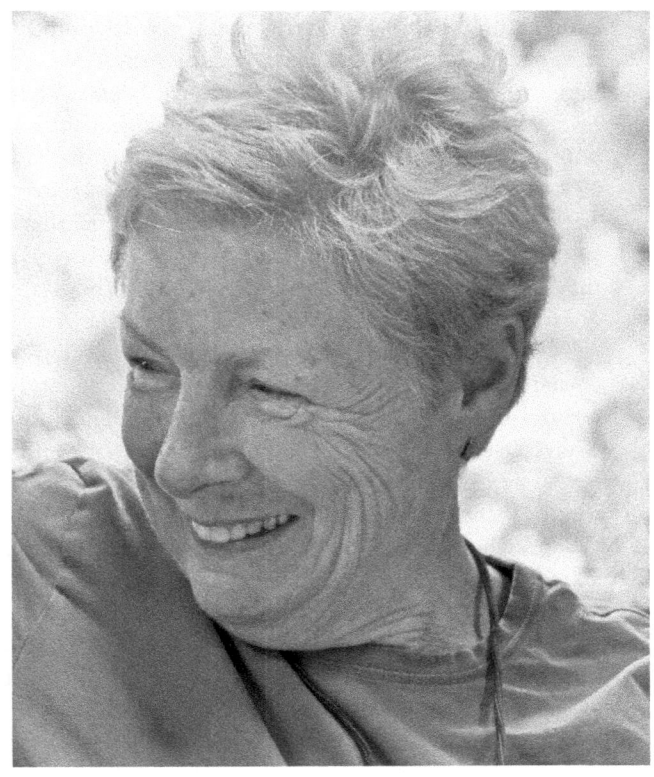

Maureen Myers.

At BI, those clinical trials were now the responsibility of Maureen Myers. She had joined BI in the spring of 1991 after a distinguished, 22-year career at the National Institutes of Health. Trained in virology at Georgetown University, Myers had worked at the National Institute of Allergy and Infectious Diseases for over a decade in antiviral research, first focusing on hepatitis, herpes encephalitis, and other life-threatening infections, and eventually rising to Assistant Director of the AIDS Treatment Program. She and John LaMontagne had created the AIDS Clinical Trials Group, and through her continued involvement with the AIDS Division, Myers understood the inner workings of the ACTG, was well connected to AIDS investigators worldwide, and knew how to direct a large, complex research program. Many on the BI project team had never worked alongside such a well-known person.[40] A no-nonsense, by-the-book administrator, Myers spoke with authority, acted decisively, and inspired confidence. Now, she applied those skills to nevirapine, setting the course of the development program, leading the clinical team, and directing the clinical trials.

Myers accompanied Cheeseman to the ACTG meeting in Washington, DC, in July, where Cheeseman formally presented the data from the single-dose safety clinical trial. Although her talk attracted a large and interested audience, the other drugs in nevirapine's class (Janssen's TIBO compounds and Merck's "L" compounds) were still further along in development.[41] The TIBO compounds had been in clinical trials for over a year. Although they were potent inhibitors of reverse transcriptase in laboratory assays, the TIBO compounds had limited oral bioavailability in people. To overcome that problem, the investigators had given twenty-two AIDS patients one of the TIBO compounds intravenously.

After about two months of treatment, the drug produced a modest reduction of HIV in the patients' blood.[42] Janssen was planning to test two newer TIBO compounds in an effort to find a better drug. Similarly, Merck had been studying its two "L" drugs, which were also reverse transcriptase inhibitors, in clinical trials for almost a year.[43] The first "L" drug was poorly absorbed in patients, and the investigators had recently turned to the other drug, L-679,661, which showed better absorption in sixteen HIV-infected patients. Merck had already begun a new and larger clinical trial, similar to BI's Christmas tree studies.[44]

Cheeseman and Richman had been treating HIV-infected adults with nevirapine in the Christmas tree studies since April, and the trial was generating great interest from all quarters. But Myers decided not to discuss the early results from those patients at the July ACTG meeting. The team had simply not collected sufficient data to draw meaningful conclusions about nevirapine's effectiveness, side effects, or appropriate dosing conditions. They did not expect to see any notable improvement until the patients had taken nevirapine for twelve weeks, which put the first disclosure of results in mid–December 1991.

The project team kept the FDA informed "almost in real time" as they gathered the results.[45] By the end of the summer, they had analyzed the data from the lower dosage groups, who had been taking nevirapine alone or in combination with AZT for three months. They were pleased that people, like the animals in the toxicology studies, reported no troublesome side effects from taking daily doses of nevirapine. But their ability to assess whether nevirapine was having a beneficial effect on the patients' HIV infections — that is, a decrease in the amount of HIV in their blood, called "viral load" — was more difficult. The available assays were imprecise, insensitive, and indirect measures of HIV, and the changes that they saw after nevirapine treatment were small and variable.[46] Every week, Myers and the project team held a teleconference with ACTG to discuss the latest findings, "looking through the fog" and trying to make sense of small changes in a small number of patients after a short period of nevirapine treatment.[47] As summer gave way to fall, they saw stronger indications that nevirapine was suppressing the patients' viral load, if ever so slightly. In the patients who received both nevirapine and AZT, the viral load seemed to be suppressed even more.

8

Patient Pressure Points

In the years leading up to that January day in 1991 when Phil became the first person to take nevirapine, AIDS advocacy groups had become increasingly more numerous, vocal, and influential. At Boehringer Ingelheim, the public relations task force knew that their plans must address not only inquiries from the media but also the intense scrutiny of AIDS advocacy groups and patients. They studied the origins of those groups, their stated objectives, and their tactics. And they monitored how federal agencies and pharmaceutical firms responded to the public pressure.

In the first decade of the AIDS epidemic, hundreds of AIDS advocacy groups had emerged. Some were large organizations with many chapters and a global reach, others served a single community. Each had its own mission and strategy. Some emphasized research. Some provided prevention, care, and treatment services. Others advocated for responsive public policies on AIDS. And still others mobilized to call attention to their plight — picketing and protesting in very public venues. But they all had two things in common: they were fiercely devoted to their cause and they were highly organized. Their message to both the federal agencies and the drug companies was simple and direct. Many new AIDS drugs were being developed, and they wanted those drugs approved and available to all patients as soon as possible. They were dying from AIDS, and any delay, literally, threatened their lives.

In its early years, the AIDS Clinical Trials Group primarily sponsored clinical trials of AZT, hoping to find ways to improve the drug's actions against HIV and minimize its bothersome side effects. But the AIDS advocacy groups wanted ACTG and other investigators to put more emphasis on finding drugs for their opportunistic infections. Short of stopping HIV, which at that time was a longshot, the most practical way to treat AIDS — and ease patient suffering — was to treat the life-threatening opportunistic infections. Most AIDS patients, in fact, died from pneumocystis pneumonia, an opportunistic lung infection.[1]

Physicians had been partly successful in treating pneumocystis pneumonia with an intravenous drug, pentamidine. Unfortunately, pentamidine caused liver and kidney damage. At San Francisco General Hospital, Bruce Montgomery, David Feigal, and Gifford Leoung thought they might be able to get better results with fewer side effects by having patients breathe an aerosol form of pentamidine, delivering the drug directly to the patient's lungs. They had previously conducted clinical trials sponsored by industry and ACTG, as well as their own independent clinical research. Drawing on that experience and driven by their desire to find a better way to treat pneumocystis pneumonia, Montgomery and his colleagues experimented with ways for patients to breathe a pentamidine-containing vapor. Encouraged by their preliminary results, the investigators forged ahead to plan a "well-controlled" clinical trial.

LyphoMed marketed the intravenous form of pentamidine under an orphan drug license from the Food and Drug Administration, and the company cooperated with the San Francisco clinicians. But from inception to completion, Montgomery and his colleagues were in charge, designing the protocol, managing the data, and handling all the other trial details. They relied entirely on physicians and clinics in the surrounding community to recruit and treat the patients — one of the first community-based AIDS clinical trials in the United States. But because they were investigating an experimental use of pentamidine, the investigators needed FDA's buy-in to proceed with the trial. And the Californians' grassroots operation lacked the polish and professionalism that FDA was accustomed to seeing in industry-sponsored trials.

Montgomery and his colleagues traveled to the FDA's headquarters in Rockville, Maryland, more than a dozen times, discussing various options for the trial, each time presenting a new and improved version of the protocol based on their previous discussions. But the Bay Area boys in their California casual attire made little progress in convincing the FDA. Ellen Cooper, the medical reviewer, politely pushed back, saying their proposed trial just did not meet FDA's standards, and cited the protocol's specific deficiencies. Finally, as they walked out of yet another frustrating session with the regulators, a LyphoMed executive pulled Feigal aside and said, "Look, if you guys want the FDA to take you seriously, you're going to have to dress the part."[2] He took the Californians to Neiman Marcus and bought all of them proper business suits.

On their next visit to the FDA, now wearing their brand-new suits, the investigators presented the latest version of their clinical trial plans. Cooper listened and again suggested numerous changes for improving the protocol, but with those changes, she said, they could start the trial. The California investigators were delighted. As they were leaving, the LyphoMed executive turned to Feigal and said, "You wouldn't have to make all those changes if I'd bought you new shoes, too."[3]

With the protocol details finally settled, Montgomery, Feigal, and their colleagues began the trial in July 1987 and quickly enrolled 400 patients.[4] Meanwhile, word of their preliminary results had spread rapidly and thousands of patients

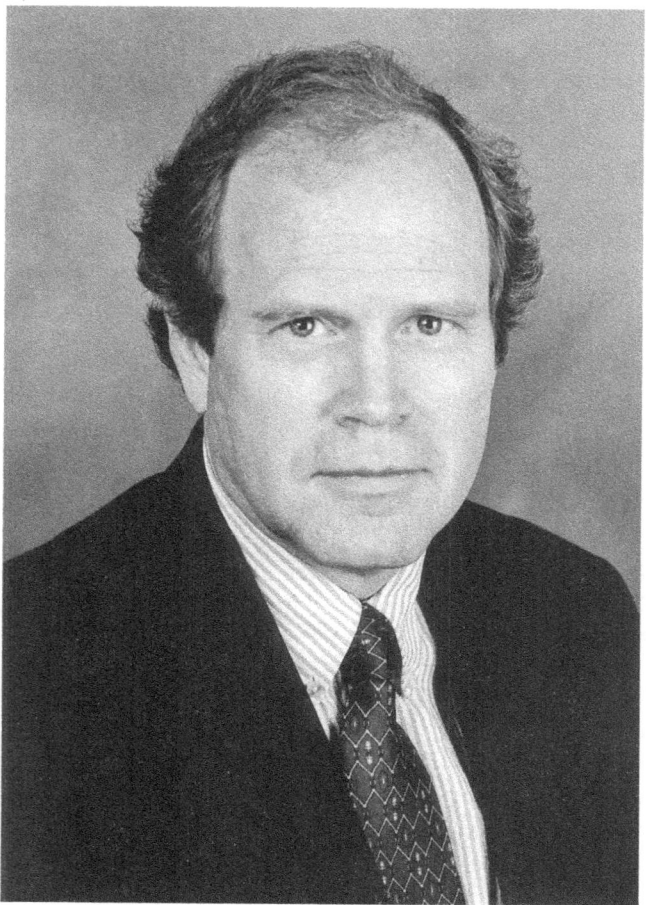

David Feigal (courtesy Food and Drug Administration, History Office).

from coast-to-coast sought aerosol treatment with pentamidine, not willing to wait for the outcome of the clinical trial. Physicians jury-rigged equipment for vaporizing pentamidine using LyphoMed's commercially available intravenous liquid. The San Francisco investigators discouraged this practice, because they had not yet worked out the optimal dosing conditions.[5] But fortunately, this renegade, off-label use did not impede the progress of the San Franciscans' controlled clinical trial. The same could not be said for ganciclovir.

* * *

Syntex began clinical trials of ganciclovir in 1984, and the preliminary results quickly convinced investigators that the drug was effective in suppressing cytomegalovirus, which causes CMV retinitis.[6] CMV retinitis is an aggressive eye infection that afflicted one in four AIDS patients, and without treatment, the infection causes blindness.[7] The well-controlled clinical trials that FDA required for ganciclovir's approval stalled for several years, while Syntex settled a patent dispute with Burroughs Wellcome over ownership of the drug. Because of the promising early results, Syntex successfully petitioned FDA to allow distribution of ganciclovir to AIDS patients under a compassionate use program until the patent issue could be resolved.

Ganciclovir worked so well in controlling CMV retinitis that within a few years, its widespread use under the compassionate use program undermined Syntex's subsequent placebo-controlled clinical trials. Physicians and patients were unwilling to participate in the trials, knowing that patients who received the placebo would go blind. Advocacy groups, with the support of their doctors and top officials at the National Institutes of Health, launched an intensive campaign, pushing for regulatory approval of ganciclovir based on their uncontrolled observations. The drug was a nuisance to take — an intravenous infusion twice a day for two weeks and then daily maintenance infusions. But as long as patients took ganciclovir, they could suppress their CMV infection and prevent blindness. They wanted the drug approved.

In 1987, Syntex used the data collected under the compassionate use program to request approval of ganciclovir. But both the FDA's Advisory Committee and the FDA reviewers rejected the application.[8] Although most of the panel thought ganciclovir worked, regulators were obligated to follow the law. Drug approvals required convincing evidence of safety and efficacy from adequate and well-controlled clinical trials, evidence that was lacking from the compassionate use experiences. To AIDS advocates, ganciclovir's rejection only added to growing frustrations about regulatory policies. Similar regulatory rigor was delaying approval of the pentamidine aerosol, which was still only midway through Montgomery and Feigal's eighteen-month clinical trial in San Francisco.

On October 11, 1988, thousands of protesters from across the country traveled to Rockville, Maryland, and swarmed around the FDA's headquarters building.[9] Citing ganciclovir as a prime example, they demanded a faster process for evaluating new drugs, expansion of drug development to include more drugs for opportunistic infections, and broadened eligibility to allow women, people of color, children, and injection drug users in clinical trials.[10] At the FDA, they blocked access to the Parklawn building's doors, walkways, and driveways. They set off a smoke bomb, plastered windows with stickers, smashed wooden police barriers, and shattered a glass door and two windows of the building. They hoisted a black banner that read, "Silence = Death" and chanted, "AZT is not enough. Give us all the other stuff."[11] One wheelchair-bound protester from Chicago told a reporter that he had been taking FDA-approved AZT but had purchased three types of experimental AIDS drugs at the demonstration.[12] For nine hours, 350 helmeted police officers with riot batons and wearing surgical gloves managed the mostly nonviolent crowd and guarded the building by standing with interlocked arms at the doors. The media reported that this was the largest protest since the Vietnam War demonstrations in the 1960s. It disrupted FDA's operations for the better part of the day, and the regulators took note.

Among them was Ellen Cooper, who watched the protesters from her office window in the Parklawn building.[13] Cooper's newly created division was responsible for regulatory approval of new AIDS drugs, the specific target of the protesters' wrath. As they shouted below, the protesters were unaware that she was already working with Syntex to resolve the ganciclovir stalemate. She was also in ongoing discussions with Bristol-Myers Squibb to accelerate development of ddI, which had entered clinical trials a few months earlier, and with Hoffmann-La Roche to facilitate ddC, which was slated to begin clinical trials shortly. Even before taking charge of the FDA's new antiviral division in February, Cooper had streamlined the agency's procedures, giving drug companies earlier and greater access to FDA officials and helping them condense their clinical testing programs. A week after the Parklawn demonstration, the FDA published regulations that formalized the procedures Cooper was already practicing.[14] Those reforms helped companies obtain the necessary data for drug approval much faster, but nothing was fast enough to satisfy the protesters, many of whom were dying from AIDS. The advocacy groups put patients above all other considerations, whereas Cooper, who had been schooled in public health, was obligated to uphold FDA's public health mandate — polarized perspectives that fueled distrust, misunderstanding, and even cynicism.

In an effort to obtain the required data for ganciclovir's approval, the National Institutes of Health and FDA restricted compassionate access to the drug, and Syntex tried to start a new controlled clinical trial in January 1989, but only eighteen people signed up.[15] On February 1, protesters voiced their displeasure of the new ganciclovir restrictions by disrupting Cooper's testimony before the Lasagna Committee, a group of eminent scientists who had been commissioned by Vice President Bush to review procedures for approving AIDS and cancer drugs.[16]

Behind the scenes, discussions continued between the FDA, the National Institutes of Health, and advocacy group representatives. LyphoMed was granted a "treatment IND" to distribute aerosolized pentamidine to patients with pneumocystis pneumonia while the FDA continued its review of the San Francisco-based clinical trial.[17] In March, FDA loosened the restrictions on compassionate access to ganciclovir.[18] But tensions grew within the agency on how to respond to the ganciclovir approval dilemma. Cooper believed clinicians who were reporting dramatic improvement in patients across the country after treatment with ganciclovir for CMV retinitis. "As a physician, I knew it worked."[19] At the same time, approving a drug without proper clinical trial data might set a precedent, opening the door for other firms to request approval of their drugs with little scientific evidence to back up their claims. Finding a way forward with ganciclovir was not clear cut, but "we couldn't stay in limbo."[20] Cooper decided to call another meeting of the Advisory Committee and follow their recommendation. On May 1–2, 1989, the Advisory Committee met and recommended approval of both ganciclovir and pentamidine aerosol.[21] FDA officially approved Syntex's ganciclovir application on June 27, 1989, based on the accumulated compassionate use data. LyphoMed received approval of pentamidine aerosol two weeks earlier, based on the outcome of Montgomery and Feigal's community-based trial.[22]

Anthony Fauci, Director of the National Institute of Allergy and Infectious Diseases, the institute that managed the ACTG network, maintained that Syntex's mistake had been in failing to conduct proper clinical trials concurrently with its ganciclovir compassionate use program.[23] To prevent this problem in the future, he supported a concept called parallel track, which patient advocates had been formulating and discussing with AIDS researchers for more than a year.[24] The objective of the parallel track was to provide access to an investigational drug with proven safety for people who were ineligible for clinical trials and had no reasonable treatment alternatives.[25] The idea gained momentum during the 5th International AIDS Conference in Montreal in June 1989, where advocacy groups gathered to hold a major demonstration. With conference registration restricted to scientists, the demonstrators' plan was only to picket outside the convention center in full view of the media and arriving delegates. But when the doors opened, they streamed into the building through sheer force of mass and boarded the escalators to the upstairs auditorium. Suddenly, the leaders of the New York contingent of ACT UP and AIDS Action Now! (Canada's largest AIDS advocacy group) saw an opportunity not to be wasted and commandeered the stage along with several hundred fellow protesters.

With a microphone thrust into his hand, Tim McCaskell, the leader of AIDS Action Now!, by default, opened the conference "on behalf of the people living with AIDS in Canada and around the world."[26] As the registered delegates began filling the auditorium for the official opening ceremonies, Conyers Thompson of ACT UP read the demonstrators' "Montreal Manifesto," a declaration of the universal rights and needs of people with HIV/AIDS, first in English and then again in French.[27] Then, the protesters settled into front row seats, which had been reserved for dignitaries including Canadian Prime Minister Brian Mulroney, whose opening speech was delayed by an hour.[28]

The activists continued to make their presence felt throughout the Montreal Conference. In one session, Ellen Cooper had been invited to explain the FDA's progress in grappling with the regulatory issues surrounding AIDS drugs: the use of placebos in clinical trials, how to determine that the drug works, and when to grant expanded drug access.[29] But her presentation was interrupted by shouting from outraged activists in the audience. One of them, John Bowen, had participated in the original AZT clinical trial and by random selection had been assigned to the placebo group. Because the trial's rules required him to discontinue treatment with the drugs that were controlling his opportunistic infections, he unfortunately developed pneumonia during the trial. Most frustrating of all, after the trial's conclusion he was denied AZT under compassionate use, because his white blood cell count was too low.[30] He felt he had been used. He did his part by participating in a clinical trial, but when he subsequently needed compassion and treatment, "you just let me go."[31]

In a series of meetings before and during the Montreal conference, Fauci met with Jim Eigo from ACT UP, Martin Delaney from Project Inform, and other advocacy group representatives to discuss their parallel track proposal.[32] While he still supported the carefully designed, controlled clinical trials that were sponsored by the ACTG, Fauci used a speech in San Francisco a few weeks after the Montreal conference as his opportunity to publicly announce his support for the parallel track concept. "We have to be creative and flexible so that we can provide increased access to promising drugs to patients who cannot participate in clinical trials."[33] Fauci had not discussed this new perspective with his colleagues at the National Institutes of Health or officials at the FDA, but he ensured that key AIDS reporters would be covering the speech, and they publicized the parallel track concept worldwide.[34]

Through the summer of 1989, many AIDS advocacy groups added their support to Eigo and Delaney, who continued to press the idea of a parallel track in intensive negotiations with Fauci, Cooper, and officials from Bristol-Myers Squibb, the manufacturer of ddI.[35] The ongoing and planned ACTG trials of ddI excluded many people who wanted to take the drug (a less toxic cousin of AZT) but did not meet the trials' stringent enrollment criteria, making it an attractive candidate for testing Eigo and Delaney's new concept. Government officials and Bristol-Myers Squibb executives, to the delight of the patient advocates, were receptive to implementing a parallel track program for ddI. Cooper understood the advocacy groups' motives but was concerned that the parallel track would slow down enrollment in the controlled trials and ultimately delay drug approval. Bristol-Myers Squibb managed to accommodate the advocacy groups without disrupting its clinical trials through careful drug management and creative application of two existing but underutilized FDA provisions, a treatment IND and an open label safety study.[36] Starting in October 1989, the company offered ddI to those who did not qualify for the ongoing clinical trials, and thousands of people took advantage of the program.[37]

Cooper continued to solicit input from all stakeholders and interpreted regulatory requirements to fit these new and rapidly evolving situations. Away from the bombast of the public demonstrations, she met frequently with representatives from the advocacy groups and engaged in "real communications."[38] They learned from each other and came to a common understanding on how to accelerate the review and approval of new drugs. To her external critics, Cooper had adapted, from an adversary to an ally.[39] Within the FDA, she exemplified a new generation of federal regulators, willing to bridge the chasm that AIDS exposed.[40] Never hesitant to make tough-minded decisions, she did her homework, listened intently, and demonstrated a flexibility that earned her the admiration of coworkers and critics alike. "There were changes that they insisted on, and we made them."[41] Clinical trials began to accommodate a wider range of patients, and within the agency she facilitated drug approvals while remaining an unwavering steward of public health.

In December 1990, when Cooper announced her decision to leave FDA's antiviral division, the news made headlines and reverberated throughout the scientific and advocacy communities.[42] Many, from the FDA Commissioner to leaders of various advocacy groups, urged her to reconsider.[43] But like Sisyphus, she had been pushing FDA's AIDS boulder uphill for six years, the last three as Director of the division. The government's chief spokesperson on AIDS drug policy, she had been the lightning rod for an unsympathetic and unsupportive administration. Patients, researchers, physicians, and even her colleagues at the government's laboratories and clinics across town all aligned to challenge the agency she represented, urging faster access to investigational AIDS drugs.[44] But she could only act on the drugs that researchers presented to the FDA for consideration, and aside from AZT and ddI, none of them — so far — had done much good against this dreaded, implacable virus.

With grace, finesse, determination, and a clear vision of federal regulators as facilitators, not obstructionists, Cooper had navigated her division through its stormiest days. She had been constantly in the public spotlight, often caught in the crossfire, since 1985. Although it would take more than a year to replace her, she left the division in good hands, having personally recruited and mentored most of her staff of sixty young professionals, setting in motion many reforms that served as models for official FDA policies, and building a rapport with consumers that led to giving patient advocates a seat at the table of FDA advisory boards.[45]

* * *

As patient advocates learned more about drug development from Cooper and others at the FDA, they soon acknowledged the limits of the agency's regulatory reach. Cooper had opened the spigot for faster regulatory approval, but there simply was no backlog of drug candidates flooding through.[46] The pipeline of new AIDS drugs was fed not by FDA but by AIDS research and clinical trials, most of which were funded by the National Institutes of Health in nearby Bethesda, Maryland. Patient advocates wanted a voice in designing those clinical trials.[47] They knew all about AIDS because they were afflicted with it, and they knew all about the limitations of the current drugs because they were taking them. In addition, the ACTG trials were funded by tax dollars, and they were taxpaying citizens, with the right to say how those tax dollars were spent. They were frustrated that despite one billion dollars of government-funded AIDS research, too few drugs were being tested, and it still took too long to get those drugs to people who were sick.[48] They wanted ACTG to drop unnecessary restrictions and enroll more HIV-infected people in the trials. To them, clinical trials were a form of healthcare — healthcare that was otherwise denied to them and that they thought they were entitled to.[49]

In November 1989, ACTG responded to the advocacy groups' complaints by forming the Community Constituency Group, a working group that allowed advocates to attend the ACTG meetings, voice their concerns, and be part of the process.[50] But the Community Constituency Group was only advisory, and its members could not vote or alter the ACTG's decisions. Some ACTG-affiliated investigators were receptive to the advocates' suggestions, and they began including more women and minorities in the clinical trials. But a small group within the ACTG retained control, and they could not be persuaded to conduct more clinical trials in inner-city communities where AIDS was spreading fastest.

The advocates wanted more than a seat at the table, and their frustration led to a demonstration by more than 500 protesters at the National Institutes of Health on May 21, 1990.[51] Twenty-one protesters managed to reach and occupy the office of Daniel Hoth, director of the AIDS Division of the National Institute of Allergy and Infectious Diseases, the institute that sponsored the ACTG network. Those sit-in demonstrators were arrested, along with 61 others, on trespassing charges. Most were fined $50 and released without incident, but they had made their point.

* * *

A month later, during the 6th International AIDS Conference in San Francisco, a delegation from BI witnessed firsthand the influence wielded by the advocacy groups. The day before the conference's official opening ceremonies, over a thousand demonstrators met at the United States Immigration and Naturalization Service offices to protest the government's travel policy barring people with HIV infections from entering the United States.[52] The Conference organizers, acknowledging the protesters' objections, announced that they would not hold future conferences in a country that restricted the entry of HIV-infected travelers.[53] (No major international AIDS conferences were scheduled in the United States until President Barack Obama officially lifted the travel ban in 2010.[54])

Every day throughout the Conference, protesters held demonstrations in the streets and outside the official Conference sites: the Marriott Hotel and the Moscone Convention Center. The demonstrators blanketed the Conference venues with posters, leaflets, and press packets. Inside the Convention Center, many delegates and speakers wore red arm bands in a show of solidarity with those protesting outside. As a consequence of the demonstrators' initiatives in Montreal the previous year, representatives of the advocacy groups received, for the first time in the annual Conference's history, official passes to attend the sessions in San Francisco. Some of their leaders were invited to address the Conference, and their rhetoric was emotionally charged. It had been almost ten years since the first clinical reports describing AIDS symptoms appeared in the medical literature. Despite intensive efforts by thousands of researchers, meaningful progress was hard to find. Some within the AIDS community questioned whether AIDS was really caused by a virus (HIV), and whether AZT really worked. Patience was growing thin, and for many of them, time was running out.

Jay Lipner exemplified the distressing situation that many of them faced. The Manhattan lawyer volunteered his time to win insurance coverage and wider access to experimental drugs for AIDS patients, and he had tangled with Cooper on more than one occasion — two strong-willed people divided by a common cause.[55] He had come to San Francisco to attend the International AIDS Conference but spent several hours each day in his hotel room infusing himself with ganciclovir through an implanted catheter.[56] Because AZT and ganciclovir both suppressed bone marrow, AIDS patients could not take both drugs, and they faced the cruel decision of choosing either their eyesight or a longer life.[57] Like most people, Lipner chose his eyesight, and he traveled everywhere with his ganciclovir IV kit. Boxes of saline solution, needles, plastic tubes, and bandages cluttered his hotel room. He died the following year.[58]

At the closing ceremonies of the San Francisco AIDS Conference, Health and Human Services Secretary Louis Sullivan's speech was drowned out by shouts, chants, whistles, and air horns. To the audience, which included demonstrators and media people along with many sympathetic delegates, Secretary Sullivan personified an insensitive government and a baseless travel policy. He doggedly read all of his prepared remarks, but his audience heard none of it.[59]

In August 1990, the Lasagna Committee issued its recommendations on approval procedures for new AIDS and cancer drugs.[60] The committee sided with the advocacy groups and urged further streamlining of the initiatives that Cooper had fostered at the FDA. A drug that improves the quality of a patient's life, the panel said, is just as important as one that prolongs life.[61] The committee recommended that AIDS drugs should be approved without waiting for completion of the lengthy clinical trials that were required to establish an improved clinical outcome and long-term safety. Although earlier approval, based on limited data, could expose patients to greater risks of unknown side effects or to drugs that might eventually prove to be ineffective, the panel argued that AIDS patients with no alternative therapy were entitled to decide for themselves. And many patients said they were willing to take the risk.[62]

Events were escalating toward a nasty confrontation when Fauci stepped in and advised the ACTG investigators to accommodate the advocates with more than a seat at the table.[63] In November 1990, the twenty-four-member Community Constituency Group, which included activists, people with HIV, women, African Americans, Latinos, HIV-infected mothers and mothers of HIV-infected children, people living with hemophilia, and ex-injection drug users, became voting members of all ACTG committees, including its powerful Executive Committee.[64] From that point, citizen and advocacy group involvement increased throughout the ACTG. Due to their influence, the ACTG-sponsored clinical trials that followed, including those involving nevirapine, were overhauled to encompass a wider range of participants and more creative, but still scientifically driven, trial designs.

* * *

Among those wanting faster progress and willing to take greater risks was Elizabeth Glaser. She had become infected in 1981 via a blood transfusion only months after the first cases of AIDS were reported and long before anyone thought to screen blood donors for HIV. At a trim 5 feet 2 inches, Elizabeth had always been fit and competitive. In school, she played field hockey, volleyball, basketball, and tennis. As an adult, she regularly played tennis and skied.[65] She had remained symptom-free and unaware of her infection until her daughter, Ariel, became ill and was diagnosed with AIDS in May 1986.[66] Michael Gottlieb, who had published the first clinical report describing AIDS, examined Elizabeth and noted only two clinical abnormalities.[67] Her white blood cell count was lower than normal, making her more susceptible to infections, and she had one, slightly enlarged lymph node.

Elizabeth began taking AZT about two years after her diagnosis, two capsules five times a day. The frequent dosing schedule made her a slave to her watch, a "constant reminder of AIDS."[68] Fearful that someone would recognize the little white capsules with the blue ring when she took them out in public, she kept her medicine in a bottle of iron tablets. In May 1989, she also began treatments with pentamidine aerosol, to protect her from pneumocystis pneumonia infection. About once a month, she sat alone in a small room for her pentamidine treatments, breathing the "disgusting and distasteful air" for thirty minutes.[69] Every six weeks, she went to Gottlieb's office for blood tests to check her white blood cell count and to monitor signs of AZT's side effects — anemia and liver damage were their greatest concerns.[70] Gottlieb predicted that Elizabeth had a thirty percent chance of becoming ill within three years, but when she reached that three-year milestone, she was still medically stable.[71] Then, just three months later, her white blood cell count dropped by one-third to a seriously low level.[72] Although the cell counts can vary, hers never moved upward, and she became increasingly tired, "a nagging sense of exhaustion."[73] By October 1989, she was also losing muscle tone, and Gottlieb's laboratory tests confirmed that AZT was damaging her muscles.[74] For almost two years, she had taken a high daily dose of AZT without experiencing the serious bone marrow suppression, anemia, vomiting, or diarrhea that prevented many patients from taking the drug. But now, she also had to stop taking it.

Fortunately, Gottlieb was able to offer an experimental drug as an alternative, ddI. Although Bristol-Myers Squibb was still conducting clinical trials, the company had made ddI widely available to HIV-infected individuals under its compassionate use program and Elizabeth signed up.[75] She read through the long list of reported side effects (inflamed pancreas, abnormal liver function, numbness and nerve damage, among other things) but with no other alternatives, she felt "lucky to be a ddI guinea pig."[76] Elizabeth followed her doctor's recommendations, but she also embraced good nutrition, Chinese herbs, acupuncture, and psychotherapy. She would maintain her health in every way she could. Two days a week, she did sit-ups, steps, and cross-country ski simulation. And she pumped iron.[77] By November, she had adjusted to ddI, fortunately did not experience any of the drug's long list of side effects, and was again medically stable. Despite her low white blood cell count, she was symptom-free and felt great.[78] But she knew she had not slain the dragon, only pushed it back a bit. Her crusade, now conducted openly on the world stage, was long from finished and she used every ounce of her renewed energy to press for more pediatric AIDS research.

* * *

The BI public relations task force was keenly aware that advocacy groups were not only targeting government agencies and laboratories but also the pharmaceutical industry. The most aggressive protesters had breached drug company security, occupied rooms, chained themselves to desks, disrupted employees' work, and even used bomb threats to call attention to their cause.[79] Although the demonstrators' approach was unconventional and sometimes confrontational, they definitely raised public awareness. But their aggressive tactics, amplified by media coverage of their public demonstrations, often contrasted sharply with their private demeanor. Their primary goal was to reach and influence the industry decision makers responsible for AIDS drug development. "Demonstrations are a last resort."[80]

Never before had drug companies faced a patient group that was so organized, vocal, and politically astute, or patients who knew so much about their disease and its treatment.[81] These advocacy groups knew firsthand the difficulties that the AIDS community faced. They were talking to regulators about streamlining the drug approval process. And they understood the merits and limitations of the drugs in development — an impressively sophisticated aspect of their advocacy. As a result, companies unaccustomed to communicating directly with their consumers during drug development got a quick education in how do to it.[82]

The protest at the National Institutes of Health was the last large demonstration orchestrated by the AIDS advocacy groups in the United States.[83] By 1991, the wall between the companies developing AIDS drugs and the patients they sought to treat was softening. And of all the companies engaged in AIDS drug development, Bristol-Myers Squibb received the most accolades for cooperation. The company took the initiative, engaging in an open dialogue with advocacy groups, incorporating community sites in its clinical trials, sharing clinical data quickly with the AIDS community, and making ddI readily available to thousands of patients, like Elizabeth Glaser, through its expanded access programs.[84]

Shortly after BI announced its clinical trials with nevirapine, executives from Bristol-Myers Squibb offered to meet with BI and share their experiences.[85] Representatives from the two companies met in Ridgefield, and the visitors from Bristol-Myers Squibb passed along their insights on regulatory issues, clinical trial strategies, and interactions with advocacy groups. The candid but cordial discussion immensely aided the BI attendees who were just stepping into a spotlight that had scorched their industrial counterpart and competitor for years. The meeting confirmed that AIDS drug development was unique and communication with advocacy groups could be challenging, but everyone was driven by the same sense of urgency and they could all benefit from working together. The advocacy groups strongly influenced AIDS patients, endorsing the clinical trials they thought were worthwhile, discouraging participation in trials conducted by drug companies that had not considered their input, championing experimental drugs that had produced good clinical results, and opposing drugs that had come up short.

The first step in BI's coalition building with advocacy groups was simply to start a dialogue. The BI public relations task force was in the process of organizing a plan for these interactions when they received a letter from Bill Snow, representing the New York Treatment and Data Committee of ACT UP, the AIDS Coalition to Unleash Power. Like other advocacy groups, ACT UP was aware that BI had recently begun clinical trials with nevirapine. ACT UP representatives attended the ACTG committee meetings, where BI's clinical trials had been discussed.[86] They considered nevirapine a promising and potentially lifesaving drug and wanted to learn more about BI's clinical plans. In exchange, Snow offered to share their insights and suggestions from the patient's perspective. ACT UP did not want nevirapine's development delayed by planning, regulatory, or patient enrollment problems, and they could help.

Although the BI public relations task force had not fully vetted its list of advocacy groups, ACT UP was as good a place as any to start their dialogue, and Terri Pascarelli took charge of the arrangements. Pascarelli had joined the research and development division of

BI in 1980 with a background in pharmacy. She then moved into sales and marketing after earning her master's degree in business administration.[87] As the Group Manager of Policy and Issues Analysis, she had been serving as an advisor to the BI public relations task force. Over the next two months, Pascarelli and Snow negotiated a detailed agenda and arrangements for a face-to-face meeting between the two organizations.

On May 28, 1991, the small BI contingent, including Pascarelli, Jay Merluzzi, and Maureen Myers, drove to New York City for the ACT UP meeting, which was held at the Parker Meridian Hotel in midtown Manhattan. They had an uneasy feeling walking into the conference room, not quite knowing what to expect, a churning mixture of emotions rooted in media reports of violent demonstrations and images of emaciated patients in the final stages of AIDS.[88] For all but Myers, this was the first time they had confronted the people they sought to help, passionate people, desperate people, people with a mission, people who rejected every excuse and grabbed every ray of hope. To BI's relief, the tone of the meeting, though not collegial or confrontational, was at least civil. Merluzzi and Myers summarized the preclinical nevirapine data and the team's current clinical trial plans, but they stopped short of discussing the clinical results.[89]

The ACT UP representatives pressed hard for expanded clinical trials, demanding that nevirapine be made available to as many people as possible, as soon as possible. Regardless of BI's progress and plans, they said, the nevirapine clinical trials were not large enough or moving fast enough. Specifically, they pressed for greater involvement of advocacy groups in the design of the clinical trials, initiation of community-based trials in addition to those sponsored by ACTG, addition of a New York clinic as a site in the ongoing clinical trials, and BI's cooperation in adding a nevirapine treatment group to an upcoming ACTG trial of Merck's "L" drug.[90]

The ACT UP representatives also pointed out that they had identified at least three places where underground supplies of nevirapine were being manufactured and distributed.[91] They asked BI to test samples of those supplies to determine their purity and confirm that the bootlegged drug had been made correctly. They also asked BI to establish communications with

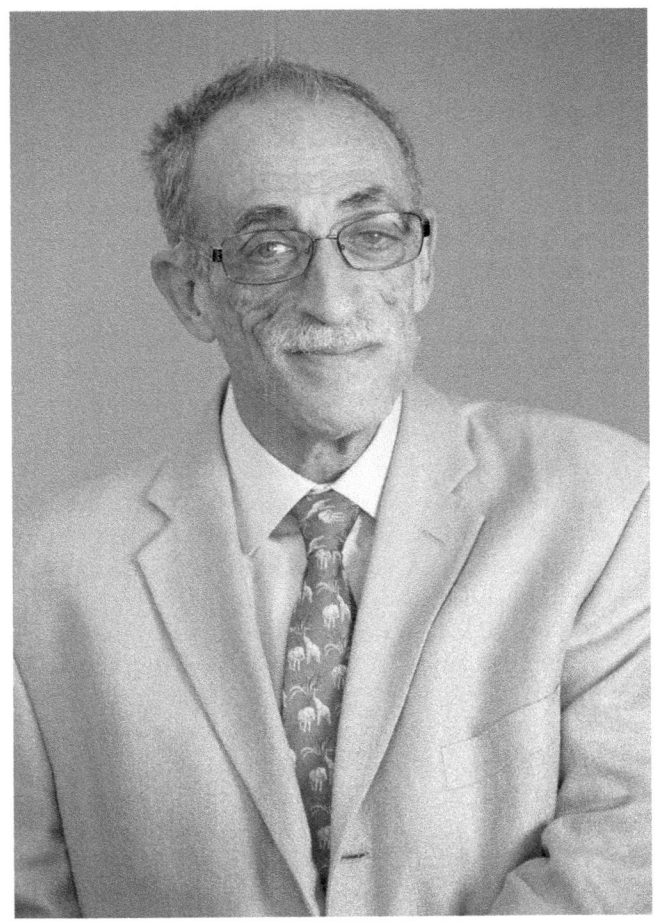

Bill Snow.

physicians and patients using bootlegged nevirapine, so that the physicians could receive up-to-date information about how to use the drug and report their clinical experiences to the company.[92] The ACT UP representatives recognized the risks associated with using black market drugs and explained that underground production of other experimental drugs had stopped only when the properly manufactured drugs became widely available to patients through expanded access programs. Bootlegged nevirapine would be unnecessary, they argued, if BI expanded access, allowing otherwise ineligible patients to obtain the BI-manufactured drug in parallel with the ongoing clinical trials.

Although "buyers clubs" had sprung up to smuggle or illegally manufacture other AIDS drugs such as ddC and ddI, it is not clear whether underground sources of nevirapine actually existed.[93] Advocacy group newsletters reported that producing bootlegged nevirapine would be difficult, because the production method published by BI was expensive.[94] Underground chemists with sufficient expertise would first need to develop a better production method, a substantial undertaking for a drug that had not yet proven its worth clinically.

ACT UP's carrots and sticks — offering to help by suggesting clinical trial improvements and threatening to circumvent the company by producing bootlegged drug — had one objective: they wanted nevirapine. People were dying from AIDS. Nevirapine held great promise as an effective new treatment. ACT UP wanted everyone to have access to the drug as soon as possible. And they would get it, one way or the other.

The BI delegation listened to ACT UP's suggestions for alternative study designs and accelerating enrollment but saw no reason to change their ongoing trials or clinical plans.[95] Myers explained that the Christmas tree studies were going well but BI had not yet determined the correct dose and did not know what side effects the drug might cause in people.[96] BI's clinical program already incorporated the broad range of patients that ACT UP advocated, including women and specific pediatric trials. Karl Grozinger and his colleagues had made some progress in scaling up production, and the project team anticipated no significant drug supply problems. They were prepared to expand access to nevirapine, if the early clinical trial results justified it. But federal drug laws prevented them from testing, verifying, or in any other way becoming involved with the bootlegged drug.[97]

And so, the push-pull continued. Each side presented its case, like lawyers in a courtroom, more intent on justifying their respective positions than making concessions. ACT UP thought BI had a beneficial drug but was imposing unnecessary barriers for AIDS patients to get it. BI thought it was already doing all it could, following rules to protect patient welfare and ensure data integrity, and avoiding reckless mistakes that would cause costly setbacks. Debate points were matched one-for-one, but nothing changed.[98] The meeting ended in stalemate.

For BI, the meeting had been stressful and at times uncomfortable, but they had taken a crucial first step. "You never get a relationship unless you have a conversation. It was the right thing to do."[99] For ACT UP, the meeting was frustrating. They were dealing with "novices" who were more concerned about protecting themselves than addressing the needs of AIDS patients.[100] True to its mission, the ACT UP committee intensified its efforts, "scrambling to get the [nevirapine] clinical stud[ies] on track."[101] Snow sent a follow up letter to Pascarelli, repeating ACT UP's list of issues but now demanding action. In addition, Snow and his colleagues sent a letter to Anthony Fauci, Director of the National Institute of Allergy and Infectious Diseases, who had jurisdiction over the National Institutes of Health's AIDS program and the ACTG's clinical trials. They asked Fauci to exert his influence and coordinate efforts between his institute, the FDA, and BI to start long-term, large scale clinical testing of nevirapine within six months and to incorporate nevirapine into the ACTG-sponsored trials of Merck's "L" drug.[102]

Pascarelli and Snow exchanged phone calls throughout the summer.[103] Snow persisted in asking BI to disclose more of the nevirapine clinical data, provide drafts of the clinical trial designs for public discussion and revision, take steps to start large scale clinical trials, and permit widespread access to nevirapine as soon as the Christmas tree studies concluded. Pascarelli held firm in sharing only information that had been presented and discussed publicly at the ACTG meetings.

Having made no progress with Pascarelli, Myers, and Merluzzi, Snow only became more determined and escalated his demands. In August 1991, he appealed to BI's senior executives in a detailed and well-reasoned, if partisan, letter.[104] In ACT UP's view, BI's clinical program was still not aggressive enough or complete enough, and Snow repeated the list of ACT UP's demands. ACT UP preferred to work with BI — citing successful ACT UP interactions with Bristol-Myers Squibb and Merck — and remained receptive to a cooperative relationship, but they would not hesitate to "do what we have always done to get pharmaceutical companies' attention" to improve and speed up drug development.[105] Snow sent copies of the letter to officials at the ACTG, the Gay Men's Health Crisis, Project Inform, the *AIDS Treatment News*, and science reporters at the *Wall Street Journal* and *New York Times*, hoping that disclosure of the stalled talks to a broader audience might loosen BI's entrenched position. But with little progress to show for its efforts, the ACT UP Treatment and Data Committee soon shifted its attention to "the larger and more sophisticated companies" whose drugs were moving faster.[106]

* * *

After this somewhat shaky start, BI's relations with advocacy groups grew more productive, a natural convergence of the advocates' increasingly sophisticated, constructive tactics and the maturation of BI's clinical trials with nevirapine. Myers, who had established professional relationships with the leaders of many advocacy groups when she was Chief of the AIDS Treatment Program at the National Institutes of Health, continued to foster those relationships after joining BI. She recognized that working with well-educated, well-connected, and well-organized advocacy groups was a critical success factor for any company developing an AIDS drug and that rapid enrollment in the nevirapine clinical trials depended on the favorable opinion and endorsement of those groups. Over the next few years, as data emerged from the nevirapine clinical trials and with the assistance of Hill & Knowlton, a public relations firm with strong ties to the AIDS community, Myers regularly met with patient advocates and publishers of AIDS-related newsletters.[107] Whenever the BI team had new information or changed the direction of the clinical program, they updated the advocacy groups. Those meetings not only informed the AIDS community but also provided a forum for their comments, input that helped the BI team understand the disease and treat it more effectively.[108]

As 1991 drew to a close, the results from the Christmas tree studies were quickly circulated not only within BI and the ACTG network but also to the various advocacy groups. And those results, although not entirely unexpected, were disappointing and dampened everyone's enthusiasm for nevirapine.

9

Resistance Is Futile — Or Not

The project team sat in stunned silence, listening to the events that led to the death of a patient in the Christmas tree study. Never before had the acoustic ceiling tiles, cloth-covered walls, and carpeted floor of the Pharmacology Conference Room in Boehringer Ingelheim's Research and Development building soaked up so much sound. The normally animated, sometimes jovial, and always outspoken scientists hung on every word as the details slowly sunk into their disbelieving, analytical brains. How could it be that a patient in the very first treatment group of the first Christmas tree study died after taking nevirapine for only four weeks? All of the animals in the toxicology studies had been fine, even after taking much higher doses of nevirapine for considerably longer periods. No one in Sarah Cheeseman's first clinical study had reported anything more serious than an occasional headache.[1] But this Christmas tree patient had developed meningitis and a brain inflammation.[2] Fluid from a spinal tap revealed that those problems were caused by a chickenpox infection, a diagnosis that was later confirmed in the autopsy. The pathologist saw nothing that linked the patient's brain damage and death to nevirapine. It seemed to be a straightforward case of chickenpox-gone-rogue in a person whose immune system had been weakened by AIDS. Still, it was a sobering moment for the project team.

For most of the laboratory scientists in the room, nevirapine was the first of their drugs to make the transition from the laboratory to testing in people. They had high hopes that it would perform as impressively in patients as it had in their laboratory experiments. Now, this one patient reminded them, with a certainty none of them could ignore, that the people who were enrolling in their clinical trials were not healthy. They had lost weight. All of them had weakened immune systems. Some suffered from opportunistic infections or Kaposi's sarcoma, a form of skin cancer. If they had taken other AIDS drugs, they were not satisfied with the results and probably experienced unpleasant side effects. They signed up for this clinical trial because they hoped nevirapine would work better. No one wanted to make their condition worse.

But some patients would get worse. And some would die. AIDS was deadly, and the project team was not yet sure whether nevirapine would help. They hoped it would. But as they proceeded with the clinical trials, they monitored the patients even more closely, prepared to deal with the unexpected, not just the clinical improvement they wanted.

* * *

As the Christmas tree studies continued throughout 1991 and the data rolled in, the project team got a clearer understanding of nevirapine's effects in people. Fortunately, none of the remaining patients in the two Christmas tree studies reported serious side effects, and the team turned its attention to the blood sample analysis, which would tell them whether nevirapine was working. At that time, the only way clinical investigators could monitor the extent of a person's HIV infection, called viral load, was an assay that measured p24, an HIV protein. For various reasons, including a lack of assay sensitivity, p24 could not always be detected in HIV-infected people, but anyone whose blood contained a measurable amount of p24 was indisputably infected.[3] Investigators hoped that decreased p24 in the patient's blood indicated that the drug was also suppressing HIV, but they could not be sure.

Despite the assay's limitations, the BI project team did not have long to wait. After patients had taken nevirapine for one week, p24 in their blood rapidly dropped, indicating that viral load had decreased. As the doses of nevirapine increased, p24 decreased accordingly. In patients who had taken nevirapine in combination with AZT, p24 levels dropped even more. It was an exciting finding. The team had demonstrated that nevirapine suppressed HIV in people, and in fact, it worked faster than any of the AZT-like drugs.[4]

Unfortunately, the effect of nevirapine on viral load did not last. After four weeks of nevirapine treatment, the p24 levels started increasing and by eight weeks, the patients' viral load had returned to the levels that had existed before nevirapine treatment began. By December 1991, the project team's initial enthusiasm about nevirapine's dramatic and rapid effect in the Christmas tree studies had faded. Their stocking contained a lump of coal. It did not come as a surprise, really, but it was still disappointing. Over the preceding two years, their own laboratory results and the results of other researchers had pointed to a potential problem, which threatened to limit the value of all AIDS drugs. The problem was something called resistance.

* * *

It is the nature of microbes to adapt when threatened with something that might harm them. An antimicrobial drug may work initially, but bacteria and viruses such as those that cause hepatitis, tuberculosis, and influenza readily adapt, find ways to resist the drug's effect, and continue to thrive despite drug treatment. Anyone familiar with infectious diseases knew that resistance was a fundamental property of microbes, and scientists used it to guide their search for newer, better drugs.[5]

Consequently, it should not have come as a surprise when Doug Richman and scientists from Burroughs Wellcome reported that HIV could adapt and thrive in patients despite AZT treatment.[6] Within six months, the HIV in the patients' blood had mutated to a resistant form, and AZT was no longer able to control the patients' AIDS symptoms. To address this problem, scientists intensified their efforts to find new AIDS drugs—hopefully ones that were powerful enough to suppress the AZT-resistant form of HIV.

Jay Merluzzi's team thought nevirapine might be such a drug. Prior to starting clinical trials, they asked Richman to assess nevirapine in his cell-based laboratory assays. They were pleased when he reported that nevirapine suppressed not only original, "wild-type" HIV but also laboratory samples of the virus that had become resistant to AZT.[7] Richman's laboratory findings meant that nevirapine might work in patients who had become resistant to the effects of AZT treatment. But Merluzzi's team worried that nevirapine, like AZT, might induce resistance if patients were treated with it for a long time. So, they asked Richman to conduct additional laboratory experiments in parallel with their preclinical development studies. Would nevirapine cause the virus to mutate into a resistant form of HIV, just as AZT had done? And if so, how quickly would it happen?

The project team got the answers just after Cheeseman started the first clinical trial with nevirapine.[8] In his laboratory, Richman repeatedly exposed HIV-infected cells to nevirapine, and after only a few passages the virus became resistant to the drug. It meant that nevirapine, like AZT, would probably be useful in patients for only a limited time. But Richman also delivered some good news. AZT could suppress the nevirapine-resistant form of HIV. This meant that nevirapine and AZT might give patients a logical treatment alternative. If they became resistant to AZT, they could switch to nevirapine, and vice versa.

It was even possible that giving the two drugs together would work better than treatment with either one alone. The principle of combination drug treatment to overcome single-drug resistance was first introduced in the 1950s to treat tuberculosis. That success led to combination drug treatment of many other bacterial infections.[9] Martin Hirsch, an infectious disease expert at Harvard University and Massachusetts General Hospital, was among the first to explore the possibilities of suppressing HIV with drug combinations. He tried all sorts of combinations in his laboratory experiments.[10] When Richman's laboratory reported that resistance limited the effectiveness of AZT, Hirsch began combining AZT with other agents, attempting to restore its antiviral effect. Some drug combinations worked better than others, but none worked well enough for a lasting effect. Hirsch had the right idea, but he needed better antiviral drugs to prove the point. In that regard, Richman had the advantage, because he had access to nevirapine.

When Richman combined nevirapine and AZT in his laboratory experiments, the drug combination proved to be synergistic. The two drugs administered at the same time profoundly suppressed HIV proliferation — much greater suppression than predicted from the single-drug effects.[11] The hope that nevirapine and AZT might be synergistic in patients was the reason the BI project team included this drug combination in the design of the Christmas tree studies.

But despite the project team's optimism that nevirapine would work in patients, viral resistance loomed as a potential problem. If HIV could mutate and become resistant after exposure to nevirapine in Richman's laboratory experiments, it was likely that HIV-infected patients would also become resistant to it.[12] So, when the Christmas tree studies started, the BI team asked Richman to collect blood samples from his patients, as well as samples from Cheeseman's patients who enrolled at the University of Massachusetts in Worcester, and look for resistant forms of HIV. Throughout the summer and fall of 1991, the BI project team anxiously awaited Richman's results.

* * *

When nevirapine was selected for development, Bob Eckner's research team regrouped. Eckner turned his attention to studying other viruses and transferred leadership of the HIV research team to Peter Grob.[13] Grob, a biochemist, was well suited to his new assignment. He had extensive research experience in virology and had been involved with drug development activities at Ayerst before joining BI in 1987.[14] While Maureen Myers and John Tiso guided the nevirapine project team, Grob set a new objective for his research team: finding a backup compound. If nevirapine failed during the clinical trials — something no one wanted but everyone realized might happen — Grob's team was expected to have an alternative compound ready to go.

The research team found it hard to improve on nevirapine's pharmaceutical properties, but Grob, Karl Hargrave, and the rest of the team addressed two of nevirapine's shortcomings. Their backup compound should inhibit both the HIV-1 and HIV-2 forms of reverse transcriptase, and they wanted a compound that was even more potent than nevirapine.[15] When Richman reported his laboratory results showing nevirapine-induced resistance,

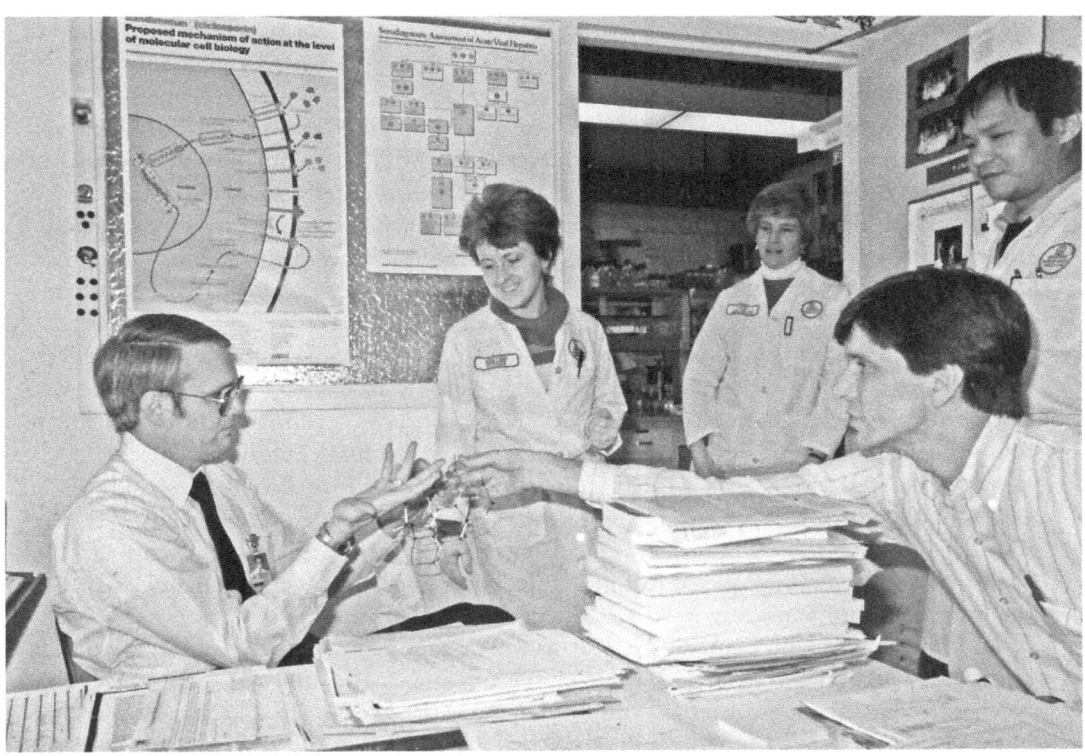

Members of the research team at Boehringer Ingelheim discussing the chemical structure and enzyme binding of nevirapine: (left to right) Karl Hargrave, Kris Eckner, Sue Goldrick, Mark Skoog, and Cheng-Kon Shih (courtesy Robert Eckner).

Grob's team shifted priorities and focused on creating a backup compound that would either not induce resistance or be potent enough to inhibit the mutant virus.[16] Julian Adams, the medicinal chemistry director, and Johanna Griffin, BI's director of molecular biology, met almost daily to monitor the progress of their departments in creating and assessing compounds that might prove to be a suitable backup to nevirapine.[17]

To make the backup compound, they needed to know much more about the AIDS virus, the reverse transcriptase enzyme, and how the enzyme became resistant when it was exposed to nevirapine. With Adams inspiring development of innovative chemical probes,[18] the help of Joe Wu's suntan lamp experiments,[19] the collaborative efforts of other BI biochemists including innovative crystallization work by Tom Warren,[20] and contributions by Richman's staff, Tom Steitz at nearby Yale University,[21] and other researchers, Grob's research team compiled a detailed and accurate picture of how nevirapine bound to and inhibited HIV-1 reverse transcriptase at the molecular level.[22]

* * *

Richman and the BI scientists submitted a manuscript reporting their laboratory findings on the nevirapine-resistant form of HIV, but that paper was not due to be published until December 1991.[23] The week of Thanksgiving, Merck announced that their drug, L-697,661, which was in the same class as nevirapine, also caused HIV to mutate and become resistant to drug treatment. In clinical trials, all patients developed a resistant form of HIV after only six to twelve weeks of treatment with the "L" drug.[24] In further laboratory experiments, the Merck scientists found that this mutant HIV was also resistant to nevirapine and to Janssen's TIBO compound.

On the same day that the Merck results were published, the BI project team finally received the results from Richman's analysis of samples taken from nevirapine-treated patients in the Christmas tree studies.[25] Of the sixty patients who had enrolled in the trials, Richman had evaluated blood samples from only ten patients. But those samples contained nevirapine-resistant strains of HIV, and in some patients the resistance had developed after only four weeks of nevirapine treatment. After eight weeks of treatment, all ten patients developed nevirapine-resistant HIV.[26]

Emergence of resistance in patients was the first major setback in the nevirapine development program. Up to this point, the team had become accustomed to seeing nevirapine easily glide over every hurdle, even the ones that cause most experimental drugs to fail. It was a potent inhibitor of HIV reverse transcriptase. In the first clinical safety study, nevirapine performed just as well as it had in the animal studies: it produced fewer and milder side effects than AZT or the other experimental AIDS drugs. It was also well absorbed and lasted long enough to justify a convenient once-a-day dosing schedule in people.[27] The chemists had faced no significant technical difficulties in producing high-quality batches of the drug, and they had formulated suitable tablets on their very first attempt.

Unfortunately, the patients' viral load, which dropped so rapidly and dramatically, bounced back after a few weeks of nevirapine treatment, and now the team knew why. Nevirapine quickly suppressed the natural, wild-type HIV, accounting for the initial decrease in p24 (the HIV-related protein) in the patients' blood. But as the virus mutated over the next few weeks into a form that was resistant to nevirapine, the p24 levels began to rise, indicating that HIV was again proliferating. Sadly, nevirapine induced viral resistance very quickly — much more quickly than AZT-induced resistance. And that threatened to end the development of nevirapine.

The clinical resistance results raised ethical concerns about treating people with a drug that the project team knew was not working, and they reacted immediately.[28] They reported their findings to FDA officials, who became concerned that treating patients with nevirapine might be worse than no treatment at all.[29] Nevirapine's beneficial effects were short-lived, and nevirapine-induced resistance might reduce the effectiveness of other AIDS drugs in the long run, leaving the patient with few treatment options. In addition to the FDA officials, Myers held discussions with BI's clinical investigators and the ACTG, who all agreed that BI should stop enrolling new patients in the clinical trials.[30] Patients who were already enrolled and receiving nevirapine were given a choice of several alternative AIDS treatments.[31]

The day before Thanksgiving, BI publicly announced it had halted the clinical trials of nevirapine as a single agent, in view of the resistance data.[32] Media reaction was swift. The *Wall Street Journal*, *New York Times*, and various wire services reported the story, quoting Richman, who confirmed that nevirapine-induced resistance "happened very quickly."[33] Spokesmen representing patient advocacy groups called the resistance findings "extremely disappointing."[34] Because of the announcements by Merck and BI, reporters pressed Janssen to comment on its TIBO compounds. Caught off guard by the news, Janssen stated that it would begin monitoring for possible viral resistance, but the company intended to continue clinical trials with the TIBO compounds.[35]

* * *

In the midst of all this activity, Myers and her clinical group, Pascarelli and her marketing group, and Tiso and his project management group all moved to new quarters on BI's Ridgefield campus. For years, they had occupied a rented wing of Union Carbide's corporate headquarters building, one mile away in Danbury. In the fall of 1991, those departments moved to BI's new Administration Office Building. Situated atop the highest peak on the wooded estate, the low-slung, semi-circular building commanded a panoramic view of the R&D laboratories and Grozinger's new pilot plant below and the Connecticut countryside beyond. Inside, the new occupants welcomed the building's abundant natural light— an essential element of all German office architecture—but found the unconventional numbering of floors, wings, and pods illogical and disorienting.[36] Many office workers planned extra time when heading to a conference room for a scheduled meeting, anticipating that they would make at least one wrong turn along the way.

The new occupants also missed the Union Carbide building's covered parking and dreaded the avalanches of icy snow that silently slid off the new building's massive metal roof and crashed to the ground with earthshaking thuds. But the proximity fostered more frequent interactions between the R&D-based scientists and the administration building-based clinical team, now a shorter drive apart.[37] Tiso shifted the project team's meetings from the windowless Pharmacology Conference Room in the R&D building to a newer, windowless conference room in the hilltop office building.

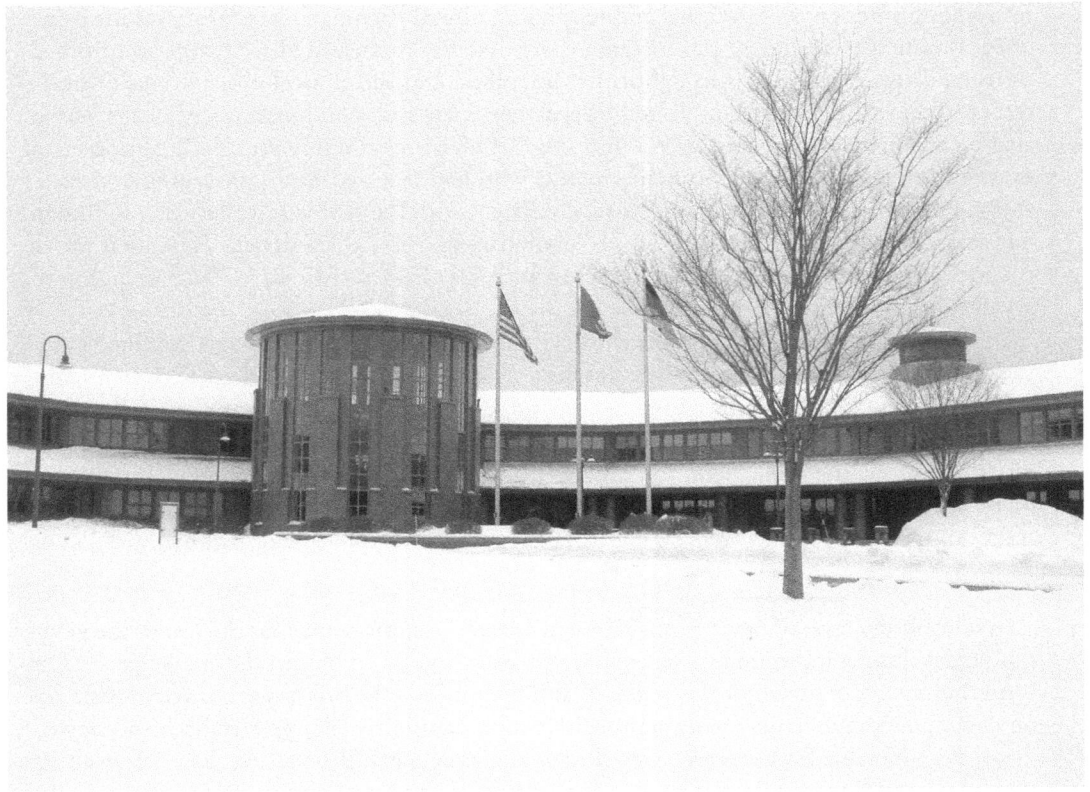

Boehringer Ingelheim's Administration Office Building in Ridgefield, Connecticut, displaying the American, German, and Connecticut state flags (courtesy Pamela Strode).

* * *

Shortly after Richman observed resistance to nevirapine in the patients' blood samples, Griffin organized an off-site meeting at a resort in Troutbeck, New York. They needed to reassess the nevirapine development program. "It was a sad day."[38] Many of the scientists thought the rapid development of clinical resistance doomed the development of nevirapine.[39] Some of BI's clinical investigators agreed. They acknowledged that the drug had proven to be a good research tool — demonstrating that non-nucleoside drugs could inhibit HIV reverse transcriptase — but nevirapine would not have a place in therapy, because of the rapid resistance.[40]

From the beginning, Alan Rosenthal had championed nevirapine as a standalone therapy for AIDS, and the project team directed all of its early efforts toward that objective. Now, everyone in the room at Troutbeck knew nevirapine could not be successful as a single-drug treatment. Rosenthal acknowledged nevirapine's undeniable limitations, saying "if we have to pull the plug, we will."[41] Merluzzi's heart sank. For three years, he had worked non-stop on this project, meeting and mastering every obstacle that threatened the team's success. They had become accustomed to solving problems, and their confidence in nevirapine steadily grew. Now, they were facing yet another obstacle, one they had anticipated for a long time but had hoped would be small and manageable. Unfortunately, it was big, onerous, and potentially, a fatal flaw.

Behind the scenes, Adams, Griffin, and Jim Wright had been discussing the clinical resistance findings with Rosenthal and reminding him of Richman's laboratory results using drug combinations.[42] Infectious disease experts like Richman and Hirsch were accustomed to using drug combinations to fight other microbes, and the clinical observations of nevirapine-induced resistance simply reinforced their view that combinations of drugs would also be required to suppress HIV infections.[43] Indeed, nevirapine and AZT appeared to exert an impressive one-two punch. Patients who had received both nevirapine and AZT showed the greatest decrease in viral load, consistent with the synergistic effect that Richman had observed with the two drugs in his laboratory assays. At Troutbeck, Rosenthal broke the meeting's somber mood by announcing with his characteristic flare, "We are going to go ahead with double therapy."[44]

Rosenthal intended to continue the nevirapine clinical trials but along a modified path, the trail that had been blazed by tuberculosis treatment forty years earlier. Richman's laboratory results gave BI's clinical investigators sufficient justification to continue testing nevirapine in combination with AZT, and that branch of the Christmas tree study continued on schedule. At the same time, the project team revised the protocol of the international clinical trial, which was enrolling HIV-infected patients in Australia, the Netherlands, and Italy. All of those patients were switched to the same nevirapine-AZT regimen.

* * *

The observation of nevirapine-induced resistance set the course for the rest of the nevirapine development program, and the project team "totally embraced the challenge."[45] But until they gained more clinical experience and determined the full impact of viral resistance on nevirapine's usefulness, the team proceeded more cautiously. They scaled back and slowed down the timetable for the toxicology studies and drug batch production. The 52-week rat toxicology study was well underway and would continue, but the team delayed starting the 52-week dog toxicology study. The dog study required a substantial amount of drug and investment in resources. A 500 kilogram (about 1100 pounds) batch of nevirapine, which was being produced at BI's chemical plant, would remain on schedule, but the team postponed plans to start the next 500 kilogram batch.

Grob's research team and Myers's clinicians forged a closer working relationship to share information and tackled the resistance issue collaboratively. To design the next clinical trials, the clinicians needed to know what was happening. To understand what was happening, the project team needed to make sense out of the viral load data. And to make sense out of the viral load data, the scientists needed to understand the interactions between nevirapine and the virus that led to resistance at the molecular level. The clinicians provided patient blood samples, and the laboratory scientists intensified their efforts in analyzing them. But the clinical sampling was fragmentary, the laboratory methods were experimental, and the results of their analysis were often contradictory. Several times each week, Adams, Myers, Griffin, and David Hall met to share and review their latest data, discuss ways to unlock the virus's secrets, and decide what to do next.[46] Over many months, they gradually learned how nevirapine interfered with HIV at the molecular level and made discoveries that helped guide Grob's team to find a backup compound. In addition, their efforts, supplemented by their close collaborations with Richman, Sullivan, Steitz, and other key research laboratories, greatly contributed to the scientific community's understanding of how HIV mutated and what could be done to overcome drug resistance.[47] These findings, which the BI team quickly published, benefited all HIV researchers.[48] "We held nothing back."[49]

At the 8th International AIDS Conference in Amsterdam in July 1992, BI presented four papers describing the laboratory and clinical data on nevirapine, including nevirapine-induced resistance.[50] Two years earlier in San Francisco, the BI delegation had merely taken notes. The next year in Florence, BI scientists had only presented laboratory data, which hardly made a ripple, except for Joe Wu's suntan lamp experiments. In Amsterdam, BI's nevirapine, Janssen's TIBO compounds, and Merck's "L" drugs were fully acknowledged by the Conference attendees as promising new AIDS treatments. But the issue of viral resistance was also a major theme of the Conference, and it posed a serious challenge for all three companies. Some Conference attendees felt that continuing to use a drug after resistance emerged did not benefit the patient, and they advocated switching to other treatments. While acknowledging the difficulties that viral resistance posed, BI publicly reaffirmed its commitment to continuing nevirapine development.[51] Only long-term clinical testing would determine whether or not nevirapine represented a successful approach to treating AIDS. BI had begun those longer clinical trials and would see them through.

* * *

As a resident in internal medicine at San Francisco General Hospital in the 1980s, Diane Havlir found herself at the center of an epidemic that looked hopeless. "Every night, ten or more patients would come in with advanced AIDS, but we had very little to offer them."[52] That experience led her to pursue a clinical fellowship in infectious diseases at Case Western Reserve University and her first academic post at the University of California in San Diego, with Doug Richman as her mentor. When Havlir arrived in San Diego, Richman was already working with BI, staging the Christmas tree studies, and he invited Havlir to join the project as a clinical investigator. To Havlir, nevirapine represented an exciting new approach to treating AIDS, and she leapt at the opportunity. It was her first experience with clinical trials.

Throughout the fall of 1991 and into 1992, Havlir was intimately involved in recruiting patients for the Christmas tree studies at UCSD. To her, these patients were not numbers on a chart but real people with names and faces and fears. And despite their "tough predicament," they showed "real courage."[53] They knew the nevirapine treatments, as designed, would probably not help them, but the results of the trials might help others who were suffering. While Richman and his laboratory staff focused on characterizing nevirapine-induced resistance, Havlir managed the patients. Together, they worked with the BI project team and the investigators at the University of Massachusetts and the other clinical sites to feel their way through the increasingly complex challenges that nevirapine presented. In a dynamic, interactive collaboration, the clinicians poured over each new clinical and laboratory result, discussed its significance, formulated a plan of action, and adjusted their treatment paradigm accordingly. Slowly but surely, as they continually modified their dosing schedules and evaluated the corresponding results, they saw more clearly how to optimize nevirapine treatment. Their goal was to find a dosing regimen that would suppress p24 indefinitely, thinking that the permanently suppressed virus would not mutate to a resistant form. If nevirapine could achieve those effects, it stood a good chance of being a valuable AIDS drug.

First, they tried an alternating course of therapy, giving patients nevirapine for one week, then switching to AZT for three weeks, and repeating the sequence for up to three months. Unfortunately, this alternating drug schedule did not prolong the suppression of p24 and did not prevent the development of nevirapine-induced resistance.[54]

Next, they examined whether resistant virus would return to its nevirapine-sensitive state after they stopped drug treatment. If so, then perhaps repeated cycles of nevirapine treatment would be effective. Unfortunately, this cycle of dosing and drug holidays also failed. The patients who had taken nevirapine still had high levels of nevirapine-resistant virus in their blood more than two months after ending their drug treatment.[55]

Finally, they tried brute force. In Richman's cell-based laboratory experiments, nevirapine could shut down resistant strains of HIV if he overwhelmed the cell cultures with enough drug. According to their calculations, the clinicians thought they could give patients a sufficiently large dose of nevirapine to overwhelm and shut down the virus in the patient's blood, even in its mutated form.[56] This strategy of

Diane Havlir (© majedphoto.com 2013).

simply increasing the drug dose to overcome viral resistance had not been possible with AZT, ddI, or ddC, because high doses of those drugs produced intolerable side effects. Fortunately, patients in the nevirapine Christmas tree studies had not experienced anything more serious than occasional sleepiness, headaches, diarrhea, and fever.[57] And it was not clear that those effects had been caused by nevirapine. After all, many people get headaches and are sometimes sleepy, whether they are taking an experimental drug or not. Many patients in the nevirapine clinical trials experienced no side effects at all. Based on their experience with nevirapine so far, the clinical team was confident that patients could safely take higher doses of the drug.[58]

Havlir and a team of clinical investigators conducted a small clinical trial of twenty-one patients, all of whom were given daily doses of nevirapine twice as large as that given to previous treatment groups. As expected, the patients' viral load decreased significantly after about three weeks of treatment and the virus mutated into its resistant form.[59] But despite this mutation, the double dose of nevirapine was able to keep p24 suppressed for up to six months.[60] Havlir went further, tripling the dose of nevirapine in some patients, who also showed a sustained suppression of p24, but the effect was no greater than in the double-dose group.[61]

It was a major achievement. The BI team had demonstrated, for the first time, that it was possible to overwhelm HIV and keep it suppressed despite its attempts to resist. Viral resistance, they concluded, was a relative rather than an absolute hurdle. When Maureen Myers and the BI clinical team met with Havlir and the other clinical investigators in the summer of 1992 to review the data from patients receiving the doubled dose, they concluded that there was still hope for nevirapine.[62] The clinical trials would continue.

Later studies using a more accurate way of assessing viral load would show that nevirapine did not actually deliver a knock-out punch.[63] Although the double dose of nevirapine had suppressed p24, HIV was still viable and continued to proliferate. To stop viral proliferation, patients would need to take an extremely high dose of nevirapine. Unfortunately, the project team had reached the maximum dose of nevirapine that patients could tolerate. A side effect that they had seen occasionally in earlier patients proved to be a major menace when patients took the double dose of nevirapine.

10

A Rash Decision

Stuart, a 31-year-old man who had been diagnosed with HIV, began taking a treatment regimen that included nevirapine and AZT, but ten days later he was admitted to the hospital with a 103° fever and a life-threatening form of skin rash called Stevens-Johnson syndrome.[1] Tender, red blotches covered his chest, back, palms, and soles of his feet. In addition, he had painful ulcers in his mouth and crusty lesions on his lips. His eyes were inflamed and he was sensitive to light. Stuart's doctors quickly ruled out other explanations for his symptoms including herpes, syphilis, and lung disease and concluded that Stuart was having a reaction to his AIDS medication. They stopped his AIDS treatment and gave him drugs to relieve his pain and treat the skin rashes. Within two days, Stuart showed signs of improvement, and after twelve days in the hospital he was discharged. Stuart's doctors monitored his recovery for more than six months. During that time, he did not take nevirapine or AZT, and he had no further skin rash episodes. Stuart's doctors thought that nevirapine had caused his skin rash, but because he was taking several AIDS drugs and they did not probe his case further, they could not prove with certainty that nevirapine was the cause.

* * *

From the time Boehringer Ingelheim began the Christmas tree clinical trials, the project team had received reports of skin rashes in patients taking nevirapine. Eleven of the 62 participants in the Christmas tree trials developed a rash, but that was far fewer than the number of patients who complained of headaches and sleepiness. In all but two cases, the investigators thought that the skin rash was probably due to other drugs that the patients were taking, rather than to nevirapine. But their views changed when they doubled the nevirapine dose to overcome the resistance problem in the clinical trial headed by Diane Havlir.

Soon after the first few patients began taking the double dose, Maureen Myers received reports that the patients were experiencing side effects. The types of side effects, such as headaches, sleepiness, diarrhea, and skin rashes, were similar to those reported by patients who had taken lower doses of nevirapine. But everyone was surprised at the number of patients who developed skin rashes, as well as the severity of those rashes.[2] The red blotches primarily affected the face, chest, and back, sometimes the arms and legs, and typically appeared within the first two weeks of nevirapine treatment. Two patients described a stinging sensation in their skin. In addition to the skin rashes, patients often had a fever and sometimes complained of muscle pain. Overall, almost half of the patients treated with the double dose developed some type of skin rash. In most cases, the rash was mild or moderate, but two patients experienced a severe skin reaction.[3] And about one-quarter of the patients voluntarily withdrew from Havlir's trial because of the skin rash problem.[4]

Throughout the spring of 1992, Myers monitored the status of these patients through weekly teleconferences with Havlir and the other clinical investigators, discussed how to interpret the skin rash results, and "recalibrated the risk-benefit."[5] They set ground rules for managing severe rashes and experimented with the dosing regimen to determine whether nevirapine had caused the skin rashes.[6] They stopped dosing with nevirapine to see if the rash would go away. It did. In some patients, the skin rash reappeared when they resumed the nevirapine regimen, but in other patients who continued taking nevirapine, the rash faded away on its own.[7] The investigators examined skin samples but saw no direct tissue damage.[8]

By the summer of 1992, the investigators and BI project team had gathered enough data to draw some preliminary conclusions. The skin rash was probably caused by nevirapine. Taking into consideration nevirapine's ability to lower viral load, the rapid emergence of resistance, and potential side effects, the team concluded that the doubled dose was the best balance between safety and nevirapine's antiviral effect.[9] But the skin rash problem clouded the BI team's plans and discouraged people from enrolling in the nevirapine clinical trials. The skin rash was at best annoying, affecting far too many people taking nevirapine, and at worst it was potentially life-threatening. The team had to find a way to minimize it.

While pouring over the clinical data, Myers, Havlir, and the other investigators saw an interesting trend. In their eagerness to ramp up the nevirapine dose and overcome resistance, they had invited some people in the Christmas tree study to join Havlir's trial and switch to the doubled dose. Other people were recruited specifically for Havlir's trial and received the doubled dose from the beginning. The people who ramped up to the doubled dose in a stepwise fashion appeared to be less prone to developing skin rashes than those who started treatment with the double dose.[10] The team also remembered that the skin rash, if it appeared at all, usually appeared in the first two weeks of nevirapine treatment.

To assist the clinicians, the project team's laboratory scientists conducted additional experiments on nevirapine's pharmaceutical properties. Jim Wright, who knew the nevirapine tablet formulation better than anyone, and Michael Lamson, a scientist in Jim Keirns' pharmacokinetics department, studied the data on the tablet's performance under various experimental conditions. They demonstrated that the tablets would dissolve better, enter the bloodstream more efficiently, and be less likely to cause a skin rash if the patient split the double dose, taking one tablet in the morning and another tablet in the evening, rather than both at once.[11]

Putting these observations together, Myers and the clinical investigators defined an optimized dosing regimen. Patients would start by taking one tablet of nevirapine daily for two weeks. If the patients showed no skin rash or other drug reactions, they doubled their dose to two tablets per day.[12] The stepwise dosing schedule allowed investigators to identify patients susceptible to skin reactions early. The patients who developed a rash continued taking one tablet for another two weeks to see if the rash would clear on its own. If so, the patient's dose was then increased to two tablets per day. If the skin rash persisted, the investigators discontinued nevirapine treatment and directed the patient to an alternative drug regimen. Using the lead-in dosing schedule, fewer patients experienced a rash, it was usually mild, and in most cases it quickly cleared, allowing patients to continue nevirapine treatment.[13] But then, investigators began reporting another side effect of nevirapine, potentially more serious than the skin rashes and, ultimately, the most troublesome drawback of nevirapine therapy.

* * *

Four years after being diagnosed with an HIV infection, 61-year-old Stefano began taking AZT and ddI.[14] After about 18 months of this two-drug regimen, Stefano's HIV infection appeared to be getting worse despite treatment, and his doctors switched from the AZT-ddI regimen to another drug regimen that included nevirapine.[15] During the two-week lead-in nevirapine regimen of one tablet per day, Stefano experienced a 103° fever, joint and stomach pains, and vomiting. He was admitted to the hospital, and his doctors immediately saw signs that pointed to a problem with his liver. The whites of Stefano's eyes had a yellowish tinge indicating jaundice, and his belly was swollen. They ordered a series of tests, which confirmed that Stefano's liver was enlarged and not functioning properly. Many things can damage the liver, but the doctors systematically ruled out all of the usual causes. Stefano had not been infected by any of the viruses or parasites that typically cause hepatitis.

Then, Stefano gave the doctors another clue. After three days in the hospital, he developed an itchy skin rash on his face, chest, and back. At this point, the doctors stopped treatment with nevirapine and the other AIDS drugs, gave him fluids, and treated the skin rash. Within two weeks, Stefano's symptoms eased. His liver slowly and steadily recovered, and his skin rash disappeared. After 30 days, Stefano was discharged. The doctors resumed his AIDS drug treatment, but they replaced nevirapine with an HIV protease inhibitor.[16] When they checked Stefano's progress one month later, none of his liver or skin rash problems had reappeared. They concluded that nevirapine was responsible for both side effects, but they did not conduct any further testing to prove nevirapine was the cause.

* * *

In the Christmas tree studies, a few of the patients developed mild changes in liver function.[17] In Havlir's trial with the doubled nevirapine dose, about one-third of the patients experienced the same mild changes.[18] A few patients developed major changes in liver function, but the investigators usually found that the problem was caused by something other than nevirapine. In San Diego, one of Havlir's study participants was an HIV-positive woman who had no AIDS symptoms when she enrolled in the trial. After starting treatment with nevirapine, the woman developed a skin rash and "her liver enzymes went through the roof."[19] Havlir stopped the nevirapine regimen, thinking that nevirapine was potentially responsible for both side effects, but she also pursued other possible explanations. After an anxious period of waiting, the hospital laboratory confirmed that the woman had a hepatitis A infection. This infection was likely due to a simple case of food poisoning and accounted for the abnormal liver function results. Once the woman recovered from the food poisoning, her liver function returned to normal, and Havlir concluded that nevirapine was not the cause after all.

Myers and the clinical investigators noted each change in liver function and monitored the patients throughout the clinical trials, but they were not unduly concerned. Patients with HIV infections have immune systems that are not functioning normally, and they are less able to fight a variety of opportunistic infections. Among the most common and serious opportunistic infections are those that damage the liver, particularly in drug users, who often become infected with both HIV and hepatitis C from using dirty needles. About one-third of the deaths of patients with HIV infections are related to liver disease.[20] Myers and her colleagues concluded that the changes in liver function seen after nevirapine treatment simply reflected the natural progression of AIDS, as the patient's immune system weakened and opportunistic infections invaded the liver.

On the other hand, the BI team knew that many drugs, including nevirapine, are metabolized by the liver. When the liver is exposed repeatedly to a drug, it typically responds by ramping up its metabolic machinery to meet the challenge — a process called autoinduction. The liver usually acclimates in a few days or weeks, and then settles into functioning at a slightly higher metabolic rate. So, the liver function changes that the investigators were seeing might simply have been the liver's natural process of adjusting its metabolic machinery to handle the large daily doses of nevirapine. The project team did not know whether the liver function changes were symptoms associated with AIDS or were caused by nevirapine. But, like the skin rashes, the team closely monitored patients for changes in liver function.

As the clinical trials proceeded, a few patients always showed changes in liver function. Eventually, the BI team collected enough data to conclude that nevirapine was responsible. In a few cases, these changes led to liver toxicity and required hospitalization, as in Stefano's case. Fortunately, they found that the two week lead-in dose of one tablet daily followed by the standard regimen of one tablet twice a day reduced not only the skin rashes but also the likelihood of liver dysfunction.

* * *

Throughout the course of the clinical trials, the project team extensively analyzed the data, wanting to understand how nevirapine might be causing skin rashes and liver toxicity. They carefully examined each case and meticulously documented the clinical condition of each patient. But there were no easy answers. The side effects did not correspond to the dose of nevirapine or the amount of drug in the patient's bloodstream. Some patients tolerated relatively high doses of nevirapine for a long time without any side effects. Others were quite sensitive, showing a severe skin reaction or liver function changes during the lead-in dosing phase.[21]

To address the skin rash problem, Myers convened a panel of international experts and developed guidelines for both the classification and management of nevirapine-induced rashes.[22] In addition, the project team instructed investigators to be especially cautious about giving nevirapine to people who already suffered from liver disease or a chronic hepatitis infection. They did not want to cause more damage to a liver that was already unhealthy. Clinicians learned to start nevirapine treatment gradually, watch for signs of skin and liver problems, and if those side effects occurred, make adjustments to minimize patient discomfort.

That was good advice for all of the AIDS drug regimens, because skin rashes and liver toxicity were not unique to nevirapine. Other drugs in nevirapine's class (i.e., the non-nucleoside reverse transcriptase inhibitors) also caused rashes, and the AZT-like drugs could also cause liver damage. Although the BI team would learn much more about nevirapine's side effect profile in the coming years, what was becoming clear, as the clinical trials proceeded, was that nevirapine did not produce some of the most troublesome side effects associated with other AIDS drugs, such as bone marrow toxicity, pancreas inflammation, nerve damage, and mood disorders.[23] Unlike those drugs, nevirapine appeared to be safe enough to give to pregnant women and children.

11

The Road to Prevention

On October 30, 1982, Arthur Ammann confidently walked to the podium in a crowded auditorium at the University of California in San Francisco.[1] The audience had gathered there for one of the first national conferences on the AIDS epidemic, and he was going to present a case that would shatter their notions about how people contracted AIDS. Ammann, who was Director of Pediatric Immunology and Clinical Research at the university's medical center, was widely recognized as a leader in his field and had introduced a number of innovations during his decade of leadership, including a pediatric bone marrow transplant program. He told his audience that in April, a 29-year-old woman, who worked as a prostitute and was an injection drug user, was admitted to the medical center in labor.[2] She had previously been treated for thrush, a fungal infection in her mouth, and had a slightly low white blood cell count, but otherwise she was healthy. She delivered a 5-pound baby girl without complications.

At two months of age, the baby developed an oral and vaginal yeast infection, which was successfully treated with antifungal medication. But when she was five months old, the infection returned, and she also suffered from an enlarged liver and spleen. By various measures of her blood, her immune system was weakening. At the time of Ammann's presentation, the girl was six months old and had again been admitted to the hospital with a fever and cough. A lung biopsy revealed that she had pneumocystis pneumonia, and Ammann began treating her with antibiotics. Despite treatment, she died a month later. Her mother had previously borne two other daughters, each by a different father, and the three children did not live together. Both of the older half-sis-

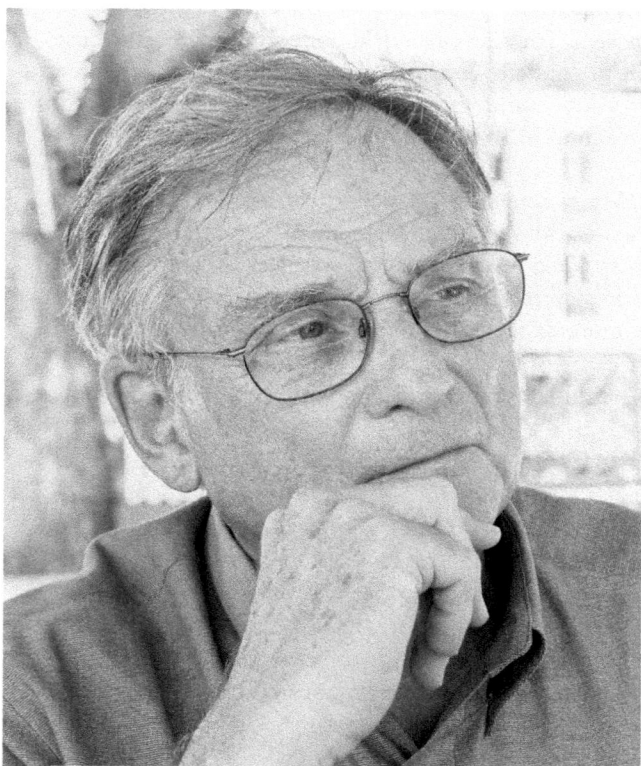

Arthur Ammann.

ters also had an unexplained immune deficiency, and one of them had also died of pneumocystis pneumonia.

Ammann ran the only immunology laboratory in northern California, and physicians frequently consulted him on cases of immune deficiency in both children and adults.[3] He told his audience that he was increasingly seeing similarities in the symptoms of patients in both age groups, similarities that suggested AIDS was not caused by lifestyle, drugs, or a genetic defect. The three half-sisters were not in any of the high-risk categories — homosexual contact, drug abuse, or hemophilia — and yet they most likely had AIDS. Although no one at the time knew what caused AIDS, the early onset of immune deficiency in these infants pointed to an "AIDS agent" that had been transmitted from mother to child either before or during birth.[4] Ammann thought the agent was probably a virus.

* * *

Fascinated by these interesting clinical cases, Ammann changed the direction of his pediatric immunology research from rare genetic disorders to studying the syndrome that was becoming increasingly common in children, AIDS. One day, Michael Gottlieb called and invited him to Los Angeles to meet with a woman who wanted to start a foundation to promote pediatric AIDS research.[5] Gottlieb would identify the woman only as a person who had become infected with HIV through a blood transfusion and whose daughter and son had subsequently also become infected. Ammann agreed to respect the woman's privacy and made the clandestine trip. In Los Angeles, Gottlieb introduced him to Elizabeth and Paul Michael Glaser. Elizabeth's foundation was little more than a concept, but Ammann was impressed by this intelligent woman, whose eyes missed nothing and whose lilting voice conveyed her passion and iron-willed determination with New York-accented precision. He agreed to join her inner circle of scientific advisors.

At her initial meetings in Washington, DC, with legislators, policy makers, and government scientists, Elizabeth Glaser was surprised to learn that they were unaware of the issues regarding pediatric clinical trials and that there was no spokesperson for pediatric AIDS.[6] Investigators had conducted a handful of AIDS clinical trials in children, but no one up to that time had commissioned a study on maternal transmission of the AIDS virus.[7] Following her interviews with the *Los Angeles Times* in 1989 and CBS's *60 Minutes* in 1990, Elizabeth continued a very active — and now very public — campaign to raise awareness and funds for pediatric AIDS research. She consulted the growing roster of health experts on her Foundation's board, boldly asking the difficult questions and emphasizing topics that many considered taboo.[8] Leaving behind her favorite sneakers and donning her "Washington wardrobe" to make the best impression, she continued to walk the halls of Congress and visited researchers at the National Institutes of Health, challenging and inspiring them all to do more.[9] She was encouraged when two presidential commissions recommended detailed, aggressive, and comprehensive steps to combat AIDS through increased funding for healthcare, antidiscrimination legislation, and accelerated approval of new drugs.[10] But the Republican-dominated White House shelved both reports. Convinced that support for people with AIDS would come only from a change in federal leadership, she traveled to New York City in July 1992 to address the Democratic National Convention.[11]

The rowdy, raucous convention hall fell silent — the delegates transfixed with tears welling up in their eyes — as she recounted her story: becoming infected with HIV through a blood transfusion, unknowingly passing the virus to her daughter, Ariel, through breastfeeding, and three years later, still unaware that she was HIV-positive, becoming pregnant again and infecting her son, Jake, probably during childbirth.[12] In recalling Ariel's final days, when her daughter could neither walk nor talk, Elizabeth told the delegates, "She taught me to love, when all I wanted to do was hate. She taught me to help others, when all I wanted to do was help myself."[13]

Elizabeth had a personal stake in wanting to block transmission of HIV from an infected mother to her child, and it became the central mission of her Pediatric AIDS Foundation.[14] One-third of all infected mothers passed the AIDS virus to their children, and Elizabeth wanted to know why some babies became infected and others did not.[15] She asked Ammann to convene a think tank meeting, bringing together prominent researchers to discuss mother-to-infant HIV transmission.[16] They represented diverse areas of science and their freewheeling discussion generated new ideas and creative approaches to the questions Ammann posed.

Elizabeth listened intently, curled up with her customary ankle socks and sneakers in an overstuffed chair at the back of the room. She knew these researchers would need to work together to untangle the multifaceted puzzle of HIV transmission. At the end of the meeting, Elizabeth, whose smile dominated her petite frame, stood up and said, "Clearly this is something that one person can't do alone. We have to do it as a group. Who's in?"[17] The researchers rallied around her, defined a research plan, and proposed a budget. They called it the Ariel Project, a five-year, forward-looking research program aimed at identifying the biologic and clinical factors associated with HIV transmission, or lack of transmission, from mother to child.[18] Elizabeth knew the Foundation needed a full-time administrator to oversee the Ariel Project, coordinate the fifteen participating institutions, and ensure that the investigators met the project's research objectives on schedule. Ammann, who was an experienced academic and industrial research administrator, was the obvious choice. After thinking it over, he agreed, and in July 1992, Ammann joined the Pediatric AIDS Foundation full-time as Director of Research.

* * *

The summer of 1992 was a time that called for bold leadership, a time for scientists to push an agenda without being reckless, seize responsibility without worrying about the consequences, and get the job done. Julian Adams, a chemist by training but also a scientist with wide-ranging interests and an even broader vision, was one such leader. In July, at the 8th International AIDS Conference in Amsterdam, Adams wandered into a session devoted to issues of AIDS in developing countries and listened as presenters showed statistics on the high rate of HIV transmission to newborns in Africa.[19] The data resonated with Adams, a father with newborns at home, and he began thinking about ways to limit HIV transmission during childbirth. Nevirapine, with its good safety record in the early clinical trials and its attractive pharmaceutical properties, struck Adams as a logical choice for testing whether HIV infections could be prevented by pretreatment with an AIDS drug. Realizing that intentionally exposing people to HIV was unacceptable, Adams mentally constructed a comparable laboratory experiment. He envisioned pretreating laboratory animals with nevirapine, then exposing them to HIV, and watching to see whether they became infected. With the theoretical experiment still on his mind, Adams pitched the idea during a chance meeting with David Ho, who was also attending the Conference.[20] Ho had trained under Martin Hirsch at Harvard and was now studying HIV at Aaron Diamond AIDS Research Center in New York. He confirmed that Adams's idea was a logical way to test whether nevirapine could prevent HIV infection, and the two collaborated on the experiment soon after they returned home.

During nevirapine's preclinical development, Adams had explored various animal models of AIDS. Among other things, the patent examiners wanted direct evidence that Boehringer Ingelheim's compounds improved AIDS symptoms. They had not been convinced by the data showing that nevirapine and its chemical cousins inhibited an HIV-related enzyme (reverse transcriptase) and prevented HIV proliferation in cell-based laboratory assays. Unfortunately, HIV selectively targets humans, and animals do not develop the debilitating and lethal symptoms of AIDS. This dilemma — not being able to improve AIDS symptoms in symptom-free animals — bogged down the patent's approval for years.[21]

Despite the inability to produce AIDS symptoms in animals, Adams and Ho knew that chimpanzees shared enough genetic similarity with humans to be a suitable species for their experiment. Chimpanzees rarely develop AIDS symptoms, but they exhibit the same blood-borne biochemical characteristics of a human HIV infection and for that reason had been used to test some of the early HIV vaccines.[22] Adams and Ho made arrangements to conduct their experiment using a few chimpanzees housed at the primate facility maintained by New York University in nearby Tuxedo, New York.[23]

* * *

In November 1992, Joep Lange traveled from Geneva, Switzerland, to Washington, DC, on an important mission. He wanted to speak with Maureen Myers, who was attending a meeting of the AIDS Clinical Trials Group, about a new clinical trial with nevirapine. Like Adams, Lange had been disturbed by the raging AIDS epidemic in Africa, especially the surge of HIV infections in newborns, and like Adams, he thought nevirapine was the right drug to prevent those infections.

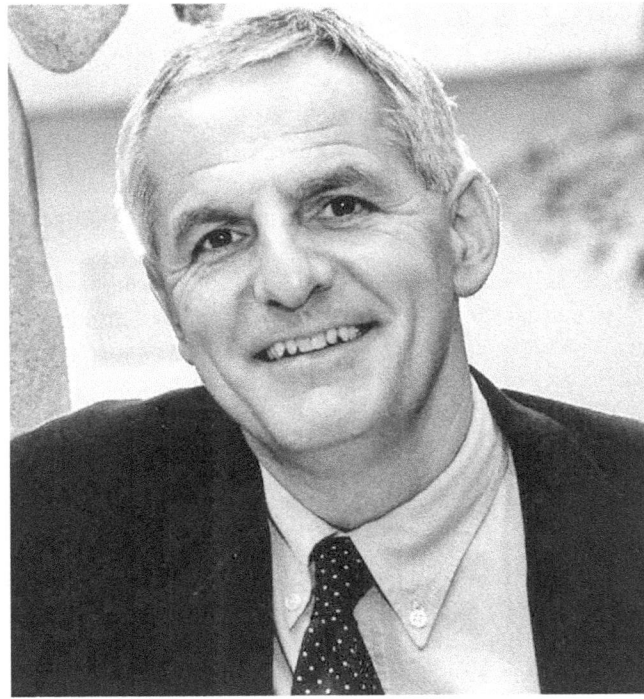

Joep Lange.

As a young Dutch investigator fresh out of medical school when AIDS emerged around the world, Lange had been at the right place at the right time. Amsterdam's enlightened lifestyle spread HIV through both sexual transmission and intravenous drug use, generating a large number of early AIDS cases. Most physicians in the Netherlands referred their AIDS patients to the Academic Medical Centre at the University of Amsterdam, a pioneering AIDS clinic, and Lange was one of the physicians heavily involved in their clinical care. By 1984, Lange's experience qualified him as a contributor to the Amsterdam Cohort Study, which was a collaboration between academic and governmental organizations in the Netherlands and one of the first systematic studies to examine the clinical course of AIDS. Delving deeper into AIDS research, Lange began laboratory investigations to identify the biological markers of HIV infection, for which he earned a Ph.D. degree in 1987.

Three years later, Lange became director of the National AIDS Therapy Evaluation Centre and was responsible for coordinating clinical trials at twenty Dutch hospitals that were caring for HIV-infected patients. His pioneering work as an HIV researcher and his clinical insight made him an obvious choice when Boehringer Ingelheim's project team began searching for consultants to assist with the nevirapine clinical trials. He participated in BI's first meeting of international consultants in San Diego to plan the international clinical program and then spearheaded the clinical trials of nevirapine in the Netherlands.

In July 1992, Maureen Myers arranged another meeting of BI's clinical consultants prior to the 8th International AIDS Conference in Amsterdam. As the investigators explored ways of overcoming nevirapine-induced resistance, Lange actively supported BI's plans, contributing ideas for the study designs and facilitating those new clinical trials in the Netherlands. Lange and the BI team both benefited from this close working relationship.

But Lange's star was still rising. "The real problem was in Africa" and his first trip to Africa was "a watershed event."[24] The World Health Organization estimated that ten million people were infected with HIV, representing one in every 250 adults in the world, and 5000 new cases were appearing every day.[25] The viral infection had become a worldwide pandemic, with an increasing portion of HIV-infected people suffering from AIDS symptoms, and virtually all AIDS patients were expected to die within a few years of diagnosis. Lange enthusiastically accepted an invitation from the World Health Organization to lead the newly created Clinical Research and Product Development branch of its Global Program on AIDS. He moved to Geneva, Switzerland, and immediately set out to do on a global scale what he had been doing in the Netherlands.

Among the most alarming trends at that time was the rapidly rising rate of HIV infections in women and children. Globally, women represented nearly half of all the new cases of HIV infection, and not surprisingly there was a corresponding increase in the number of HIV-infected children born to them.[26] Disturbed by those trends, Lange declared HIV infections in women and children a priority for his office at the World Health Organization. He rapidly took steps to address the issue and was willing to devote the bulk of his budget to it.

In October 1992, Lange invited John Sullivan to attend a meeting at the World Health Organization headquarters in Geneva to discuss the global AIDS epidemic with a group of physicians who represented a number of African countries.[27] The African physicians were dealing with HIV infections and AIDS cases on a scale far beyond any other region, and they were most disturbed by the rapid rise of HIV infections in infants. In the western, industrialized world, physicians had resources and, increasingly, treatment options to comfort patients and delay AIDS symptoms, if not prolong life. But the resources and treatment options available to physicians in sub–Saharan Africa were severely limited. During the Geneva meeting, to illustrate the magnitude of their challenges, one African physician reached for the large, elegant water pitcher sitting in the center of the conference table, poured a glass of water, and holding it in front of him said, "We can't do that in my country."[28] He had no ornate water pitchers at home or large conference tables to set them on. Most communities did not have running water, and for some, clean drinking water was hard to find. To Sullivan and the other western physicians sitting around the table, this simple demonstration gave new meaning to "resource-limited settings." They realized that the drugs and medical practice they took for granted would not work in Africa. Treatment regimens needed to be extremely simple in countries where clean water was a luxury.

Together, the physicians explored ideas for a clinical trial, aiming for the simplest, shortest, and most effective way to give an AIDS drug to mothers and infants. From observations that Sullivan and other clinicians had recently made, they knew that three-fourths of HIV-infected infants, like Ariel and Jake Glaser, became infected during childbirth or via breast milk after birth.[29] The physicians thought they might be able to prevent a baby from becoming infected if they treated the mother with an appropriate AIDS drug during labor and continued treatment of the mother and baby for a short time after delivery, during breastfeeding. Sullivan and Lange, as BI consultants and investigators on the clinical trials of nevirapine, had been impressed with the drug's clinical performance so far. They thought that nevirapine's pharmaceutical properties made it an attractive choice for the mother-to-child transmission study, and the physicians who gathered in Geneva designed the clinical trial specifically with nevirapine in mind.

With this plan for the nevirapine clinical trial in his briefcase, Lange then flew to Washington, DC, where the AIDS Clinical Trials Group was meeting at the Omni Shoreham Hotel. On Wednesday, November 4, 1992, Lange and Sullivan met with Myers, David Hall (the project statistician), and other members of the BI team to discuss the clinical trial outlined at the World Health Organization meeting. Lange needed BI's cooperation to use nevirapine as the drug treatment in this clinical trial, of course, and the BI team expressed interest. Although Lange saw the greatest need in African countries, where HIV infection was spreading and affecting large numbers of women and children, he explained that this treatment idea, for social and ethical reasons, should first be studied in a developed country, preferably the United States. (The infrastructure at American clinics easily accommodated clinical trials and could efficiently deliver trustworthy results. In addition, well-established federal regulations ensured that the rights of the study participants would be protected.) But for that, Lange needed, in addition to BI's support, the cooperation of the ACTG, whose network of American investigators was the most experienced at conducting AIDS clinical trials. And before regulatory authorities would allow such a clinical trial, the investigators would need to conduct a preliminary study to show that nevirapine was safe in pregnant women and newborns. It was a complicated, convoluted, and precarious process, but Lange was determined.

Lange's next stop was a meeting with David Feigal. Feigal had served as an investigator on various AIDS clinical trials, including the pivotal trial that supported approval of pentamidine aerosol for preventing pneumocystis pneumonia. He had also served as a member of FDA's Antiviral Drugs Advisory Committee from its inception, grappling with all of the issues surrounding rapid approval of the early AIDS drugs. In January 1992, he had moved from California to become Director of FDA's Antiviral Drug Products Division, the post that Ellen Cooper had vacated more than a year earlier. Lange wanted to know how FDA officials would view data collected in clinical trials conducted in a third world country. Because Feigal also served as an advisor to the World Health Organization, he knew that running a clinical trial in Africa required adjustments to the monitoring and oversight procedures, but he was willing to accommodate those changes. To Feigal, Lange's proposal "made a lot of sense."[30] He knew that patients tolerated nevirapine better than AZT and that it had better pharmaceutical properties. He encouraged Lange and Myers to stay in touch as they proceeded and to work out the details of the clinical protocol with the FDA's assistance.

On Thursday, Lange's traveling road show moved to the Pediatric Core Committee of the ACTG, where the committee members' discussions concentrated on the issue of HIV transmission from mothers to infants. The committee saw Lange's proposed clinical trial as a valuable way to resolve some important questions about HIV infections in children. They enthusiastically discussed ways in which the ACTG network might assist, including scheduling the preliminary clinical trials in the United States using ACTG resources.

Later on that drizzly, gusty day, Lange, Sullivan, and Myers drove down Connecticut Avenue from the Shoreham Hotel to the Pan American Health Organization building, which housed the Global Program on AIDS, the parent unit of Lange's branch of the World Health Organization. Lange's branch was new and the mother-to-child clinical trial was among the first he had proposed. The visitors learned that the World Health Organization had previously worked with industry to develop other new drugs for use in remote areas of the world. The most recent successful example was the collaboration between the World Health Organization and Merck to develop ivermectin for river blindness.[31] River blindness is caused by a parasitic worm that penetrates the skin after bites from infected black flies and reproduces thousands of larvae, which travel through the lymph system and concentrate in the eye.

Merck conducted clinical trials of ivermectin over a seven year period in twelve African countries, treating hundreds of thousands of river blindness patients. The drug was highly effective and well tolerated in a once-per-year dosing schedule, easily transported and stored without refrigeration, and therefore unusually convenient for disease management in even the most remote corners of the world. Consequently, the World Health Organization and Merck joined forces, sponsoring a program for widespread, community-based distribution and monitoring of ivermectin treatment throughout Africa and later also in Latin America.[32]

HIV is a much different microbe than a parasite, AIDS is a much different disease than river blindness, and nevirapine is a much different drug than ivermectin. As Myers sat and listened to the discussion on that gray November day, the whole thing sounded daunting: setting up clinical trials in third world countries where BI had no research infrastructure, coordinating the interests and requirements of multiple governmental and non-governmental organizations, and ultimately establishing distribution procedures for the drug in remote communities that had few healthcare providers. Despite all these potential obstacles, the idea of preventing transmission of HIV from mother to child was compelling both scientifically and altruistically, and Myers kept that idea alive.

Two weeks later, Myers presented to the BI project team a summary of her discussions with Lange, the ACTG, and the World Health Organization, including the proposed protocol of the mother-to-child transmission clinical trial. The project team knew, as did Lange, that this trial could not start until they successfully completed the required preliminary studies. The first of these was a set of studies to examine whether the drug caused reproductive damage in pregnant and newborn animals. The team's toxicologists had already conducted those studies and reported that they had seen no harmful effects that would limit the subsequent clinical trials.[33] But the preliminary clinical trial that Lange and Sullivan wanted to conduct in the United States (and that the ACTG was willing to support) generated extensive discussions at BI.

* * *

In parallel with the BI project team's toxicology studies, Adams managed to start his chimpanzee study. Predictably, the control chimpanzee developed an HIV infection, which the scientists confirmed by the usual blood tests. The animals that received nevirapine before and shortly after exposure to HIV also initially registered changes in their blood, confirming that they had been exposed to the virus. But over the following weeks, HIV quickly disappeared from their blood. The investigators monitored the chimpanzees for years and continued to observe the same results: a steady-state HIV infection in the control chimpanzee and no evidence of HIV in the animals pretreated with nevirapine.[34] It was an outcome that pleased the experimental animals as much as the investigators. Because the chimpanzees had been exposed to HIV, even though most of them remained virus-free, they could not be used for other experiments. They retired and comfortably lived out their days on a generous BI pension.[35]

The results of Adams's chimpanzee study established that nevirapine pretreatment, at least under experimental conditions, could prevent HIV infection. The two most common situations where such treatment was needed were accidental HIV exposure to healthcare workers from needle sticks and HIV transmission to babies from their HIV-infected mothers. The chimpanzee study provided justification for both uses, but everyone was most interested in establishing nevirapine's ability to prevent HIV infection in infants.

In December 1993, Lange, Sullivan, and Doug Richman — all experienced investigators in BI's ongoing clinical trials — gathered in Ridgefield to discuss the clinical program and the nevirapine development strategy. During the meeting, Adams presented the results from the first eight months of his chimpanzee study.[36] The clinicians were impressed by the results, immediately realized their significance, and urged BI in the strongest possible terms to conduct clinical trials to determine whether nevirapine would also prevent HIV transmission from mothers to newborns.[37]

Myers backed the investigators' enthusiasm for the mother-to-child clinical trial, and the project team explored how to incorporate it into the overall nevirapine development plan. But the team was already quite busy, managing the fast-track development of nevirapine for treating adults, upholding their promise to the FDA to conduct comparable pediatric clinical trials, overcoming the challenges of nevirapine-induced resistance, probing the causes of the skin rash and liver toxicity side effects, coordinating their efforts with the ACTG network, and mindful that all of these activities were being scrutinized under the watchful eye of multiple regulatory agencies, patient advocacy groups, and the patients themselves. Besides, the question about whether it was possible to prevent mother-to-child transmission of HIV was already being addressed by an ongoing, ACTG-sponsored clinical trial using AZT.

* * *

In 1987, Art Ammann and Cathy Wilfert were among the pediatricians attending a meeting in Philadelphia organized by Surgeon General C. Everett Koop, a pioneer of pediatric surgery, to discuss the growing problem of pediatric AIDS.[38] All of the pediatricians were facing a distressing and unfamiliar situation in their practices, and they felt helpless to cope with it. Childhood infections rarely required hospitalization. But when children needed hospital care, they were treated for a while, usually recovered, and then returned home. Not so with pediatric AIDS. Those children needed intensive hospital care, they usually got progressively worse, and there was little that doctors could do except watch them die.[39] Hospital wards everywhere were admitting children terminally ill with AIDS. Like other pediatricians, Wilfert, who was based in North Carolina, saw her pediatric AIDS caseload increasing. HIV spread in the Southeast chiefly through heterosexual transmission, aggravated by injection drug use and transmission to the partners of drug users. Each year,

Duke University Medical Center was seeing fifty to seventy babies who had become infected by their mothers, and the pediatric AIDS cases were piling up year after year.[40]

But Wilfert came to Koop's meeting with an exciting new idea. She had seen the dramatic improvement in adult AIDS patients who were treated in the first clinical trials of AZT at Duke, and she was leading the ongoing clinical trials of AZT in HIV-infected children.[41] Wouldn't it be better, she thought, if you could treat the babies with AZT before they were born? Perhaps early drug treatment could prevent HIV infection altogether. She had noted with interest the results of a study just published by Ruth Ruprecht at the Dana Farber Cancer Institute, proving that AZT given to pregnant mice could penetrate into the unborn pups.[42] Wilfert proposed conducting a clinical trial in HIV-infected pregnant women to test whether AZT could also penetrate into their unborn babies and prevent mother-to-child transmission of HIV.[43] At that time, AZT was not the best drug for such a study. It was the only drug.

Soon after the pediatricians' meeting with Koop, Wilfert, who led the Pediatric Core Committee of ACTG, submitted her idea to the protocol committee for review, but it received a chilly reception.[44] Some members of the committee considered her proposed trial unethical. Physicians were concerned about drug-induced birth defects, and they had been discouraging HIV-infected women from taking AZT during pregnancy.[45] Certainly, AZT produced severe reactions in some people, including bone marrow suppression, liver toxicity, and muscle wasting. Some critics remembered the thalidomide incident in the 1960s, in which several thousand children had been born with deformed arms and legs after their mothers had taken thalidomide during pregnancy. Other critics cited the more recent diethylstilbesterol episode. Young women were developing cervical cancer because their mothers had taken that drug during pregnancy — a problem that took a generation to manifest itself. What if AZT caused those sorts of problems?

In addition, no one yet knew when and how HIV was transmitted from mothers to infants. The Ariel Project had not yet started, and none of the studies that would eventually determine the timing of HIV transmission from mothers to their babies had yet been

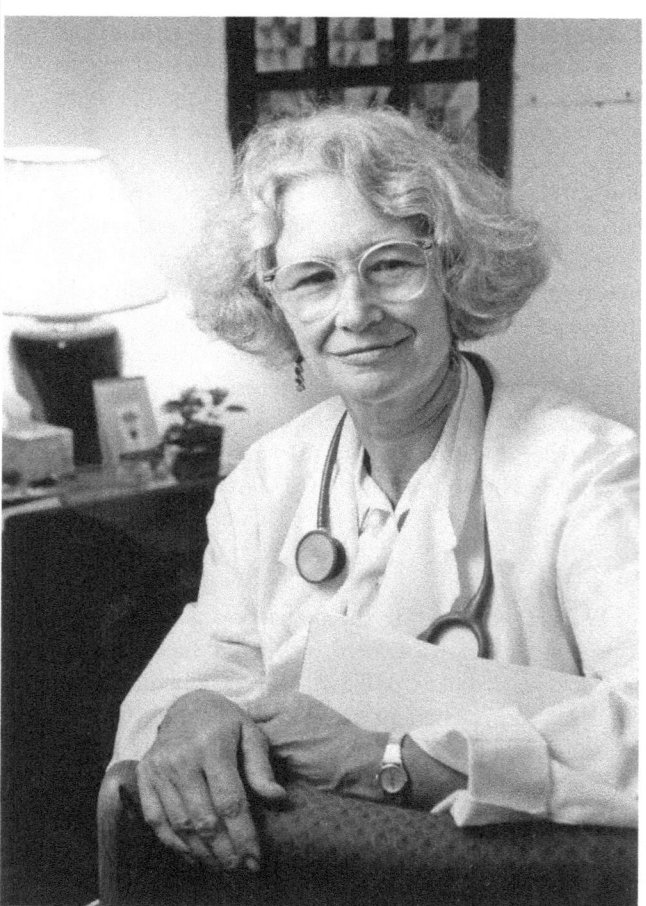

Catherine Wilfert (courtesy Elizabeth Glaser Pediatric AIDS Foundation).

conducted.[46] The virus might invade the mother's womb right after conception, before any drug could be given. Also, only one in three babies born to HIV-infected mothers became infected, and investigators had no method for determining which babies were vulnerable. Was it wise to expose seventy percent of babies to AZT unnecessarily in order to protect the thirty percent who needed it?

Finally, Wilfert somehow needed to overcome the practical barriers to such a study. Most women at that time did not know their HIV status and were not required to take an HIV test. To protect patient privacy, the researchers who tracked the spread of AIDS had resorted to pooling blood samples from fifty people and only tested the pooled blood for HIV.[47] Increasingly, healthcare workers on maternity wards were requesting transfers, fearing that sooner or later their daily exposure to the blood and other body fluids of women during childbirth would infect them with HIV. But even in the face of that potential risk, pregnant women still had the right to refuse HIV testing. Could Wilfert recruit women for her trial, given that most people did not want to know their HIV status?

Despite all these difficulties, Wilfert and a small group of like-minded physicians persisted in championing the idea. The protocol committee, headed by Edward Connor, held numerous discussions within the ACTG and with FDA officials to debate the issues, negotiating the delicate balance between the benefits of preventing HIV infection versus the risks of causing permanent, perhaps debilitating, birth defects. Slowly, the idea gained momentum, but designing a study that satisfied all the critics was not easy.[48] Connor's committee had no direct evidence to guide them in choosing an optimal dosing regimen, assuming that such a regimen even existed. So, their study design was driven by a desire to deliver maximal drug exposure at minimal risk to the baby.[49] Not knowing when HIV transmission occurred, they assumed that it could occur at any time throughout pregnancy, which meant starting AZT treatment as soon as possible. But they also wanted to minimize the chance of causing birth defects. Because most birth defects occur in the first trimester, they decided to begin giving AZT to the pregnant women at fourteen weeks and continue the regimen through the remainder of pregnancy. In addition, they decided to give a constant intravenous infusion of AZT while the mother was in labor, to ensure that she maintained a high level of drug in her body, and hopefully some of the drug would reach the baby before and during childbirth. Finally, they decided to give the baby AZT for six weeks after birth. The cutoff was somewhat arbitrary, but they hoped that six weeks would be sufficient time for any of the mother's residual virus to clear from the baby's body. After years of debate and delays, the ACTG reached a consensus, and the study, which was designated ACTG 076, finally started in April 1991.[50]

Still, the AZT regimen used in the ACTG 076 trial, although devised rationally, "was a shot in the dark" and many were skeptical whether AZT — or any drug — would work.[51] AZT was inherently short acting, making it a nuisance to take, and no one had worked out the optimal dosing schedule for women. To ensure adequate drug exposure, the pregnant mothers took doses of AZT five times a day, and the newborns received AZT by mouth four times a day. Given the less-than-ideal pharmaceutical properties of AZT, the risks of drug-induced side effects in individuals when they were most vulnerable, and the uncertainty of how HIV was transmitted, BI's hesitation to conduct a comparable trial using nevirapine was justified. If AZT failed to prevent HIV infections in newborns — and that was the most likely outcome — nevirapine probably would not work, either.

Sometimes, proceeding in the dark and aiming an arrow at the elusive, mythical dragon trumps all the rational arguments for not proceeding. Sometimes, the stakes are so high and the status quo is so unacceptable that taking aim in any direction is better than not shooting at all. The investigators of the ACTG 076 trial strained to see a ray of light in the darkness, took aim with more conviction than confidence, and hit the dragon right between the eyes. The results of the clinical trial, announced in February 1994, were impressive, beating the investigators' most optimistic expectations. The long, inconvenient dosing regimen of AZT reduced the risk of HIV infections in infants by two-thirds.[52] Within months, the United States Public Health Service published guidelines for using AZT to prevent HIV transmission from mothers to infants, based on the study's findings.[53] Public and private organizations immediately launched AIDS prevention programs, implementing the new health service guidelines nationwide. Within a year, the rate of HIV infections among infants born to HIV-infected mothers dropped by almost half and soon fell to less than two percent in the United States.[54]

* * *

In April 1995, Maria was admitted to the University of Massachusetts Medical Center.[55] She was in labor and had already made arrangements for her newborn fraternal twins to be adopted. Everything seemed normal and routine until a few days later when the doctors reviewed Maria's hospital laboratory results. Although she had no AIDS symptoms, Maria was infected with HIV, and the doctors were concerned that she might have also infected the twins during childbirth.[56] Had they known about Maria's infection earlier, the doctors would have given her AZT during the final stages of pregnancy and throughout labor, according to the newly established Public Health Service guidelines. But it was too late for that. As a precaution, they began treating the twins, Jason and Jane, with a five-week regimen of AZT—hoping that AZT would block any virus circulating in their blood from taking root.

The doctors continued to monitor Jason and Jane after completion of the five-week AZT regimen. By most measures, they were normal babies, and they had healthy immune systems. Unfortunately, both Jason and Jane soon developed a high viral load of HIV.[57] They were only ten weeks old, but suddenly the course of Jason and Jane's lives changed from that of carefree youngsters to a lifetime of doctor's appointments, drug treatment, and constant vigilance to keep their HIV infections in check.

* * *

Despite its success in wiping out HIV transmission from mothers to babies in the United States, Europe, and other wealthy nations, the AZT dosing schedule established by the ACTG 076 trial was too complicated, expensive, and impractical for use in developing countries, where healthcare during pregnancy was limited and treatments needed to be both simple and inexpensive.[58] And as Maria's case illustrated, failing to follow the complete AZT regimen in both mothers and babies greatly diminished the drug's ability to work. Nevirapine offered an attractive alternative, and Lange, Sullivan, and others continued to champion clinical trials using nevirapine in pregnant women and newborns in sub–Saharan Africa, where more than 500,000 children, primarily infants born to HIV-infected mothers, became infected each year.[59] Myers communicated frequently with Lange and other international clinicians and offered comments on the design of these clinical trials. But within BI, the idea failed to gain any traction. As the team continued testing HIV-infected adults at lightning speed, the clinical trials that might prove the efficacy of nevirapine to prevent HIV infection in infants languished for years.[60]

By this time, a number of researchers had produced data indicating that up to seventy percent of mother-to-child transmissions of HIV occurred during labor and delivery.[61] This observation led them to think that a shorter and more manageable drug regimen might work as well as the cumbersome AZT regimen used in the ACTG 076 trial. If so, they would be able to prevent HIV infections in areas of the world where simple but effective drug regimens were desperately needed. Unable to obtain nevirapine, which was still an experimental drug controlled by BI, investigators redesigned their clinical trials of these short-term regimens with the only available alternative, AZT.

In 1996, investigators from the United States Centers for Disease Control and Prevention and two Bangkok hospitals collaborated on a placebo-controlled clinical trial in Thailand to examine the value of a short-term AZT regimen.[62] This experimental regimen started later in pregnancy, required less frequent dosing, involved no intravenous infusions, and required no infant treatment. And it worked. The Thai short-term AZT regimen reduced the rate of infant HIV infections by half, compared to the placebo group. The Centers for Disease Control and Prevention estimated that this simpler, less expensive AZT regimen could prevent thousands of infant HIV infections in developing countries.[63]

Also in 1996, Lange, now having returned to the University of Amsterdam, led a team of Dutch investigators to examine another short-term drug regimen in pregnant women in Tanzania, South Africa, and Uganda. To provide extra protection, the investigators paired AZT with 3TC, a second-generation AZT-like drug that had recently been approved.[64] This PETRA study (short for Promoting Evaluation, Teaching, and Research on AIDS) was sponsored by the United Nations AIDS agency, supplemented with funds from the Australian, Italian, and Swedish governments, and showed that only a few doses of AZT/3TC given during labor and for one week after the baby's birth reduced HIV transmission — the shortest effective regimen yet discovered. Unlike the Thai study, most of the African mothers in the PETRA study breastfed their infants. Concerned that the babies might still become infected through their mothers' milk, Lange continued to follow the babies in the PETRA study for 18 months after birth.[65]

* * *

Although investigators were making steady progress streamlining the AZT regimens, they still argued that nevirapine's pharmaceutical properties made it an attractive, and potentially better, option for preventing mother-to-child transmission of HIV. Despite the encouraging evidence from Adams's chimpanzee study and Myers's full-throated support, BI instead focused on the ongoing clinical trials of HIV-infected adults. Recent laboratory experiments using a new treatment strategy had bolstered the project team's confidence in nevirapine's therapeutic value to treat adult AIDS patients. They called the new drug regimen "convergent combination therapy."

12

The Trifecta

In February 1993, newspapers and wire services reported that laboratory workers had succeeded in wiping out HIV infections.[1] Using a combination of three drugs in their laboratory experiments, researchers at Massachusetts General Hospital could prevent the virus from infecting healthy cells as well as clear HIV from cells that had already become infected.[2] They called the phenomenon convergent combination therapy, and the report raised hopes in an increasingly impatient AIDS community that a cure had finally been found.

* * *

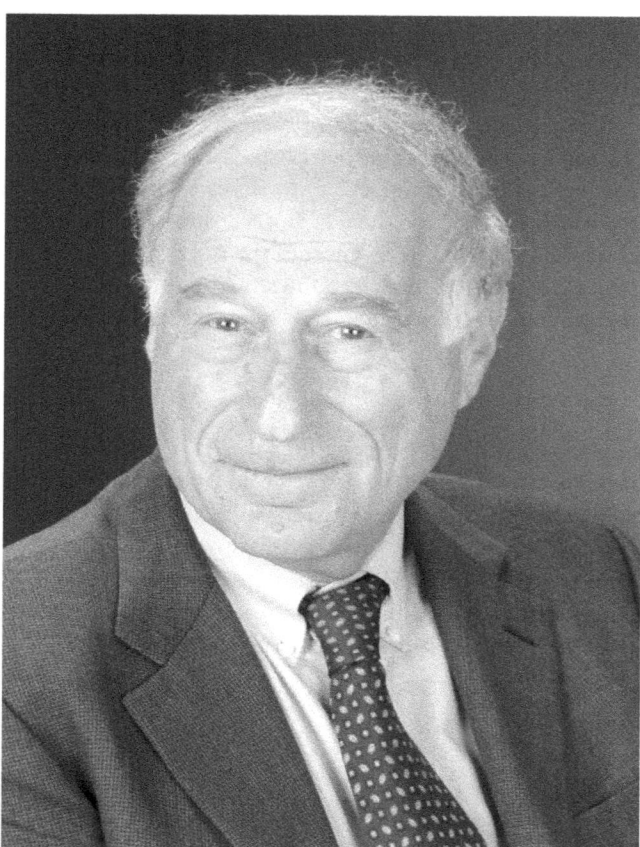

Martin Hirsch.

As a youngster, Martin Hirsch wanted to be a veterinarian — until a visit to a pig farm changed his mind. Instead, he attended Johns Hopkins University Medical School, where a chance opportunity to conduct some immunology research set the course for the rest of his career.[3] After postdoctoral training at the University of Chicago, the Centers for Disease Control, and the National Institute for Medical Research in London, Hirsch arrived in Boston in 1969 to start a clinical and research fellowship in infectious diseases at Massachusetts General Hospital and Harvard Medical School. Two years later, he joined the Harvard faculty. Throughout the 1970s, Hirsch conducted a series of insightful studies describing how viruses cause disease and then applied that knowledge in clinical trials. His ability to translate laboratory observations into innovative medical practices resulted in new treatments for herpes and cytomegalovirus infections. In the 1980s, Hirsch turned his attention to AIDS. He became director of HIV/AIDS activities at Massachusetts General Hospital and director of Harvard's AIDS Clinical Trials Unit, one of the first clinical centers in the newly created ACTG network. Initially, Hirsch and his team concentrated on identifying the locations in the body that harbored HIV. They found the virus in the brain, spinal cord, nerves, and cerebrospinal fluid, findings that helped explain the mental, movement, and sensory losses experienced by many AIDS patients. Hirsch also found infectious virus in the genital secretions of both men and women, confirming that HIV could be transmitted to both sexes.

In 1985, Hirsch's laboratory began exploring drug combinations to stop HIV proliferation, an approach that had been successful in treating other stubborn diseases such as tuberculosis, bacterial endocarditis, and cancer. The early years were frustrating, but as better AIDS drugs emerged, Hirsch's laboratory experiments succeeded more frequently. "Two drugs worked better than one, and three drugs worked better than two."[4] Encouraged by these laboratory results, Hirsch became an early advocate for clinical trials of AIDS drug combinations. While attending the 5th International AIDS Conference in Montreal in 1989, Hirsch and a couple of colleagues brainstormed their ideas during dinner at a French restaurant.[5] They sketched the design for a drug combination clinical trial on a dinner napkin. Then, Hirsch, a charter member of the AIDS Clinical Trials Group, took the concept that he and his colleagues had drafted and presented it to the ACTG. Wanting to build on this basic idea, Hirsch's ACTG colleagues asked him to draft a Master Protocol, a document that could serve as the blueprint for clinical trials using various AIDS drug combinations.

At the July 1991 meeting of the ACTG in Washington, DC, a subcommittee discussed Hirsch's draft of the Master Protocol and their options for appropriate drug combinations. AZT, ddI, and ddC each caused side effects, and combining them might produce intolerable side effects that would offset any therapeutic benefit. Hirsch proposed using nevirapine, a potentially more attractive choice, as a pilot drug to test the Master Protocol. But at that time, Boehringer Ingelheim had just begun the Christmas tree clinical trials and had not yet established nevirapine's safety, effectiveness, or optimal dosing conditions. Hirsch continued to craft his Master Protocol and moved forward with a scaled-back clinical trial that examined the two-drug combinations of AZT, pairing it with either ddI or ddC.[6]

* * *

Meanwhile, Yung-Kang Chow, a student in the MD-PhD program at Harvard, was conducting his research project in Hirsch's laboratory, studying whether drug combinations could overcome viral resistance. HIV readily mutated in the presence of a single AIDS drug, eventually resisting the drug's effects and continued proliferating. But Chow reasoned that there was a limit to how much the virus could mutate and still function. He decided to choose drugs that would gang up on the virus by targeting the same critical point in the virus's life cycle, the reverse transcriptase enzyme. Put in enough drugs, all converging to inhibit this single enzyme in slightly different ways, and the drugs would either do their job (inhibiting the enzyme) or force the enzyme to shape-shift into a completely dysfunctional form. Either way, the virus would be shut down. Chow called this idea convergent combination therapy.

For nine months, Chow methodically compiled evidence in his laboratory assays to support his ideas about convergent combination therapy. His data seemed to prove that the combination of AZT, ddI, and Merck's "L" drug forced the enzyme to mutate into such a deformed shape that HIV could not survive. In his cell-based assays, the three-drug combination stopped the spread of the viral infection, and eventually HIV disappeared from his cultured cells altogether. In some of his experiments, Chow substituted BI's nevirapine for Merck's "L" drug, and it worked just as well. This was not surprising, because all of the non-nucleoside inhibitors, such as nevirapine, the "L" drug, and Janssen's TIBO compounds, induced an identical form of viral resistance. But none of the other AIDS drugs or various drug combinations that Chow tried reduced HIV infection like the three-drug combination of AZT, ddI, and the "L" drug (or nevirapine).

Chow and Richard D'Aquila (Chow's immediate mentor in Hirsch's laboratory) presented their preliminary results at the 8th International AIDS Conference in Amsterdam in July 1992.[7] Although scientifically intriguing, the paper generated only mild interest and no publicity. Many researchers were exploring novel ideas about how to attack the AIDS virus, but most of those ideas never advanced beyond the laboratory. Chow's ideas seemed radical, and this critical audience had been fooled many times before. Clinicians, reporters, government regulators, advocacy groups, and patients all wanted better AIDS treatments, but they would remain skeptical until they saw proof that those treatments worked in HIV-infected people.

Shortly after returning from Amsterdam, Chow, D'Aquila, and others in Hirsch's laboratory completed their experiments and submitted a manuscript to the prestigious scientific journal, *Nature*. In September, Chow traveled to Ridgefield and presented his data to the BI scientists, showing that the combination of nevirapine, AZT, and ddI could knock out HIV infections under laboratory conditions — the most dramatic antiviral effect that the BI scientists had ever seen.[8] Excited and intrigued by Chow's data, Peter Grob's research team tested two- and three-drug combinations in their laboratory assays to confirm Chow's result, and they began looking for BI compounds that might work even better than nevirapine.[9] In parallel, Maureen Myers continued discussions with Hirsch on the design of the ACTG Master Protocol. They had known each other from the beginning of the ACTG network, when Myers worked at the National Institutes of Health creating the AIDS Division and Hirsch served as the ACTG's first Executive Committee chairman. Now, Myers directed BI's clinical trials with nevirapine and had engaged Hirsch as a BI clinical consultant.

* * *

At the ACTG meeting in Washington, DC, in November 1992, Hirsch's colleague, Richard D'Aquila, delivered a presentation on the convergent resistance hypothesis, citing Chow's data as justification for a comparable clinical drug regimen. Hirsch, with Myers's backing, presented the latest version of his clinical trial Master Protocol and received general support from the ACTG committee.[10] Plans moved forward to start an ACTG-sponsored trial in early 1993, based on D'Aquila and Hirsch's design and using nevirapine in the triple-drug combination. But the BI project team first needed to address some important safety questions about nevirapine.

The Food and Drug Administration had approved Bristol-Myers Squibb's ddI, making it, along with AZT, readily available for use in the proposed clinical trial, but nevirapine was still an experimental drug. The Christmas tree studies confirmed that nevirapine could be given safely in combination with AZT, but the BI team had not examined the safety of a nevirapine-ddI combination. The risks of undesirable drug interactions from a three-drug combination of nevirapine, AZT, and ddI had also not been assessed.

Within a month of the ACTG meeting, BI started a small clinical trial at the University of Alabama in Birmingham to study the safety of various combinations nevirapine, ddI, and AZT in HIV-infected adults.[11] The investigators quickly established that the three-drug combination was safe and produced acceptable blood levels of all three drugs. The BI team therefore decided to continue treating these patients to establish long term safety of the drug combinations. They also hoped to gather some preliminary evidence indicating that the three-drug regimen suppressed the patients' viral load of HIV, as Chow's experiments predicted.

Jim Wright knew the BI team would face another complication when they gave ddI as part of a drug combination. Patients were instructed to take ddI with an antacid, because the drug otherwise broke down quickly in stomach acid.[12] Unfortunately, the absorption of nevirapine depended, in part, on the stomach's acidic environment. If nevirapine was taken at the same time as ddI, the antacid would likely interfere with nevirapine's ability to dissolve and be absorbed into the bloodstream. One day, Wright decided "to have a little fun" and wheeled a cart of flasks into the project team meeting to demonstrate these stomach acid properties.[13] He dissolved a sample of nevirapine in a liquid that simulated stomach acid, creating a clear solution. When he added the antacid solution containing ddI, the mixture turned cloudy, and white particles of nevirapine drifted to the bottom of the flask like flakes in a snow globe. It was the first, and probably the only, experiment ever conducted in BI's new office building, but Wright had convincingly demonstrated the problem.[14] In the clinical trial, patients would need to take their doses of ddI and nevirapine at different times of the day, allowing time for the stomach's acid to adjust, before and after antacid treatment.

* * *

By January 1993, the ACTG Master Protocol was finally approaching consensus approval, after years of refining and adjusting a multitude of details to satisfy the diverse views expressed in numerous discussions with BI and the ACTG. This first clinical test of the triple-therapy idea was an ambitious undertaking for Hirsch, BI, and the ACTG, and they had prudently considered every aspect of the protocol. Everyone agreed that this clinical trial needed to be large enough, designed well enough, and conducted carefully enough to produce convincing data. The triple therapy idea might work, it might not work. Either way, Hirsch, the BI team, and the ACTG all wanted to make sure that the final data left no doubts about the study's outcome. There was a lot at stake.

Despite Hirsch's vast experience in HIV research and AIDS clinical trials, this trial might fail to deliver the results that Chow's laboratory experiments predicted. After all, the highly touted scientific "breakthroughs" of many previous laboratory studies had not translated to successful clinical trials. For BI, this study represented the most ambitious clinical trial of nevirapine conducted to date, and it came at a particularly critical time. The BI project team had been constantly adjusting their plans, reacting to each new clinical revelation, and struggling to define a niche for nevirapine in the realm of AIDS therapeutics.[15] And in the process, the AIDS community's enthusiasm for nevirapine had dampened considerably. BI was having "an extremely hard time keeping the drug in clinical trials."[16] Many patients dropped out and opted to sign up for clinical trials of more promising experimental AIDS drugs. The triple-therapy trial was yet another attempt to demonstrate nevirapine's therapeutic value. For the ACTG, officials faced the administrative challenges of coordinating patient treatment with three drugs manufactured by three different drug companies and harmonizing the work of participating clinical investigators who were spread literally from coast to coast.

Then, on February 18, 1993, the lengthy deliberations, the constant tweaking of the study protocol, and the long stretches of slow progress between ACTG meetings suddenly ended. Chow and Hirsch's research paper, which had been submitted the previous July, was finally published in *Nature*.[17] And Chow's concept of convergent combination therapy "took the antiretroviral world by storm."[18] Major newspapers, wire services, AIDS newsletters, and the editorial pages of scientific journals all carried the news that the research group in Boston had made a major breakthrough, one that might roll back, if not eliminate, AIDS. Reporters hounded Chow and Hirsch for interviews, and the 31-year-old graduate student's photo was published in the *New York Times* and *Scientific American*.[19] They earnestly and humbly tried to downplay speculation about their results, repeatedly pointing out that the real value of their findings would need to be proven by further testing in clinical trials. Similarly, the press release issued by Massachusetts General Hospital, one of the oldest, most prestigious, and conservative hospitals in the country, included multiple cautions about not misinterpreting or overstating Chow's results, emphasizing those cautions with underlined and bold-faced type.[20]

But nothing could dampen, much less stop, the surge of optimism this news generated in the hearts of an increasingly desperate public. For more than a decade, researchers had spent billions of dollars conducting brilliant science, but little of it had translated into new AIDS drugs. The AIDS pandemic was spreading—thousands of people were becoming infected every day, and most of them were doomed to die for lack of an effective treatment. The public's anxiety about AIDS was heightened by the recent deaths of tennis champion Arthur Ashe and Russian ballet star Rudolf Nureyev.[21] Jonas Salk's much-touted AIDS vaccine had failed, as had the Concorde study, in which AZT failed to delay the onset of AIDS symptoms or prolong the lives of HIV-infected people.[22] The 9th International AIDS Conference, held later that year in Berlin, would be remembered as the most disheartening leg of the AIDS scientific marathon, littered with many disappointments and setbacks.[23] In the face of this prevailing mood of despair and confusion,[24] Chow's convergent combination therapy represented the first good news people had heard in a long time—perhaps the best news since the discovery of AZT.

The public's enthusiasm vastly accelerated the pace of ACTG's plans for the triple-drug clinical trial. A few days after the *Nature* paper appeared, the ACTG group gathered for their sixteenth meeting at the Ramada Renaissance Techworld Hotel in Washington, DC, and everyone rushed to finalize the plans for the triple-drug clinical trial. They chose nevirapine, AZT, and ddI as the three drugs for the study. Even though Chow had generated more data with Merck's "L" drug, nevirapine and the "L" drug appeared to produce the same results in Chow's laboratory tests, and many of the ACTG investigators favored nevirapine based on their experience with it in previous clinical trials. The trial would be jointly sponsored by the ACTG, Boehringer Ingelheim (the maker of nevirapine), Burroughs Wellcome (the maker of AZT), and Bristol-Myers Squibb (the maker of ddI). D'Aquila and Hirsch, colleagues at Massachusetts General Hospital, headed the clinical team, which included nine other clinical centers around the United States.[25] A total of 200 HIV-infected adults would be recruited and divided into two groups. One group would receive daily doses of AZT and ddI, a drug combination that Hirsch and his colleagues had proven to be superior to AZT in their earlier clinical trial—the trial that had been designed on the restaurant napkin in Montreal.[26] The other group would receive daily doses of the triple-drug combination: nevirapine, AZT, and ddI. Chow's theory predicted that the triple-drug regimen could suppress HIV indefinitely, so the investigators decided to continue the drug treatment for 48 weeks, a period of time much longer than any individual AIDS drug was known to work. The trial medications were coded, and no one knew which treatment regimen was being given to each patient. Consequently, until the codes were broken at the end of the one-year treatment period, no one would know whether nevirapine, in the triple-drug combination, worked better than the AZT-ddI regimen.

When the news media reported plans for the triple-drug clinical trial, BI was besieged with inquiries from the anxious but hopeful AIDS community.[27] Following the ACTG meeting, Myers headed a team that spent two months touring the country, meeting with patient advocates and publishers of AIDS-affiliated newsletters.[28] Their goal was to communicate BI's plans for developing nevirapine, manage the public's expectations about the triple-drug combination clinical trial, and provide a forum for dialogue.[29] The only people who had taken the triple-drug regimen were those in the small study at the University of Alabama in Birmingham. Some patients in that study had been treated for five months without notable side effects, but it was too early to assess whether the triple-drug therapy had worked. Myers repeatedly reminded her audiences that BI was exploring many ways of using nevirapine alone and in various other combinations, not just Chow's triple-therapy idea.[30] As the nevirapine program moved forward and results became available, she reassured the advocacy groups that BI would continue to inform them and solicit their input.

A week after Chow and Hirsch's *Nature* paper was published, another press release hit the newswire, announcing a corresponding three-drug clinical trial, using L-697,661 (one of Merck's "L" drugs) in combination with AZT and ddI.[31] This clinical trial, sponsored by Merck, involved only three clinical sites, would proceed more cautiously, and would follow the patients half as long as D'Aquila and Hirsch's ACTG-sponsored trial.[32] Chow had generated most of his laboratory data using the "L" drug in his triple-drug experiments, a sound rationale for conducting clinical trials with these same three drugs. Although Merck had abandoned development of L-697,661 due to resistance and had turned to another "L" drug, the company had decided that Chow's data justified further clinical trials to examine whether the original "L" drug would work better when combined with AZT and ddI.

Enrollment opened in the D'Aquila-Hirsch clinical trial in May 1993. Suddenly, after months of declining interest in nevirapine, everyone wanted to get into this trial. Within a few weeks, ACTG doubled the number of patients who were allowed to enroll in the trial to a total of 400 and expanded the number of clinical sites from ten to sixteen. Ten to twenty people competed for each slot in the clinical trial, and the investigators set up waiting lists and lotteries to parcel enrollment fairly.[33] By July, only a couple of months after the trial started, the investigators had filled all 400 slots.

* * *

The publicity surrounding the D'Aquila-Hirsch clinical trial raised the hopes of many desperate AIDS patients and their families, including the parents of a little boy in New York City.[34] David had become infected with HIV through a contaminated blood transfusion in the late 1980s, a condition unnoticed until he began suffering the symptoms of AIDS.[35] He had been treated with AZT, which worked for a while. Then, his parents sought treatment with the newer, AZT-like drugs, but soon those drugs also failed to work. David was now about the same age as Ariel Glaser when she had been hospitalized and, like her, his condition was deteriorating for lack of any alternative treatment. When the news of the miraculous triple-drug regimen reached David's father, he was determined to get it for his son, no matter what it took. Through David's physicians and other contacts in New York, his father tried to get a supply of nevirapine for him. Unfortunately, they explained, nevirapine was still an experimental drug and could only be obtained from BI, the company that made it. And BI could only dispense nevirapine according to rules laid down by the FDA.

On a Friday in the spring of 1993, David and his father got in the family car and made the ninety-minute drive north to Ridgefield, reaching the gates of BI in early afternoon. Inside the high wrought iron fence that surrounded the wooded estate, BI's assembly line was cranking out thousands of nevirapine tablets every hour, all destined for patients in the ongoing clinical trials. David's father demanded just a few of those tablets for his son, and he refused to leave until he got them. But like all drug companies, BI did not conduct clinical trials on its campus and did not have the facilities to evaluate David's condition or monitor his treatment. The nearest clinic where BI was sponsoring clinical trials with nevirapine was the University of Massachusetts in Worcester.

When John Sullivan's phone rang late on that Friday afternoon, he was wrapping up another busy week of work, reviewing the latest data from his laboratory studies of HIV, monitoring his own patients, and watching with great interest nevirapine's role in the new triple-drug clinical trial. The caller was Alan Rosenthal, who described the drama unfolding outside BI's gates and asked Sullivan whether he would be willing to see this patient. Sullivan readily agreed.[36] After some tense negotiations, David's father packed up his son and drove north another two hours to Worcester, Massachusetts, where Sullivan and his colleague, Katherine Luzuriaga, were waiting.

Although Sullivan and Luzuriaga had been conducting nevirapine clinical trials from the beginning, the Worcester site was not one of the sixteen sites in D'Aquila-Hirsch's triple-drug trial. And unfortunately, that trial was enrolling only adults. They were discussing plans for a comparable triple-drug combination trial in children, but that pediatric clinical trial would not officially start for another year. The University of Massachusetts team had only one remaining option in David's case. They were required to petition BI and ask the company to grant "compassionate use" of the drug, outside the normal clinical trial procedures. They worked into the weekend, evaluating David's condition, completing all the paperwork, and obtaining signatures from the appropriate hospital officials within twenty-four hours. The clinicians at BI, accustomed to handling calls from clinical investigators at all hours, were standing by, quickly processed the request through the appropriate regulatory channels, and authorized the University of Massachusetts team to proceed. Consequently, under the compassionate use mechanism, David became the first pediatric patient to receive the nevirapine triple-combination therapy.[37]

* * *

Many AIDS experts, including those who respected Hirsch and believed Chow's results, openly worried that patients, the media, and the public in general were overreacting to Chow's convergent combination theory.[38] Despite Hirsch's best efforts to downplay the significance of the laboratory experiments, many people were taking the findings out of context, a false optimism that might lead to disappointment and even be dangerous. The news of previous "breakthroughs" had put vulnerable patients on a rollercoaster, buoying them up with unrealistic hope and then inevitably dashing those hopes when the real news fell short of their expectations. Investigators worried that some patients might abandon proven drug treatments to try this unproven regimen. While they acknowledged and supported the triple-drug clinical trial as a critical test of the convergent combination idea, they cautioned that the impressive laboratory results might not be confirmed in clinical trials. And they pointed out that the nevirapine-AZT-ddI regimen was not the only idea being explored by clinical investigators. The ACTG was sponsoring other drug combinations in clinical trials without the bluster and bravado that the nevirapine/AZT/ddI combination had generated.

BI never publicly endorsed Chow's concept of convergent combination therapy.[39] To dampen the hyped up, worldwide speculation, the company held a rare news conference in Ridgefield.[40] BI spokesmen expressed doubts that the triple-drug regimen would produce the same results in people as Chow had seen in the laboratory. The BI team was continuing a full range of ongoing clinical trials, confident that they could boost nevirapine's effects by pairing it with AZT or one of the other new AIDS drugs, but not promising a cure. Like everyone else, they were awaiting the results from all of the clinical trials and would not speculate in the meantime. But inside BI, the project team had shifted into overdrive.

* * *

The speed with which D'Aquila-Hirsch's triple-drug combination trial was proceeding and the renewed public interest in nevirapine caused the BI project team to reexamine its development plans. If everything continued to go well, they expected nevirapine would be introduced to the market before 1996. Among other things, they realized that the drug still needed a brand name. The trademark registration process normally took about two years to complete, and the project team worried that they might actually complete the development program before they finalized a registered trademark. The team reviewed a list of possible brand names that had been presented by their marketing representative and indicated their preferences: Viramun (debating whether it might alternatively be Viramune), Virune, Revune, Bixir, and Novirep. Various BI stakeholders evaluated and shuffled those names, and the company continued the methodical process of registering the trademarks internationally.

* * *

Chow's published results tipped the balance in another clinical trial initiative that had been brewing for some time. Many drug companies were developing AIDS drugs, each designed to attack the AIDS virus in a slightly different way. Some drugs, such as AZT, ddI, and ddC, had been more successful than others, but the limited duration of clinical benefit strongly suggested that no single drug could stop HIV. Chow's findings reinforced the views of many investigators who increasingly advocated using drug combinations. But those drug combinations most likely were products manufactured by competing drug companies. If AIDS treatment was to advance, those companies would need to find a way, despite their legendary concerns about trade secrets and government-imposed regulatory constraints, to collaborate, "share information early [and] figure out which drugs will work best together."[41]

The notion of an industry collaboration originated with two Merck executives, Roy Vagelos and Edward Scolnick.[42] When they floated the idea with their counterparts at other companies involved with AIDS drug development, some executives were willing to consider collaborating but others raised a number of concerns. Not fazed by the difficulties, Vagelos and Scolnick persisted in fostering the idea in many behind-the-scenes meetings and informal discussions. Finally, the same week that Chow's research paper was published, the fifteen major drug companies most active in AIDS research, including Boehringer Ingelheim, Burroughs Wellcome, Hoffmann-La Roche, Bristol-Myers Squibb, and Merck came together to form the Inter-Company Collaboration for AIDS Drug Development.[43] Although their goal — to facilitate more rapid development of drugs to fight HIV — was admirable, they struggled to reach a consensus on how to do it. These were self-assured leaders more accustomed to leading subordinates than cooperating with demanding people who were not only their peers but also their competitors. Occasional gnashing of teeth and more than a few bulging neck veins characterized those early discussions, as their legal advisors whispered in their ears, reminding them not to violate the United States' antitrust laws or the European Union's competition law.[44] But within a few months, they hammered out an acceptable and legally compliant agreement to work collaboratively on clinical trials, share data, and, where appropriate, share drug supplies to expedite combination regimens of AIDS drugs.

After the ground rules for the collaboration had been settled, senior clinical and scientific representatives from each company met regularly to exchange information. Despite the large number of participants (usually thirty to forty people, half of whom were lawyers), the group managed to make steady progress.[45] This unique industry collaboration expedited more efficient clinical trials of drug combinations and facilitated development of standardized laboratory assay methods for measuring HIV viral load and immune system function.[46] Over the next few years, Maureen Myers and Johanna Griffin represented BI in these discussions, and nevirapine factored significantly in the drug combination clinical trials sponsored by this collaborative group.[47]

* * *

In addition to the flurry of activity to test Chow's convergent combination therapy in clinical trials, researchers rushed to their laboratories to see if they could independently reproduce and expand upon Chow's intriguing laboratory findings. The most distinguished of these research teams were at Burroughs Wellcome, the makers of AZT, and at Merck, the makers of the "L" drugs.[48] Within a few months, both groups had recreated Chow's experiments, but unfortunately neither group observed the dramatic results that Chow had reported. They could not eliminate HIV from infected cells with the three-drug combination, as Chow had claimed. The resistant virus, instead of mutating itself to death, was in fact still viable. These new reports by Merck and Burroughs Wellcome lent support to those who had tried to temper the hype surrounding Chow and Hirsch's original publication. The contradictory experimental results needed to be explained, and it fell to Chow to sort things out.

Chow returned to the laboratory, reviewed his experiments, and re-examined his biological samples. He discovered that he had made a mistake.[49] His virus samples contained additional mutations than the ones he had originally observed. Also, he realized that he had not monitored his HIV-infected cells long enough. Eventually, the virus in those cells mutated to a form that could resist the triple-drug combination. Chow, D'Aquila, and Hirsch quickly acknowledged these errors in a follow up letter that was published in *Nature*.[50] They also presented their corrected findings in July 1993, at the 9th International AIDS Conference in Berlin, adding another layer of bad news to so many other failures reported at that Conference.[51] In addition to the failed attempts to produce a vaccine and the poor performance of AZT in the Concorde trial, investigators at the Berlin Conference also reported disappointing results of the first large clinical trial of a drug combination. This trial examined the combination of AZT and ddC and showed that the two-drug regimen was more toxic and no more effective than AZT alone.[52] Those who had enthusiastically embraced Chow's convergent combination idea and thought that a three-drug combination might eliminate HIV infections now had good reason to doubt the approach. Perhaps, these combination regimens would only increase the side effects of drugs that were already known to be toxic individually.

When Chow and the other laboratories disclosed the errors in his original work, the news created another publicity blitz, making the front page of the *New York Times* and generating the same over-reaction as his original finding.[53] The news, along with the failure of the AZT-ddC combination clinical trial, forced a critical review of the D'Aquila-Hirsch triple-drug clinical trial. Just as suddenly as people had climbed up the rollercoaster tracks hoping that combination therapy would save them, the rollercoaster had plummeted and shattered their faith in this new treatment regimen. All of the patients had now enrolled and begun treatment, but should D'Aquila and Hirsch continue their trial for the entire one-year treatment period? The ACTG committee discussed the matter, and most investigators, including the critics of Chow's original findings, said yes. Triple-drug therapy was still a good idea and needed to be tested — it just might not be the cure-all that people hoped it would be. The clinical trial would continue as planned, but the ACTG committee sent a letter to all participants in the study, notifying them of the new and less-optimistic laboratory findings and inviting them to discuss this information with their study physician. After considering their options, 341 people decided to stay in the trial.[54]

One year was a long time to wait for an answer to the triple-drug treatment regimen — an outcome that was now less certain than everyone had hoped — and the newsletters of AIDS advocacy groups carried numerous editorials urging investigators to pursue additional studies that would get answers sooner.[55] They wanted patients who were deteriorating on other therapies switched to the triple-drug regimen and greater access of experimental drugs to patients who did not qualify for the clinical trials. At BI, expanded access was an option that had been looming in the background for a long time. Now, it surfaced again with greater urgency, driven not only by pressure from patient advocacy groups but also by the possibility that the outcome of the D'Aquila-Hirsch triple-drug clinical trial would put nevirapine on an even faster track, requiring more drug supplies and reducing their control over development of a promising but still experimental drug.

13

Supply and Demand: Getting to PICNIC

Ordinarily, chemists at drug companies are able to improve the yield and streamline production to deliver the drug supplies required for clinical trials. But AIDS drugs were not ordinary, and there was nothing ordinary about those clinical trials. Desperately ill patients demanded greater and earlier access to experimental AIDS drugs, and that created greater and earlier stresses on drug production.

Anthony Fauci, the Director of the National Institute of Allergy and Infectious Diseases, was instrumental in promoting a "parallel track," which was first proposed by several advocacy groups in 1989.[1] They wanted wider distribution of experimental drugs to HIV-infected people who had no therapeutic alternatives or did not qualify for ongoing clinical trials, a distribution track that would run in parallel with, but separate from, the official clinical trials.[2] The parallel track program, which the Food and Drug Administration announced in July 1989 and published as a new policy on May 21, 1990, increased the demand for experimental AIDS drugs at a much earlier stage of development, a time when they had only shown the "promise" of working based on limited animal and clinical testing.

While the proposal for a parallel track system was making its way through the government's review process, drug companies improvised expanded access programs. In 1989, Bristol-Myers Squibb took advantage of existing FDA provisions to offer ddI to patients who could not tolerate AZT, had failed to benefit from AZT treatment, or were not eligible to participate in the ongoing ddI clinical trials.[3] Hoffmann-La Roche launched a similar expanded access program to distribute ddC.[4] Thousands of patients received ddI or ddC through these programs.[5]

By the time nevirapine entered clinical trials in January 1991, the FDA was encouraging all companies, including Boehringer Ingelheim, to incorporate expanded access in their development plans for new AIDS drugs.[6] Throughout 1991, expanded access was always included in the BI project team's discussions when they reviewed and revised the nevirapine development plan. Included in the discussion, that is, but not incorporated in the plan. Certainly, distributing nevirapine to patients through an expanded access program was consistent with BI's corporate values as a caring pharmaceutical company and the actions of other companies developing AIDS drugs. But expanded access was the project plan's fifth wheel — not really needed, not really wanted, perhaps adding some value, but always threatening to pull the team's development plans off course.

In executing their expanded access programs, Bristol-Myers Squibb and Hoffmann-La Roche learned bruising lessons, which the BI team heeded. So many people participated in Bristol-Myers Squibb's expanded access program (more than 20,000 overall) that the company had difficulty recruiting patients for its clinical trials, delaying collection of critical data needed for regulatory approval of ddI.[7] Hoffmann-La Roche's ddC was known to cause nerve damage and other serious side effects, and some critics questioned widespread distribution of ddC before sufficient data from controlled clinical trials had established proper treatment conditions. They worried that the lack of close oversight put patients in the expanded ddC program at unreasonable risk.[8]

During the early days of the nevirapine clinical program, the project team constantly juggled their plans to match the delivery of Karl Grozinger's drug batches. Their highest priorities were the ACTG-sponsored clinical trials, long term toxicology studies, and formulation development work. But BI's international clinical consultants were also eager to begin clinical trials in other countries. And then there was the allocation for the expanded access program, the biggest potential drain on their drug supplies. Without expanded access, the team could keep nevirapine development on a fast track. With expanded access, they would have to ration drug supplies for their clinical trials and other key studies. Unsympathetic patient advocacy groups, especially the New York unit of ACT UP, kept up the pressure through the summer and fall of 1991, urging BI to move forward with an expanded access program as soon as possible.[9]

At the same time, AIDS community clinics and patient advocacy groups were urging Maureen Myers and the BI clinicians to include a Large Simple Trial in the BI clinical plan and to schedule the start of that trial soon. The basic idea was to enroll and treat a very large number of patients — perhaps up to 10,000 — regardless of the state of their health or the other drugs they were taking.[10] In the opinion of those AIDS groups, a Large Simple Trial helped both the patients and the drug company. Thousands of HIV-infected people would have access to the experimental drug, and the large trial would allow the drug company to determine whether the drug worked in a relatively short time, facilitating its approval. ACT UP offered suggestions on how BI should design such a trial with nevirapine.[11]

Myers asked her clinical team to solicit input from BI's independent consultants and experts in the ACTG and the FDA. All of them saw advantages to a Large Simple Trial. Investigators were finding it increasingly difficult to conduct traditional clinical trials in the United States because those trials restricted the use of other medications while the patients were in the trial. A shorter trial would be more attractive to those patients. The Large Simple Trial would also generate extensive data characterizing the drug's side effects. But the Large Simple Trial also posed challenges. Managing the trial, with its large number of patients and widely distributed clinical sites, would be much more difficult than the well-structured trials BI was conducting under the ACTG umbrella. Also, investigators in other countries were less enthusiastic about this type of trial, and the team would likely be limited to enrolling patients at American clinics. Predictably, the FDA took a middle-of-the-road position on the issue. A Large Simple Trial was acceptable to federal regulators, but only if BI had collected sufficient data from previous clinical trials to ensure that the drug was reasonably safe.

Pressed by public sentiment, the project team conducted an exercise to forecast how much drug would be needed for the Large Simple Trial, as well as how many patients might opt to request nevirapine through an expanded access program. Jim Wright, whose job was to monitor the delivery dates of Grozinger's drug batches and coordinate production of the tablets and liquid suspension, took all of the drug supply requirements, converted those requirements into tablet totals and liquid volumes, and proposed how to allocate the tablets and bottles of liquid most efficiently.[12] To cover all of the team's needs, Wright estimated that the chemists would have to double their planned drug batches and deliver one ton of nevirapine within the next year.[13]

Two factors prevented the team from pursuing expanded access and the Large Simple Trial beyond a paper and pencil exercise. Grozinger and his colleagues in BI's large-scale chemical plant had made progress in scaling up production of nevirapine to batches of 100 kilograms (about 220 pounds) or more. But the project team continued to add trials to the clinical plan, along with new toxicology studies and Wright's formulation activities to support them. The chemists' output and delivery schedule were just sufficient to keep up with this demand. They simply could not produce more batches to support an expanded access program or a Large Simple Trial — at least for the moment.

The second factor was the observation, late in 1991, that nevirapine induced viral resistance. Interest in nevirapine by patients and advocacy groups evaporated as quickly as it had appeared. While those groups still advocated rapid and efficient clinical trials to sort out the value, if any, of nevirapine, they were no longer insisting that BI implement an expanded access program quickly. The project team's priorities shifted to address the resistance issue. Now faced with designing different clinical trials to cope with viral resistance and less certain whether nevirapine would be good enough to overcome resistance, the project team pulled back its aggressive plans for large drug batches. Instead of the one ton that Wright had projected, the chemists produced about half that amount, sufficient to support the modest list of ongoing clinical trials but not much more.

* * *

In parallel with supplying nevirapine for the Christmas tree studies, the first international clinical trials, and the first pediatric clinical trials, Karl Grozinger and Julian Adams had been spearheading efforts throughout 1991 to improve their methods and make batches of nevirapine more efficiently, safely, and in higher yields.[14] As the list of clinical trials grew and the demand for expanded access continued, they examined every aspect of Grozinger's original method and explored alternatives that would work better for industrial-scale production.

Grozinger's original laboratory method required seven, sequential chemical reactions to produce nevirapine as the final product. That seven-step process worked reasonably well for small batches in the chemistry laboratory, kilogram-sized batches in Grozinger's pilot plant, and even batches of one hundred kilograms in BI's chemical plant. But to make larger batches for a possible expanded access program as well as for commercial use, the chemists needed to improve their methods. One of the chemicals used in a key reaction step was not available from chemical suppliers in large quantities and had to be produced by the BI chemists. The chemical reaction to produce this key material generated an uncontrollable amount of heat and could only be performed safely in a chemistry laboratory.[15] A few near-accidents in the laboratory convinced the chemists that this method could not be used on a large scale. An explosion was certain and would be catastrophic. So, the chemists abandoned this method and tackled the production of nevirapine from an entirely different angle. The new method would use chemicals that were readily available, solvents that were environmentally friendly, and reaction conditions that were safe and efficient.[16] Using guidelines defined by the FDA, the starting point for the official production of nevirapine was a chemical called CAPIC.[17] In a three-step process, the chemists first converted CAPIC to an intermediate chemical called PICNIC and then through another intermediate step to nevirapine.[18]

Their commitment to move forward with this new method depended on whether

Myers and the clinical team could successfully address the resistance problem. If not, they would not need large batches of nevirapine produced by any method. On the other hand, if the clinicians could overcome resistance by doubling the nevirapine dose, then the chemists would be asked to produce even larger batches. Wright's original calculations had assumed that patients would be taking the dose established in the Christmas tree studies. Doubling that dose meant that the chemists would need to produce twice as much of the drug.

Adams wanted to avoid the problems of other AIDS drug makers, who had resorted to lotteries because their drug supplies had not kept pace with demand. He made his own calculations, and he knew in detail the effort required to produce large drug batches.[19] To supply the fast tracked clinical trials and the anticipated, but still uncertain, commercial drug supplies required considerable planning. It took 14–16 months to produce a ton-sized batch. Despite the uncertainties about the future of nevirapine in June 1992, Adams knew he could not afford to wait. He traveled to Europe to meet with BI's chemical manufacturing group. On his own initiative, he placed a $2.4 million order for one ton of nevirapine.[20] Knowing that he did not have signature authority to cover this order, Adams informed Alan Rosenthal, his boss, as soon as he returned to Ridgefield. After only a moment's reflection, Rosenthal simply said, "Don't ever do that again." Adams replied, "I hope I don't have to."[21]

The ups and downs of drug supply and demand continued through 1992. When the clinicians observed that they could overcome viral resistance by increasing the dose of nevirapine, the project team asked the chemists to speed up production. But within a few months, the problems with nevirapine-induced skin rashes caused the project team to slow down again, as they sorted out whether they could adjust the dosing schedule in a way that reduced the likelihood of skin rashes. The new dosing schedule (a two week lead-in dose of one tablet, followed by a long-term daily dose of two tablets) again put nevirapine on the fast track, and the project team again asked the chemists to ramp up production. During this period of uncertainty, the chemists stuck with Grozinger's original method to make their drug batches. But Grozinger and Adams continued to refine their improved production method and were prepared to implement it as soon as the project team sorted out the direction of the clinical program.

The chemists and formulation scientists were especially relieved when the toxicologists filed the worker safety reports for nevirapine. They were now routinely handling buckets of nevirapine in their efforts to supply drug for the clinical trials and large toxicology studies. Not knowing the drug's side effects, they had been wearing head-to-toe body suits with a self-contained respirator. The toxicologists' assessment of the worker safety data confirmed that nevirapine was safe to handle in bulk quantities and allowed them to shed their bunny suits in favor of less cumbersome laboratory coats, goggles, and gloves.[22]

* * *

Waiting not-so-patiently on the sidelines while the project team grappled with the issues of expanded access, a Large Simple Trial, viral resistance, and skin rashes were the toxicologists. They knew that the 52-week dog toxicology study was required both to support the clinical trials and for regulatory approval. Because it would take nearly two years to conduct the dog study, analyze the data, and complete the final study report, they risked holding up the entire development program if they delayed much longer. But the investment in drug supplies, resources, and number of animals was significant, and no one on the project team wanted to make such a large and expensive commitment until they were confident that the nevirapine clinical trials would continue. Every time the clinical results caused a setback, the dog toxicology study was delayed. When the clinical program got back on track, the dog toxicology study was put back on the schedule. Despite the uncertainty, the toxicologists continued their preparations and worked out procedural details. They wanted to make sure there were no mistakes once they actually started the 52-week study. Among the problems they encountered in their shake-down experiments was the large variation in how individual dogs reacted to drug treatment. Determining the cause of these unexpected differences, which turned out to be due to dogs bred by different animal suppliers, caused further delays in setting a start date for the definitive study.

As time went on, the lack of long-term safety data from the 52-week dog toxicology study became critical to nevirapine's development. When patients completed their treatment in the Christmas tree studies, they were allowed to continue receiving nevirapine under an "open label extension" study, and the earliest of those patients had now been taking the drug for about a year. To comply with FDA requirements, the team needed to collect long-term safety data in animals. Otherwise, they could not continue treatment of the patients. So far, the toxicologists had produced data showing that nevirapine was safe in rats and dogs treated for three months. They had also recently completed the 52-week toxicology study in rats with similar results. But the FDA also required 52-week safety data from a second species. BI's promise to conduct the 52-week dog study had so far satisfied the FDA officials, because the risk to patients was small compared to the potential therapeutic benefits. But that balance between risk and benefit was rapidly shifting as more patients wanted to continue treatment.

* * *

Delivery of a 430 kilogram (about 950 pounds) batch of nevirapine in mid–1992 at first appeared to ease the need for setting priorities and delaying new studies. But when Jim Wright inspected the batch, he saw something unusual: a smattering of tiny specks that had not been present in the previous batches. The specks were too small and too few to be detected when the chemists performed their highly sensitive quality control tests, but the specks' bright blue color stood out against the off-white nevirapine powder.[23] Using a microscope, Wright and his analytical colleagues teased out a few of the specks and determined that they were cobalt chloride, a relatively harmless chemical commonly used in chemical production.[24] Nothing in the nevirapine manufacturing process could explain the appearance of cobalt chloride, and none of the previous batches contained it.[25] The blue specks were finally traced back to a filter or related equipment used to dry the bulk batch of nevirapine. Minute specks of cobalt chloride had clung to the equipment after the production run of another drug immediately preceding its use for the nevirapine batch and caused the contamination.[26] The procedures for cleaning equipment between production runs were revised accordingly, and the problem never resurfaced.

But the blue specks in the delivered batch were an impurity, and they had to be removed from the nevirapine before it could be used in any animal or human studies. Rather than proceeding with their planned campaign to make batches using Grozinger and Adams's new production method, the chemists concentrated their efforts on extracting the little blue specks from the contaminated batch. Once again, the project team was forced to set priorities. The BI team's entire program relied on just-in-time delivery of drug supplies, and any setback, no matter how small, disrupted their aggressive timetable.[27] They allotted the small amount of drug remaining in their inventory to resupply the ongoing clinical trials, and once again the 52-week dog toxicology study was delayed.

By the end of 1992, Grozinger and Adams were finally ready to test their new production method on a large scale. They worked with their colleagues in BI's chemical plant to prepare a test batch of 100 kilograms (about 220 pounds). The test went well and the chemists began planning full-scale production with this new, improved method. The project team again felt confident in making more ambitious clinical plans. Myers and the ACTG were continuing to make progress with the design of the triple-drug combination trial, and the team again discussed plans for expanded access. Wright calculated that to supply 6,000 patients with the doubled daily dose under an expanded access program would require about one ton of nevirapine per year.[28] If drug production proceeded smoothly, the chemists would be able to ramp up their batches to supply both the project team's clinical trials and an expanded access program. With those clinical programs in mind, Grozinger, Adams, and the project team started discussing plans for production and delivery of five tons of nevirapine.[29]

The newly purified batch of nevirapine, which had been made using Grozinger's original method — now without the little blue specks — arrived in early 1993, just in time for Wright and his colleagues to make tablets for the start of the triple-drug combination clinical trial. This batch was large enough to also supply drug for the 52-week dog toxicology study. But Grozinger reported to the project team that the chemists at the chemical plant were in the middle of producing a 500 kilogram (about 1100 pounds) batch of nevirapine using the new, improved procedure. The toxicology study could start right away with drug made by the old method, or the toxicologists could wait a few months for the batch of nevirapine produced by the new, improved method. All things considered, the toxicologists opted to wait.

Construction of the state-of-the-art toxicology wing adjoining the R&D building in Ridgefield was now nearing completion. For many BI employees, the value of the new toxicology facilities was offset by some sadness at losing the historic Manor House, which had been demolished to make room for the new wing. But the Ridgefield toxicology laboratories greatly enhanced the drug development capabilities of the project team, who could now conduct a full range of preclinical studies under one roof. The 52-week dog study would be the first major toxicology study conducted there. The toxicologists prepared a detailed schedule for the study and had been allowing the dogs to acclimate to their new surroundings while they awaited drug delivery. The timing was tight. If they could not start the study by November 1993, the dogs would be too old to start the one-year dosing schedule, and ordering a new set of younger animals would cause another delay.

Then, one morning in August 1993, as the production chemists were nearing completion of the 500 kilogram batch, Grozinger and Wright received some disheartening news when they arrived at their desks.[30] During one of the production steps, a buildup of pressure in the reaction vessel tripped the safety valve, like a cask of fermenting wine venting gas, causing release of a large yellow cloud into the air outside the chemical plant. No one was injured, but production stopped while plant officials investigated the incident, determined the cause, and planned a course of action. Within a month, the plant managers reengineered their procedures to limit the volume of ingredients in the reaction vessel and established additional process controls to prevent future incidents.[31] They resumed production, salvaging as much material as they could from the 500 kilogram batch and, in parallel, applied their new safety procedures to the five ton production plan.

The first 59 kilograms of nevirapine salvaged after the plant incident arrived in time for the toxicologists to begin their long-delayed 52-week dog toxicology study in November 1993. Altogether, the chemists salvaged enough of the reaction mixture to produce about

300 kilograms of the intended 500 kilogram nevirapine batch, and Wright used most of it to make tablets for the clinical trials. The triple-drug combination study had doubled in size, from 200 to 400 patients, and other large clinical trials had also started or were being planned.

Having optimized nevirapine production, Grozinger, Adams, and their chemistry colleagues turned their attention to manufacturing nevirapine on an industrial scale. For some time, they had been considering the addition of a second manufacturing facility to ensure that nevirapine supplies would not be interrupted. The recent incident at BI's chemical plant reinforced the wisdom of a backup plan. After considering various options, they decided to engage Boehringer Ingelheim Chemicals, Inc., a sister company to Boehringer Ingelheim Pharmaceuticals, Inc., located in Petersburg, Virginia.[32] BI Chemicals would need to set up equipment and train staff to produce nevirapine batches that were identical to those that had already been produced. Together, the project team and representatives from the two chemical plants prepared a plan to produce the five tons of nevirapine stipulated by the project team, while simultaneously helping BI Chemicals to qualify as the second production site. The plan ensured that BI would have sufficient capacity to produce multi-ton quantities of nevirapine to meet the expected demand not only for the project team's planned clinical trials and expanded access but also for commercial production.

Starting in January 1994, chemists at BI's original chemical plant began cranking out standard 200 kilogram (about 440 pounds) batches of nevirapine, the first two of which were turned over to the project team for use in the remaining toxicology studies and clinical trials. They also shipped one ton of the CAPIC starting material to BI Chemicals so that the chemists in Petersburg could begin practicing their production method.[33] Within a few months, the Petersburg chemists successfully completed several 200 kilogram nevirapine batches of their own, and Wright used those batches to make tablets for the ongoing clinical trials.[34] From the beginning, Wright's goal had been to use a nevirapine tablet formula so simple that he could "take it, granulate it, and press it" efficiently and with a low probability of failure.[35] The R&D production line was now routinely turning out 10,000 perfect nevirapine tablets per hour.[36]

By the end of 1994, coinciding with the completion of the 52-week dog toxicology study and completion of the one year dosing schedule of the triple-drug combination clinical trial, the chemists had fully implemented their procedures for large-scale production of nevirapine. The Petersburg chemists had successfully produced a total of one ton of nevirapine, most of which was used by the project team to continue the nevirapine development program. In addition, BI's original production site produced and stockpiled more than two tons of nevirapine, providing a generous inventory for the project team's future needs. They also took another sizable lot of the CAPIC starting material and converted it to three tons of PICNIC. Rather than moving forward to produce nevirapine, they stockpiled the PICNIC, allowing the team to determine when and where it should be used to make future batches of nevirapine.

Getting to PICNIC—tons of PICNIC—had been a long, hard journey, marred by unanticipated setbacks and more than a little frustration. But now, the project team's larder was brimming with enough nevirapine to supply anything on their wish list, even the expanded access program. Whether there would be a sufficient demand and whether the three tons of PICNIC would ever be converted into nevirapine tablets depended on the outcome of the triple-drug combination clinical trial. Disclosure of those results was only weeks away.

14

Surrogates and Accelerated Approval

When people develop a rare lung infection called pneumocystis pneumonia, when their skin sprouts purplish-brown blotches of a rare form of skin cancer called Kaposi's sarcoma, when their bodies cannot fight usually non-threatening infections such as tuberculosis, influenza, bronchitis, or fungal infections, when their lymph glands are swollen, when they suffer from hepatitis and an enlarged liver, when their muscles waste away from poor appetite, excessive vomiting, and an irritated gut, and when their minds are clouded so they cannot follow a conversation, think clearly, or walk unassisted, the diagnosis is easy.[1] They have AIDS. But what if an otherwise healthy person has a fever, muscle aches, and nausea, all of which go away in a few days? Are those symptoms due to HIV or simply a case of the flu?

HIV is sneaky. It cannot be detected for weeks after it infects a person, who may in the meantime donate blood, have unprotected sex, or breastfeed. The virus swims through the bloodstream of its victims, burrowing deep inside their bodies, proliferating, and waiting for a chance to infect somebody else. With only temporary flu-like symptoms or no symptoms at all, people infected by HIV continue to lead a normal life, unaware that they are infected unless they specifically take a test for it. Silently, the virus and the person's immune system continue waging a clandestine battle, often for a decade or more, a battle that in most people the virus wins. And when AIDS symptoms finally do appear, they emerge slowly, unpredictably, and perhaps intermittently, mimicking a dozen harmless ailments. Only later, after the person's immune system has surrendered, are the symptoms of AIDS unmistakable.

Clinicians needed a way to identify HIV infections before the obvious signs and symptoms of AIDS appeared, and investigators wanted an objective way to assess whether their experimental drugs were working. They needed to count something, and that something needed to correlate with the stage of the disease: a representative, "surrogate" marker that confirmed the presence of HIV and corresponded to how much of the virus had infiltrated the person's body.

Scientists with well-equipped laboratories could isolate and identify HIV, but those laboratory procedures were laborious, expensive, and required special precautions to protect the laboratory workers from becoming infected. For diagnosing and monitoring HIV infections in routine medical practice and in clinical trials, physicians used a simpler and safer assay. That simple assay measured p24, a protein unique to HIV. Early clinical trials, including Boehringer Ingelheim's Christmas tree studies, measured p24 as a marker of HIV in the patient's blood. But the p24 assay was not very sensitive, and in the latter stages of AIDS, when patients were the sickest, the p24 assay gave misleading results. Consequently, although the BI project team had seen decreases in p24 after treatment with nevirapine in the Christmas tree studies, they were not certain whether those decreases really corresponded to a decreased viral load and a beneficial drug effect.[2]

During the time that the BI project team was conducting the Christmas tree studies, scientists were developing a number of newer, more sensitive, and more reliable HIV assays. These assays measured viral RNA, the genetic material stored in HIV's nucleus. Scientists thought HIV-RNA more accurately reflected a person's viral load. Chiron, Roche, the AIDS Clinical Trials Group, and others were simultaneously developing versions of the HIV-RNA assay, each of which had advantages and disadvantages as a surrogate marker assay for use in clinical trials.[3]

Besides direct measures of viral load, clinicians also considered using a surrogate marker that was an indirect measure of HIV-induced damage: the state of an infected person's immune system. HIV attacked many tissues and organs but it specifically targeted white blood cells. One particular type of white blood cell, called the CD4 lymphocyte, was especially vulnerable, and the loss of CD4 cells signaled the inability of the immune system to fight infections. Investigators noticed that when the CD4 cell count dropped, HIV-infected patients suffered opportunistic infections and began to develop the symptoms of AIDS. The CD4 cell count in a normal, healthy adult is around 1200.[4] When Elizabeth Glaser discovered that she was infected with HIV, her CD4 count was 210.[5] Physicians knew less about the normal CD4 counts in children or the significance of changes in CD4 levels in HIV-infected children. But they agreed that low CD4 counts were not good.[6] Ryan White's CD4 count was 25 when he was first diagnosed with AIDS.[7] Ariel Glaser's was only 4.[8]

* * *

To approve any experimental drug for commercial use, regulatory agencies, including the Food and Drug Administration, required strong clinical evidence that the drug worked. A drug intended for life-threatening diseases such as AIDS needed to prolong life or decrease the severity of life-threatening symptoms. The clinical trials of AZT satisfied this regulatory requirement. Investigators showed that fewer patients died in the AZT treatment group than in the placebo control group. AZT also reduced the number and severity of AIDS-related symptoms, compared to the control group.[9] The benefits of AZT treatment were so obvious that the investigators stopped the clinical trial early and offered AZT to all patients who had been taking the placebo. Based on this conclusive evidence, FDA quickly approved the drug.

But showing a clinical benefit of the experimental AIDS drugs that followed AZT was more difficult. Clinical trials could no longer be designed like the AZT trials. Now that a beneficial drug was available, namely AZT, withholding treatment from patients in the control group (by giving a placebo) was considered unethical. Instead, all clinical trials following AZT's approval compared the effects of the experimental drug to a control group receiving AZT. Clinical trials to demonstrate prolonged life or reduced AIDS symptoms under these conditions needed to enroll larger numbers of patients and took years to complete.

The politically active AIDS community pressed regulators to rely more heavily on laboratory assays as the basis for drug approvals, arguing that changes in surrogate markers could indicate much quicker that the drug was working than actual improvement in the patient's symptoms. Unfortunately, in the late 1980s, Ellen Cooper, director of the FDA's antiviral division, felt there was "no single surrogate marker that is sufficiently well validated to substitute by itself for the more definitive clinical endpoints in controlled efficacy trials."[10] The only surrogate markers for AIDS at that time were CD4 cell counts, an indirect measure, and p24, a component of HIV that did not correspond to the patient's disease status.

The Lasagna Committee, which had been commissioned by Vice President George H.

W. Bush, spent two years holding discussions, hearings, and deliberations on the issue and in August 1990 sided with the advocacy groups.[11] Using surrogate marker data to speed the process of drug approval, the panel said, was "morally, ethically, and scientifically justified," because the alternative for many AIDS patients was no therapy at all.[12]

When David Kessler arrived as the newly appointed FDA Commissioner in December 1990, he supported the Lasagna Committee's recommendations.[13] A pediatrician who had worked in the Bronx in the 1980s, Kessler understood the impact of AIDS on public health, and one of his first directives as commissioner was to ask his staff to formulate a strategy for faster approval of AIDS drugs.[14] They settled on the notion of "conditional approval," a procedure for conditionally approving new AIDS drugs based on measurements of a surrogate marker that was a proven indicator of the disease and corresponded to the patient's health status. This shortcut approval would make AIDS drugs available to physicians and their patients much sooner than traditional approval. But Kessler's regulators recognized that long-term clinical trials were still the only direct way to establish that the drug improved the patient's clinical symptoms. Their proposal included provisions for pulling a conditionally approved drug from the market if the results of those longer trials did not live up to expectations.[15] Although Kessler championed this streamlined approach, the concept of conditional approval needed to be vetted through a lengthy federal review process before it became official FDA policy.

The first test of the conditional approval idea came with Bristol-Myers Squibb's ddI. After successfully gaining expanded access of ddI for patients who did not qualify for the drug's clinical trials, Martin Delaney of Project Inform continued lobbying regulatory officials. Throughout 1990, he orchestrated a series of increasingly aggressive tactics — letters of support from various advocacy groups and Congressional leaders, consensus statements, petitions, and ultimately a highly publicized multi-city press conference — urging the FDA to use its existing authority to facilitate early approval of ddI.[16]

Enrollment in Bristol-Myers Squibb's well controlled trials, which were being conducted through the ACTG, was lagging behind schedule, and in Delaney's mind, this was causing an unacceptable and unnecessary delay in the drug's approval.[17] He wanted the company to compile its fragmentary surrogate marker data from the early ddI clinical trials and submit it for the FDA reviewers' consideration and, hopefully, approval.[18] The FDA reviewers did not want to be an obstacle, but they needed guidance from experts — HIV researchers, ACTG officials, and advocacy experts — on how to interpret the surrogate marker data and a consensus on what changes in these markers corresponded to the patient's clinical outcome.[19] They felt that an increase in CD4 cell count, a measure that had become increasingly common in AIDS clinical trials, was not sufficient and could be misleading, unless it could be combined with other convincing data. Some HIV/AIDS experts disagreed, arguing that an increase in CD4 cell count should be proof enough.

Delaney obtained assurances from Bristol-Myers Squibb that the company would submit its application for ddI's approval after the FDA's Antiviral Drugs Advisory Committee, a panel of independent experts, held discussions to seek a consensus on the surrogate marker issue.[20] The Advisory Committee met in February 1991 and, based on data from the original clinical trials with AZT, agreed that there was a relationship between CD4 cell counts and clinical outcome.[21] If the CD4 count increased, it was a sign that the drug was having a beneficial effect on the patient's immune system and general health.[22] But the individual committee members' opinions varied widely on the strength of this relationship, some characterizing it as weak and others as very strong.

On April 2, 1991, Bristol-Myers Squibb submitted its New Drug Application, requesting approval for ddI. The submitted data for assessing whether the drug worked came from a hodgepodge of early clinical trials that collectively enrolled only 170 patients — too few to be representative of the general AIDS population — and the studies were uncontrolled, used a variety of dosing schedules, and employed several formulations, none of which was the formulation proposed for the marketed product.[23]

On Thursday, July 18, 1991, the Antiviral Drugs Advisory Committee met at the Holiday Inn in Bethesda, Maryland, to review the data and make an impartial recommendation to the FDA on whether ddI should be approved.[24] Bristol-Myers Squibb used a non-traditional method to analyze the CD4 counts of the patients who received ddI. The FDA's statisticians analyzed the same data using traditional analysis methods. Unfortunately, neither analysis procedure yielded conclusive evidence that the drug worked, and "the committee was alarmed."[25] Some committee members described experiences from their own medical practices, in which individual patients had shown marked improvement after ddI treatment. But much as they all wanted the drug to work, scientific evidence from these early clinical trials was lacking. For twelve hours in the hotel's hot and stuffy Versailles Ballroom, the committee poured over the eclectic data from every possible angle but made little progress. Those early trials simply had not been designed to provide definitive evidence that the drug worked. They retired to their hotel rooms late that night, disheartened and troubled by the thought that they could not, in good conscience, recommend approval of ddI.

But the next morning, the FDA analysts presented additional data for the advisory committee's consideration. In the months leading up to the advisory committee meeting and in an unprecedented move, the FDA had requested data from several ongoing ACTG clinical trials of ddI, and the National Institutes of Health, which was sponsoring the trials, cooperated in sharing it.[26] The ACTG trials had been designed according to FDA's traditional standards for assessing clinical outcome (that is, looking for changes in AIDS symptoms and evidence of prolonged life) but were scheduled to continue for at least six more months. Relying on incomplete surrogate marker data from these ongoing trials, the FDA's interim analysis indicated that ddI produced a modest increase in CD4 cell counts.[27] This small improvement was not enough to justify drug approval according to the traditional criteria, but many of the committee members believed the CD4 increase was real evidence of ddI's benefit and liked the idea of a conditional approval. Conditional approval would allow Bristol-Myers Squibb to market ddI while they all awaited the final outcome of the ongoing ACTG clinical trials.

Unfortunately, the committee chairman explained that conditional approval was not an option. Although Kessler and his staff had been formulating this alternative procedure within the agency, it had not yet been posted in the Federal Register or publicly vetted through the government's review process. The scope of the advisory committee's recommendations were dictated by the FDA's current regulatory boundaries for drug approvals and only permitted a choice between "approval" and "disapproval" — nothing in between. The advisory committee faced a heart wrenching dilemma: vote for approval despite the lack of "traditional" clinical data to back it up, or vote against approval despite evidence from the CD4 surrogate marker analysis suggesting that ddI worked. Constrained by these two choices, five panelists voted to recommend approval, two voted against approval, and one member abstained.[28] Afterwards, the committee members worried that the vote did not accurately reflect their views. They were comfortable with a conditional approval but not a full, traditional approval of ddI.[29]

The advisory committee's endorsement of CD4 as a surrogate marker in February and their majority recommendation for approval of ddI in July influenced the FDA reviewers. The reviewers were also influenced by the very large number of people who had received ddI through Bristol-Myers Squibb's expanded access program, which provided a large body of safety data on the drug. And they were certainly aware of the strong sentiment marshaled by Martin Delaney among the AIDS community and healthcare workers who wanted the drug approved despite less-than-impressive clinical data.

The FDA's approval of ddI on October 9, 1991, marked a major turning point in the way AIDS drugs were evaluated. For the first time, a drug had been approved based on surrogate marker data, rather than the traditional evidence showing that the drug made a real improvement in patients' clinical symptoms.[30] The FDA still required completion of the ongoing ACTG clinical trials, and those trials provided definitive proof that ddI delayed AIDS symptoms when the results were analyzed in 1992.[31] But Kessler said that the agency now recognized surrogate marker data as "an important tool to speed promising drugs to people who desperately need them."[32]

Kessler continued discussions within the FDA to formulate the new policy for rapid drug approvals based on surrogate marker data. Insurance companies only reimbursed approved drugs, and "conditional" status did not meet their standard definition of an approved drug.[33] To clarify matters, the new FDA guidelines called the program "accelerated approval," a term that neutralized the reimbursement issue. FDA posted the new accelerated approval program for public comment on April 15, 1992 and published the final rules on December, 11, 1992.[34] In the meantime, the agency accepted surrogate marker data to justify the benefits of Hoffmann-La Roche's ddC and granted accelerated approval of ddC on June, 19, 1992.[35]

* * *

In 1993, the ACTG investigators who had just started the D'Aquila-Hirsch triple-drug combination clinical trial using the nevirapine/AZT/ddI regimen decided to measure surrogate markers (CD4 and HIV-RNA) as well as traditional clinical outcome endpoints (delayed onset of AIDS symptoms and prolonged life).[36] The one-year duration of the triple-drug trial would allow enough time for the investigators to determine whether the changes in surrogate markers corresponded to changes in AIDS symptoms and, hopefully, prove that those surrogate marker changes reflected the course of the patient's disease. At BI, the project team was staging two controlled clinical trials to confirm the therapeutic value of the nevirapine/AZT combination.[37] These trials would rely on surrogate marker assays and were intended to support BI's request for accelerated approval, but the team needed to select appropriate surrogate markers and use appropriate assays to measure them.

The FDA had accepted CD4 cell counts as a surrogate marker for evaluating ddI and ddC, drugs in the AZT class. But none of the drugs in nevirapine's class (i.e., the non-nucleoside reverse transcriptase inhibitors) had been presented to the FDA for approval, so the BI team was uncertain whether the FDA would accept CD4, p24, or HIV-RNA as a surrogate for nevirapine's therapeutic effects. In the spring of 1993, Maureen Myers, David Hall, and others from BI met with the FDA to discuss the issue of surrogate markers.[38] The FDA officials agreed with BI's proposal to use HIV-RNA as a measure of viral load and CD4 cell counts as a measure of immune function.

Because accelerated approval of nevirapine would be based almost solely on this surrogate marker data, the project team needed to conduct all aspects of the surrogate marker analysis flawlessly. Critical decisions needed to be made on where, when, and how the patients' blood samples would be processed in the surrogate marker assays, and those decisions required input from scientists who knew the intricacies of laboratory technique, clinicians who knew how to handle human blood samples, and data managers who knew how to keep track of the results. Sorting out all of those details fell to a surrogate marker task force led by Johanna Griffin, the head of BI's molecular biology department in Ridgefield.[39]

In 1993, surrogate marker assays for HIV-RNA and CD4 had barely matured beyond experimental laboratory techniques. Few commercial laboratories had the trained staff, equipment, and laboratory safety procedures required to process large numbers of blood samples from HIV-infected people.[40] And each of those laboratories had adopted different methods for assaying surrogate markers, different capacities for the number of samples they could assay at one time, and different sized facilities for storing samples.[41] The BI task force had to select the right assays, not knowing which assay methods would be most successful.[42] And they had to select the right commercial laboratory without having prior experience with any of them. The Inter-Company Collaboration meetings, where experts from various pharmaceutical companies freely shared ideas and discussed their progress in developing new HIV assays, proved to be a valuable forum and helped the BI task force to narrow their choices.[43] They sent representatives to inspect each facility on their short list, meet the laboratory staff, and evaluate first-hand how the laboratory conducted its work. Following these site evaluations, the task force invited representatives from the commercial laboratories to BI for more extensive discussions.

As he had done with so many other aspects of the nevirapine project, Jim Wright tagged along with the task force, attended their frequent meetings, and listened to their discussions. He knew nothing about surrogate marker assays, and handling blood samples was not his job, but he was fascinated by the logistics of organizing, shipping, and tracking large numbers of clinical samples.[44] He bought books on how to sample blood and used the knowledge gained from his years as an analytical chemist to map out procedures for sample handling. After the task force selected the commercial laboratories, Wright urged his colleagues to conduct a series of preliminary tests using mock samples.[45] He wanted to make sure that every aspect of their proposed sample handling procedures worked before they started processing real samples from the clinical trials.

They assessed the volume of blood needed for the assays, finalized the sample preparation procedures, determined the shipping conditions, and subjected blood samples from volunteer donors to various freeze-thaw cycles and storage conditions.[46] After that, Wright devised a dry run to follow the samples through every step of their handling procedures from drawing blood at the clinic to assaying and data reporting at the commercial laboratory. Using duplicate blood samples, this dry run assessed the clinic's sample collection procedures, the shipping courier's performance, the laboratory's ability to assay the samples, the elapsed time to report the assay results, and the ability to repeat all these steps and get the same results.[47] The success of these practice runs reassured the task force, and they proceeded to implement their plans for surrogate marker testing of samples collected in the clinical trials.

Another issue the task force addressed was viral resistance. Patients who took nevirapine rapidly developed resistant strains of HIV. When patients took nevirapine in combination with other AIDS drugs, the virus mutated in different ways. The project team, as well as the FDA reviewers, wanted to understand these patterns of viral resistance, and the agency asked BI to include an analysis of the various mutations in the protocols for the controlled clinical trials. Peter Grob's research team had worked with Myers and the clinical team to define the molecular characteristics of nevirapine-induced resistance using blood samples taken from patients in the Christmas tree studies. Now, the BI scientists would also isolate and characterize HIV from nevirapine-treated patients in the upcoming controlled clinical trials. They would determine whether patients with resistant virus responded to nevirapine treatment, whether changes in the surrogate markers corresponded to various resistant forms of the virus, and whether the amount of resistant virus correlated with the dose of nevirapine.

By the fall of 1993, the task force had chosen the commercial laboratories that would be doing the surrogate marker and resistance assays, worked out the details for sample handling, and decided on the procedures for storing the data. They had chosen the best and most reliable assays then available for measuring the HIV-RNA and CD4 surrogate markers, but all of their work was still a gamble. While they were conducting their trials, newer assays and perhaps different surrogate markers would probably emerge and be adopted as better predictors of AIDS. So, in addition to assaying the samples for viral load and CD4, the task force arranged to store the patients' blood samples for possible re-analysis by these new, yet-to-be-introduced methods.[48]

Grappling with technical issues such as surrogate marker assays, solving biological mysteries such as viral resistance, and striving to satisfy regulatory requirements for rapid drug approval usually dominate the time and attention of pharmaceutical project teams. If they are to succeed in delivering an acceptable new drug in a reasonable time, they must focus on those technical details and become experts in the numbers game. Numbers dominate their work and push all thoughts of individual patients to the back of their minds. In addition, privacy regulations prevent drug company personnel from knowing the identity of the patients participating in their clinical trials. Project teams never know the patients' names, never see their faces. So, as the observations from individual patients accumulate into mounds of data, aggregating the symptoms, side effects, and laboratory results of hundreds or thousands of cases, the project teams see only numbers: sterile, impersonal numbers that they group into categories and analyze with detached, academic accuracy. They become intrigued with manipulating the numbers and solving the scientific puzzle, a clinical Rubik's cube, forgetting that those numbers were measurements taken from people who have feelings, hopes, and an overpowering desire to get well.

But the project teams that worked on AIDS drugs did not forget. And certainly not the BI project team that was developing nevirapine. Often woven into their team discussions and never far from their minds were the patients who were dying—horrible, agonizingly slow and excruciating deaths that continued to dominate newspaper headlines. They were reminded daily that the virus was spreading and anyone who became infected had little hope of surviving. They may not have known the patients' names nor had any personal contact, but they tracked each case, monitoring vital signs, viral load, and clinical status, conjuring up a mental portrait of each person as vivid as any photo. They reveled at each report that a patient was improving and doggedly investigated each patient who showed signs of failing treatment. They were "sitting on an important weapon" and knew the importance of finding the right dose, the right time to start treatment, and the right treatment conditions.[49] "We did not want to foul up."[50] Their determination got them out of bed early each morning, got them through each grueling day, and made them linger at their desks late into the evening. And the next day. And the next.

* * *

Throughout 1994, Myers and the BI clinical team closely monitored the activities of the FDA and its advisory committees in parallel with the progress of BI's controlled clinical trials. In most of these trials, nevirapine was being given in combination with AZT.[51] In some cases, nevirapine was paired with ddI or ddC. The results of these controlled clinical trials were similar to the Christmas tree study results: drug treatment decreased viral load, and some patients exhibited a skin rash or changes in liver function. The surrogate marker data collected in these trials met the FDA's current requirements for accelerated approval. With each passing month, the project team gained confidence that they could compile a convincing set of surrogate marker data showing that nevirapine, in combination with AZT or perhaps ddI, was an effective treatment for HIV-infected adults. But would they be able to make the same case for accelerated approval of nevirapine to treat HIV-infected children?

15

To Peds or Not to Peds

In August 1982, attending physicians in pediatric hematology at the University of California Medical Center in San Francisco decided it was finally time to consult Art Ammann on a case that had been baffling them for months.[1] Their patient was a little boy who had been born by Cesarean section on March 3, 1981, a slightly premature but otherwise healthy six pounds, four ounces.[2] Because of an Rh factor incompatibility, which had been diagnosed during the mother's pregnancy, the baby developed jaundice and was given a series of blood exchange transfusions over the first four days of his life. He remained in the hospital for two months, during which he received whole blood, packed red blood cells, and platelets from eighteen donors. When he was discharged in May, he appeared to be doing well, but in July he developed an enlarged liver and spleen.

Through the summer, the little boy's growth and development were normal, but starting at six months of age, his rate of development slowed and he began losing weight. At seven months, he was hospitalized with an ear infection and was given antibiotics. He subsequently developed thrush, a fungal infection in his mouth, which persisted despite antibiotic treatment. At ten months, he experienced episodes of vomiting and diarrhea, and the doctors diagnosed hepatitis. At 14 months, he was again admitted to the hospital, this time suffering from thrush, enlarged lymph nodes, bloody stools, and a swollen liver. He also had a number of blood abnormalities: low platelet and red blood cell counts and a weakened immune system.

After reviewing the medical history and performing a physical examination, Ammann suspected that the boy might have some form of immune system deficiency along with other infections. He recommended a culture of the patient's bone marrow. Three months later, the results of the bone marrow culture revealed that the boy had a rare infection caused by *Mycobacterium avium-intracellulare*. At 18 months of age, the boy was readmitted to the hospital to treat the *M. avium* infection. But despite aggressive antibiotic treatment, the *M. avium* infection persisted. Other tests showed a disturbing pattern of immune system abnormalities: elevated levels of antibody and decreased cellular immunity. To Ammann, the boy's jumble of symptoms, the *M. avium* infection, the sluggish response to treatment, and abnormal immunity tests were all too familiar. He had seen the same pattern of abnormalities in dozens of men living in San Francisco. He told the boy's attending hematologist, "It looks to me like this baby has AIDS."[3]

Over the next two months, the boy had recurring low platelet and red blood cell counts, and the doctors supplemented his feeding with an intravenous infusion of liquid nutrients, along with intravenous antibiotics. But despite all of these treatments, his immune system continued to weaken and he developed pneumocystis pneumonia. The boy was two years old when he died, primarily from pneumonia and the *M. avium* infection.[4]

Like the case of the prostitute's daughter whom Ammann had seen a few months earlier, this was a puzzling case. The little boy had none of the risk factors for contracting AIDS. His parents were heterosexual, non–Haitians and had no history of injection drug use — the known AIDS high-risk factors. In addition, both parents and his older brother were in good health and had no family history of immune deficiency.

To solve the mystery of how the boy had contracted AIDS, Ammann called the Centers for Disease Control and told them he had treated a child who might have acquired AIDS from a blood transfusion. Harold Jaffe, who had been investigating new cases of AIDS at the CDC, flew to San Francisco to investigate. Joined by Herbert Perkins from Irwin Memorial Blood Bank and Selma Dritz from the San Francisco Health Department, Ammann and Jaffe painstakingly cross-referenced every blood donor whose blood had been given to the baby boy with the names of AIDS patients who had been reported to the San Francisco Health Department.

They discovered that one of the boy's platelet transfusions had come from blood donated by a man who had subsequently died from AIDS. The 47-year-old Harvard graduate belonged to a socially prominent San Francisco family, was a member of the prestigious Pacific Union Club, and worked as an international trade consultant.[5] He regularly donated blood and was in good health when he made the fateful donation on March 10, 1981. The next day, his platelets were extracted and transfused into the baby boy at the University of California Medical Center.[6] Eight months later, the trade expert complained of fatigue and decreased appetite, and he had swollen lymph nodes. In December 1981, he entered the hospital with a fever, shortness of breath, and pneumocystis pneumonia. Although antibiotics helped for a while, he progressively lost weight, suffered several opportunistic infections including thrush, and developed encephalitis. He died on August 6, 1982.[7]

Jaffe and Ammann's case gave the scientific community the first solid proof that a contaminated blood transfusion could lead to AIDS. HIV had not yet been isolated, but this was the second time that Ammann's astute observations had provided sound evidence that AIDS was caused by a virus. The prostitute's daughter had most likely contracted AIDS from her mother who also suffered from AIDS, and the baby boy had no possible means of contracting AIDS except through a blood transfusion that had come from a donor who also suffered from the disease. Unfortunately, Ammann's observations were not unique. Pediatricians across the United States were seeing children with puzzling and unexplained immune system weakness, a syndrome similar to the AIDS symptoms in adults. And like the older patients, the children's condition worsened despite all the pediatricians' efforts.

* * *

When John Sullivan arrived at the University of Massachusetts in Worcester in 1978, he set up his laboratory in the university's newly established medical school to study how the immune system responds to viral infections. During his medical training, he had studied the viruses responsible for measles and influenza, but in his new laboratory he focused his attention on the Epstein Barr virus, the virus responsible for mononucleosis. The medical center managed a large number of children with hemophilia, and when some of them developed AIDS symptoms, Sullivan approached his clinical colleagues. He wanted to collaborate with them to study how these children with weakened immune systems responded to infections with the Epstein Barr virus.[8] After the virus responsible for AIDS was identified in 1984, Sullivan expanded his research to also study how the immune system responds to HIV infections, particularly in children.

Meanwhile, Cathy Wilfert was also seeing children with unexplained immune deficiencies at Duke University in Durham, North Carolina. A graduate of Stanford and Harvard, Wilfert joined the Pediatrics Department at Duke in 1969.[9] She quickly gained a reputation among students and faculty as an intelligent, insightful, and effective teacher, who was equally comfortable mentoring residents and coaching track.[10] Her responsibilities at the medical center included running the virology laboratory, and she had studied a number viral diseases — polio and Rocky Mountain spotted fever, among others.[11] By 1983, Wilfert and her husband had already raised eight children in their yours-mine-and-ours marriage when she saw her first pediatric case with the now-familiar but then-bewildering symptoms. Over the next few years, as chief of pediatric infectious diseases, she admitted hundreds of children with the same symptoms to Duke University Hospital. Wilfert and her colleagues took care of them as best they could, treating the children's infections in the intensive care unit. But unable to determine the cause of their illness or find an effective treatment, Wilfert watched them die. "It was horrible to live through the first years."[12] Later, when the blood test for HIV became available, Wilfert's laboratory finally confirmed that these children had died from AIDS.

Three years after admitting its first pediatric AIDS patient, Duke was designated as one of the first three pediatric centers in the National Institutes of Health's new AIDS Clinical Trials Group network. Wilfert had already begun the first pediatric clinical trial with AZT, sponsored jointly by ACTG and Burroughs Wellcome, and when the ACTG formed its Pediatric Core Committee, she became its first chairman.[13] The pediatric network of ACTG quickly grew to more than thirty clinical sites throughout the United States, but the number of pediatric clinical trials was limited both by the relatively small number of HIV-infected children and by ACTG's preference for conducting clinical trials of new drugs in adults.[14]

* * *

Never one to accept excuses when actions were needed, Elizabeth Glaser continued her personal mission, campaigning for pediatric research in general and pediatric AIDS research in particular. She wanted to protect her son and all HIV-infected children from AIDS. Jake Glaser was born with HIV in 1984, an infection that was discovered 18 months later when his sister, Ariel, first developed AIDS symptoms.[15] Jake was a healthy toddler, but everyone worried that he would become sick and suffer the same fate as his older sister. As a precaution, Jake's pediatrician did a developmental workup when he was five.[16] The results of the three-hour evaluation indicated that his intelligence and muscle coordination were normal for his age. As Jake grew, this baseline information would serve as a reference for assessing his physical and mental development.

Unlike his sister, Jake continued to thrive, a healthy and athletic boy showing no signs of AIDS. And unlike many HIV-infected children, he had been flung into a very select world.[17] While others faced fear and stigma, he benefited from a supportive family, an extensive network of friends, and teachers who treated him no differently than his classmates. They all knew his HIV status, because of his mother's very public pediatric AIDS campaign, but they made a point of taking it in stride, were open-minded, and helped him keep a positive outlook. When he reached the age at which his sister had developed AIDS symptoms, Jake's doctors began testing his blood more frequently, from every twelve weeks to every six weeks, looking for changes in his immune system.[18] One time, his CD4 count dropped, but then it bounced back and he remained stable and strong.[19] When he was eight years old, even though he still showed no AIDS symptoms, the doctors decided to start drug treatment. He went to UCLA Medical Center and over the next few days they phased in his drug regimen of AZT and ddI.[20] Every morning and evening after that, his parents gave him his medicine, and every day at lunchtime, he would go to the school nurse for another dose. The liquid drugs tasted horrible, and because they also "tore your stomach up," he guzzled tons of Maalox.[21] Elizabeth knew the discomfort that he was experiencing all too well. She had taken AZT until her body could no longer tolerate it, and she was taking ddI alongside her son. She constantly impressed on him the importance of taking his meds. "They may taste bad and be hard to swallow, but you need to take them."[22] And all the while, she kept urging researchers and government officials to make better and safer drugs for HIV-infected children.

The Food and Drug Administration allowed the labels for drugs to include statements regarding pediatric use only if those statements were backed up by data from pediatric clinical trials.[23] Instead of conducting the necessary pediatric trials, many manufacturers chose to collect only adult clinical trial data and label the drug for use only in adults. Pediatricians could still legally prescribe these drugs for off-label use in children through the "practice of medicine."[24] But Elizabeth and her advisors at the Pediatric AIDS Foundation knew that the lack of data from pediatric clinical trials posed problems for treating children, especially those with AIDS. From a biological perspective, children are not just little adults. Their bodies have not matured, and they often handle drugs differently than adults.[25] From a disease perspective, children were vulnerable to HIV in different ways than adults. HIV hindered a child's physical growth and brain development. Loss of brain function was more common in children than adults, whereas pneumocystis pneumonia, the hallmark symptom of AIDS in adults, occurred less frequently in children.[26] Those differences suggested to Elizabeth, her advisors, and many other experts that they needed different AIDS drugs for children, or at least, they needed to know the best ways to use AIDS drugs in children. Relying on the experiences from adult clinical trials to treat children with AIDS might be misleading, or even dangerous.

At a time when the ACTG was sponsoring thirteen pediatric clinical trials, Elizabeth and her

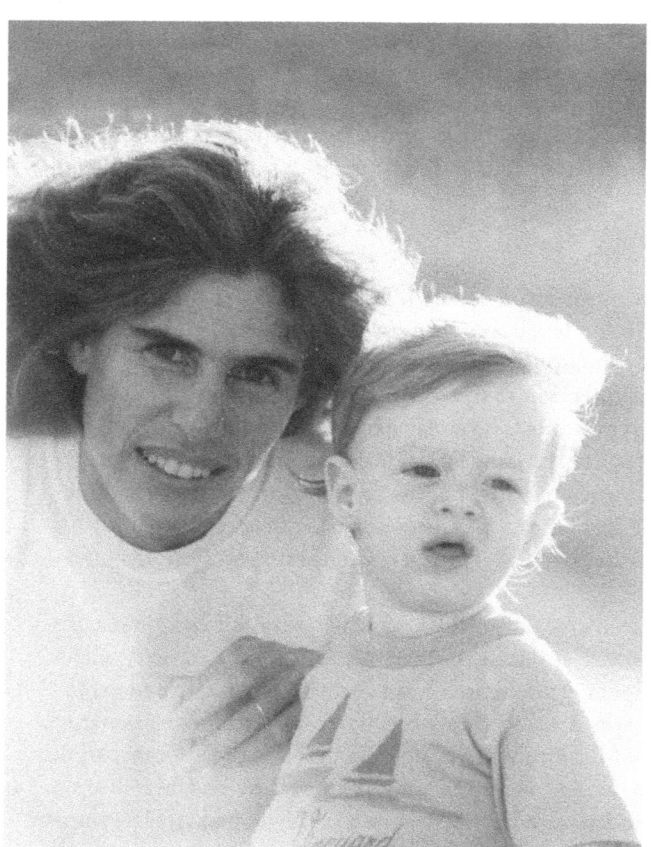

Jake Glaser with his mother, Elizabeth (courtesy Elizabeth Glaser Pediatric AIDS Foundation).

advisory board thought investigators should be conducting at least twice that many.[27] Within the ACTG, pediatricians were also pushing for more autonomy and control of the pediatric clinical program, and the ACTG reorganized to create separate adult and pediatric governing bodies. In conjunction with the reorganization at ACTG and through Elizabeth's lobbying, Congress increased appropriations and established specific earmarks for pediatric clinical trials in the National Institutes of Health's budget in the early 1990s.[28]

Most of the ACTG-sponsored pediatric trials focused on AZT and the other drugs in its class (ddI, ddC, and d4T). Those trials were aimed at optimizing the treatment regimens for children, but the AZT-like drugs had shortcomings as pediatric AIDS drugs. Based on their experiences, investigators like Wilfert outlined the desired, although perhaps unattainable, properties they wanted in an ideal drug to treat pediatric AIDS.[29] It had to penetrate all parts of the body, including the brain. It needed to have a longer half-life and be better absorbed than the AZT-like drugs. It needed to be especially safe and well tolerated, because children would need to take it for a lifetime. The formulations needed to be easy to take and taste good. Finally, because they knew resistance developed to the AZT-like drugs, pediatricians wanted alternative drugs that could be given alone or in combination to children who became resistant to their current therapy. It was a tall order. But when Sullivan and Boehringer Ingelheim presented their first protocols for nevirapine to the ACTG, Wilfert and her colleagues saw the drug's potential advantages as a treatment for pediatric AIDS.

* * *

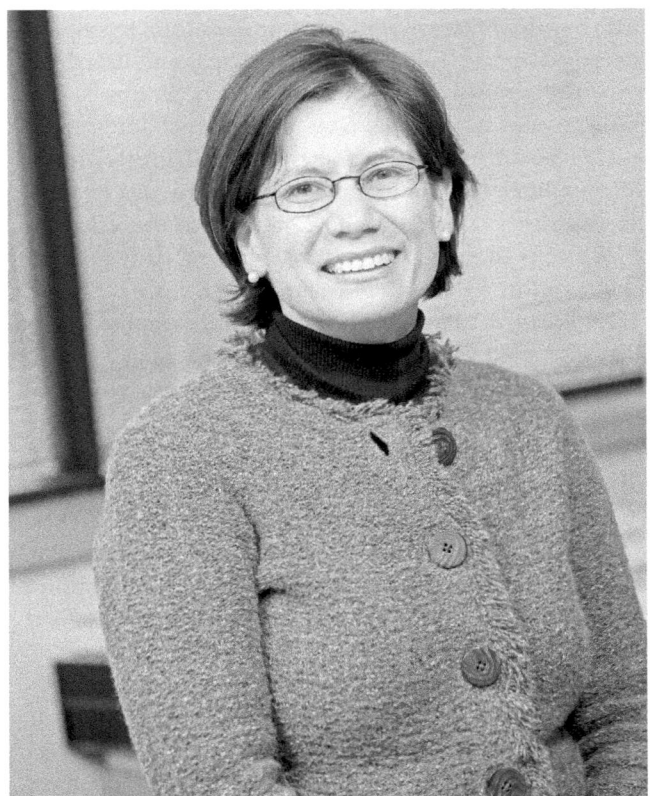

Katherine Luzuriaga.

In the summer of 1991, less than five months after the adult clinical trials started, Sullivan moved ahead with the first pediatric trial of nevirapine at the University of Massachusetts in Worcester.[30] Sullivan was the principal investigator on the pediatric trials sponsored by ACTG and BI at the university, and he encouraged Katherine Luzuriaga, a young investigator in his research group, to play a key role. After her residency in pediatrics at Tufts University, Luzuriaga moved to the University of Massachusetts and was working as a research fellow under Sullivan when his laboratory first observed nevirapine's ability to suppress HIV proliferation in infected cells. In 1990, she joined the medical school faculty in pediatrics, and Sullivan invited her to help develop the clinical protocols for the first nevirapine pediatric trials. Drawing on their clinical and research expertise, Sullivan and Luzuriaga moved smoothly between the laboratory and clinic in the early days of nevirapine's development, using their laboratory observations to understand how best to use the drug in their patients and using nevirapine's performance in the clinical trials to understand how the virus worked and the timing of HIV infections.[31]

The nine children who enrolled in Sullivan and Luzuriaga's first trial ranged in age from nine months to 14 years. Seven of them, like Jake Glaser, had been infected by their HIV-infected mothers and two, like Ryan White, had hemophilia and had received HIV-contaminated blood products. Sullivan and Luzuriaga gave each of the children a single dose of nevirapine, and none of them developed any side effects. They were off to a good start.

* * *

From 1991 through 1994, the nevirapine pediatric clinical trials tagged along behind the adult trials. In a natural, almost unconscious manner—and typical of most things in life—the adults led, the children followed. At the BI project team meetings, the pediatric trials were never first on the agenda. Often, they were not discussed at all.[32] The team concentrated on their increasingly high-maintenance adult program, which zigged and zagged in response to each new revelation in the clinical trial results. And those complications made the pediatric trials even more challenging for the inexperienced BI team. But the pediatric clinical trials kept going, driven by strong hints from federal regulators about the importance of pediatric data, supported by a small but dedicated subgroup of project team members at BI, championed by enthusiastic investigators like Sullivan and Luzuriaga, and urged on by the passionate persistence of parents, pediatricians, and patient advocacy groups.[33]

After the University of Massachusetts team successfully treated the first children with nevirapine and determined that the drug posed no safety concerns, the BI project team authorized the next pediatric trial of nevirapine. This time, Sullivan and Luzuriaga headed a team of pediatric investigators at five medical centers, and they intended to use a dosing schedule comparable to the protocol for adults in the Christmas tree study: a daily dose of nevirapine to groups of children for six months.[34] By early November 1991, three children had enrolled in this junior version of the Christmas tree trial. Then, the project team received news from the ongoing adult trials that disrupted their plans.

Blood samples taken from adults in the Christmas tree study contained a resistant form of HIV, and this observation forced the BI project team to re-examine the entire clinical program, including the pediatric trials. The three children had taken nevirapine for only ten days, but out of an abundance of caution and until they could figure out what to do, the project team halted the pediatric trial. The team also indefinitely postponed new batches of the liquid suspension formulation, which Amale Hawi had scheduled to produce for the upcoming pediatric trials. Hawi had stockpiled about 20 gallons of the liquid formulation, which was sufficient to meet the team's immediate needs. They would not need any more of it, unless the team decided to move ahead with the pediatric program. Hawi advised the team that if they did resume the pediatric trials, she would need time to prepare fresh supplies. Each batch took about six weeks to produce.[35]

The project team grappled with how to restructure the development program and what to do, if anything, with the pediatric trials. If viral resistance to nevirapine developed so rapidly in adults, would the same thing happen in children? Probably. They were considering changes to the adult clinical protocols to overcome the viral resistance problem by increasing the dose of nevirapine. Knowing that children had not shown side effects after a single nevirapine dose at the University of Massachusetts and three children had tolerated nevirapine for ten days without difficulties, could they safely increase the daily dose they were giving to children? Possibly.

After two months of deliberations, the project team resumed the stalled pediatric trial — with some modifications. They revised the pediatric protocol and increased the nevirapine dose more than ten-fold higher than the dose they had given to the first three children.[36] Based on their calculations, this new dose was equivalent to the adult-strength tablet of nevirapine and should be sufficient to overcome viral resistance.[37] The clinical investigators enrolled six children and treated them daily with this new dose level for six months. Confident that the pediatric trials were back on track, the project team asked Hawi to resume production of the liquid suspension formulation so that the new batch would be ready in the summer of 1992. Hawi ordered a big mixing bowl and other equipment. Starting with experimental-scale batches of 10 liters (about 3 gallons), she ramped up production to 40 liter batches and later, batches of 90 liters (about 24 gallons).[38]

By the spring of 1992, the project team had completed analysis of blood samples taken from the nine children who had received a single dose of nevirapine in Sullivan and Luzuriaga's first pediatric study. They discovered that children were able to flush nevirapine from their bodies more efficiently than adults. In order to compensate for this rapid clearance, the BI team realized that the daily dose the children were receiving in the ongoing pediatric trial was probably not sufficient to overcome viral resistance. So, they adjusted the protocol again, increasing the daily nevirapine dose to a level roughly corresponding to the two tablets per day that they were giving to adults.[39]

Sullivan, Luzuriaga, and their colleagues enrolled four children and started giving them this higher daily dose of nevirapine. But in the adult clinical trials, which were further along in using the doubled nevirapine dose to overcome resistance, a new problem appeared: frequent reports of skin rashes.[40] Concerned that children would also develop a skin rash on the newly adjusted high dose, the project team changed the pediatric trial protocol again. Instead of giving the high dose of nevirapine all at once, they asked the investigators to ease the children into nevirapine treatment, similar to the two-step adult schedule. The children received the lead-in dose of nevirapine for four weeks. Then, the investigators increased treatment to the full, high daily dose, giving the liquid formulation in equal parts twice a day for the remainder of the six month trial.[41] Eleven children were treated with nevirapine using this two-step dosing schedule.[42]

Like many of the adult clinical trials of nevirapine, this pediatric trial was sponsored by the ACTG, and during her regular trips to Washington, DC, Maureen Myers reported on the status of the frequently amended pediatric trial protocol. At the ACTG meeting in November 1992, Myers and the clinical investigators discussed whether the newly adjusted high dose of nevirapine would be sufficient to suppress HIV in children. They hoped that it would, but Luzuriaga wanted to give the children AZT in addition to nevirapine. BI had already collected data from laboratory experiments and from the Christmas tree studies in adults showing that the combination of nevirapine and AZT seemed to work better in suppressing viral load than nevirapine or AZT alone.

The project team wanted — indeed, they were obligated — to determine the safety of nevirapine in children. Adding other drugs to the study would make it more difficult to distinguish side effects caused by nevirapine versus something else. The ongoing pediatric trial, in which children received daily doses of nevirapine for six months, certainly would demonstrate the drug's safety, but it might not be sufficient — if it was given alone — to suppress the children's HIV infections. Collecting clear-cut safety data was important, but Luzuriaga, Myers, the BI project team, and the ACTG also wanted to make sure that they gave the children a treatment that had the best chance of suppressing HIV infections. The data that the project team had already collected from adults in the Christmas tree studies gave them reasonable assurance that the risks associated with the drug combination were low. And the benefit might be great.

So, in December 1992, the protocol of the pediatric trial was modified again.[43] For the first two months, the investigators administered only nevirapine to the children and closely monitored them for signs of drug-induced side effects. After that and for the remainder of the six-month trial, the children continued receiving their daily doses of nevirapine but they were also offered AZT. Altogether, Sullivan, Luzuriaga, and their colleagues administered this drug combination sequence to seventeen children.[44]

The data from the junior Christmas tree pediatric trial revealed no surprises, even though it involved a small number of children overall, and the different treatment conditions in the frequently modified protocol made conclusions difficult. Similar to the adult trials, nevirapine suppressed HIV-associated p24 in the children for a short time. The combination of nevirapine and AZT seemed to work a bit better and suppressed p24 longer than nevirapine alone. The children rapidly developed resistant forms of the virus, and the lead-in dosing schedule reduced the likelihood of producing skin rashes — results that also paralleled the adult trial findings. In fact, the only notable difference from adults was that children, especially very young children, more efficiently eliminated the drug, and the investigators increased the dose of nevirapine proportionately to compensate for this rapid clearance.[45]

Based on the data they had gathered, Sullivan, Luzuriaga, and the BI project team concluded that children would respond to nevirapine similar to adults. They planned the remaining pediatric clinical trials using the same dosing schedules and drug combinations that BI was either already using or planning to use in the adult trials, adjusting only for the size and age of the children. But the pediatric trials attracted little of the BI project team's attention. By the end of 1992, Martin Hirsch had gained significant support for his ideas about triple-drug combinations, and nevirapine was the most attractive drug to combine with AZT and ddI. Over the next few months, ACTG and the BI project team refined the protocol of the triple-drug combination clinical trial in adults. When Chow and Hirsch's data were published in February 1993, announcing their theory about convergent combination therapy, Hirsch, the ACTG, and BI rushed to start the triple-drug combination trial in adults, buoyed by a tidal wave of public enthusiasm and optimism that an effective treatment for AIDS had finally been found.

* * *

Unfortunately, the triple-drug therapy came too late for David, the boy whose father had stood outside the gates of BI demanding nevirapine. After securing compassionate use authorization for David to receive the triple-drug regimen, Luzuriaga began his treatment and monitored his progress.[46] Over the following weeks, David experienced no side effects from the combined drugs, but unfortunately this new treatment regimen did not improve his symptoms, and his health continued to worsen. For all its virtues and its promised benefits when coupled with other AIDS drugs, nevirapine could not slay the dragon in David's battle against AIDS.

David's heartbreaking situation and ultimate death underscored a growing clinical problem: HIV-infected children who had not responded to AZT treatment or who had become resistant to AZT needed alternatives. These children suffered from an AIDS syndrome that developed rapidly, ruthlessly, and fatally.[47] Despite the poor condition of children like David who had advanced disease, Chow's convergent combination therapy of nevirapine, AZT, and ddI just might work, if investigators could find the right treatment conditions. In conjunction with the BI project team, the ACTG devised a pediatric protocol with these children in mind, using the triple-drug regimen of the D'Aquila-Hirsch adult trial as a guide. They called it the pediatric salvage study — a treatment regimen to salvage children from the downward spiral of AIDS after an AZT-like drug had failed.[48]

Luzuriaga at the University of Massachusetts and Sandra Burchett at Boston Children's Hospital shared responsibilities as co-chairs of this team of investigators.[49] Like the D'Aquila-Hirsch adult trial, the pediatric salvage study would be blinded. That is, nevirapine and its matching placebo were coded, and the children and the investigators would not know who received nevirapine until the end of the trial. The placebo liquid, which would look and taste the same as the nevirapine liquid, would be given to children in the second group who received only AZT and ddI, so that their treatments looked identical to the group receiving nevirapine, AZT, and ddI.[50] It took time for Hawi and her colleagues to work out the recipe for the placebo liquid, and the trial could not start until it was available.

Like the adult triple-drug combination trial, the pediatric salvage study would be large, one of largest pediatric trials ever undertaken with any AIDS drug.[51] More than 400 children would be enrolled and treated for at least one year. The chemists needed to produce about 18 kilograms (about 40 pounds) of nevirapine, which Hawi would convert into about 475 gallons of the liquid suspension formulation. And Hawi would need to make about the same amount of the placebo liquid.

* * *

Sullivan and Luzuriaga's first pediatric study with nevirapine lagged only a few months behind the first adult clinical trial. But over the next few years, the project team sharpened its focus on collecting adult data, and the pediatric clinical trials lagged further and further behind. As the lag grew, the BI project team debated whether to seek approval for using nevirapine in children. The adult data would be available first, allowing them to proceed with regulatory approval for adult treatment. On the other hand, the pediatric data would permit labeling the drug for use also in children but would delay regulatory approval by many months.

Complicating the situation was the uncertainty surrounding all pediatric AIDS trials. The team simply did not know how much pediatric data the regulatory reviewers would require in the future, when the nevirapine pediatric trials concluded. The FDA's approval of AZT for pediatric use had been based on data from a relatively small number of children. But regulators were charged with protecting the welfare of children. For the newer AIDS drugs, including the nevirapine-containing combination regimens, the FDA reviewers might require much more safety data before allowing pediatric use in the drug's label. Whether BI would request approval of nevirapine for use in children depended on how much pediatric data the regulatory reviewers would require — which no one knew, including the reviewers, until the actual data were available — and how fast the team could compile it. So far, the BI project team had collected very little.

Finally, with their current equipment and resources, Hawi and her colleagues were able to prepare enough of the liquid formulation to supply the ACTG-sponsored pediatric clinical trials, even those that were not part of BI's development plan.[52] Increasingly, the ACTG protocols included nevirapine, often as a reference treatment in its clinical trials of other experimental AIDS drugs. To meet these requests for drug supplies, Hawi set up a continuous production schedule that eventually delivered 1800 liter (about 475 gallon) batches of the liquid formulation, one after the other.[53] But the BI project team had not made plans for production of the large amounts that would be needed for a full pediatric development program. That would require significant planning and a much greater investment in resources.

Weighing these various factors — the rapid progress of the adult clinical trials, the uncertainty of regulatory requirements for a pediatric indication, and the resources required to scale up the liquid formulation — and wanting to ensure the success of nevirapine's development overall, BI decided in the fall of 1993 not to include the liquid formulation in its plans for nevirapine approval. The project team continued to support the ongoing pediatric trials, and if those trials yielded good results, the team was prepared to reevaluate and accelerate the pediatric program. But BI's first priority was to seek accelerated approval of nevirapine tablets for adults. The big pediatric salvage study stalled.

* * *

By 1993, pediatric AIDS had become a pressing healthcare issue — the leading cause of death in the United States for children 1–5 years of age.[54] Children who had become infected by their mothers in the 1980s were now developing the unmistakable symptoms of AIDS. Other children who had been infused with HIV-contaminated blood or blood products prior to the start of blood bank screening in 1985 were also developing AIDS. And yet, most pediatricians still knew very little about pediatric AIDS and even less about how to treat it.

When Jamie was eight years old, her parents were contacted by her doctors and asked to come in "to discuss some things."[55] Five years earlier, Jamie had received blood transfusions during open heart surgery to correct a heart defect. Now, the hospital was informing all patients like Jamie that their transfused blood might have contained HIV and was offering to test them. Jamie had quickly recovered from her operations and became a robust and active little girl, even failing to catch chickenpox when her older sister contracted it. Because she had always been healthy, her parents at first opted not to have her tested. Then, a few months later, Jamie unexpectedly developed several strep throat infections, and her parents decided to go ahead with the test.

When the test results came back, the doctor surprised her parents with the unexpected news that Jamie was infected with HIV. He leaned back in his chair, relaxing his hands behind his head, and casually told them that their daughter had two years to live. He had no treatment to offer them. At that time, no one lived with HIV. But a nurse advised them to explore clinical trials as a way to access the new experimental AIDS drugs. Jamie's parents asked her to add Jamie to the waiting list. In the meantime, they put on brave faces and showered their love and affection on a daughter they thought they would soon lose.[56] They told Jamie that she had a bug in her blood. She asked if the bug meant that she needed another heart surgery. When they said no, she was relieved. "It didn't faze me."[57]

When Jamie was ten years old, her parents were finally informed that their daughter qualified for a pediatric clinical trial.[58] Jamie was accustomed to doctor's appointments, blood tests, and the other procedures included in her regular heart checkups. But now, she would be going to a different hospital and seeing a different set of doctors. Her parents knew that it was time to tell her what this "bug" really meant. Realizing that Jamie had not understood the gravity of an HIV infection, her parents took her to the hospital and asked a nurse to help them. Jamie sat with the nurse who again talked about the bug in her blood. Jamie's calm reaction changed when the nurse explained that HIV was the virus that causes AIDS. Jamie had seen television reports of people dying from AIDS. Now, she made the connection, and she started to cry. "It was horrible" and she was terribly upset.[59] But a short while later, the little girl who had already seen more of hospitals and doctors than most children bravely told her parents, "You can tell my sisters now."[60] They already knew.

Jamie's parents were overjoyed when she was accepted in the pediatric trial, because they viewed clinical trials as their only option. Yes, their daughter would be taking an experimental drug. But for the first time, she would be receiving treatment, and she would be under the care of experts who knew a lot about AIDS. Jamie was among the first children to receive ddI, and it "was a huge change in our lives."[61] Her mother followed the detailed instructions for Jamie's medication, down to the minute. Three times a day, her mother took the ddI solution out of the refrigerator, measured the proper amount, and gave it to Jamie precisely two minutes after she had swallowed a large gulp of antacid — always careful that Jamie had not eaten anything for an hour before or after her medicine.

Nearly every month, Jamie and her mother made the one-hour drive from their home in Gettysburg, Pennsylvania, to the clinic for a full day of laboratory tests and other medical evaluations. Despite being poked and prodded in a marathon of procedures, Jamie enjoyed going to the clinic. Everyone made her comfortable and she could spend special time with her mom. Afterwards, they would go shopping.

Jamie saw some of the same children on her regular visits to the clinic. "Some were sicker than I was."[62] Occasionally, she would ask about one of them, only to learn that the child had died since her last visit. It was sad and upsetting news, and she knew their parents must be devastated. But she was grateful that her parents had always given direct answers to her questions. When she asked whether she was going to die, they said, "[We] don't know, but we are going to do everything that we can to keep you healthy."[63]

Jamie took ddI for several years, but eventually it outlasted its usefulness. Like so many other children who had reached the end of AZT or ddI's usefulness, Jamie had few therapeutic alternatives.[64]

* * *

As this critical need for new pediatric AIDS drugs grew, the ACTG continued to explore new options. And they continued to discuss the pediatric salvage study, which would use the triple-drug combination of nevirapine, AZT, and ddI. As originally proposed, the pediatric salvage study was large, lengthy, and expensive. With such a huge investment of resources at stake, the ACTG considered a number of design changes to ensure the trial's success. In the fall of 1994, the ACTG finally decided to proceed with the first step of their newly configured protocol. They authorized a pilot study in which Luzuriaga, Burchett, and their colleagues would enroll just enough children with advanced disease and treat them just long enough to collect preliminary data on the effects of the triple-drug combination.[65] If the results of this pilot study were encouraging, ACTG would invest the resources to conduct the full-blown, one-year trial.[66]

Myers and the BI project team participated in these discussions with the ACTG, provided supplies of the nevirapine liquid and matching placebo, and conducted laboratory tests to ensure the quality and consistency of the drug supplies.[67] But because pediatric trials were no longer a priority at BI, the project team's contingency plans for the pediatric program sat on a shelf. Whether they implemented those plans depended on a number of factors, the most important being the outcome of the ongoing adult clinical trials.

For nearly four years, the project team had been accumulating data that, in general, raised their confidence in nevirapine. Some of the data was anecdotal, most of it was supportive, but so far none of it was definitive. Throughout 1994, the project team had designed and started several large, long-term clinical trials to treat HIV-infected adults with nevirapine, in combination with AZT or ddI. Those trials would eventually provide definitive data. But the first convincing evidence of nevirapine's value would come from D'Aquila and Hirsch's triple-drug combination trial in HIV-infected adults. The team had been waiting to see those results for more than a year. When the treatments for each patient were decoded, the data were analyzed, and the results of that trial were announced in November 1994, the pediatric trials would be pushed even further down the priority list.

16

And the Winner Is ...

It was an unusually short but memorable meeting. On November 15, 1994, the nevirapine project team gathered in a conference room in Boehringer Ingelheim's Administration Office Building, as they had done every month for the past several years. But unlike so many of their previous meetings, when they had wrestled with a long list of vexing and urgent issues, the agenda on this Tuesday afternoon consisted of only two items. First, the toxicologists reported that they had completed the one year dosing schedule for the much-delayed 52-week dog toxicology study. They were still dissecting the animals and conducting the microscopic analysis, which would take many more months to complete, but so far they were encouraged by the results. Long-term treatment with nevirapine had not produced any unexpected side effects in the dogs. The project team was relieved that this dog toxicology study — so long in the planning and so long in its implementation — was finally nearing completion. But they were even more interested in the second agenda item.

Maureen Myers updated the team on the status of the D'Aquila-Hirsch triple-drug clinical trial. In July, the last of the 341 patients had completed the one-year treatment period. Over the next few months, the staff at the AIDS Clinical Trials Group had compiled the data. Each patient's treatment in the blinded trial had been decoded, and the ACTG statisticians had been analyzing the data. The three drugs used in the trial were owned by three different drug companies, and the ACTG officials planned to send the analyzed results simultaneously to all three of them. They were all anxious to know whether the triple-drug regimen could wipe out HIV. Myers told the team that she expected the ACTG officials would be sending the study results to BI on the following day. The ACTG also planned to issue a press release publicly announcing the study results one day after the three companies had been notified.

* * *

At noon on Wednesday and right on schedule, Myers received the fax from ACTG, a one-page executive summary of the D'Aquila-Hirsch clinical trial results.[1] The statisticians would not complete their detailed analyses for several more months, but the key study findings were clear.[2] Initially, the blood of patients who received the two-drug combination of AZT and ddI contained less HIV-RNA (indicating a decreased viral load) and an increase in CD4 cell counts (indicating improvement in the patients' immune system). This result was similar to the outcome of several previous clinical trials in which patients received the AZT/ddI regimen for a short time. Unfortunately, the beneficial effects of AZT/ddI quickly faded and by the end of the one-year trial, the patients' viral load and the CD4 counts were worse than they had been at the beginning of the study.[3]

The triple-drug regimen worked better. By adding nevirapine to AZT and ddI, the patients' HIV-RNA was suppressed lower and their CD4 counts were higher than those who received the combination of AZT and ddI.[4] Although these beneficial effects also faded over time, patients in the triple-drug group still had lower HIV-RNA and higher CD4 counts than the AZT/ddI group at the end of the one-year trial. These results confirmed the beneficial effects of nevirapine that investigators had seen in BI's earlier and smaller clinical trials, as well as Hirsch's long-held conviction that three drugs worked better than two. The triple-drug trial's results also contributed to the growing body of evidence favoring nevirapine's approval. But the triple-drug regimen did not produce the knockout punch that Chow had demonstrated in his original laboratory experiments. Chow's convergent combination theory predicted — and the investigators hoped — that the triple-drug regimen would wipe out HIV, reduce the patients' AIDS symptoms, and prolong their lives. Unfortunately, it did not.

Unlike the hoopla surrounding the publication of Chow's original convergent combination theory and the enthusiasm surrounding the launch of the D'Aquila-Hirsch triple-drug clinical trial, the release of the trial's results generated little interest. Various newsletters of patient advocacy groups reported the results to the AIDS community but downplayed the value of triple-drug regimens.[5] This was just another disappointing clinical trial that failed to deliver a breakthrough. As had become customary in BI's public statements, Myers was also careful not to overstate the trial's outcome, calling it "definitely a positive trend."[6]

Once again, Myers reached out to patient advocacy groups, explaining the insights gleaned from this latest trial and soliciting input, comments, and support for the next clinical trials in the nevirapine development plan.[7] The advocacy groups expressed concern that the triple-drug regimen had not reversed AIDS symptoms or prolonged life, and they remained skeptical about nevirapine's value as an AIDS treatment. But Myers assured them that the BI team was planning long-term clinical trials specifically to determine whether nevirapine in combination with other AIDS drugs could slow disease progression or reverse the symptoms of AIDS.

* * *

After ACTG started the D'Aquila-Hirsch triple-drug clinical trial in 1993, BI sponsored several other trials to answer specific questions about nevirapine's effects. Three of these were small trials in which a combined regimen of nevirapine and AZT was given to patients for six months.[8] In addition, the team wanted to expand the scope of the international clinical trials and, specifically, to examine the triple-drug regimen in an international setting. Myers invited the lead investigators who had conducted the early international trials with nevirapine to Ridgefield for an investigators meeting: Joep Lange from the Netherlands, David Cooper from Australia, and Stefano Vella from Italy. Joining them for the first time was Julio Montaner from Canada. Myers had first met Montaner in the fall of 1991 when she and David Hall traveled to Vancouver to see Canada's largest AIDS clinical center. Myers and Montaner were intellectually well matched and quickly struck a professional alliance. Montaner was impressed by nevirapine and wanted to participate in the clinical trials. Myers was impressed by the Canadian site, but BI's ongoing clinical trials were already in the hands of senior, internationally-recognized clinical investigators. She assured Montaner that if nevirapine survived the early clinical trials, BI would expand the clinical program, perhaps including his Canadian site. Now, three years later, he was finally getting his chance.

Although Montaner was the youngest and least experienced of the investigators, the international group asked him to take the lead in developing the clinical protocol and conducting the new triple-drug trial. He had conducted numerous clinical trials in Canada, but this was his first time leading an international trial. He enthusiastically seized the opportunity. The investigators incorporated into this new protocol all that the BI team had learned from the preceding clinical trials regarding nevirapine dosing, choice of surrogate markers, length of treatment, and other factors that would maximize the value of combined treatment with nevirapine, AZT, and ddI. Not surprisingly, the BI team wanted to enroll patients similar to those who were being treated in D'Aquila-Hirsch's ACTG-sponsored triple-drug trial, which at the time was still ongoing. To qualify, those patients had to be "treatment experienced." That is, they had already received treatment with an AZT-like drug for at least six months. By the early 1990s, most AIDS patients in the United States had taken AZT as their initial treatment. When they no longer responded to AZT, which always happened, they needed alternatives. Consequently, ACTG focused on clinical trials that would offer these patients viable alternatives, and the ACTG-sponsored clinical trials of new drugs, including nevirapine, often limited enrollment to treatment-experienced patients.

But Montaner and the other international clinical investigators argued strongly that their new clinical trial should instead enroll "treatment naïve" patients. They were convinced that the nevirapine-containing triple-drug regimen would work, but their best chance of proving it was in HIV-infected people who had never been exposed to AIDS drugs and had not developed any viral resistance. In the back of his mind, Montaner linked this situation to the clinical cases he had often discussed with his father, a tuberculosis specialist. Over and over, the elder Montaner advised his son that "you have to hit a magic number" of combined drugs to stamp out an infectious disease.[9] In the case of tuberculosis, appropriately

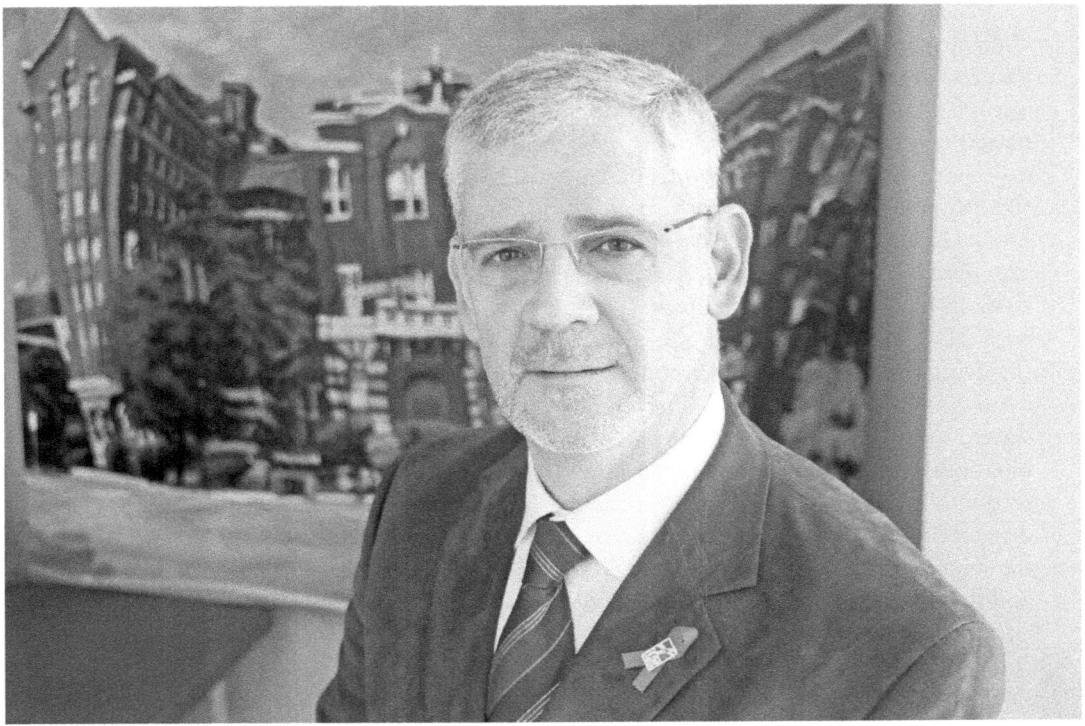

Julio Montaner.

combined drugs result in a cure, but improperly applied and less aggressive treatment can be disastrous. As a young clinician in 1956, he had received a limited but insufficient shipment of the antibiotic, streptomycin. With too little drug available to treat too many patients, he asked his department head for guidance and was told to give the drug to the person who needed it the most. His most desperate patient was a young girl with tuberculosis-related meningitis. He gave her the precious sample of streptomycin, and she made a remarkable recovery. But it only lasted for a day. Without any more streptomycin available, she quickly deteriorated and did not survive. Insufficient drug, Montaner advised his son, only lets the disease come back with a vengeance.[10]

No one thought they could cure AIDS, but the younger Montaner and his international colleagues hoped the right drug combination under the right treatment conditions would produce a sustained suppression of viral load. They wanted a tight, clean trial. To give nevirapine the best chance of success, they insisted on enrolling only treatment-naïve patients.[11] And they finally got their way. Montaner christened the resulting trial INCAS, an acronym comprised of the four countries participating in the study, and a subtle reference to the Indian tribes of his native South America. The INCAS trial began in the fall of 1994, while the ACTG statisticians were completing their analysis of data from the D'Aquila-Hirsch triple-drug trial. The Canadians not only enrolled a sizeable portion of the patients in the INCAS trial, they also conducted the surrogate marker analyses of HIV and CD4 on all of the patient samples.[12] This well controlled and efficiently conducted trial would be nearing completion when the FDA reviewed nevirapine for approval.

* * *

Meanwhile, Myers and her BI colleagues continued to participate in the Inter-Company Collaboration for AIDS Drug Development, the group of fifteen pharmaceutical companies that was meeting regularly to expedite clinical trials of experimental AIDS drugs. Throughout 1994, the Inter-Company Collaboration held numerous discussions on the design of a master clinical protocol for studying drug combinations. Nevirapine, as the most advanced experimental drug in its class of non-nucleoside reverse transcriptase inhibitors, factored significantly in these discussions. In addition, the rapidly emerging class of HIV protease inhibitors was also attracting a great deal of interest among investigators. The most advanced experimental drug in this class was Hoffmann-La Roche's saquinavir. After a series of discussions within the Inter-Company Collaboration committees, industry representatives met with FDA officials to finalize the master protocol.[13] They settled on a large clinical trial involving twenty medical centers and 225 HIV-infected adults who had not been previously treated with any AIDS drugs. This clinical trial, which the investigators dubbed ICC 001, started in February 1995, and the patients were treated for one year with various drug combinations including nevirapine.[14] In July 1995, the Inter-Company Collaboration started a second clinical trial, ICC 002, again including nevirapine as a key element of the triple-drug regimens.[15] Although the data from the ICC trials did not arrive in time to support the regulatory review of nevirapine, these trials helped the BI team understand the utility and limitations of various nevirapine-containing drug combinations.[16]

* * *

By 1994, Elizabeth Glaser could see tangible progress as well. In February, the ACTG 076 trial had proven that HIV transmission could be prevented by giving AZT to pregnant women and newborns. The new AZT regimen had been adopted as the standard treatment in the United States and other developed countries for HIV-infected pregnant women and immediately lowered the number of babies infected with HIV. The Ariel Project, sponsored by her Pediatric AIDS Foundation, was well underway, studying the factors responsible for HIV transmission from mothers to infants.[17] And through her persistent lobbying efforts, federal funding had been specifically earmarked for pediatric AIDS research and clinical trials.

She had navigated the halls of Congress, the FDA, and the National Institutes of Health with ease, a private citizen with a public persona, sharp mind, and passionate mission. Long after her CD4 count had dropped to zero and even as her characteristic energy began to wane, she continued to press the power brokers, never leaving a meeting without a firm commitment from them: the follow up steps, the action plan, or the starting date of a new program. The advisors on her Foundation's boards were also accustomed to her familiar challenge to all of their proposals: "How is that going to help people like me and my children?"[18]

But physically, she became weaker. Her few public appearances were exhausting, and she was noticeably frail. She spent most of her time at home in Santa Monica rather than the Foundation's office, which now sported fourteen desks and twelve employees.[19] Her sunny bedroom overlooked her vegetable garden and accommodated a constant stream of family, friends, and foundation colleagues. With her increasingly raspy voice, Elizabeth still challenged them, convinced that the next dollar spent in the next minute could be the moment of breakthrough.[20] Sometimes, her mind wandered but her resolve never wavered.

The few AIDS drugs available to her, AZT and ddI, had provided temporary relief, but they could not stop or reverse the inevitable onslaught of AIDS. She was increasingly distracted by pain and no longer able to follow even a modest exercise routine, but one day she mustered enough strength to get up and dance to rock-and-roll music.[21] On another day, to the amazement of her doctors, she put on her sneakers and walked around the block, twice.[22] At a time when house calls had become extinct, the Glaser home was filled with doctors, all keeping a watchful eye on their patient, champion, and friend. In November, they were finally able to secure one of the new HIV protease inhibitors, still an experimental and unproven AIDS drug.[23] Stretched out on the sofa in her living room, she ceremoniously took her first dose and remained optimistic. Simultaneously on the opposite coast, the news of nevirapine's value in the D'Aquila-Hirsch triple-drug clinical trial was announced, triggering a flood of new clinical trials using the powerful new three-drug regimens.

Unfortunately, the news came too late for Elizabeth. Two weeks later, on December 3, 1994, Elizabeth Glaser died. The dragon had won another round. For more than ten years, she had fought to maintain her health and that of her children. For six years, after the death of her daughter, Ariel, she had reached out to researchers, physicians, politicians, neighbors, friends, celebrities, journalists, and ordinary people with her story, her hopes, and her plans to help those who had HIV, especially poor people, gay people, people of color, and most of all, children. A strange spokesperson, she admitted, "for such a group: a well-to-do white woman."[24] But she organized them and inspired them until her cause became their cause, her courage became their strength, and her loss only reinforced their determination. No one knew that December, as the world mourned the loss of yet another tireless crusader who had vowed to live life "fully right up until the end"[25] and as the BI project team shifted into overdrive to obtain nevirapine's regulatory approval, that the paths of Elizabeth Glaser's Pediatric AIDS Foundation and Boehringer Ingelheim's nevirapine were slowly but surely converging.

* * *

The BI project team was pleased that the D'Aquila-Hirsch triple-drug clinical trial had signaled a more effective drug regimen for treating AIDS, and they were pleased that nevirapine had played a key role in proving the point. They also felt that these results, combined with the data from their earlier clinical trials, were sufficient to qualify for fast-track approval of nevirapine. Even though they had not yet demonstrated that nevirapine was able to delay the onset of AIDS symptoms or prolong the life of HIV-infected people, their clinical trials had consistently shown the impact of nevirapine on surrogate markers of AIDS, such as decreasing viral load and increasing CD4 cell counts. Regulatory approval of ddI and ddC had been based primarily on this type of surrogate marker data. Would the FDA reviewers consider such data sufficient for nevirapine?

17

Oh, Canada!

When Pamela Strode joined Boehringer Ingelheim in February 1994, she found the nevirapine program flying in the middle of the AIDS whirlwind. It had tremendous momentum but was being buffeted and blown in all directions. Jay Merluzzi, followed by John Tiso, had successfully led the nevirapine team through four hectic years, facing, tackling, and conquering the problems of drug supply, viral resistance, skin rashes, and possible liver damage. The D'Aquila-Hirsch triple-drug clinical trial was more than halfway through its one-year treatment schedule. Maureen Myers and her clinical coworkers had collected enough information from the earlier clinical trials to raise their confidence in nevirapine as part of a treatment regimen, if not as a standalone AIDS drug. And several key decisions had already been made: BI would not pursue regulatory approval of nevirapine to prevent mother-to-child transmission of HIV, would delay seeking approval of the liquid formulation for use in children, and would focus exclusively on gaining approval of nevirapine to treat HIV-infected adults.

The project team was following the same fast track that had led to accelerated approval of AZT, ddI, and ddC, but nevirapine was the first example in a new class of AIDS drugs (the non-nucleoside reverse transcriptase inhibitors). In many ways, nevirapine was different from the AZT-like drugs, and no regulatory guideline or precedent existed for approving drugs like it or the emerging HIV protease inhibitors, which represented another new class of AIDS drugs. Should nevirapine follow the recently established path for approving the AZT-like drugs, or did a new drug class require different or additional criteria for registration? The AZT-like drugs, despite their wide use through expanded access programs and accelerated approval, had made little impact on AIDS. By 1994, many experts and patient advocates were questioning the lax criteria for accelerated approval, and the FDA was holding formal meetings with them, listening to their wide range of ideas, and reconsidering the criteria for accelerated approval of AIDS drugs.[1] Despite the uncertainty surrounding the regulatory requirements, the BI project team had already set a goal of submitting the nevirapine New Drug Application to the FDA by the end of 1995 — about eighteen months away. Strode, as the team's new regulatory affairs representative, had to figure out how to make that happen.

Pam Strode brought to BI relevant regulatory experience from Bristol-Myers Squibb, where she had supported the company's regulatory interactions leading to the successful approval of ddI. She also assisted with the development of stavudine (often abbreviated as d4T), which Bristol-Myers Squibb had just submitted for FDA review and would soon become the fourth AIDS drug approved for use in the United States.[2] Strode's regulatory work at Bristol-Myers Squibb had been unremitting. It would be no different at Boehringer Ingelheim.

Wasting no time, she leaped onto the nevirapine express train and took stock of the project team's progress. The hodgepodge of accumulated clinical data reflected the team's efforts to stay on track despite all the twists and turns they had faced: the breakthroughs in HIV research and nevirapine's performance in patients. They had struggled to find the right treatment regimen, conducting more than a dozen clinical trials — some using nevirapine alone, others studying dual therapy with AZT or alternating between nevirapine and AZT, and some exploratory trials using a range of doses and dose schedules. "Things changed every six months."[3] They had collected lots of bits and pieces but not enough data under the same conditions to support regulatory approval.

By 1994, BI was sending a constant stream of nevirapine information to the FDA: final study reports, new protocols, safety updates, and updated investigator brochures, among other things. Strode made sure that each of these documents had been checked and rechecked for accuracy, completeness, and compliance with FDA's requirements.[4] But she went beyond the usual interactions, using each document as an opportunity to talk to and build a personal rapport with her counterpart at the agency, the FDA project manager assigned to the nevirapine program. She also shared with him her running list of questions and responses. The list, some items initiated by the BI team and others initiated by the FDA review team, was her personal reference, but the FDA project manager appreciated having this handy reminder of their interactions. Strode conscientiously alerted the project manager to real and possible changes in the BI team's activities, especially those rare occasions when she anticipated the team would miss a deadline. Their frequent conversations created a relationship of mutual trust and opportunities to spot possible regulatory issues, which she passed along to her team.[5]

Monitoring the latest regulatory trends, Strode closely followed the progress of other AIDS drugs that were seeking regulatory approval, read reviews of FDA presentations, and noted the advances in surrogate marker development.[6] She also continued her practice, begun at Bristol-Myers Squibb, of attending AIDS conferences, FDA Advisory Committee meetings, and any other forum where FDA representatives discussed their views. Strode and Myers often traveled together, including international trips, specifically noting any comments by regulatory officials that would impact nevirapine's development. Advocacy groups frequently participated in these same forums, a constant reminder of the urgent need for new AIDS drugs. Patients could not afford to wait, and Strode and Myers, who stayed in close contact with many of the advocacy groups, were determined to prove nevirapine's worth to regulators as fast as possible. Together, they devised an efficient, bare-bones clinical and regulatory strategy. "We didn't cut any corners but we rounded off a lot of corners."[7]

Strode focused on the clinical trial issues and coordinated her activities with Patricia Watson, her regulatory colleague, who worked with the BI chemists to transform nevirapine from an experimental drug to a commercial product.[8] How much nevirapine should they put into each commercial tablet? They decided to continue with their standard clinical dose of 200 milligrams. What color should the tablets be? The marketing director wanted them to be green, his favorite color. They opted to keep them white. What shape should the tablets be? They decided on oblong tablets scored with a grove across the middle. How many tablets per bottle? They settled on sixty tablets, which gave patients a one month supply of nevirapine at the standard dose of two tablets per day. The push to make these decisions early was driven by the need to collect data showing that the commercial-style tablets had a shelf life of at least twelve months. To meet their target date (at the end of 1995) for the New Drug Application, Jim Wright and his colleagues needed to begin analyzing the tablets for stability no later than September 1995, which meant he had to put the tablets on the shelf and start the twelve-month clock for stability testing no later than September 1994.

*   *   *

At the end of 1994, encouraged by the results of the D'Aquila-Hirsch triple-drug trial, the project team shifted into "NDA mode."[9] Their target date for submitting the nevirapine New Drug Application to the FDA was now only a year away, and they had still plenty of work to do. From her regulatory experiences at Bristol-Myers Squibb, Strode knew better than anyone else on the BI project team — most of whom had never prepared a New Drug Application — that the challenges before them were daunting. In addition to the completed triple-drug trial, several other controlled trials were nearing completion. But each of those clinical trials had used slightly different treatment conditions, and the team still did not have enough data to define the optimal nevirapine regimen. In addition, they had to address the skin rash problem. In the early trials, skin rash was a frequent and serious problem. Shifting to the staggered, lead-in dosing regimen seemed to reduce the severity and frequency of rashes, but they had not yet collected enough data to prove the point. Bits and pieces, all pointing in the same direction, suggested that nevirapine was a good drug for its proposed use. But stitching together this crazy quilt of mismatched data for registration might take the same creativity, perseverance, and passion that had produced the AIDS Memorial Quilt, which so prominently blanketed the Mall in Washington, DC, each fall.

While they all awaited the results from the ongoing clinical trials, Strode worked with the team to organize the other available data for inclusion in the registration submission. She advised and guided Peter Grob, the leader of the HIV research team, who organized the laboratory assay data, Jim Keirns's staff who compiled the reports of their studies describing nevirapine's bioavailability and half-life, and Laura Andrews's colleagues who continued writing the toxicology study reports.[10] Without the benefit of blackberries, cell phones, or laptops, Strode kept in touch with everyone by email or by phone, often referring to her handy list of office and home phone numbers so she could reach them, day or night.[11]

Strode also found a room in a quiet corner of the Administration Office Building where she could begin compiling the New Drug Application, a room that industry insiders call the War Room. The no-frills storeroom had shelving bolted to the walls, a couple of rectangular tables and, importantly, a photocopy machine. Behind its locked door, the War Room guarded the accumulating documents that would eventually comprise the New Drug Application. The first reports and summaries to arrive came from Grob's, Keirns's, and Andrews's colleagues. Strode carefully reviewed each one, ensuring that the information was complete and in a form that would facilitate the FDA reviewers' assessments. When the documents passed her scrutiny and had been approved by the appropriate departmental reviewers, she passed them along to her colleagues in the regulatory operations group. They cataloged the documents in FDA-required, color-coded yellow, white, and orange binders and stored them on the War Room shelves.

*   *   *

Myers, Strode, and the rest of the project team knew that they needed to conduct additional clinical trials with nevirapine even after accelerated approval in order to obtain full, "Traditional Approval." Because the clinical trials to determine whether a drug actually provides a real improvement in patients (that is, a favorable "clinical outcome") can take many years, FDA's regulations permitted an earlier approval of drugs to treat serious diseases and to fill an unmet medical need, based on early trial data. FDA would grant approval of a drug based on such early data, on the condition that post-marketing clinical trials would be conducted to verify the anticipated clinical benefit. And, those large, long-term clinical outcome trials (aimed at verifying the clinical benefit) needed to start before they submitted the New Drug Application for Accelerated Approval. So, along with preparing the application for Accelerated Approval, the BI project team began orchestrating the clinical outcome trials for Traditional Approval.

The AIDS Clinical Trials Group was also interested in proving that the new triple-drug regimens improved the patients' clinical symptoms. Together, the ACTG and BI designed a clinical outcome trial of more than 1200 patients, divided into groups that compared nevirapine in a three-drug combination with various two-drug combinations without nevirapine.[12] The design of clinical outcome trials was open-ended. Patients would continue receiving their assigned drug regimen until a pre-determined number of the patients died, at which time the investigators would compare the number of survivors in each treatment group. This was the first time the ACTG had sponsored a clinical trial using the patients' survival as its main objective.[13] It had already started by the time Strode arrived at BI, and it would continue for more than three years.[14] The project team decided to use it as one of their clinical outcome trials. But the patients who enrolled in this trial had CD4 cell counts less than 50, and some critics felt that no combination of AIDS drugs could improve the survival of patients who were already so sick.[15]

Myers and the project team arranged a second clinical outcome trial, which they managed independent of ACTG. This trial, which started in 1995, would enroll more than 2200 HIV-infected adults, who were given either the three-drug combination of nevirapine, AZT and 3TC, or the two-drug combination of AZT and 3TC.[16] Most of the patients in this BI trial had CD4 cell counts greater than 50, and most had been previously treated with AIDS drugs. Like the ACTG trial, the BI trial would follow the patients for two years or longer and monitor emerging AIDS symptoms.

* * *

Having launched the long-term clinical outcome trials, the BI team returned to their top priority, obtaining Accelerated Approval. Scientists had made rapid progress in defining and measuring robust surrogate markers, and the FDA reviewers preferred to base Accelerated Approval on data from the newer, and presumably more reliable, HIV-RNA assays of viral load, rather than the older viral assays such as p24 or indirect surrogate markers such as CD4 cell counts. Nevirapine was far along in development and most of the nevirapine clinical trials relied on surrogate marker data using "old" assays.[17] No one, including the FDA, wanted to delay approval of a potentially valuable drug simply because the older assay techniques had become obsolete, but everyone agreed that the new assay methods were better indicators of how well an AIDS drug worked.

This dilemma was resolved, in part, by FDA's Antiviral Drugs Advisory Committee, which agreed to discuss BI's situation in a closed session in April 1995.[18] After reviewing the accumulated data from the nevirapine trials, the committee concluded that the trials' surrogate marker results met the requirements for accelerated approval. But their views were only advisory, and everything could change when the ongoing clinical trials were completed. At that time, the Advisory Committee would meet again and they, along with the FDA officials, would review all of the results before making a final decision.

* * *

Another detail that remained unresolved was the trade name for nevirapine. Among the names on the short list — Viramune (or Viramun), Virune, Novirep, and Revune — Viramune, had been percolating through the international registration process for more than a year. In July 1995, it became apparent that Viramune™ would be acceptable as an international brandname. BI's version of nevirapine tablets as well as the liquid suspension formulation would be called Viramune.

Also in the summer of 1995, the project team received news that came unexpectedly and was somewhat disappointing. All along, they had assumed that nevirapine would be marketed by BI's sales force. Instead, the company decided that the responsibility for launching and selling Viramune in the United States would transfer to Roxane Laboratories, a pharmaceutical subsidiary of BI located in Columbus, Ohio.[19] Roxane, which mainly sold products for palliative medical care, was already marketing Marinol, a synthetic form of marijuana used to control nausea, stimulate appetite, and treat the muscle wasting of AIDS patients.[20] It was a thin connection to AIDS, compared with the heavy-hitting drugs that BI and other companies were developing to directly knock out the AIDS virus. But Roxane's marketing expertise with Marinol in the AIDS community trumped the BI sales force's experience, which was limited to visiting physicians to discuss BI's drugs for heart and lung diseases.[21] The BI project team in Ridgefield continued to manage the nevirapine clinical trials, but the sales force at Roxane Laboratories would handle the product's market launch and subsequent marketing activities.

* * *

In August 1995, Strode and other members of the project team traveled to Rockville, Maryland, for their official pre-NDA meeting with the FDA.[22] Throughout nevirapine's development, FDA officials had reviewed the protocol of each study before it started and received a final report describing the results after each study concluded. Individually, these reports provided one or a few pieces of information about nevirapine. Now, the FDA reviewers considered whether all of these reports collectively met FDA's standards for Accelerated Approval. The pre-NDA discussions spanned two days, during which the regulators asked BI to prepare a detailed accounting of the skin rash observations in addition to the submitted reports.[23] But in the end, the regulators said the accumulated nevirapine data seemed sufficient for submission, and the two sides agreed on a plan and format for the New Drug Application. (One formatting agreement was to combine the Clinical and Statistical sections of the application into one, which ensured that the FDA's medical and statistical reviewers would see identical information in an identical format.) Nevirapine was one step closer to accelerated approval.

Up to this point, the speed of nevirapine's development had been governed by things that could not be compressed. Chemical reactions and drug processing in the manufacturing plant were constrained by the laws of chemistry and physics. Dosing animals in the 52-week toxicology studies could not be completed in less than a year. Likewise, the dosing regimens for patients each took six months or a year to complete, as defined by the clinical protocols. But now, bulk drug supplies were sitting in storage and ready to be used, the toxicology study reports had been written, and the data from the clinical trials using surrogate markers were in the final stages of being analyzed. All that remained was paperwork. The rate-limiting factor in obtaining FDA's approval was how fast the project team could work to complete and submit the New Drug Application. And they knew that every hour of every day that they spent preparing the application, a hundred people died from AIDS.[24]

Through the fall and early winter of 1995, Strode continued to advise and guide the project team, monitoring their progress with each section of the New Drug Application. Within the regulatory affairs department, she orchestrated the process of incorporating those sections into the final application format, checked for inconsistencies and missing items, generated and circulated endless drafts for review by the team and BI's senior management, and page by page — alongside her colleagues in the regulatory operations group — built the New Drug Application. Red binders containing the chemistry data, manufacturing procedures, and details of the nevirapine formulation joined their color-coded neighbors on the War Room shelves.

As she compiled the documents, Strode maintained her communications channel with the FDA project manager, resolving details of the application package. Sometimes the issues and questions required a broader conversation, including members of the BI project team and the FDA reviewers assigned to nevirapine. After one of those teleconference discussions, which had gone especially well, David Hall, the BI team's statistician, noticed a figurine perched on a file cabinet along the wall of the conference room. The small wooden figure, made out of reeds tied together in the shape of a rather dowdy duck, seemed to have brought them good luck. Soon afterward, the team held another teleconference with the regulators, which also went well and again with the ugly duck looking on. From then on, the team adopted the duck as their lucky charm, and Strode made sure it attended all of the team's pivotal discussions.[25]

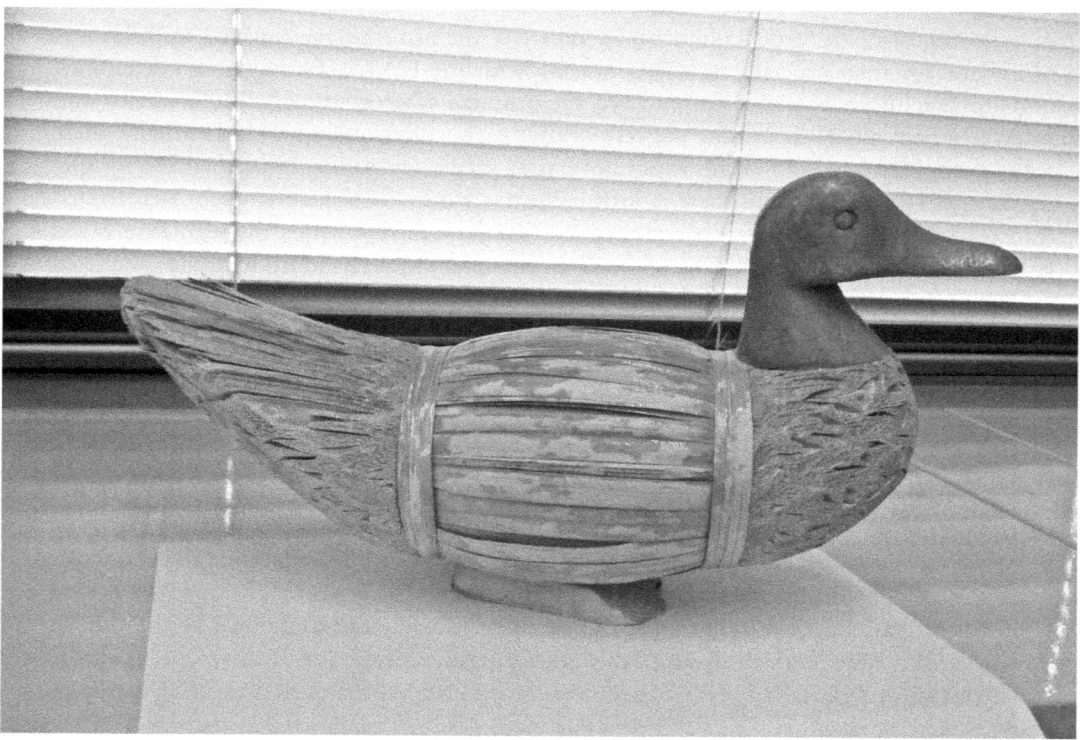

The duck that served as the nevirapine project team's unofficial mascot (courtesy Pamela Strode).

* * *

Guiding the nevirapine data analysis activities was Mike Tsianco, who had joined BI a year before Strode, also relocating to Ridgefield from Bristol-Myers Squibb. Initially, he advised Hall, the project team's statistician, sharing the lessons he had learned while preparing Bristol-Myers Squibb's applications for ddI and d4T. But soon, Tsianco was drawn directly into the team's discussions, spending more and more of his time on nevirapine and leaving him little time to run his department. Faced with the choice, he transferred his departmental responsibilities to a colleague and for the next nine months worked full time on the New Drug Application alongside the project team.[26]

Days turned into weeks, and weeks turned into months, as Tsianco, Myers, and Strode tackled the largest, most challenging part of the application: analyzing and compiling the data from thirty clinical trials.[27] The clinical team members worked nonstop. Housed together in one pod of BI's Administration Office Building, they were constantly in each other's offices, sharing information, checking details, and resolving questions.[28] They were just steps away from Tsianco's data management and statistics group, and Strode's regulatory affairs group was just down the hall. That wing of the building never closed. Clinicians, statisticians, and data managers who had routinely been working sixty-hour weeks now put in twelve to fifteen-hour days, seven days a week.[29] They passed their drafts from desk to desk, supported and guided, day and night, by their three leaders. Myers took the day shift, Strode worked through the evening/early morning hours, and Tsianco worked the graveyard shift. Throughout the day, the authors generated documents and submitted them to Strode, who reviewed them overnight, providing her feedback in emails that were waiting for them the next morning.[30]

In short order, Myers, Tsianco, and Strode forged a close working relationship. Each Friday afternoon they met to discuss and coordinate strategic issues regarding the clinical part of the application. Sometimes, when the meetings were long, they would break away and conclude their discussions off-campus. "It helped to get out," a rare opportunity to glimpse the luminescent fall foliage and breathe the crisp Connecticut air.[31] They would seek a quiet corner of some lonely bar and in that relaxed setting continue mapping out the application. Interspersed with these weekly discussions, Myers and Strode made frequent trips to keep abreast of the latest issues on AIDS drugs and to attend face-to-face meetings with FDA officials — their lucky duck always traveling in Strode's suitcase.

That year, winter arrived early and hit hard. Connecticut endured two back-to-back eighteen-inch snow storms and persistent, penetrating arctic winds.[32] But the project team kept working, reviewing briefcases of documents at home when they could not make it to the office. Their trips to the FDA were productive, but "just getting to Washington was difficult."[33] On one trip, their return flight was canceled due to weather, and they wound their way up Interstate 95 in a rented car with their lucky duck in the trunk.[34]

Through the holidays, Strode tracked critical documents, coordinated report deadlines, and staggered schedules, giving workers a breather after they turned in their assignments. The team took a few hours to celebrate the holidays, but work on the New Drug Application rarely stopped, and their pace never slowed. The lights in the building on the hill burned late into the night, every night. Everyone, whether officially on the team or not, understood the goal and did what they could to help.[35] Administrative assistants and support staff pitched in to handle the paperwork. Computer technicians rescheduled their shutdowns and computer upgrades to accommodate the team. The facility managers responded at all hours to unlock the building's doors and admit team members. "The emotion was palpable throughout the whole company."³⁶ Drafts flew back and forth in a syncopated cadence of emails, phone calls, reviews, and revisions until each document was ready for signature. Day after day, night after night, they slaved away, oblivious to the wind, rain, sleet, and snow outside, oblivious even to a massive January snowstorm that shut down the whole state, except for the BI workers preparing the nevirapine New Drug Application. Weary staff and managers alike trudged with paper-laden briefcases through the snowy, windswept, and dimly lit parking lot in the wee morning hours, often finding their cars glazed with ice, chipping away at frozen door locks with numbed fingers, a final indignity to already over-taxed minds and bodies.

Steadily, through February 1996, the green and light brown binders containing the clinical reports and statistical analyses joined their neighbors on the War Room shelves. Next, the team wrote the product label (the instructions and other information that is inserted in all prescription drug packages). While the company observed the Presidents Day holiday, a small dedicated team was at work, manually cross-referencing every key statement in the product label to the corresponding study reports and data that supported those label statements. After final edits and writing the cover letter describing the intensions of the New Drug Application, the final pages were incorporated, the last round of management reviews were completed, the last page numbered, the last binder labeled, and the official

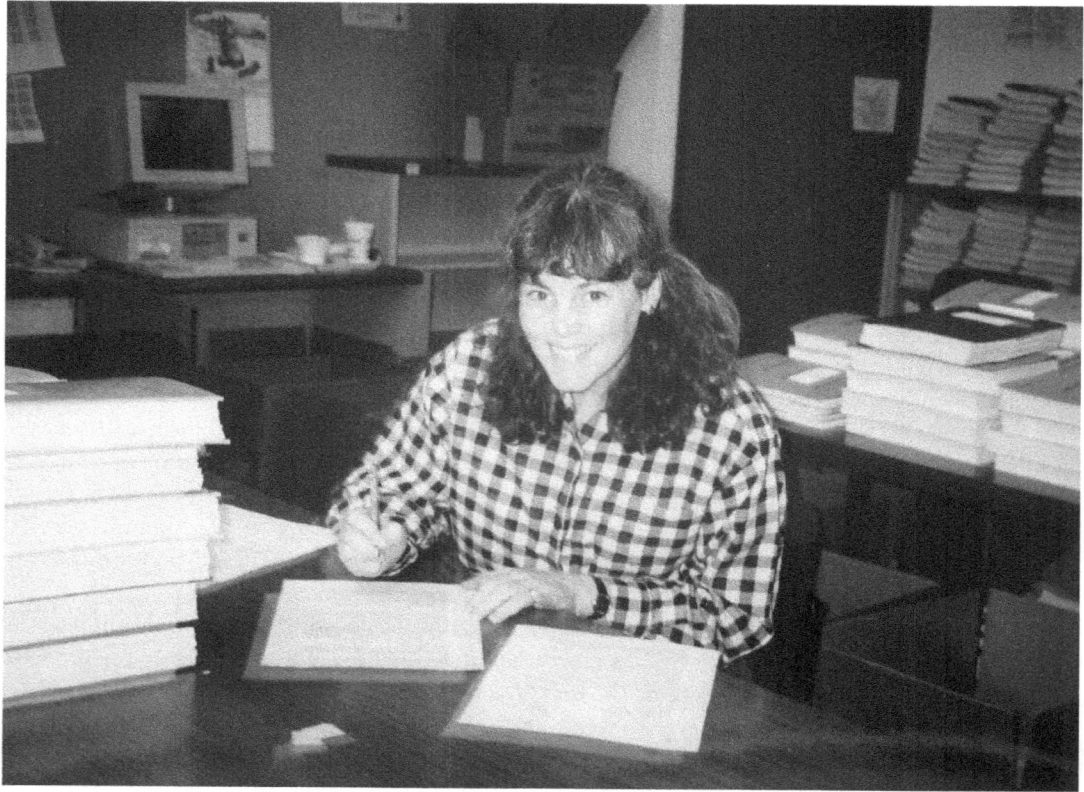

Pamela Strode signing the cover letter for the nevirapine New Drug Application in the Boehringer Ingelheim War Room.

version of the New Drug Application was signed and photocopied one last time. The shelves of the War Room sported a rainbow of 239 binders, each two inches thick, comprising the nevirapine New Drug Application — small by industry standards.[37] Next to them was a duplicate set of volumes in blue binders for the FDA's archive and another partial set for the FDA's field inspectors. Strode's staff had also prepared a fourth, complete copy of the application for BI's archives. Altogether, nearly a thousand volumes of official documents and supplementary materials crammed the War Room.

On Thursday, Strode called "all hands on deck," and employees throughout the company put aside their daily work, reported to the War Room, and rolled up their sleeves.[38] Under Strode's supervision, they packed the binders, each box carefully labeled with its contents, numbered sequentially, taped shut, and logged into the corresponding bill of lading. They then transported the boxes to the building's loading dock for safekeeping overnight.

At 5:00 A.M. on Friday, February 23, 1996, the sealed boxes were stacked in a cargo truck at the loading dock. The plain, simple truck, which was built to handle ordinary freight, somehow seemed an unfitting way to transport such an important set of documents to the FDA. Strode gave the truck driver specific instructions, insisting that the boxes arrive at the Parklawn Building in Rockville, Maryland, before the end of the day, complete with a signed bill of lading and date-stamped to confirm delivery to FDA's Document Control Room — Strode taking personal pride that the application's official submission date would be the same as the shipping date.[39] At first light, Strode and her hardworking colleagues stood on the loading dock and watched the truck pull away, disappearing into the morning fog. Unlike the arctic temperatures and biting winds that had dogged them all winter, that morning felt positively balmy. Exactly six years and two weeks after nevirapine had been selected for development, the duck had flown.

That evening, the extended project team, exhausted though they were, took time to celebrate their accomplishment at a blow-out party in Myers's home. For years, they had subsisted on little more than coffee and adrenaline. Now, their work was finally in the hands of FDA, their desks were cleared of everything except the drafts destined for the shredding bins, and they received no more emails from Strode — least of all at 2:00 A.M.. Nothing left to do except enjoy that exhilarating moment. As the alcohol flowed, their bleary-eyed celebrations stretched late into the night, with some exhausted revelers slumped over Myers's kitchen table. On Saturday morning, she discovered one lingering guest asleep on the living room floor.[40]

* * *

On Monday, Strode was back at her desk, with the first FDA request regarding the New Drug Application already waiting for her. To supplement her frequent conversations with the FDA project manager and to facilitate the transfer of documents for the FDA's review, Strode had established a secure email line between BI and the FDA — not a trivial task in the early days of electronic communication.[41] She and the project manager emailed queries and documents back and forth, cutting costly hours and days out of the FDA's review time, then followed up with formally submitted hardcopies.

Two weeks after shipping the New Drug Application, Strode submitted the first of 31 amendments. Some amendments provided the FDA reviewers with updated information as it became available, and others clarified or addressed questions from the reviewers about information in the original application.[42] The New Drug Application included data from eighteen clinical trials that profiled the safety of nevirapine and ten clinical studies that addressed specific characteristics of the drug's bioavailability, half-life, interactions with other drugs, and formulation comparisons.[43] But the medical reviewers were most interested in the results showing how well nevirapine worked in HIV-infected adults. The Christmas tree studies and two other early clinical trials, which had tested nevirapine alone or in combination with AZT, produced supportive and encouraging data, but these studies enrolled only small numbers of patients and treated them for a relatively short time. The most impressive data on nevirapine's therapeutic effects came from the large, D'Aquila-Hirsch triple-drug trial, sponsored by ACTG. The FDA reviewers agreed with the ACTG's and BI's conclusions that nevirapine combined with AZT and ddI worked better than treatment with the two-drug combination of AZT and ddI.[44] But they wanted assurance that this observation could be repeated. The project team hoped that the INCAS trial, another clinical trial that was treating HIV-infected adults with the triple-drug regimen, would confirm the D'Aquila-Hirsch trial results. But the INCAS trial was still ongoing, and the project team did not have time to wait for the results before deciding to submit the New Drug Application.

* * *

In January 1996, while Strode was putting the finishing touches on the New Drug Application, Julio Montaner, the Vancouver-based lead investigator on the INCAS trial, got some disheartening news. He had traveled to Washington, DC, to attend the Conference on Retroviruses and Opportunistic Infections, and during a break in the sessions, he met with Mark Wainberg to discuss progress on the INCAS trial. Wainberg, a native of Montreal, had studied at McGill, Columbia University in New York, and Hebrew University in Jerusalem before returning to Montreal to join the faculty at McGill and the research staff at Jewish General Hospital. Following a sabbatical in Robert Gallo's laboratory at the National Institutes of Health, Wainberg had been the first researcher in Canada to study HIV and among the first in the world to describe drug-induced HIV resistance.[45] When Montaner began the INCAS trial in 1994, he asked Wainberg, Canada's most prominent virologist, to assay the patients' blood samples for the presence of HIV.

It was a time when the various assays for surrogate markers of viral load were still experimental, none yet proven to be sensitive enough or reliable enough to be representative of HIV's true activity in patients. Wainberg's technique, which was among those on the leading edge of science, measured the "time to viral culture positivity." In a laborious and expensive procedure, Wainberg's laboratory technicians incubated the blood samples and measured how long it took — up to three or four months — for HIV to reappear in the culture. The more potent AIDS drugs caused a longer delay in the reappearance of HIV in the culture medium.

Wainberg told Montaner that in many of the blood samples from patients in the INCAS trial, he could not get the virus to grow, even after long incubation periods. The result was too good to be true, and instead of being overjoyed, both men were very concerned. They immediately assumed something must be wrong with the blood samples, potentially ruining the entire clinical trial. The news hit Montaner like "a cold shower."[46] They needed to check all of their procedures and resolve this problem quickly. Both men followed up with their staffs as soon as they returned home. In Vancouver, Montaner and his clinical laboratory workers scrutinized every aspect of their blood collection and handling procedures but found no technical errors. Likewise, Wainberg's assay methods were faultless. Both laboratories were doing everything correctly.[47] They began to think, guardedly, that perhaps Wainberg's results were correct after all. Perhaps nevirapine really had suppressed HIV so low that he could not detect it.

Coincidently, Montaner had been contacted about the same time by Roche Molecular Systems, asking if his laboratory would test a new HIV assay kit Roche was developing as a commercial assay of viral load using the new HIV-RNA method.[48] With Myers's and Wainberg's knowledge and support, Montaner directed his laboratory to re-assay the blood samples. The Roche assay detected HIV in all of the patients' blood at the start of the trial, but less and less as they progressed in their treatment. All of the blood samples were still blinded, only identified as belonging to treatment group A, B, or C. But all three groups were receiving a two- or three-drug regimen, two of those regimens included nevirapine. Most importantly, Montaner's results with the Roche assay mirrored Wainberg's findings. The samples had not been mishandled. Rather, the assay results indicated that the drug regimens were substantially reducing HIV, even below detection. It was not bad news. It was good news, very good news.

* * *

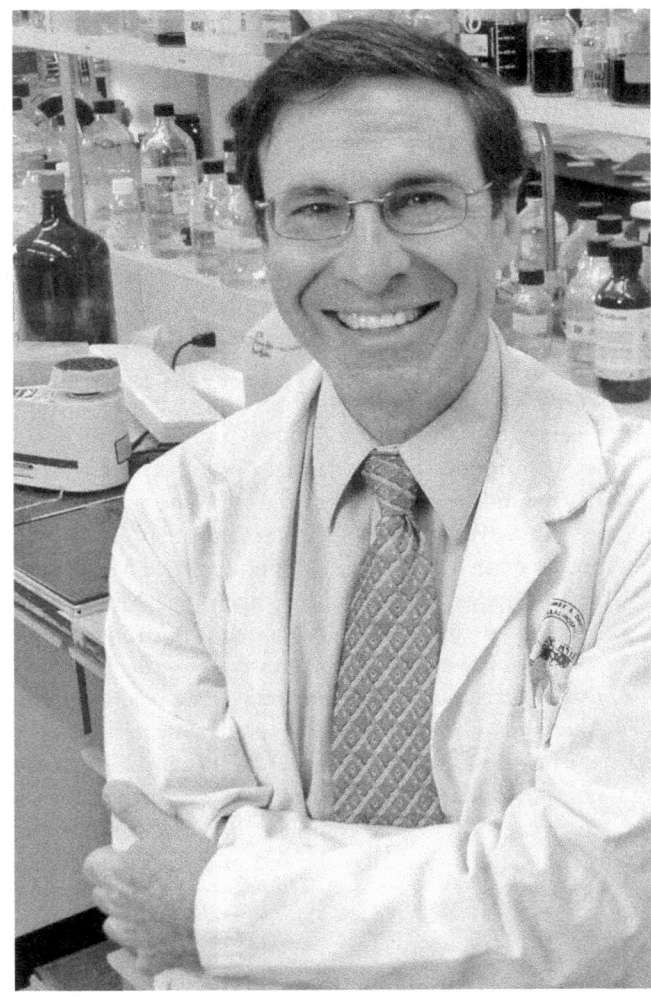

Mark Wainberg.

Among Montaner's patients in the INCAS trial was a 42-year-old man who had become infected with HIV as a result of intravenous drug use.[49] Aside from his cocaine addiction, Colin was healthy and had no AIDS symptoms.[50] But his low CD4 cell count of 425 indicated that his HIV infection was already damaging his immune system.[51] Colin began the triple-drug regimen of nevirapine, AZT, and ddI in March 1995. After two weeks, his viral load (measured by the HIV-RNA assay) decreased below the detection limit of the assay. Throughout the rest of the trial, Colin's blood remained free of HIV.

* * *

At the beginning of 1996, the HIV/AIDS scientific community buzzed with renewed optimism. In the three years since the dismal International AIDS Conference in Berlin, scientists and clinicians had steadily pushed through one barrier after another, reaching the threshold of drug regimens that would revolutionize the treatment of HIV infections and AIDS. A new generation of AZT-like compounds, exemplified by Glaxo Wellcome's 3TC, and the HIV protease inhibitors, exemplified by Hoffmann-La Roche's saquinavir, were all yielding impressive results. One day, Diane Havlir stood at the fax machine as the results of the Merck 035 trial came over the wire. A decade earlier as a resident in internal medicine, she had nothing to offer the AIDS patients who streamed into San Francisco General Hospital every night and crowded the hospital wards. Five years later, as a new Assistant Professor at the University of California in San Diego, she conducted her first clinical trial under Doug Richman's mentorship, investigating an exciting new drug called nevirapine. Later, she led the team of clinical investigators who characterized nevirapine's major weaknesses: rapid development of resistance and a life-threatening skin rash. Combination drug regimens were the obvious next step in the search for effective ways to tackle AIDS, and Havlir was an investigator on the first nevirapine triple-drug trial, led by Richard D'Aquila and Martin Hirsch. Although that trial did not live up to everyone's expectations, Hirsch had the right idea, and the results pointed investigators in the right direction.[52]

Now, five years after her first clinical trial, Havlir was an experienced clinical investigator. She had conducted clinical trials with a number of experimental AIDS drugs and was accustomed to seeing progress and setbacks in equal measure. Merck's HIV protease inhibitor, indinavir, was another new investigational drug offering hope to the increasingly skeptical AIDS community. And the Merck 035 trial was another attempt at triple-drug therapy, combining indinavir with AZT and 3TC. Havlir stared at the fax printout in disbelief. It had been sent to all of the Merck 035 trial investigators including Havlir and summarized the trial's results. The indinavir-containing triple-drug regimen had suppressed HIV below detection for a full year. It was the best outcome of an AIDS clinical trial that anyone had ever achieved and the first evidence that, perhaps, they could suppress HIV indefinitely. Still staring at the fax, Havlir was elated and thought, "Everything is going to be different from now on."[53]

Investigators presented preliminary results from the Merck 035 trial and many other recently completed trials at the Conference on Retroviruses and Opportunistic Infections in Washington, DC, in January 1996, a preview of the more comprehensive clinical results that would be presented at the 11th International AIDS Conference, scheduled to be held in Vancouver in July 1996. Realizing that "everything that was exciting was [going to be] presented in Vancouver," Montaner urged Myers and BI's clinical collaborators to showcase nevirapine at the Vancouver meeting.[54] Montaner's and Wainberg's preliminary analysis had shown that nevirapine-containing drug regimens could wipe out viral load, clinical results that were just as impressive as with the other new AIDS drugs. Unfortunately, the INCAS trial was still in progress at medical centers in Italy, the Netherlands, Canada, and Australia. The trial was not due to conclude until May, and the treatment groups would not be unblinded until April.[55] With only Montaner's preliminary results from the blinded samples available, Myers submitted an abstract for the Vancouver meeting.[56] She and Montaner knew they could complete their analysis of the unblinded data before their presentation in July and hoped that the full analysis would confirm their expectations of nevirapine's value.[57]

* * *

On March 18, 1996, Strode, Myers, Hall, and other key members of the BI team met with the FDA reviewers in a post-NDA-submission meeting to discuss the progress of the

FDA's review of the nevirapine New Drug Application.[58] In the course of the meeting, BI informed the reviewers of their preliminary analysis of the INCAS trial data and the abstract that had been submitted for the Vancouver meeting. The reviewers expressed interest in seeing any additional data to support the New Drug Application, especially measurements of HIV-RNA and CD4 from early analysis of the INCAS trial data.[59] The reviewers were looking for confirmation that the beneficial effects of nevirapine seen in D'Aquila-Hirsch's ACTG-sponsored trial could be repeated.

It was an unusual request but an important, perhaps critical, issue. The INCAS trial's results would, hopefully, strengthen BI's request for nevirapine's approval. But the INCAS trial was blinded, and not all of the patients had completed their one year of treatment. If the statisticians decoded the assigned treatment groups now, they would ruin the trial. On the other hand, nobody wanted to hold up nevirapine's approval by waiting until the INCAS trial finished.[60]

Fortunately, all of the patients had been treated for at least six months, and by applying special rules and precautions, Hall and the other BI statisticians could analyze unblinded data collected during the first six months of each patient's treatment.[61] Over the next three weeks, they analyzed six months of data from 151 patients — mostly from the Canadian medical centers — and Strode compiled the information in a major amendment, which she submitted to the FDA on April 12.[62] During the next six weeks, she submitted thirteen more amendments and faxed a half-dozen corrections, clarifications, and comments on BI's proposed packaging and label for the drug.[63]

* * *

As is customary, the FDA had asked its Antiviral Drugs Advisory Committee, an external panel of HIV/AIDS experts, to review BI's data and make an independent recommendation whether FDA should grant accelerated approval of nevirapine. In the weeks leading up to the advisory committee meeting, which was scheduled for early June, Strode, Myers, and Tsianco again directed the project team's preparations. They compiled a briefing document, largely written by Strode and edited by Myers and Tsianco, and sent it to the committee members in advance, so that the committee could prepare questions that they wished to direct to the company and to FDA. Although the INCAS trial data had not been included in BI's original New Drug Application, FDA allowed the team to present it at the advisory committee meeting.

The Advisory Committee could ask about any and all aspects of the nevirapine data in the briefing document, and the BI team was determined to answer every question thrown at them. Strode and Myers, who would present a summary of the nevirapine data package, rehearsed their presentations in front of team members, external experts, and advocacy representatives, who advised and helped them prepare for every contingency. In addition to the 35 mm slides that accompanied Strode's and Myers's prepared remarks, the team produced an extensive set of backup slides, all cross-referenced for rapid retrieval. Myers, who was an accomplished public speaker and would field the most questions, took no chances. She prepared speaker notes that were cross-referenced to her slides and covered each strategically planned point of her presentation.[64] And then they drilled each other, again and again, fine-tuning their prepared remarks and practicing their responses to every possible question the committee might ask — each answer supported by corresponding backup slides.

The BI delegation arrived in Washington, DC, the day before the scheduled Advisory Committee meeting. One last time, they rehearsed, now with their senior management present. Anticipating that they might need to make some last minute changes to their slides, Strode had identified an outside slide service near their hotel and arranged for "rush" production of new 35 mm slides at a cost of $200-$300 per slide, depending on complexity. As a result of the final rehearsal, a few new slides were created and rushed through production. Photocopies of the new slides were also produced for the slide reference binders that would be given to each member of the Advisory Committee and FDA review team. At 10:00 P.M., the BI team gathered in Strode's hotel room and under the supervision of the manager who had created the new slides, they formed an assembly line, removing and replacing the affected pages in the binders of the slide hardcopies.

On the morning of June 7, 1996, the BI delegation arrived at the Quality Hotel in Silver Spring, Maryland, to attend the Antiviral Drugs Advisory Committee meeting. With the ugly-lucky duck snuggled in her briefcase, Strode began the day-long meeting by describing the claims that BI was seeking for Viramune (nevirapine) Tablets.[65] Myers then summarized the results of the clinical trials, showing that treatment with nevirapine in double- and triple-drug regimens worked better than the corresponding drugs without nevirapine. She also commented on the status of the two large clinical outcome trials, both of which were in progress and were aimed at determining whether nevirapine would delay the onset of AIDS symptoms and prolong life.[66] The Advisory Committee peppered Myers and the BI team with questions, some for clarification, some challenging, and some probing. In each case, Tsianco whispered into his headset, instructing an assistant to pull up the appropriate slide, and the designated BI team member answered the question, supported by a projected slide showing a graph or table of results, just as they had rehearsed. "It ran like clockwork."[67]

Satisfied with the discussion, the committee chairman opened the meeting for public comments, and three AIDS advocacy representatives stepped forward to speak.[68] They were united in their support of nevirapine, explaining that some of the highly touted HIV protease inhibitors did not penetrate the brain, whereas nevirapine did, an important consideration for the patients whose AIDS symptoms resulted from brain damage.[69] Martin Delaney of Project Inform pointed to the large number of studies conducted with nevirapine, saying "the professionalism in which the data has been presented" went far beyond the content in applications of other approved AIDS drugs.[70] He noted that serious side effects, such as pancreatitis, neutropenia, myopathy, and neuropathy, "are very common among people right now using the other drugs" and reported that "most of the folks that we hear from suggest that nevirapine has been a pretty easy ride," producing at most a skin rash and occasionally changes in liver function.[71]

After lunch, hampered by a faulty thermostat that was unable to overcome suburban Washington's sweltering summer heat and a false fire alarm that threatened to evacuate the hotel, the committee members pressed on. They deliberated at length about which AIDS drugs could be safely combined with nevirapine. Multi-drug combinations increase the risk of side effects, and nevirapine had only been tested in combination with a few other drugs. They did not want their concerns to delay the approval of nevirapine, but they strongly recommended additional safety studies. (That recommendation led to scheduling a multitude of small clinical trials pairing nevirapine with a wide range of other AIDS drugs to assess drug interactions and side effects.[72])

The other significant outcome of the committee's discussions was loosening the criteria for nevirapine treatment. In February, BI's New Drug Application requested accelerated approval to use nevirapine in patients with advanced infection and who were deteriorating despite treatment with other AIDS drugs.[73] Most of the clinical data, including the results of D'Aquila-Hirsch's ACTG-sponsored triple-drug trial, had been obtained from HIV-infected adults who were "treatment experienced." But the results of the INCAS trial, which the FDA reviewers had requested for additional evidence of nevirapine's clinical benefits, showed that the same triple-drug regimen worked even better in HIV-infected adults who had not previously taken any AIDS drugs.[74] In half of the patients receiving the nevirapine-containing triple-drug regimen (including Colin), Montaner and Wainberg could find no detectable HIV-RNA, an effect that lasted throughout the one-year treatment period.[75] Suddenly, after years of probing numerous treatment strategies, the INCAS trial had generated data that was "dramatically positive, opening up many new options for nevirapine's use" and BI requested broadening the claims on the drug's label.[76]

The Advisory Committee agreed. Based on the INCAS results, they thought that nevirapine could be given to HIV-infected adults whose immune system or clinical condition was worsening, regardless of the previous treatments they had received.[77] Julio Montaner and his Canadian colleagues, who had followed nevirapine's development from the very beginning with great interest and who had waited years to participate in the nevirapine clinical trials, made a critical contribution just when it was needed most. The INCAS clinical trial not only confirmed the results of the earlier trials but, in fact, produced a better outcome. A patient advocate and clinical investigators alike wondered how many people could have been saved if this triple-drug regimen, as it was used in the INCAS trial, had been discovered a few years earlier.[78]

Now, it all came down to the Advisory Committee's vote, and the BI team's confidence rose as the chairman polled each committee member. The controversy, uncertainty, and caution that had dominated the Committee's reviews of earlier AIDS drugs were absent from their deliberations over nevirapine. On the contrary, they praised BI "not just for a very clear and balanced presentation," but also BI deserved "commendation for the perseverance in developing this drug," despite the setbacks caused by rapid development of viral resistance and the emergence of skin rashes and liver problems in some patients.[79] In addition, they praised the BI team's thoroughness and scientific contributions, noting that "the development of this drug has also taught us a lot about the virus itself and pathogenesis, not just issues in drug development."[80] In an unprecedented move, the Advisory Committee's eight members voted unanimously to recommend accelerated approval of nevirapine.[81]

The meeting ended at 2:00 P.M., hours earlier than scheduled, and in the midst of the excitement of winning the Committee's positive vote, Strode had to step away and contact the company's travel agency. Revised transportation arrangements needed to be made — the old-fashioned way, before smart phones and the internet — for the large BI support team, as they made their way back to their respective destinations in New York and New England. The BI team's high spirits continued throughout the shuttle flight to New York's LaGuardia airport. "We were elated."[82] When Strode and Myers boarded their limousine for the one-hour drive to Ridgefield, they discovered a bottle of champagne, a gift from a BI executive congratulating them on a job well done.[83] But the FDA reviewers would have the final word on whether nevirapine received Accelerated Approval.

* * *

A series of teleconferences, faxes, and emails via the secure line followed over the next two weeks between BI and the FDA to hammer out details of the drug's label, stability data, and packaging. The week of June 17 was particularly hectic for Strode, and her rapport with the FDA project manager — already strong — became even stronger. On Tuesday she submitted two amendments, on Wednesday she sent three amendments, and on Thursday she filed two more, one of which was a very important letter. In the letter, BI officially made the commitment to conduct and complete a series of clinical trials as a follow up to FDA's accelerated approval. Among them were the ongoing clinical outcome trials to verify nevirapine's clinical benefit by demonstrating a delay of the onset of AIDS symptoms and prolongation of the life of HIV-infected adults.[84] At 10:00 P.M. on that Thursday evening, the FDA Medical Reviewer sat with the nevirapine paperwork strewn across her bed and called Strode at home to discuss final labeling comments and questions over the phone.[85]

On Friday, June 21, 1996, Pam Strode drove to the office through the persistent fog and drizzle that had enveloped Ridgefield all week. Unlike the constant stream of discussions and documents that consumed her time on the preceding days, Friday was unusually quiet. Late in the afternoon and just as the sky began to clear on the longest day of the year, her phone rang. The FDA project manager said that a fax was on its way to Ridgefield. At 4:45 P.M., Strode heard the familiar whirring next door in the fax room. The dormant fax machine began its warm up cycle, readying itself to print the incoming document as Strode watched and waited. Finally, it began to print the most important facsimile of its mechanical life.

The fax was a letter from David Feigal, the director of FDA's Antiviral Division. Reading down the first page while the second sheet was still printing, Strode let out a shout. The letter detailed numerous follow up steps and obligations that BI would need to fulfill as its part of the deal, but the only sentence that mattered was "the application is approved effective on the date of this letter."[86] The FDA reviewers agreed with their Advisory Committee that the accumulated clinical data, especially the new results from the INCAS trial, justified expanding nevirapine's use, as part of a drug combination, for all HIV-infected adults who needed treatment.[87] They had completed their assessment of BI's application in a short 119 days, a record for BI covering review, negotiation, and an advisory committee meeting, and Viramune was the ninth drug the agency had approved for the treatment of AIDS. Strode had already prepared an expansive distribution list for an email, which she issued after filling in the placeholder blanks in her message for the date and time of Viramune's accelerated approval. Her message also thanked everyone for their hard work, expressed the hope that Viramune would benefit many of those living with AIDS, and assured them that "it was all worth it."[88]

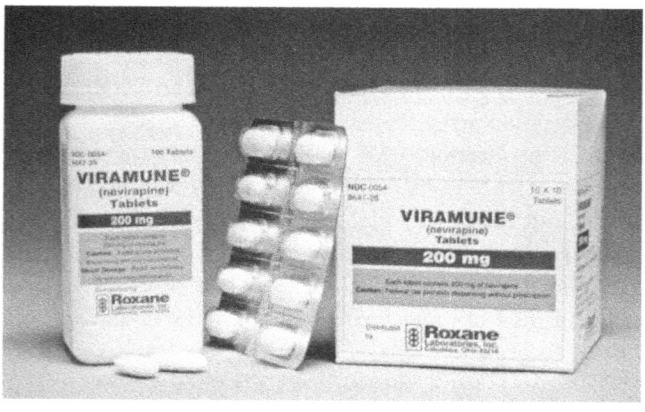

Viramune (nevirapine) tablets, originally distributed under the Roxane Laboratories label. A few years later, when Roxane shifted its business to concentrate on generic drug distribution, Viramune distribution reverted to Boehringer Ingelheim (courtesy Pamela Strode).

Viramune's approval was a major accomplishment for BI, especially the scientists, clinicians, and staff in Ridgefield. It was the first drug discovered at that facility to achieve regulatory approval, which coincided with the 25th anniversary of the founding of BI's American affiliate. Manufacturing personnel quickly shifted to commercial production, rolling out large batches of nevirapine at BI Chemicals in Petersburg, Virginia, and formulating and packaging

Viramune tablets at the BI manufacturing plant in Danbury, Connecticut. In August, Roxane Laboratories in Columbus, Ohio, began distributing the tablets to wholesalers, hospitals, and pharmacies throughout the United States.[89]

Nevirapine's rapid approval left little time for developing an extensive expanded access program.[90] HIV-infected adults in the United States could now obtain a prescription for Viramune from their physician. Unfortunately, many people were not able to get health insurance, were denied insurance coverage, or had their policy dropped altogether when they tested HIV-positive and sought treatment. BI launched an assistance program for those patients.[91]

Strode immediately turned her attention to seeking approval of Viramune in other parts of the world. Regulatory affairs specialists in each of BI's worldwide offices handled the applications for their respective countries. But as the international team member for regulatory strategy on nevirapine, Strode was directly in touch with her colleagues regarding each of these submissions.[92] BI took advantage of procedures established by the European Agency for the Evaluation of Medicinal Products to submit one application that permitted marketing Viramune in all European Union countries. But the format and content of the European application differed from the FDA application, and Strode spent two weeks working alongside her European colleagues to revamp the information.[93]

During that year, Strode made nearly three dozen domestic and international business trips related to Viramune: FDA meetings, AIDS conferences, investigator and advocate meetings, and meetings with other health authorities.[94] When their flight to Australia for the Australian Drug Evaluation Committee meeting was unexpectedly cancelled, Strode, Myers, Tsianco, and the team made their presentation to the committee—the equivalent of FDA's Advisory Committee—by telephone from Myers's home at 2:00 A.M..[95] As the months went by and the various registration applications were reviewed, Viramune was systematically approved by regulators in the European Union, Australia, New Zealand, Switzerland, and eight Central-South American countries. The BI team continued to accumulate data from 42 clinical trials and preliminary results from additional trials, all demonstrating that nevirapine, when used in combination with other AIDS drugs in optimized dosing regimens, reduced viral load to a level below the limit of detection of the most sensitive assays then available.[96]

* * *

In a few short months, from November 1995 to July 1996, the trajectory of AIDS took a sharp turn, leading to a vastly improved standard of care for HIV infections.[97] After more than a decade of frustration, false starts, wrong turns, setbacks, and dashed hopes, scientists had learned how HIV affects the immune system, researchers had developed a reliable HIV test for measuring viral load, and clinicians had found treatment regimens that reduced the virus to undetectable levels in the blood of infected patients. AIDS was rapidly making the transition from a deadly disease to "a chronic, manageable disorder, like diabetes."[98] Scientists established that HIV-RNA reliably correlated with HIV disease progression, and this measure of viral load quickly replaced CD4 cell counts as the standard surrogate marker of HIV/AIDS.[99] In conjunction with this scientific observation, FDA approved the first diagnostic kit for measuring HIV-RNA—the same kit Montaner had used to assay the INCAS blood samples—allowing every physician to routinely monitor a patient's viral load, not just the investigators who were conducting clinical trials.[100]

At the FDA, David Feigal, the Director of the Antiviral Drug Products Division, had created four teams, which worked in parallel to keep pace with all of the AIDS drugs undergoing clinical trials. Instead of a single medical officer, he assigned multiple reviewers to each application, putting all fifteen of his physicians to work and declaring, "Everybody does reviews."[101] Despite strong personalities, differing work styles, and massive blizzards that paralyzed the eastern seaboard that winter, everyone in the Division was committed to facilitating the drug companies' progress and issuing the accelerated approvals as fast as they could. "It was a very interactive process."[102] Feigal's decision makers attended the Advisory Committee meetings, and he asked the drug companies to bring their decision makers to the meetings, as well. Together, they hammered out the details of the product labels as soon as the Committee made its recommendations.[103] In those few months bridging 1995 and 1996, the FDA approved five AIDS drugs — more drugs than had been approved in the previous ten years: Boehringer Ingelheim's nevirapine, Glaxo Wellcome's 3TC, and three HIV protease inhibitors, Hoffmann-La Roche's saquinavir, Abbott Laboratories' ritonavir, and Merck's indinavir.[104]

* * *

The newly approved drugs gave investigators many choices for creating drug regimens to treat AIDS, and new clinical trials of various three-drug regimens soon confirmed and surpassed the results of the INCAS and Merck 035 trials. There was nothing magical about using three drugs. Some clinical trials yielded good results by combining four AIDS drugs. The number of drugs mattered less than choosing the right combination, drugs that reinforced and complemented each other's actions, shutting down HIV's ability to proliferate and minimizing the chances of inducing resistance or causing harmful drug interactions. Nevirapine had proven to be a key component of these early drug regimens. But the HIV protease inhibitors also worked well in combination with other drugs,[105] even though they did not fit Chow's original convergent combination theory. Theories mattered less than clinical success, and the accumulated success of many clinical trials all pointed to a new standard of treatment for HIV/AIDS. The recipe typically was a three-drug regimen: a "backbone" of two AZT-like drugs and either a drug in the nevirapine class (the non-nucleoside reverse transcriptase inhibitors) or an HIV protease inhibitor. Investigators would soon refer to this triple-drug recipe as Highly Active Anti-Retroviral Therapy. By driving HIV below detection indefinitely, these triple-drug regimens also might delay progression of AIDS symptoms and death.[106]

Investigators were careful not to call this new treatment approach a cure, but for the first time in a long time, they were optimistic about controlling, if not eliminating, a nasty virus.[107] Before HAART, AIDS patients taking the one- or two-drug regimens of AZT-like drugs had a life-expectancy of about two and a half years.[108] The number of people dying from AIDS in the United States had steadily increased, year after year, peaking at 51,000 deaths in 1995.[109] After HAART was introduced, those numbers began dropping in the United States and in other regions where the triple-drug regimens were implemented. As long as patients continued to take their combined drug regimen, they could keep the virus suppressed. For the first time, people with HIV infections could look forward to leading a relatively normal life.

These impressive results prompted David Ho, an investigator at the Aaron Diamond AIDS Research Center in New York, to go one step further. Ho advocated treatment with HAART as soon as a person became infected, "hit HIV early and hard."[110] According to his calculations, early and aggressive HAART treatment would prevent the virus from taking root, and after several years of such treatment, patients could theoretically eliminate the last remnants of HIV from their bodies — essentially curing them.[111] Ho backed up his theory with sound data and accurate calculations, but investigators soon made clinical observations that challenged his idea. Colin, one of Montaner's patients in the INCAS trial, was a case in point.

When Colin enrolled in the INCAS trial, his plasma viral load was 2142 copies per milliliter, a modest HIV infection.[112] Within two weeks of beginning treatment with the nevirapine triple-drug regimen, his viral load dropped below detection and it remained there for the rest of the one-year clinical trial. When the INCAS trial concluded in June 1996, Montaner continued to prescribe a HAART regimen and periodically monitored Colin's viral load, which remained below detection for another year.[113] Then in October 1997, Colin was found unconscious following a suspected cocaine overdose and rushed to the emergency room. Lack of oxygen to Colin's brain before he reached the hospital greatly dimmed hopes for his recovery, but his condition temporarily stabilized in the intensive care unit. Colin had taken his triple-drug regimen up to the time of his last clinic visit in August 1997, and at that time Montaner detected no HIV in his blood. But sometime after that, and certainly during the three weeks that Colin lay unconscious in his hospital bed, he had not taken the AIDS drugs. Montaner recognized this as an opportunity to test Ho's eradication theory. The triple-drug regimen, which had suppressed Colin's viral load below detection for more than two years, should have been sufficient to eradicate the virus, according to Ho's theory. After obtaining permission from Colin's family, Montaner drew a sample of Colin's blood in the hospital and discovered that Colin's viral load was a whopping 123,036 copies per milliliter.[114] Only a few weeks after discontinuing treatment with his HAART regimen, Colin's HIV infection had re-emerged with a vengeance. Other investigators reported similar findings, indicating that HIV could hide in "latent reservoirs" that even the most powerful drug regimens could not reach. They could lock up the dragon in a deep, dark dungeon, but it lurked behind the bolted door, ready to squeeze through the smallest crack and unleash its revenge the moment the dungeon's defenses lapsed.

* * *

As Montaner had predicted, all of these advancements were reported at the 11th International AIDS Conference in Vancouver in July 1996, called the "eradication conference" by some and the "Woodstock of AIDS conferences" by others.[115] Certainly, it was the "coming-out party for HAART regimens."[116] But the approval and clinical benefits of nevirapine, the first drug in its class of non-nucleoside reverse transcriptase inhibitors, was all but lost in the shuffle, as one investigator after another stepped to the microphones in Vancouver, reported impressive findings with other triple-drug regimens, and speculated that HIV eradication, though still elusive, was now within reach.

After the Vancouver conference, investigators shifted their attention to practical matters such as reducing the handfuls of pills that AIDS patients needed to take and finding multidrug combinations with the fewest side effects. The early HAART regimens frequently produced side effects, which at best were bothersome and at worst were intolerable. Drugs in the AZT class could suppress bone marrow, damage nerves, and cause an inflamed pancreas, especially if the drugs were used in high doses for a long time. The HIV protease inhibitors could cause nausea, vomiting, diarrhea, and a build-up of fat called a "buffalo hump." And all of the AIDS drugs could cause changes in liver function, sometimes serious liver toxicity. Next to these problems, nevirapine, with its reputation for causing skin rashes — even a life-threatening form of skin rash in a small fraction of patients — held its own. Patients who could not tolerate the side effects of the HIV protease inhibitors often found nevirapine an attractive alternative.[117]

Officials at the National Institutes of Health's Division of AIDS were justifiably proud of the contributions they had made, through their ACTG network, toward nevirapine's successful development. Noting nevirapine's attractive pharmaceutical properties, they speculated that the drug might be useful in other medical situations, specifically for preventing mother-to-infant HIV transmission.[118] ACTG-sponsored clinical trials exploring that idea were already underway.

18

Into Africa

The more John Sullivan learned about nevirapine, the more convinced he became that it could prevent HIV infections in newborns. While the Boehringer Ingelheim project team focused on compiling nevirapine data from the adult clinical trials for submission and approval of its New Drug Application, Sullivan continued to discuss his ideas for prevention clinical trials with ACTG's Pediatric Core Committee. In 1995, the program priorities of the BI project team and the ACTG pediatrics committee finally converged on one small clinical trial. The trial would examine the safety, bioavailability, and half-life of nevirapine in pregnant women and newborns. For the BI team, the results of this trial would support expanding nevirapine's approved use in HIV-infected adults to include pregnant women. For Sullivan and the ACTG, this trial was a necessary preliminary step toward their ultimate goal. Before starting a clinical trial examining nevirapine's effects on HIV transmission from mother to child, they needed to determine the drug's safety in pregnant women and infants.

Sullivan led a small group of ACTG investigators, enrolling HIV-infected pregnant women who resided in the United States and Puerto Rico.[1] In addition to safety, they monitored the blood levels of nevirapine in the mother and newborn. When Sullivan and his colleagues gave a single dose of nevirapine to the mothers during labor, they saw, as expected, the same bioavailability and half-life of nevirapine in the mothers' blood that they had seen in earlier clinical trials of adults. As they had hoped, some of the nevirapine also transferred through the placenta to the baby, and the drug continued to circulate at a therapeutic level in the baby's bloodstream for about four days after birth. Encouraged by these results, Sullivan made one adjustment to the dosing schedule. In addition to the single dose of nevirapine to the mother during labor, the investigators also gave a single nevirapine dose to the baby two or three days after birth. The booster dose prolonged the therapeutic level of nevirapine in the baby's blood for more than a week. Best of all, this single-dose regimen did not produce skin rashes or any other nevirapine-induced side effects in the mothers or babies.[2]

In this small, simple experiment, Sullivan and his colleagues not only confirmed nevirapine's safety but also established a simple dosing regimen that would be used in many future clinical trials. A single dose of nevirapine given to the mother during labor followed by a single nevirapine dose to the baby shortly after birth produced a sustained amount of drug in the baby's blood for more than a week.

* * *

When the FDA's Antiviral Drugs Advisory Committee met in June 1996 to make their recommendations for accelerated approval of nevirapine, they also asked for an update on the pediatric clinical trials, including the potential use of nevirapine for preventing mother-to-child transmission of HIV. At the meeting, Sullivan presented his results, obtained a year earlier, showing that nevirapine's pharmaceutical properties made it "a natural" for preventing HIV infections in babies born to HIV-infected mothers.[3] Because nevirapine rapidly moved from the mother through the placenta to the baby during labor, Sullivan predicted that the drug would protect babies as they slid through the birth canal, the time when they were most likely to become infected with HIV.[4] Nevirapine also made its way into the mother's breast milk, and Sullivan thought that the drug might also protect the babies during breastfeeding, despite the presence of HIV in the mother's milk. If the single-dose nevirapine regimen worked as Sullivan predicted, it would be much more convenient than the long-term AZT regimen for preventing mother-to-child transmission of HIV.[5] For years, Sullivan and Joep Lange had been championing a clinical trial to prove that point.

* * *

Despite all the hopes expressed at the 11th International AIDS Conference in Vancouver in 1996 that "we had turned the corner"[6] on AIDS therapeutics, the new triple-drug regimens had actually created two worlds of HIV infected people, worlds that were sharply divided by economics. The new drug regimens cost $16,000 a year, and only wealthy, insured people could afford them.[7] In developing countries, where most HIV-infected people could barely pay their living expenses, few could afford simple antibiotics to prevent and treat opportunistic infections, let alone the new AIDS multi-drug combinations. And untreated adults meant that HIV was being transmitted to babies at an alarming rate, threatening to lower the life expectancy in some countries by decades.[8] The only hope for people in those countries was to remain uninfected. A positive HIV test was "the end of the line."[9]

Florence Ngobeni was one of the mothers who received that devastating test result.[10] On September 10, 1996, just a few months after news of the triple-drug regimens swept through the convention center in Vancouver, Florence gave birth to her first daughter. Nomthunzi Ngobeni had her mother's eyes, and to Florence, she was the most beautiful girl in the world. Although this should have been a happy time for the Ngobeni family, Florence's husband suddenly fell ill and died three months later. By December, Nomthunzi also became ill, coughing and losing weight.[11] Florence took her to Chris Hani Baragwanath Hospital in Soweto, South Africa, where both mother and daughter were tested for HIV, and both tested positive. Unfortunately, the doctors told Florence that they had no AIDS drugs to treat children, and both mother and baby were discharged. At home, Florence comforted Nomthunzi, always holding her close because she "cried endlessly and was in so much pain."[12] Every few days, Nomthunzi would take a turn for the worse, and Florence called an ambulance. But at the hospital, there was nothing the doctors could do. As the weeks rolled by, the cycle of trips in and out of the hospital continued. Florence watched helplessly as her daughter fought the dragon and slowly slipped away. Five-month-old Nomthunzi died on February 27, 1997.

Losing Nomthunzi changed Florence's life forever. She was a gorgeous 22-year-old, tall and slim as a model, but she felt only grief. For the next two years, she was chronically depressed, crying frequently and unable to eat or sleep. In Africa, AIDS was a secret disease. Many people did not understand it, and many denied that it existed. "To even mention AIDS was seen a curse."[13] Making matters worse, some people blamed Florence for her husband's death, thinking that she had given him AIDS. "It's very easy to blame women when times are bad."[14] Others refused to associate with her. At home, she was surrounded by reminders of her husband and daughter, but the rooms were hollow and silent, the same emptiness she felt inside.

Florence desperately wanted to escape the unhappiness that her house forced on her. Psychiatrists and therapists were not available to most South Africans, but she found comfort in talking and sharing her feelings with friends and colleagues. They stood by her, encouraged her, and helped her through her depression. Like Elizabeth Glaser and so many other women who had lost children to AIDS, she was determined to fight — a mother's fight. She would not give in to the disease that had taken her daughter and would affect her as well. "I chose to stand up and help others who were in my same situation."[15]

During high school, she thought about becoming a counselor and had taken a ten-day training course. Two years later and now HIV-positive, she approached her new friends at Chris Hani Baragwanath Hospital about counseling. Despite her lack of a university degree, they worked out a job for Florence, and she began counseling HIV-infected patients and mothers who had lost children to AIDS. Armed with only her irresistible smile, she befriended her clients, told them about losing her daughter, and welcomed them into her home. They sang together, cried together, prayed together, and shared their stories over plates of comfort food. "There were no boundaries" between counselor and client.[16] She told them about HIV and explained how the virus spread, but there were no drugs and no programs to help HIV-infected women who wanted to protect their babies. After counseling sessions with people who had lost a child to AIDS, Florence would retreat to a secluded room and cry. Every day, she witnessed needless deaths, so many deaths, and "it felt like it was only getting worse."[17]

* * *

John Sullivan had been keenly aware of the need for simple, effective AIDS drugs in the developing world since his discussions with Lange at the World Health Organization in Geneva in 1992. But despite his experience in conducting clinical trials and his enthusiasm for nevirapine as the appropriate agent to prevent mother-to-child HIV transmission, he lacked the wherewithal to launch clinical trials with single-dose nevirapine in the countries where it would do the most good. Then, one day he received a request from Dhayendre Moodley, a young investigator at the University of KwaZulu-Natal in South Africa. Moodley had been impressed with Sullivan's HIV research and asked if she could visit his laboratory. With Sullivan's assistance, Moodley received a fellowship from Elizabeth Glaser's Pediatric AIDS Foundation and spent several weeks working in Sullivan's laboratory.[18] Always a gracious host, Sullivan invited Moodley to stay with his family during her visit.

Moodley's brief fellowship was the first step in a longstanding and prolific collaboration between Sullivan and the University of KwaZulu-Natal. Moodley and Sullivan stayed in touch, and Sullivan soon made plans for his first trip to Africa. Not realizing the travel requirements in apartheid South Africa, Sullivan's first attempt was halted at the airport for lack of a proper visa.[19] A few weeks later, having sorted out his visa, he successfully landed in Durban, South Africa, and Moodley reciprocated his hospitality, inviting him to stay at her home. The invitation struck Sullivan as nothing unusual. But Moodley, who is of Indian descent, was considered "colored" by the apartheid government, and her home was in a segregated section of the city. The comings and goings of a white man raised eyebrows among Moodley's neighbors.

Sullivan was impressed with the staff and facilities during his visit and returned to the University of Massachusetts confident that he had finally found a way to move forward with his clinical trial plans. Triple-drug regimens had not yet been implemented in South Africa, and the AIDS epidemic was spreading virtually unchecked in the continent's second-most populous country. Thousands of infants were infected at birth by their HIV-infected mothers for lack of a feasible drug regimen. It was the perfect place to test whether single-dose nevirapine would prevent mother-to-child transmission of HIV. But launching the trial would not be easy or fast. Similar to Lange's unsuccessful attempts several years earlier, Sullivan had difficulty convincing the BI team to support clinical trials in Africa, and funding mechanisms for international clinical trials through the National Institutes of Health had not yet been established. Still, Sullivan continued to champion the idea of single-dose nevirapine at every opportunity, and one of those discussions took place at a scientific conference in 1994, a casual conversation with J. Brooks Jackson.

* * *

In her final year of medical school, Laura Guay finally fulfilled her childhood ambition of going to Africa.[20] But instead of satisfying her wanderlust, the two-month clinical rotation in Zaire only fueled her desire to go back. A few years later, after completing her residency in pediatrics at Case Western Reserve University, Guay got lucky again. Fred Robbins, a distinguished pediatrician at Case Western and Nobel laureate for his work in isolating the polio virus, had just been awarded a grant from the National Institutes of Health to set up an international collaboration and survey HIV infection trends in Africa. He was looking for a pediatrician to head the largest of the project's four components. Guay was preparing to begin a clinical fellowship in the United States, but Robbins's offer was too tempting. She arranged to postpone her fellowship for a year and headed back to Africa in 1988.

Guay conducted her part of Robbins's project at Makerere University in Kampala, Uganda, where she was appointed a visiting lecturer and established relationships with faculty members who became longstanding collaborators. Among them was Francis Mmiro, a native Ugandan who had just been appointed Head of Obstetrics and Gynecology at Makerere Medical School. Uganda was among the most progressive African countries to address the AIDS epidemic. Unlike many of its neighbors, the Ugandan government readily acknowledged the crisis it was facing—one in three pregnant women in Uganda's urban areas was infected with HIV—and actively sought solutions to the problem, including assistance from abroad.[21] The Robbins survey project was an important first step, documenting HIV infection rates. But Ugandan authorities advised Guay not to tell patients that they were HIV-positive, fearing the

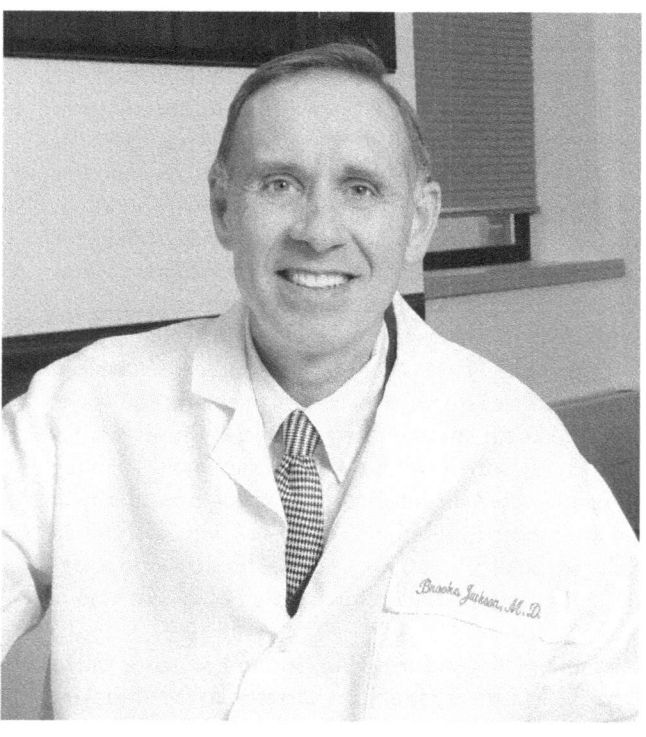

J. Brooks Jackson.

patients would become despondent and commit suicide.[22] Guay found the work interesting and wanted to see it through to completion. Unfortunately, at the end of her one-year commitment, much remained to be done. She cancelled the American clinical fellowship that she had deferred and stayed in Uganda two more years.

The HIV investigative work introduced Guay to new career options, and she returned to Case Western Reserve in 1991 to pursue a fellowship in pediatric infectious diseases. The fellowship kept her busy with laboratory and clinical responsibilities, but she also stayed in touch with her Ugandan colleagues. After completing her fellowship, Guay wanted to continue in pediatrics, but no pediatrics positions were available at the university. Instead, she accepted a position in pathology under J. Brooks Jackson.

Jackson had arrived at Case Western Reserve in 1989 to direct clinical pathology at the University Hospitals of Cleveland, a position that included responsibility for managing the blood supply and transfusions. He had been drawn into HIV investigations in the early days of the AIDS epidemic, screening blood donors, and had developed new assay methods for detecting HIV. Within his pathology subspecialty, he had gained experience in clinical trials, investigating blood components such as the clotting factors that were used by hemophilia patients. He also served as the HIV virologist on a number of study teams conducting AIDS clinical trials.

At Case Western Reserve, Jackson attracted research funding to continue his clinical investigations, which, thanks to the Robbins grant, now had an international component. Guay returned to Kampala, Uganda, in 1994, and together, Jackson and Guay introduced the first laboratory capability in Africa for measuring viral load using the newly developed HIV-RNA assay.[23] Starting with Robbins's grant and continuing with research grants obtained by Jackson, Guay, and others, a strong international collaboration developed between the two universities. In addition to studying the natural history and prevalence of HIV, Jackson's research interests shifted more and more toward pediatric AIDS and mother-to-child transmission of HIV, influenced by Guay's pediatric expertise and her liaison with the clinical team at Makerere University.

It was at this point that the incidental discussion between Jackson and Sullivan took place. Both investigators saw the potential value of nevirapine in preventing HIV transmission from mother to infant. Jackson and Guay's studies of HIV in Uganda confirmed the desperate need for simple drug regimens to thwart the rampant HIV infections in newborns. Sullivan had completed his initial trial showing that a single dose of nevirapine to pregnant women was safe and produced therapeutic levels of the drug in both the mother and infant. The next step was to test whether the single-dose regimen prevented HIV transmission to infants. Sullivan wanted to conduct the trial in South Africa, building on his recent collaboration with Daya Moodley at the University of KwaZulu-Natal and his longstanding relationship with BI. Jackson thought the ideal setting was Uganda, where Guay had established a productive collaboration with Makerere University, but he had not conducted international clinical trials with any experimental AIDS drugs and had never worked with the BI project team. After their initial discussions about a possible collaboration, Jackson and Sullivan went their separate ways.

* * *

Following accelerated approval of nevirapine by the FDA, BI became more receptive to trials examining prevention of mother-to-child transmission of HIV. Maureen Myers and the BI project team assisted Sullivan and his team of ACTG investigators in designing and implementing a large clinical trial enrolling pregnant mothers at clinics in the United States, Europe, and several other developed countries.[24] By the time this trial started, the standard of care for HIV infections in those countries was a combination of AIDS drugs, usually a triple-drug regimen. The women who enrolled in Sullivan's BI-sponsored trial continued to take their prescribed AIDS drug regimen throughout pregnancy. Those regimens reduced the women's viral load to undetectable levels, protecting the mothers' health and minimizing the chance that they would infect their babies with HIV. Consequently, the single-dose nevirapine regimen given during childbirth did not, in fact could not, reduce HIV infection further.[25]

The situation, of course, was much different in developing countries, where mothers did not have access to triple-drug regimens, and babies continued to be infected at an alarming rate. With BI's support and cooperation, Sullivan moved ahead with his plans to conduct the single-dose nevirapine clinical trial in South Africa, using the University of KwaZulu-Natal in Durban as his base of operations. He called it SAINT, the South African Intrapartum Nevirapine Trial.[26] But the clinical centers in South Africa at that time had very limited experience in conducting clinical trials, and Sullivan made many trips to Durban to work out the trial plans with Daya Moodley and her colleagues. The study protocol underwent multiple revisions to satisfy the South African investigators, the BI project team, and various ethics committees and review boards. Sullivan also tackled a multitude of operational details: how the staff at the study sites would be trained, how the blood specimens would be analyzed, how the data would be handled, and how the drug supplies would be shipped, stored, and dispensed. Weeks stretched into months, and months stretched into years.

* * *

Meanwhile, the conversation with Sullivan kept percolating in Brooks Jackson's brain. Jackson knew that the team in Uganda was capable of conducting a clinical trial to test Sullivan's single-dose nevirapine theory, but he needed a research grant to fund the trial. And he was in luck. The National Institutes of Health had recently established the HIV Network for Prevention Trials, HIVNET. Whereas the ACTG network sponsored clinical trials of drugs to treat patients with HIV infections and AIDS symptoms, HIVNET would sponsor clinical trials aimed at preventing HIV infection. The main focus of those prevention trials was to investigate HIV vaccines, but HIVNET's mission included clinical trials to prevent HIV transmission from mothers to infants. Tapping into the new HIVNET program, Jackson mapped out the entire protocol for his single-dose nevirapine trial during an airplane flight.[27] In October 1995, the Division of AIDS at the National Institutes of Health approved his proposal, one of the first HIVNET-funded trials.[28]

With funding now secured, Jackson approached BI to request supplies of nevirapine for his trial. He could purchase Viramune (nevirapine) tablets, because that product was now on the market. But his protocol also called for giving babies the liquid suspension formulation, which had not yet been approved. Liquid nevirapine, as well as placebo supplies matching the tablets and liquid, could only be obtained from BI. The company was already sponsoring two clinical trials with Sullivan as the lead investigator (the trial based in the United States and Europe and the SAINT trial in South Africa) and felt those trials would be sufficient to determine whether single-dose nevirapine prevented mother-to-child transmission of HIV. BI told Jackson that the company was "not anxious to burden our registration package with additional studies outside of the registration plan."[29] The negotiations went back and forth for nearly a year, with Myers finally brokering a deal to provide the drug supplies to Jackson — BI acknowledged that there was prevailing "pressure to explore additional opportunities to address the world-wide catastrophe of perinatal transmission of HIV."[30]

During the negotiations with BI, Jackson moved from Case Western Reserve to Johns Hopkins University. Guay, who was still living in Uganda, also transferred her affiliation to Johns Hopkins and continued reporting to Jackson. In addition, the pediatric/perinatal unit of the Case Western Reserve-Makerere research program transferred to Johns Hopkins, creating a three-way collaboration of HIV research between the Case Western Reserve, Johns Hopkins, and Makerere Universities.

* * *

In 1996, Art Ammann left the Pediatric AIDS Foundation and founded Global Strategies for HIV Prevention, a complementary organization that addressed the medical, social, and political issues surrounding mother-to-child transmission. In September 1997, he organized a Global Strategies Conference in Washington, DC, underwritten by BI and other corporate, governmental, and non-governmental sponsors, to share the latest scientific and clinical results, promote international cooperation, and set specific goals for addressing infant HIV infections and mortality.[31] Ammann wanted to create a forum where "everyone was hearing the same thing" at the same time, and the 800 conference attendees represented a broad cross-section of investigators, physicians, and governmental decision makers from developed and developing countries.[32] The complex and expensive AZT regimen that had been established by the ACTG 076 trial had already stopped HIV transmission from mothers to infants in the United States and other countries that could afford to use it. The Conference attendees hoped that the shortened AZT regimen in the ongoing Thai clinical trial and the even shorter AZT/3TC regimen in the ongoing PETRA trial would also prove to be effective. Both of those clinical trials were nearing completion. But even these short-term regimens might be too complex and expensive in countries where pouring a glass of clean drinking water was considered a luxury.

Myers took advantage of Ammann's Global Strategies Conference to hold parallel discussions with the investigators of the South African and Ugandan clinical trials, both of which would evaluate the single-dose nevirapine regimen as a simpler alternative.[33] The investigators agreed to harmonize their study protocols to enhance the likelihood that the results would be definitive, one way or the other. Both trials were designed as blinded studies and included placebo control groups.

Ammann also arranged a small satellite meeting after his Conference to discuss the issue of drug access in the developing world, and the use of placebos in the mother-to-child transmission trials was a hot topic. Myers, representing BI, attended this meeting, along with a dozen people representing several AIDS drug manufacturers, FDA, the United Nations' AIDS program, the International AIDS Society, and investigators from several developing countries.[34] A half-dozen clinical trials were in progress in developing countries, each aimed at finding a drug regimen that was more feasible than the long-term AZT regimen, and each of those ongoing clinical trials included a placebo control group. By the mid-1990s, investigators had abandoned using a placebo group in most AIDS clinical trials. Instead, they assessed a new drug regimen by comparing it to another regimen that was known to be beneficial, a positive control group. But the long-term AZT regimen, although an acceptable positive control, was simply not feasible for the mother-to-child transmission clinical trials conducted in developing countries. Pregnant women rarely visited a clinic until they went into labor (making AZT treatment during pregnancy unworkable), and most clinics were not equipped to deliver the intravenous AZT infusion during labor or monitor the six weeks of AZT dosing to the babies after delivery. The only practical way investigators could assess the short-term alternative regimens, none of which was yet proven to work, was to compare them to a placebo treatment.

Two weeks after Ammann's Global Strategies Conference, the issue of placebos in mother-to-child transmission clinical trials reached the flashpoint. In an editorial, the *New England Journal of Medicine* claimed that giving a placebo to participants in the mother-to-child clinical trials showed "a callous disregard of their welfare for the sake of research goals."[35] The journal compared the ongoing trials in developing countries to the infamous Tuskegee Study in which poor African American men with syphilis were studied for forty years and deprived of penicillin, a known, effective, and affordable treatment. The editorial prompted an immediate, forceful, and united reaction from the scientific community. David Ho and Cathy Wilfert, the two AIDS experts on the journal's editorial board, promptly resigned in protest.[36] Wilfert's action was particularly noteworthy. She had been the driving force behind the ACTG 076 trial, and as chairman of the ACTG's Pediatrics Core Committee she had been intimately involved in designing clinical trials and addressing the issue of mother-to-child HIV transmission for years. Wilfert considered the editorial biased and "a grievous misuse of the journal's power."[37] Her name on the journal's masthead implied that she agreed with the editorial, but she did not.

Along with many others, Wilfert considered the comparison to the Tuskegee Study inappropriate. That comparison showed a lack of understanding of the way contemporary clinical trials were being conducted. Unlike the Tuskegee Study, the current trials' investigators were following widely accepted ethical principles and guidelines. Institutional review boards in the United States and in the respective developing countries had assessed and approved the study protocols, confirming that the rights of the participating women and infants were protected. In addition, the scientific communities and public health officials in the developing countries had rigorously vetted the trials, and the investigators had obtained authorization from the local governments. Also, unlike the Tuskegee Study, all of the women in the current trials knew that they might be getting a placebo rather than the experimental drug. And, the treatment of the participants in the ongoing clinical trials was consistent with the standard of care in their respective countries, where women otherwise would not receive any drug treatment during pregnancy or even know that they were infected with HIV.

The editorial, critics claimed, also had not adequately considered the needs of the developing countries where the mother-to-child trials were conducted.[38] Uganda was a typical example. Like most African countries, AIDS drugs were largely unavailable in Uganda, and there were no programs for preventing mother-to-child transmission of HIV. Many mothers delivered their babies at home, and with Uganda's limited public health, clinical, and laboratory resources, the complex, long-term AZT regimen was impractical, if not impossible.[39] Unable to pay for much-needed healthcare improvements, Ugandan authorities welcomed the financial sponsorship of external organizations like the National Institutes of Health's HIVNET program. But Ugandans ran the programs. In the words of Edward K. Mbidde, the chairman of Uganda's AIDS Research Committee, "These are Ugandan studies conducted by Ugandan investigators on Ugandans ... for the good of their people."[40]

* * *

Laura Guay, who was still based in Uganda, worked with her collaborators at Makerere University, Francis Mmiro and Philippa Musoke, and established Mulago Hospital in Kampala as the clinical site for Jackson's HIVNET single-dose nevirapine clinical trial. Mulago Hospital, the largest government referral hospital in Uganda, had the expertise, facilities, and patient population necessary to conduct the trial.[41] Its well-staffed obstetrics, pediatrics, and child health departments handled 45,000 pregnancy-related visits per year, and approximately 85 percent of the hospital admissions were HIV-related.

As a first step, Guay and her colleagues conducted a small pilot study, enrolling twenty-one pregnant, HIV-infected women at Mulago Hospital.[42] Their goal was to repeat the single-dose nevirapine regimen used by Sullivan in the United States and confirm the safety and bioavailability of nevirapine in the Ugandan mothers and newborns. The results of this pilot study were essentially identical to Sullivan's findings in the earlier American study. A single dose of nevirapine given to the Ugandan mothers during labor produced a therapeutic blood level of the drug in both the women and their newborns. The mother's breast milk also contained a therapeutic level of drug. And supplementing the infants with a single dose of the nevirapine liquid formulation within three days of birth ensured that the babies maintained a therapeutic level of drug for at least seven days. Guay and her colleagues also monitored the viral load of HIV in the mothers and examined the babies for signs of HIV infection. The study was too small to make any firm conclusions about nevirapine's effectiveness, but this simple nevirapine regimen seemed to protect the babies from HIV infection.[43] The results were certainly encouraging and justified moving ahead with Jackson's larger, controlled clinical trial.

In November 1997, after many months of discussing and refining the study protocol, Guay and Mmiro began enrolling HIV-infected pregnant women at their clinic in Mulago Hospital. The clinical trial, which was officially designated HIVNET 012, was originally designed as a large, definitive trial of 1500 mother/infant pairs. The treatments were blinded, and the women were randomly assigned to receive either the single-dose nevirapine regimen, a short-term

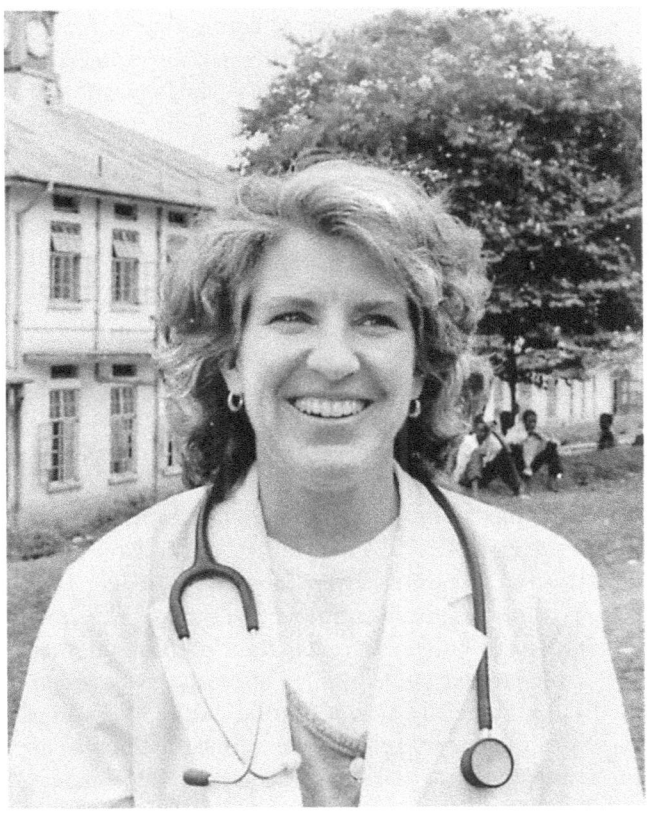

Laura Guay working in Uganda during the HIVNET 012 clinical trial (courtesy Johns Hopkins Medicine Archives).

regimen with AZT, or a comparable placebo.[44] Because neither of these drugs (given as short-term treatment regimens during labor and after delivery) had been proven to prevent mother-to-child transmission of HIV, the investigators used the placebo group to determine whether either or both of the drug regimens worked better than the control group receiving no treatment.

Then, three months later, in February 1998, the results of the Thai clinical trial were publicly announced, showing that short-term AZT treatment prevented HIV transmission in half of the newborns.[45] Because the short-term AZT regimen proved to be nearly as effective as the longer and more complex AZT dosing regimen used in the ACTG 076 trial, investigators who were studying mother-to-child transmission in several developing countries, including Thailand and Côte d'Ivoire in western Africa, immediately adopted the short-term and more convenient AZT regimen as their new standard.[46]

Having received news of the Thai study's results, Guay and Mmiro stopped enrollment in the HIVNET 012 clinical trial. Now that a short-term AZT regimen had proven to be effective, Jackson, his Ugandan colleagues, and the ethics review boards in the United States and Uganda concluded that it would be unethical to continue their trial with a placebo control group.[47] But they now faced a dilemma. To redesign the blinded trial with an ethically acceptable "positive" control group would take months. In the meantime, the HIV-infected women who had already signed up for the original trial would receive no treatment. Jackson and Guay asked the Division of AIDS at the National Institutes of Health in Washington, DC, and the ethics review boards for permission to bridge this gap by continuing their current trial as an "open-label" study. They wanted to keep using the original nevirapine and AZT treatment regimens but would eliminate the placebo group.[48] This change meant that the investigators and all of the women in the trial would know who received the short-term AZT regimen (which they now expected to be beneficial) and who received the experimental single-dose nevirapine regimen. The review boards allowed Guay and Mmiro to proceed with HIVNET 012 as a scaled-down, open-label trial, which resumed in April 1998. The investigators in Uganda intended to continue this open-label trial only until the new blinded trial could be launched.[49] In parallel, Jackson began drafting the protocol for this new trial "with an appropriate control arm."[50]

* * *

All clinical trials have their challenges. Recordkeeping may be inconsistent, patients may miss scheduled visits, and transcription errors may occur when copying information from the patient's medical chart to the trial's official data forms. Investigators face special challenges when the trial involves giving experimental drugs to women in labor and drawing multiple blood samples from infants. But the HIVNET 012 trial turned out to have more than its fair share of difficulties. Because the trial's treatments were intended to benefit only the infant (that is, prevent HIV infection in the infant, not improve the mother's health), Guay and Mmiro's staff needed to obtain permission for treatment from both the mother and father, as stipulated by HIVNET's administrative guidelines.[51] The mothers were eager to do anything that would ensure the health of their babies, including participation in a clinical trial, but obtaining permission from the fathers proved more difficult. Because of the physical distance of the fathers, fear of intense stigmatization, social and economic repercussions, and even violence against the women if their HIV status became known, the women were rarely able or willing to identify the fathers.[52] Guay's team made a reasonable effort to obtain the father's permission, encouraging the women to bring along their partners to the clinic for counseling and HIV testing. But the clinic staff made no attempt to follow up if the father failed to appear, partly because most households in Uganda at the time did not have telephones, but mostly because they felt that disclosure of the woman's HIV status would violate her right to privacy and would put her at personal risk.[53] If the father did not come to the clinic, they simply noted in their study records that he was unavailable and enrolled the woman without obtaining his consent.[54]

In cases where the mother died after delivery, Guay's staff needed to find and consult a legal guardian, who would be the responsible decision maker for the infant's follow up care during the remainder of the trial's 18-month evaluation period. But reaching out to family members for follow up of the infant would have required disclosing the mother's and the infant's HIV status, and the investigators were constrained by their respect for confidentiality of the information that the deceased mother had shared with them, including her HIV infection.[55]

In addition to these ethical challenges, Guay managed the trial under environmental conditions that were uncommon and with healthcare facilities that were more austere than in developed countries. Determining whether the experimental drug regimens caused side effects and assessing HIV-related symptoms were complicated by the presence of other diseases such as malaria and tuberculosis. A patient who develops malaria during a clinical trial in the United States would raise serious concerns, but malaria was common in Ugandan women and infants, whether they were HIV-infected or not.[56] In the HIVNET 012 trial, sorting out drug-induced side effects from pre-existing medical conditions required careful assessments.

Guay and her staff set up their clinic for the HIVNET 012 trial in an unoccupied ward at Mulago Hospital. But about halfway through the trial, they were informed, on short notice, that the building was scheduled for renovation and they needed to vacate the ward.[57] With no alternative location available, they stripped wood from the ward and built a shed on the grounds of the hospital, using plywood dividers to create eight to ten exam rooms. Because the shed had no electricity or running water, they moved their computers and data processing center to the research laboratory where the patients' blood samples were processed. Their new "offices" consisted of a row of chairs and repurposed tabletops in the hallway of another building. The delivery and postnatal wards were also moved to accommodate the renovations. The hospital relocated the delivery ward to an empty house nearby, and the study staff stored their experimental drugs in a secured cupboard in the house. On the lawn near their newly constructed shed, Guay's staff pitched two tents, which served as the waiting area and provided space for counseling, education, and demonstrations. But the heat in equatorial Africa often made the tents too uncomfortable, and the women preferred sitting under nearby shade trees, unless it was raining.

Every week, hundreds of women patiently sat under the trees or tents waiting their turn to meet with the counselors and study staff, checking in with their babies as part of the 18-month follow up period. It was a new experience for both the study staff and the patients. Guay and Mmiro's fulltime counselors and study nurses, who were experienced Ugandan healthcare workers, were accustomed to providing "episodic care," processing patients in an assembly line and typically seeing each patient only once. But in the HIVNET 012 trial, they invested considerable time with each patient, collecting medical histories, explaining the hazards of transmitting HIV, answering questions about the trial procedures, and conducting follow up visits at the patients' homes if the women were unable to come to the clinic. Unlike the restrictions Guay had faced on her first deployment to Uganda, she could now justify frank discussions with HIV-infected women because she could also offer them counseling, support, and hope.

For pregnant women, the HIVNET 012 trial was an attractive option. They wanted to enroll in the trial, because they received drugs and medical services that were not otherwise available to most Ugandans. Because of the personal attention they received, they were more willing to welcome the counselors into their homes and more likely to come to the clinic for medical needs beyond their scheduled study visits. Consequently, infant mortality among the trial participants was lower than in the general population.[58] One of the counselors' biggest challenges, in fact, was easing the disappointment of the women who did not meet the enrollment criteria for the trial and could not access the treatment, medical care, and personalized attention it offered.

Guay and her staff created secure spaces in their makeshift clinic and the laboratory to store their study records, but when the women or infants required hospitalization, Mulago Hospital employed separate recordkeeping procedures. Because the hospital did not have a standardized filing system — it consisted of "heaps of patient files in boxes" in a storage room — Guay and her staff also documented the patients' hospitalization activities using their own forms, which they kept in the patients' study file.[59] Often, those shadow files were more complete than the hospital's official records, and they served as an important backup. The edges of some of the medical records in the hospital's storeroom were nibbled by rodents or insects. At one point, a log book, which contained notes about follow up visits to the women's homes, was damaged by flooding due to a plumbing problem and also had to be transcribed.[60]

Guay closely monitored the progress of the trial, reviewing weekly reports on the number of patients tested, enrolled, and treated. She also paid close attention to the medical care of the women and infants but otherwise was unaware of the trial results. The study team in Uganda merely forwarded the data to the HIVNET data processing center in Seattle, Washington, for analysis.[61] Occasionally, though, Guay heard her staff commenting that fewer babies in the nevirapine group seemed to be infected.[62]

Meanwhile, Jackson continued to draft the protocol for the new blinded clinical trial. In addition to HIVNET 012, Mmiro was leading a team at Mulago Hospital that was participating in Lange's PETRA trial to assess the value of short-term AZT/3TC regimens for preventing mother-to-child HIV transmission. Jackson was awaiting completion of the PETRA trial, hoping that the results would confirm that AZT/3TC was an appropriate positive control regimen for his new trial.[63] Unfortunately, the PETRA trial progressed more slowly than originally planned, and in the meantime, Guay and Mmiro continued to enroll women in HIVNET 012. Then, one day in June 1999, Guay received a call from Jackson.

During a routine meeting of the Data Safety Monitoring Board (an independent panel that was charged with reviewing data in the ongoing HIVNET 012 trial to make sure there were no safety problems or other reasons to stop the trial), the panel members saw a surprising result.[64] Few investigators had given nevirapine any chance of working in the HIVNET 012 trial, fewer had expected nevirapine to work as well as the short-term regimen of AZT, and no one dreamt that nevirapine would work better than AZT. But despite all of those preconceived doubts, the data handlers had found sufficient statistical proof that the single-dose nevirapine regimen prevented HIV transmission better than the AZT regimen.[65] They immediately informed the National Institutes of Health's Division of AIDS and Jackson, who informed Guay and the study team in Uganda. It was an important finding and one that Jackson felt obligated to report to the scientific community as soon as possible. They stopped enrollment, having enrolled 626 women, and the last infant in the HIVNET 012 trial was born on June 19, 1999.[66]

Jackson knew that the report of the HIVNET 012 results needed to be backed up with rock-solid data. Using the time zone difference to their advantage, Jackson and Guay shuttled data and messages daily between Kampala, Baltimore, and Seattle, working around the clock to analyze the HIVNET 012 data. Despite the pressure to report their findings quickly, their analysis was thorough, precise, and complete. In Kampala, Guay checked every endpoint and patient outcome.[67] In Baltimore, Jackson personally checked every printout of every HIV-RNA assay.[68]

One morning, Guay was awakened by the ring of her phone at 3:00 A.M. It was 8:00 P.M. in Baltimore and 5:00 P.M. in Seattle, and Jackson was asking about a laboratory result, an infant's hemoglobin reading of 4. That reading was incompatible with life if medical measures were not taken quickly, and he asked: What happened to that baby? The study records gave no details. Guay instinctively knew the reading could not be correct, because she had tracked all abnormal laboratory results during the trial and would have remembered a number this low. To resolve the issue, Guay got up, drove through the darkened streets of Kampala, and rummaged through the study files to find the original laboratory printouts. The laboratory had spotted an error when the original test was run and repeated the assay. The baby's hemoglobin, in fact, was normal.[69]

On July 12, 1999, less than one month after the last baby in the HIVNET 012 trial was born, the statisticians and data monitors held a teleconference to discuss their preliminary findings with the trial investigators at Johns Hopkins and Makerere Universities.[70] The rate of mother-to-child transmission of HIV in the single-dose nevirapine group was nearly half of that in the group receiving the short-term AZT regimen.[71] Nevirapine's effect was especially impressive, considering that nearly all of the mothers breastfed their infants. Nevirapine protected the babies from becoming infected despite exposure to HIV, both during childbirth and through breast milk. Two days later, Uganda's Minister of Health announced the study's findings in a press release in Kampala, and later that day, HIVNET administrators at the National Institutes of Health, who had sponsored the trial, issued a similar press release in Bethesda, Maryland.[72] Both agencies hailed the single-dose nevirapine regimen as "more affordable and practical than any other examined to date" for preventing transmission of HIV from mother to child.[73]

Within weeks, news of the HIVNET 012 trial's findings reverberated around the world and set a new standard for preventing mother-to-child transmission of HIV. In developing countries where most women did not receive prenatal care, approximately 1800 newborn babies were becoming infected with HIV every day. Health authorities estimated that widespread use of single-dose nevirapine could prevent 300,000 to 400,000 babies from becoming infected each year.[74] In addition to its therapeutic benefit and convenience, nevirapine was also much less expensive. The long, complicated AZT regimen that was being given to pregnant women and newborns in the United States and Europe (based on the ACTG 076 trial) cost $815, and the short-term AZT regimen that had recently been adopted for use in developing countries (based on the Thai study results) cost $268. The cost of single-dose nevirapine for mother and infant was $4.[75]

The properties that the BI scientists built into the nevirapine molecule years earlier had now proven their worth.[76] They wanted a drug that worked rapidly and decreased viral load, and nevirapine was immediately taken up into a baby's bloodstream and mother's milk after a single dose, reaching therapeutic levels in the baby within hours and decreasing the HIV viral load in breast milk ten-fold.[77] They wanted a drug that had a long half-life, and nevirapine, unlike AZT, could be administered once to a newborn and remain at a therapeutic blood level for at least a week. They wanted a drug that was stable, and the nevirapine formulations could be stored at ambient temperature — an important consideration in developing countries.[78] They wanted a drug that was easy to manufacture, and nevirapine cost a fraction of AZT. And finally, they wanted a drug that was safe, and nevirapine, when given as a single dose, produced no side effects.

Jackson knew that many investigators, policy makers, and healthcare workers were anxious to see the final study report, and he drove his team to complete the data analysis for publication. He drafted the manuscript, incorporating the analyzed data as Guay and the statisticians completed each section. The detailed results defined nevirapine's beneficial effects more completely. By three months of age, the portion of HIV-infected babies had gradually risen in both treatment groups, due to transmission of HIV through breast milk. In the AZT treatment group, the portion of HIV-infected babies at three months of age was the same as untreated babies in the general population in Uganda. But in the group who had received a single dose of nevirapine, significantly fewer three-month-old babies had become infected.[79] Jackson circulated the completed manuscript to all of the authors and key contributors, insisting on a 48-hour turnaround for comments, and then submitted the revised manuscript for publication. Details of the HIVNET 012 trial were published in the prestigious journal, *Lancet*, on September 4, 1999, less than three months after the last baby in the study had been born.[80] In the paper, Jackson acknowledged the key contributions of Sullivan, Myers, Ammann, and Wilfert in proposing the concept for the study, designing the protocol, and supporting the trial.

* * *

Just after Guay enrolled the last patient in the HIVNET 012 trial in Uganda, John Sullivan's collaborators finally began enrolling women in the SAINT trial. For several years, Sullivan had persisted in his efforts to examine the value of a short-term nevirapine regimen. He had made many trips to South Africa, coordinating arrangements for the trial with Daya Moodley and her department head, Hoosen "Jerry" Coovadia, at the University of KwaZulu-Natal in Durban, who served as the lead investigators. With backing from BI, the cooperation of investigators at eleven hospitals in South Africa, and authorization by regulatory authorities in both the United States and South Africa, Sullivan finally had been able to make his clinical trial a reality. This large trial would enroll more than 1300 HIV-infected South African women and compare a nevirapine regimen similar to that used in the HIVNET 012 trial with a short-course regimen of AZT and 3TC that Joep Lange and his Dutch team had used in the PETRA trial.[81] Both regimens had proven to be effective in preventing mother-to-child transmission of HIV, but the SAINT trial compared the safety and efficacy of the two regimens side-by-side. Essentially, it was the definitive, controlled trial that Jackson had wanted to conduct in Uganda as the follow up to the open-label HIVNET 012 trial. Although the results of the SAINT trial would confirm the results of the PETRA and HIVNET 012 trials, it became embroiled in a controversy in South Africa that took years to resolve.

19

I Remember Montreal

Montreal in 1989 versus Montreal in 1999: What a difference a decade had made. People who attended the 5th International AIDS Conference in Montreal in 1989 remembered it for two things. The first was the insistence of advocacy groups not just to be heard but to be a full partner in the crusade to fight AIDS. It started innocently, with demonstrators intending only to picket the Montreal conference center's entrance on the opening day of the Conference. But when the doors opened, they spilled into the building, a wave of humanity propelled by the sheer force of their numbers.[1] They dominated the Conference's opening session, crashed press conferences, and sneaked into a few of the scientific sessions. The international press corps, more than a thousand strong, recorded their actions in print and video for the world to see, even though the protesters competed that week with the photo of a Chinese man staring down a row of tanks in Tiananmen Square.[2] But they made their point and would never be outsiders again.

The second memorable, although more muted, event in Montreal in 1989 was the spotlight on the widely spreading AIDS epidemic in developing countries. The conference organizers specifically invited scientists, physicians, and journalists from those countries, and those delegates set the tone for the meeting, a bleak outlook that one speaker compared to ticking time bombs that would explode within a decade.[3] Stopping the spread of HIV in their countries presented social, cultural, and economic problems never before encountered by healthcare providers, such as introducing safe-sex practices in societies where sex was a taboo subject. The Ugandan government considered it tantamount to genocide to advise HIV-positive women to refrain from bearing children.[4] And then there was the issue of cost. Investigators at the Conference reported encouraging outcomes with the aerosol form of pentamidine, which prevented pneumonia in AIDS patients, and progress toward control of HIV with AZT, the only approved AIDS drug.[5] But those drugs were prohibitively expensive in developing countries. Conference delegates were also sensitized to the changing demographics of AIDS, from a disease predominantly in gay men to a disease increasingly affecting other vulnerable individuals. Among them were women and infants. Just hinted at by the Conference speakers, but a growing concern, was the issue of HIV transmission from mothers to infants.[6]

In 1989, the protesters and representatives from developing countries were thinking more about staying alive than making history, but that Conference was a turning point. "After Montreal, the International Conference on AIDS [would] never be the same."[7] Rather than an exclusive scientific forum, future International AIDS Conferences would attempt to strike a balance between scientific, social, political, and economic issues.

If Montreal in 1989 had been a turning point, Montreal in 1999 was a launch pad. For months, Art Ammann had been planning the second Conference on Global Strategies for

HIV Prevention, a follow up to the conference that he had organized in Washington, DC, two years earlier. He scheduled updates on issues that had been raised and ongoing trials that had been discussed at the first conference: the effectiveness of short-term AZT regimens to prevent mother-to-child HIV transmission, the role of breastfeeding in spreading HIV, the safety of drugs given to pregnant women and infants, and the impact of other infections such as tuberculosis, malaria, and syphilis on transmission of HIV to newborns. Then in July, the results of the HIVNET 012 trial were announced. Ammann shuffled the Conference program to include a presentation by the trial's investigators and arranged travel grants so that key representatives of the large Ugandan study team could attend.[8] For some of them, it would be their first trip outside their country.

Ammann also knew that the broad cross-section of conference delegates gave him a golden opportunity to energize their scientific, industrial, and political constituencies. Now, they could go beyond just talking about the expanding AIDS epidemic and do something about it. He wanted to inspire this collective human capital to launch an AIDS prevention campaign, and the single-dose nevirapine regimen provided the mechanism to make that happen in the countries that needed it the most. But he knew it would take more than inspiration. The campaign would also need financial resources and someone to manage the prevention programs. In the weeks leading up to the Conference, he contacted a number of organizations and individuals who might be willing to support the effort, including the Elizabeth Glaser Pediatric AIDS Foundation.[9]

* * *

In 1996, Cathy Wilfert retired from Duke University and followed Ammann as Scientific Director at the Pediatric AIDS Foundation. In her first few years at the Foundation, she continued the activities that Ammann had started, evaluating proposals and funding research grants. She also continued Ammann's program of Elizabeth Glaser Scientist Awards, which funded individual, young investigators to do HIV/AIDS research.[10] Considerable progress had been made since the days when Elizabeth Glaser and her two friends first organized the Foundation. The Ariel Project had concluded its five-year investigation of the causes and risk factors contributing to transmission of HIV from mothers to infants.[11] In the United States, the widespread use of AZT and other AIDS drugs to treat women had virtually eliminated HIV infections in newborns, and consequently, pediatric AIDS in the United States was disappearing.[12] Elizabeth's original goal had been achieved, and the Foundation's board of directors debated what to do next. They needed a new mission. Just at that moment, they heard the announcement of the HIVNET 012 trial's results.

Ammann contacted Wilfert to ask for the Foundation's support. He envisioned a "call to action," a comprehensive program to eliminate HIV transmission to infants through drug treatment programs, maternal and infant medical care, information and education programs, and continued research for better drugs.[13] The Foundation's board enthusiastically supported Ammann's idea and made a large financial contribution toward the effort.[14] In the weeks leading up to the Montreal Conference, Ammann and Wilfert worked behind the scenes on the details of this new initiative.

* * *

Headlining the Global Strategies Conference on September 1, 1999, Laura Guay told the astounded audience in Montreal about the HIVNET 012 trial results, explaining that single-dose nevirapine prevented HIV transmission to infants.[15] The attendees also heard about encouraging progress with other short-term drug regimens, but they hailed single-dose nevirapine as the breakthrough they had been seeking. The goal of finding effective, affordable solutions to the rapidly expanding AIDS epidemic had suddenly turned from hopeful promises to actionable realities. The international delegates, particularly those from African countries, overwhelmingly embraced this news—finally there was a feasible way to prevent HIV transmission in their communities.[16] They swarmed to grab copies of the press release summarizing the HIVNET 012 trial results, some dangerously clambering across banks of escalators for a copy as they were conveyed up and down.[17] One delegate remembered thinking, "Our whole world is changed now."[18] Representatives from the Elizabeth Glaser Pediatric AIDS Foundation huddled to draft a full page ad for the *New York Times*, laying out the impact that single-dose nevirapine would have in preventing mother-to-child HIV transmission in developing countries.[19]

Ammann presented recognition awards to Sullivan for his advocacy of preventative treatments and to Jackson, Guay, Mmiro, and others on the HIVNET 012 team for their landmark trial. The delegates stood up and cheered.[20] The Ugandan musician and humanitarian, Samite, enhanced the festive mood and had the delegates singing and dancing well into the evening. The Conference delegates readily endorsed the call to action concept, which challenged foundations, governments, nongovernment organizations, and faith-based organizations to make life-saving AIDS treatments available worldwide. And single-dose nevirapine led the way, a regimen so simple, inexpensive, and effective that it broke through all the barriers that had prevented access to HIV/AIDS healthcare in resource-limited countries.[21] As the skies cleared over Montreal and the delegates dispersed on the final day of the Conference, "the idea picked up incredible momentum."[22]

* * *

The Elizabeth Glaser Pediatric AIDS Foundation expanded its mission: to prevent HIV transmission in the resource-limited countries where pediatric AIDS was still a major health problem.[23] And the Foundation provided leadership, management, and administrative oversight of the Call to Action initiative.[24] It was a monumental undertaking for an organization that at the time consisted of only three dozen people. They had limited international experience (related only to research awards), and they had to shift from an organization that distributed grants for pediatric AIDS research to a service-delivery organization.[25] Similarly, Cathy Wilfert, the Foundation's Scientific Director, had limited international experience. But she was an expert on pediatric AIDS, and, having inspired the landmark ACTG 076 trial, she knew a lot about how to prevent HIV transmission from mother to child. For Wilfert, this new challenge became a personal mission.[26] To save the children. In every corner of the world.

Within a few months, the Foundation had attracted donations from several organizations, including $15 million from the Gates Foundation, to launch the Call to Action program, and single-dose nevirapine was a key element of their multi-country initiative.[27] During his tenure at the Foundation, Ammann had established procedures to solicit and review grant proposals, as well as to manage and monitor the progress of the Foundation's funded research projects. Wilfert and the Foundation staff now applied those procedures and skills to the Call to Action program. They solicited applications from healthcare workers in developing countries who wanted to implement mother-to-child prevention programs. Single-dose nevirapine was not a requirement. The applicants could propose the AZT regimen or any other HIV prevention program, but the simplicity and low cost made single-dose nevirapine feasible in regions where other regimens were not.[28]

Wilfert felt that the only way to properly assess the fitness of each applicant was to visit the sites, meet the local champions, and address problems that might hinder implementation. "One person who didn't want to cooperate could derail the program."[29] Although she "learned as I went," Wilfert rapidly settled into her new role. Her peer reviewers quickly evaluated the first applications and awarded funds for HIV prevention programs at eight clinics in six countries. And with their finely tuned procedures, she and her staff kept going. They got new prevention clinics up-and-running within a few months of receiving an applicant's proposal, far faster than comparable government foreign aid programs.[30]

Wilfert traveled sixty percent of the time, assessing new sites, providing support for the ongoing prevention programs, and guaranteeing that the Foundation's funds reached the places where the medical services were most needed. She would not have tried to operate a clinic at Duke without seeing it, and she gave the same personal attention to the clinics in Africa.[31] Equally comfortable in the boardroom and on the playground, Wilfert shaped the Call to Action clinics' services, person by person, day by day, listening, advising, and reassuring — a sixty-something grandmother with a stethoscope around her neck. Laura Guay also visited some of the clinics and offered advice based on her experiences in Uganda.[32] They cooperated with each country's Ministry of Health, worked in concert with local customs and culture, and tapped into the existing public health system, clinics, faith based organizations, and other groups to implement the funded programs. They also respected the regulatory authorities in each country, confirming that the AIDS drugs, including nevirapine, were approved before they were used in the Call to Action programs. The Foundation provided program management and monitoring, under Wilfert's leadership. In addition, the Foundation hired a few people in each country to handle administrative, financial, and technical tasks, but local healthcare workers in the country's healthcare system ran the programs.[33]

Treatment with nevirapine or other drug regimens required knowing whether the pregnant woman was HIV-positive. Knowing that she was infected required HIV testing. And conducting HIV tests in countries where AIDS carried a significant stigma required extensive, but delicately applied, counseling. Call to Action funded all of these services, but Wilfert faced a multitude of practical challenges in implementing them. Most of the clinics had no doctor. At best, a clinical officer, comparable to a physician's assistant, was in charge. Two hundred women a day would typically be sitting in the clinic waiting to be seen by one nurse, and in most countries, nurses could not prescribe medicines.[34] Prenatal care consisted of blood pressure measurements, vitamins and iron supplements, malarial medicine, and a tetanus shot.[35] Most women visited the clinic only once or twice during their pregnancy. Nearly half of them did not visit a clinic at all, and only sixty percent delivered their babies in a healthcare facility. To have an impact under those conditions, the HIV prevention regimen had to be simple as well as effective. "One pill at the time of delivery has a much greater chance of impacting the system."[36] Wilfert worked to bundle counseling and testing on the mother's first — and perhaps only — visit to the clinic and issued nevirapine if she was HIV-positive, along with instructions for taking the drug during childbirth.[37]

* * *

As Wilfert and the Elizabeth Glaser Pediatric AIDS Foundation continued to feel their way through the fog, modern day Livingstones successfully establishing HIV prevention programs at a growing number of clinics throughout Africa, their efforts were largely ignored by the rest of the world. Ammann's Montreal Conference had generated considerable excitement among the 700 delegates, but press coverage had been comparatively light. It was going to take a bigger event with more media clout to capture the world's attention, sway policy makers, and marshal international political will. Working in his laboratories at nearby McGill University and the Jewish General Hospital during Ammann's Conference, Mark Wainberg viewed the progress of the new HIV prevention and treatment initiatives with great interest and a growing concern. Wainberg had been a co-developer of 3TC, the first of the second generation AZT-like drugs, and had also been a key collaborator on the INCAS trial, the trial that showed nevirapine-containing drug combinations could drive HIV below detection. Three years earlier in Vancouver, he had seen the overwhelming enthusiasm generated by the results of the INCAS trial and many other clinical trials of triple-drug regimens, drugs that stopped HIV in its tracks. But Wainberg also realized that the scientific and clinical advances presented in Vancouver only benefited a small fraction of the world's growing population of HIV-infected people. "Africa was not on the radar screen."[38] As the incoming president of the International AIDS Society, Wainberg had the opportunity to change that.

The International AIDS Conferences, sponsored by the Society, had never been held in a developing country, but to Wainberg, there was no more appropriate location. The International AIDS Conferences were the largest, most diverse, and most influential forum for discussing HIV/AIDS and were covered by a global press corps. Wainberg lobbied hard and steered the Society's leadership to select Durban, a port city on the eastern shore of South Africa, as the site for the upcoming Conference in 2000. Scientists are unaccustomed to making politically calculated decisions, but Wainberg considered this site selection "the most important thing I've done in my life."[39] The convenient location permitted large numbers of African healthcare professionals and health ministry officials to attend, giving them an unprecedented opportunity to tell their western colleagues about the devastation AIDS was inflicting on their continent. And the press corps would draw the world's attention to Africa, amplifying the voices of concerned scientists, investigators, and a multitude of HIV-infected people who had been muted for a decade.

Among the most eloquent of those voices was Edwin Cameron, who delivered the plenary speech on the opening day of the Durban Conference.[40] A native South

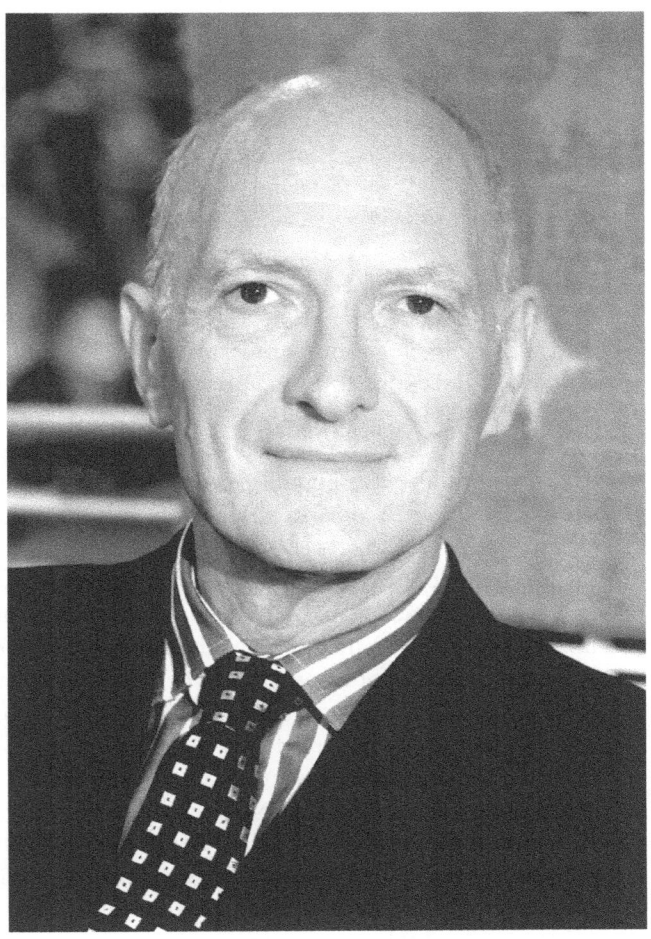

Edwin Cameron.

African, Cameron embodied the contrast between east and west, rich and poor, and life and death. On a continent in which the heaviest burden of the AIDS epidemic had been borne by women, he was a man. In a region where HIV infections were predominantly transmitted through heterosexual contact, he was proudly gay. In a country still struggling to shed apartheid and its history of racial injustice, he had been born white. And on a continent in which 290 million people survived on less than a dollar a day, he enjoyed the privileged income of an appeals court judge.

Cameron became infected with HIV in 1985, and twelve years later he developed the characteristic symptoms of full-blown AIDS.[41] Climbing a flight of stairs exhausted him, a thrush infection made his mouth rough and dry, he had no appetite, and he was losing weight. His doctor successfully treated his opportunistic infections and then prescribed AIDS drugs that had just become available in South Africa, later changing him to a daily regimen of nevirapine, AZT, and 3TC.[42] In April 1999, the judge announced his HIV status, the first and still the only government official in South Africa to do so. Fearful of a public backlash, Cameron was surprised and gratified that his announcement instead brought the AIDS issue to the forefront of public discourse in South Africa, as the revelations of Rock Hudson and Magic Johnson had done in the United States.[43]

Cameron had urged the Conference organizers to select a black South African leader to deliver the plenary speech, thinking that such a person would better represent the nation, the issues, and the impact of AIDS.[44] But no one accepted the invitation. So, Cameron, who had provided legal counsel to AIDS advocacy groups and had become a highly visible and influential spokesperson for the South African AIDS community, served to bridge the Conference's African hosts and Western visitors. He told his multi-national audience that he continued to lead a vigorous, healthy, and productive life, because his disease was controlled by his triple-drug regimen. He paid $400 per month for those drugs, a price that was beyond the reach of most Africans. Without treatment, based on the average life expectancy of AIDS patients, he would be dead. "I am here because I can afford to pay for life itself."[45] And for lack of single-dose nevirapine, he said, 5000 babies were being born every month with HIV: infections that were preventable, suffering that was preventable, and deaths that were preventable.

Cameron emphasized the social benefits that triple-drug therapy had created in addition to the medical breakthrough it represented. By transforming AIDS into a chronically manageable condition, the drug regimens had helped dispel the fear, prejudice, and stigma associated with AIDS. In areas of the world where those drug regimens had been implemented, the psychological and social changes in attitude toward HIV-infected people had been close to miraculous. Not so in South Africa, where less than two years earlier and only twelve miles from where Cameron now addressed the Convention delegates, Gugu Dlamini had been stoned and stabbed to death. The 36-year-old mother was murdered shortly after she revealed on television and radio that she was HIV-positive.[46]

For lack of access to life-saving AIDS drugs, Africans continued to suffer not only from the certainty of illness and death but also from discrimination and prejudice. Echoing predictions made at the Vancouver conference four years earlier, Cameron agreed that "of all the walls dividing people in the AIDS epidemic, the gap between the rich and the poor is most pervasive."[47] He called on international agencies, national governments, and the pharmaceutical industry to act and ensure equitable access to these drugs for all people with AIDS worldwide. It was a global economy, after all, and "how we live our lives affects how others live theirs."[48]

Cameron's impassioned speech and similar messages by a thousand other speakers at the Durban Conference were reported by the amassed journalists to their worldwide readership. Three points were indisputable and finally shocked the world into action: HIV was spreading throughout Africa at an alarming rate, AIDS drugs were desperately needed in Africa, where even the most basic medicines were not available, and politicians needed to show leadership and end the inequity in drug availability between rich and poor countries.

Among the first to act was Boehringer Ingelheim. In conjunction with the Durban Conference, BI announced in July 2000 that it would offer nevirapine free of charge for five years to developing countries for use in preventing mother-to-child HIV transmission.[49] Later that year, the Republic of Congo became the first country to take advantage of BI's nevirapine donation program.[50] Meanwhile, investigators continued to study nevirapine in prevention clinical trials in Zambia, Malawi, Tanzania, Kenya, Zimbabwe, and South Africa and confirmed the results of the Ugandan HIVNET 012 trial.[51] On October 24, 2000, the World Health Organization and the United Nations-sponsored UNAIDS agency, having determined that single-dose nevirapine was a safe and effective treatment for preventing mother-to-child transmission of HIV, endorsed single-dose nevirapine for use in general practice.[52]

In parallel, Wilfert and the Elizabeth Glaser Pediatric AIDS Foundation had been supporting the implementation of HIV prevention services within clinics throughout sub-Saharan Africa, honing their international administrative skills, and building the Foundation's reputation as a large service-delivery organization. Single-dose nevirapine was the vehicle that launched those initiatives, doubling the size of the Foundation in one year and proving that it was possible to deliver HIV prevention services to the most resource-constrained parts of the world. The Durban Conference commanded the world's attention, scaled up political will, and created the momentum that would expand the Foundation's programs at an increasingly rapid rate.

* * *

Maureen Myers and the BI project team had fully cooperated with the ACTG and HIVNET investigators who conducted the initial clinical trials aimed at preventing mother-to-child HIV transmission, offering suggestions to improve the study protocols, sharing their knowledge of the drug's properties, serving on the study teams, and donating supplies of nevirapine for the clinical trials. But BI's energy and internal resources were directed at fulfilling a closely related but separate commitment it had made to the FDA, namely, to complete the pediatric clinical trials and demonstrate that nevirapine in combination with other AIDS drugs was a safe and effective treatment for HIV-infected children.

20

The Kids' Turn

Jason and Jane's luck was about to change.[1] The adopted fraternal twins had become infected with HIV by their mother, Maria, at birth in April 1995. Although the long-term AZT regimen was the standard treatment in the United States for preventing mother-to-child HIV transmission at that time, Maria was unaware of her own infection, and the AZT regimen was started too late to prevent the twins' infections. Fortunately, their case was referred to John Sullivan and Katherine Luzuriaga at the University of Massachusetts. Sullivan and Luzuriaga had just started the first pediatric clinical trial of the nevirapine-containing triple-drug regimen, which Martin Hirsch had advocated and Julio Montaner was currently giving to adults in the INCAS trial.[2] The twins were only ten weeks old and had not developed any AIDS symptoms when they began taking the triple-drug regimen of nevirapine, AZT, and ddI.

Jane's viral load steadily dropped and became undetectable after eight weeks of treatment.[3] HIV-RNA remained undetectable in her blood for the rest of the 18-month trial. Other specialized assays (PBMC cultures and HIV antibody analyses) confirmed that the triple-drug regimen had cleared the virus from Jane's blood. Sullivan and Luzuriaga also noted other benefits of the treatment regimen. Children who are infected with HIV often do not respond to routine childhood immunizations, making them susceptible to childhood diseases like measles and mumps. But Jane received all of her routine childhood immunizations and her immune system responded normally.

Similarly, Jason's viral load quickly dropped and became undetectable after 24 weeks of treatment with the triple-drug regimen. Like Jane, his PBMC and HIV antibody tests confirmed that the drug regimen had cleared HIV from his blood. When Jason was sixteen months old, he received an influenza vaccination. Within a few weeks, HIV-RNA appeared in his blood — a small "blip" in his viral load but one that concerned the investigators. They switched his triple-drug regimen to 3TC, AZT, and ritonavir (an HIV protease inhibitor). Three weeks later, HIV-RNA again disappeared from his blood and remained undetected for the rest of the 18-month trial.

Jason and Jane's CD4 cell counts were normal for their age throughout the trial, indicating that their immune systems remained robust. Combining the results from Jason, Jane, and the other children in the trial, Sullivan and Luzuriaga confirmed Montaner's findings in the INCAS trial and concluded that the best way to control HIV in infants who became infected by their mothers was to start the triple-drug regimen within the first few weeks of life.[4]

* * *

When the Food and Drug Administration approved Viramune (nevirapine) tablets for use in adults in June 1996, the Boehringer Ingelheim project team had complete data from only nine children in the New Drug Application — far too little data to assess the benefits and risks of the drug for pediatric use. David Feigal, the Director of FDA's Antiviral Drug Products Division, urged BI to "move pediatric information into the label as quickly as possible."[5] He knew that BI had "a very full pipeline" of children in clinical trials.[6] Approximately 350 infants and children had received nevirapine, some for up to five years.[7] But the pediatric trials were at an "awkward stage" with much of the work still in progress, including the big ACTG-sponsored pediatric salvage study.[8]

Luzuriaga, Sandra Burchett, and their colleagues had begun the pediatric salvage study about the same time that Montaner and his colleagues started the INCAS trial in the summer of 1994, and they ultimately enrolled 431 children at 68 medical centers. Like the adult trials, the pediatric salvage study compared the triple-drug regimen of nevirapine, AZT and ddI with two-drug combinations.[9] Luzuriaga and Burchett's trial spanned three years and was just concluding when the BI team traveled to Rockville, Maryland, in June 1997. They met with FDA officials to discuss the requirements for expanding the Viramune label to include treatment of children.[10] On the table for consideration, in addition to the pediatric salvage study, were the final study reports of Sullivan and Luzuriaga's two, small pediatric trials, which described nevirapine's effects when given alone and in combination with AZT. More than half of the children had continued taking nevirapine, as part of a drug combination, after those trials concluded. Many had been taking nevirapine without difficulties for years.[11] The pediatric salvage study greatly increased the number of children taking nevirapine and reinforced the results of the earlier, smaller trials showing that the drug was safe. The BI team felt these trials collectively provided sufficient evidence to justify giving nevirapine to children. At the meeting, the two sides agreed on the package of data that the team should compile for the FDA reviewers' consideration.[12]

On March 13, 1998, the BI team submitted the pediatric supplement to its New Drug Application, requesting market approval of nevirapine for the same indications in children as the FDA had previously approved in adults.[13] The supplemental application consisted of 23 volumes of pediatric data describing the safety and efficacy of nevirapine, primarily from the clinical trials headed by Sullivan, Luzuriaga, and Burchett. At this point, Jason and Jane had been taking their triple-drug regimen for three years, were still healthy, and still had no detectable HIV in their blood.[14]

In April 1998, BI sent to FDA a second New Drug Application, consisting of eight volumes of chemistry data characterizing Amale Hawi's liquid suspension formulation.[15] And in July, at the request of the FDA reviewers, BI sent one more volume of information: clinical study reports and published manuscripts elaborating on the safety of nevirapine in newborns.[16] In addition, BI submitted fifteen sets of supplemental data and information in response to the FDA reviewers' requests or as a follow up to teleconference discussions, clarifying various aspects of the pediatric data.[17] The BI team and FDA reviewers traded questions and answers monthly in April, May, and June, exchanged official correspondence weekly in July, and negotiated almost daily in August and early September. On September 11, 1998, BI received the official letter from the FDA, granting accelerated approval of Viramune (nevirapine) tablets for use in children and Viramune (nevirapine) oral suspension.[18] Fast-track approval (called "exceptional circumstances") by the European regulatory authorities for pediatric use of Viramune tablets and oral suspension soon followed.[19]

Regulators on both sides of the Atlantic viewed the liquid formulation as an especially useful addition to the AIDS "therapeutic armamentarium" for physicians who were treating HIV-infected children.[20] Pediatricians agreed. They welcomed Hawi's pleasant-tasting nevirapine syrup, noting that alternative AIDS drugs, though effective, "taste terrible" and "getting kids to swallow such drugs is very difficult."[21] But the regulators also expected the BI team to continue their ongoing clinical trials and demonstrate, conclusively, that nevirapine improved the clinical condition of AIDS patients—specifically, that the drug delayed the onset of AIDS symptoms and prolonged life. In 1998, young people accounted for nearly half of all new HIV infections, and they needed AIDS drugs that were good enough and safe enough to suppress their HIV infections for a lifetime.[22]

* * *

HIV had always been an integral part of Jake Glaser's life. In his family, seeing doctors, having frequent blood tests, and taking precautions at school were routine and normal activities. He was healthy, never thought much about HIV, and certainly did not view it as a threat. As a fifth grader, he spent most of his time with friends, because his mother did not want him to see her sick. She insisted that he go out and play, rather than sit by her bed. The two French doors to her bedroom at the end of the hall in their Santa Monica home were always closed.[23] One day, though, he said screw it and ran through those doors. Elizabeth greeted him lovingly, as she always had. "It was the last time I spoke to her."[24]

A short while later, his mother died. For the first time, Jake became "scared for my own life," realizing that "this disease can kill."[25] His daily meds, which had always been a bother, now stirred up a "wild internal battle" of painful memories, physical distress, and emotional reminders of his own mortality.[26] He was a child, just entering adolescence, and his mind was a jumble of questions without answers and emotions driven by fear. It was the start of his personal journey: "Finding Jake." At first, he coped by just ignoring his pent-up emotions, instead concentrating on athletics and hanging out with friends—anything to escape the turmoil swirling in his head and tearing at his heart.

His daily schedule of drugs, instead of easing his fears, tormented him. One liquid medication was so disgusting "I couldn't keep it down."[27] His family tried every food and flavor, but nothing could mask its foul taste. Others were "huge horse pills," impossible for a child to swallow. His father would empty the capsules and fill them with sugar to let Jake practice, but "my gag reflex would kick in and I would choke."[28] Getting the medicine down was only half the battle. His stomach was often upset, and he was unable to eat. Once, his whole body broke out in a rash, and he wanted to stay home from school, very self-conscious about his appearance. As newer drugs were developed and approved for pediatric use, his drug regimens changed, but the battle between body and meds continued. Looking at those pills every day was a nagging, inescapable reminder: he had HIV, and AIDS could kill.

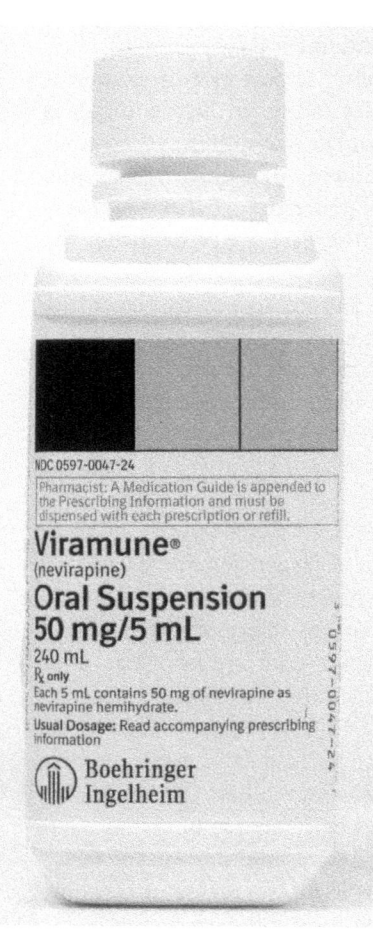

Viramune (nevirapine) oral suspension (courtesy Boehringer Ingelheim).

As a teenager, Jake learned that he had inherited the CCR5 gene mutation from his father.[29] This rare mutation accounts for the ability of some people to resist HIV infection. Although Jake was HIV-positive, the mutation probably explained his good health compared to his sister and mother. Suddenly, he felt super-human. With the right energy and taking care of his body, he "could handle this."[30] For a couple of years, he rebelled and flushed his pills down the toilet, still doing all he could to distract himself from his feelings. His family and friends sat with him every day, sometimes for hours, urging him to take his meds. All along, his father had patiently stood by him but also encouraged him to work through his built-up emotions by talking. Jake's friends, therapists, and a lot of other people also persisted in urging him to open up. Finally, as a high school junior and with their help, Jake began his long-delayed process of grieving and healing. More mature and with the curative powers of passing time, he saw his mother's fight from a new perspective. HIV became a motivating, rather than a controlling, factor in his life. He might not conquer HIV, but he would conquer the day, every day. And having endured years of insufferable pediatric meds, he wanted more and better drugs, ones that would eradicate HIV.

* * *

The day before Jamie's graduation, her high school in Gettysburg, Pennsylvania, held a special assembly. She had coordinated the arrangements for the assembly with the school superintendent, and she was the only person on the program.[31] In front of the assembled students and teachers, she bravely disclosed the secret that she had been keeping for years: she was HIV-positive. Through the 1980s and early 1990s, her family had good reason to be secretive about her HIV status. Families were stigmatized and the victims of hate crimes. Homes were threatened, and HIV-positive children were kicked out of school. Her parents had only told the gym teachers, in case Jamie was injured in gym class, and the school nurse, who supervised her drug treatment during the school day. No one else knew, not even her closest friends. When they asked about her frequent doctors' appointments, she said it was because of her heart problem — a half truth. Her infection had been caused by a contaminated blood transfusion during open heart surgery when she was a child. But most of her follow up medical care was to treat her HIV infection, not her heart.

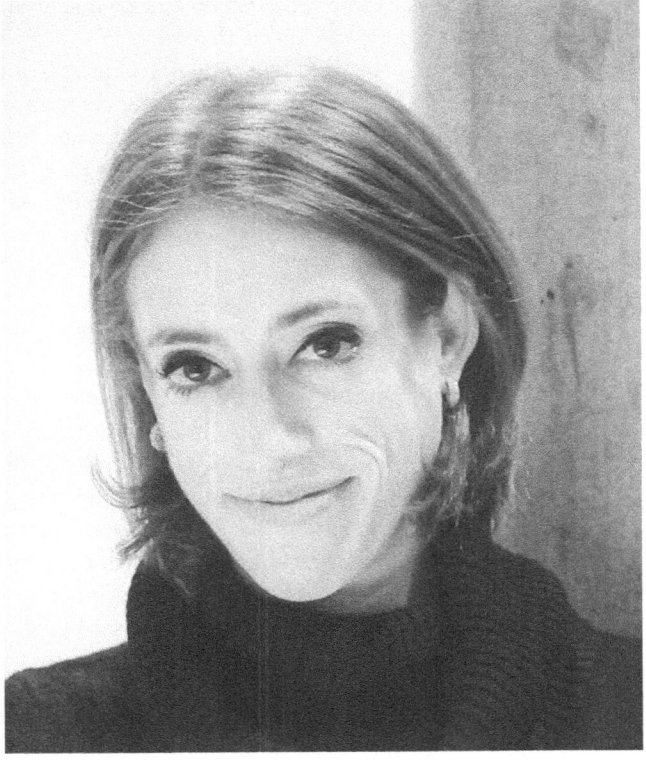

Jamie Gentille (courtesy Elizabeth Glaser Pediatric AIDS Foundation).

She had waited until her last day of high school to tell everyone, hoping to minimize the fallout if things went badly. She was leaving, in any case. But she felt a strong obligation to tell them the truth, if belatedly, because she wanted them to know that HIV was all around them. Her senior classmates would be scattering, and some, like Jamie, were headed to college. She knew as well as anyone the anguish, uncertainty, and medical nuisance that HIV infections imposed, and she wanted them to be careful. Her infection was unavoidable, but they had a choice. They could spare themselves a life like hers, shaped by constant worry, frequent clinic visits, and a lifetime of drugs.

She was still participating in clinical trials, jumping from one experimental drug regimen to another when the drugs stopped working. HAART regimens were still quite new, and she remained a participant on the leading edge of science as investigators explored the best ways to deliver these powerful new drugs to pediatric patients. She was lucky that most of them were very successful, but she knew as well as anyone what could happen when things went wrong. Years earlier, she had become "good buddies" with a boy who was also in the pediatric trials. They were the same age, they came from similar families, and because they lived near each other, the families became friends as well. Unfortunately, his parents were not as strict about giving him his medicine. They did not want to make him feel bad when he complained about the drugs' side effects. Perhaps predictably, his AIDS symptoms worsened. He died when he and Jamie were thirteen years old. Jamie chose not to go to his funeral. She did not want to remember him in a casket.[32] But she remembered him. Life was precious, and she was alive only because of well-timed research and her mother's diligence in supervising her treatment. When the high school assembly ended, Jamie's message was well received. "I'm glad I did it that way."[33]

Thousands of people in the United States — millions in the world — were becoming infected with HIV. Most of them were teenagers and young adults, and for the rest of their lives, AIDS drug regimens would govern the fine line that determined their health or lack of it. The triple-drug regimens could push HIV to undetectable levels, but those drugs often produced intolerable side effects and sometimes failed. Children like Jason, Jane, Jake, and Jamie, who would be treated for a lifetime, needed alternatives.

* * *

To gain full regulatory approval (also known as "Traditional Approval"), the BI team still needed to demonstrate that nevirapine produced a clinical benefit and improved AIDS symptoms. Both clinical outcome trials, which had been designed to provide the required proof, were well underway at the time of nevirapine's accelerated approval: one trial sponsored by ACTG in more than 1200 HIV-infected adults, and the other sponsored by BI in more than 2200 HIV-infected adults.[34] The ACTG-sponsored survival study finished first, and BI submitted the data to the FDA in December 1997, hoping that the results would be sufficient to demonstrate nevirapine's clinical benefits.[35] Unfortunately, by the time the trial concluded, its design had become outdated, making it hard to interpret the trial's "clinical endpoint" results. So, the BI project team soldiered on with the clinical outcome trial that the company was sponsoring and which had started two years later than the ACTG-sponsored trial.

In the eight years during which these two clinical outcome trials were in progress, much had changed.[36] Both trials had been designed at a time when patients had few treatment options and investigators were hampered by crude assays for measuring viral load. To prove that an AIDS drug actually worked, regulators had required the rigorous clinical outcome trials, which followed patients until their symptoms improved or their lives had been prolonged. But by 1998, physicians were routinely treating HIV/AIDS with various three-drug combinations, including nevirapine, a treatment regimen that had its own name, HAART — highly active antiretroviral therapy. HAART could suppress viral load indefinitely. In some patients, like Jason and Jane, HIV was undetectable, even with the most sensitive and sophisticated laboratory assays. Confidence in those assays, which measured HIV-RNA in the patient's blood, was so great that both investigators and regulators trusted them as an indicator of a patient's disease status.

This relationship between treatment-induced changes in HIV-RNA and clinical disease, coupled with the declining illness and death rates in patients taking HAART regimens, was shifting the FDA's views on requiring clinical outcome trials for traditional approval of AIDS drugs. Instead of requiring data showing a delayed onset of AIDS symptoms and death, the FDA reviewers would now accept "maximal and durable HIV-RNA suppression" as sufficient evidence that an AIDS drug was working.[37] For accelerated approval, the drug needed to suppress HIV-RNA for 24 weeks. For full, traditional approval, the HIV-RNA suppression needed to last at least 48 weeks.

On May 31, 2001 (Pam Strode's birthday) BI again submitted a supplemental application requesting traditional approval of nevirapine.[38] Since nevirapine's accelerated approval in adults in 1996 and the pediatric accelerated approval in 1998, BI had accumulated approximately 260,000 person-years of clinical experience with nevirapine.[39] The supplemental application consisted of data from 3003 patients in five clinical trials, including the BI-sponsored clinical outcome trial, which factored prominently in BI's claims of nevirapine's clinical benefit.[40] After consulting with the FDA reviewers, BI's statisticians had used HIV-RNA measurements for their main analysis.[41] Although they were only required to show that nevirapine suppressed viral load for 48 weeks, their analysis showed that nevirapine suppressed HIV-RNA for 96 weeks.[42] The nevirapine-containing triple-drug regimen also significantly improved CD4 cell counts throughout the two-year treatment period. Consequently, on March 27, 2002, the FDA notified BI that all of the company's commitments for required follow up clinical trials of Viramune had been fulfilled and granted traditional approval of the drug in the United States.[43] That traditional approval, although based largely on data collected from the adult trials (and extrapolated to children), also applied to the pediatric use of nevirapine.[44] Jason and Jane were seven years old, were still taking their triple-drug regimen, and still had no detectable HIV-RNA in their blood. Viramune (nevirapine) tablets had now been registered in more than 100 countries, and Viramune oral suspension for pediatric use had been approved in 90 countries.[45]

* * *

The ACTG and other investigators, in cooperation with BI, continued pediatric clinical trials, examining the effects of nevirapine in various drug combinations and under various experimental conditions.[46] The results of these trials confirmed the findings of BI's earlier pediatric clinical trials and contributed new information about nevirapine's particular value in treating children. Because nevirapine readily penetrated all organs including the brain, children grew normally, gaining weight and getting taller, rather than suffering the stunted growth and brain damage that HIV infections had inflicted on children like Ryan White and Ariel Glaser.[47]

Of course, an even better application of nevirapine was the single-dose given to mothers during labor and their babies — a simple, inexpensive, and convenient regimen that was having a profound impact around the world on preventing HIV transmission from mother to child. The FDA reviewers noted that "nevirapine has several properties which make it a potential candidate antiretroviral therapy to interrupt HIV-1 transmission" to newborns and encouraged BI to continue exploring the drug for that purpose.[48] BI was engaged in clinical trials to determine the value of the single-dose nevirapine regimen, but those clinical trials were not without controversy.

Among the most vocal critics of the single-dose nevirapine regimen was Joep Lange. Lange had been an investigator on BI's international clinical trials and a key consultant to the BI project team as they mulled and modified their plans for pediatric trials and pursued studies of mother-to-child transmission of HIV. In parallel with the HIVNET-sponsored trial of nevirapine in Uganda, Lange headed the UNAIDS-sponsored PETRA trial to explore the value of combined AZT/3TC regimens, a trial that enrolled more than 1700 pregnant women in South Africa, Tanzania, and Uganda. Although babies receiving the AZT/3TC regimens appeared to be less prone to HIV infections in the first few weeks of life, some of those babies later became infected, probably through breastfeeding, and by 18 months of age, the HIV infection rates were the same in the AZT/3TC and placebo treatment groups. The PETRA trial results were presented at the 13th International AIDS Conference in Durban, South Africa, in July 2000.[49] Following the presentation, Lange generalized the trial's findings, saying "there is no reason to believe that the loss of effect is specific" for the AZT/3TC combination.[50] Other short term AIDS regimens, such as single-dose nevirapine, would probably also suffer from the same shortcoming.

But following the PETRA presentation, Maxie Owor, representing Brooks Jackson's team of investigators from the Johns Hopkins and Makerere Universities, stood at the same podium and presented an update of the HIVNET 012 trial's results. They had continued to monitor the babies who had been given a single dose of nevirapine and found that the rate of HIV infection remained nearly half that of the babies who had received a short-term AZT regimen, even though nearly all of the babies had been breastfed.[51] The National Institutes of Health, which had funded the Ugandan study, issued a statement saying that this long-term follow up of the babies in the HIVNET 012 trial provided further evidence that single-dose nevirapine "is an effective, simple, and extremely low-cost method for preventing transmission of HIV from mother to child in developing countries."[52]

Lange's other concern was nevirapine-induced resistance. Clinical trials had firmly established that HIV resistance emerged more quickly after nevirapine treatment than with any other class of AIDS drugs. To counter and overcome the resistance problem, the BI project team had increased the dose and combined nevirapine with other drugs, triple-drug regimens that crippled the virus. Citing nevirapine-induced resistance as a troublesome limitation, Lange now openly questioned the use of nevirapine as a single agent, and as the newly elected President of the International AIDS Society, the organization sponsoring the annual International AIDS Conferences, he had an influential platform from which to speak.

Lange's concerns had merit. Resistant virus could develop even from a single dose of nevirapine, and the resulting mutant virus could have long-lasting consequences for both the mother and baby. For a mother with drug-resistant HIV, the single-dose nevirapine regimen might not work in subsequent pregnancies to protect her future newborns. In addition, the resistant virus might limit the choice of treatment regimens to ensure her own health. The commonly used triple-drug regimens in developing countries contained nevirapine and would likely work less well if the woman was resistant to nevirapine. For the babies who became infected with HIV despite single-dose nevirapine treatment, the penalty was potentially greater. They might be doomed to a lifetime — perhaps an unnecessarily short lifetime — of failed or sub-optimal AIDS treatment because they harbored drug-resistant HIV mutants. These were scientifically valid concerns, which Lange asserted should "provoke a rethinking" of the single-dose nevirapine regimen.[53] But they were only theoretical concerns.

Jackson and Guay were already addressing the resistance issue. They had amended the HIVNET 012 protocol to examine the long-term effects of the single-dose nevirapine regimen. Instead of their planned 18-month follow up period, they would follow the mothers and babies for five years, specifically looking at the impact of nevirapine on producing viral resistance and any other detrimental long-term effects.[54] Analysis of blood samples from the Ugandan clinical trial revealed that about one-fifth of the mothers developed nevirapine-resistant HIV after the single-dose regimen. Of the small number of babies who became infected despite single-dose nevirapine treatment, about half had nevirapine-resistant HIV in their blood.[55] Fortunately, the resistant virus faded over time, and after a period of months the HIV in both mothers and babies was again suppressed by nevirapine. Other clinical trials in other countries subsequently confirmed Jackson and Guay's findings.[56] Nevirapine-resistant HIV faded completely in mothers between one and two years after delivery, and in HIV-infected babies, the resistant virus was no longer detected at one year of age. In addition, single-dose nevirapine treatment was equally effective in preventing mother-to-child transmission of HIV in babies born to mothers who had previously received single-dose nevirapine during an earlier pregnancy and delivery.[57]

Those findings reassured investigators, who found they could avoid the resistance problem by simply waiting a sufficient period of time between giving the single-dose nevirapine regimen and subsequently treating an HIV-infected mother or baby with a nevirapine-containing triple-drug regimen.[58] Armed with this information, healthcare workers could balance concerns about nevirapine-induced resistance against the simplicity, efficacy, and economics of single-dose nevirapine treatment. Based on the accumulated findings, health agencies and federal officials issued statements affirming their earlier recommendations to use single-dose nevirapine.[59]

In countries with well-funded healthcare systems, most HIV-infected women were now taking highly effective combinations of AIDS drugs throughout pregnancy, virtually eliminating the likelihood of mother-to-child HIV transmission, and protection with single-dose nevirapine was not needed.[60] But in developing countries, many HIV-infected women did not seek prenatal care, the AZT treatment regimens were impractical, and HIV transmission from mothers to infants was still a problem. In those countries, simple medical solutions such as single-dose nevirapine were the only option. Through Cathy Wilfert's tireless efforts, the Elizabeth Glaser Pediatric AIDS Foundation funded 187 HIV prevention programs in eleven African countries in the first year of its Call to Action program.[61] Often starting with the single-dose nevirapine regimen to prevent mother-to-child HIV transmission, the prevention programs quickly expanded to include other critical services to pregnant women, such as HIV counseling and testing, infant-feeding education, and HIV/AIDS treatment programs.

In many countries where the Call to Action programs were operating, the countries' health ministries were also taking advantage of BI's nevirapine donation program. In the first year of the program, BI provided free supplies of nevirapine to sixteen sub–Saharan countries for use in preventing mother-to-child HIV transmission.[62] Among them was Malawi, one of the poorest countries in Africa and one that had been heavily hit by the

AIDS epidemic. A team of HIV/AIDS specialists traveled from North Carolina to establish a prevention clinic at the Kamuzu Central Hospital in the capital city of Lilongwe.[63] Having overcome many obstacles, they were working with government officials to obtain nevirapine, a critical component of the program. In the meantime, they had requested an emergency shipment of the drug from the United States. The clinic staff was still not quite ready to offer their services when they received their first patient.

She was a pregnant woman who already knew she was HIV-infected when she heard about the new program. She had taken two bus rides over three hours to reach the clinic. When she discovered the clinic was not open, she went to the staff's administrative office, fifteen minutes from the clinic, and was waiting in the outer office at 7:30 in the morning, already in labor. The office staff immediately transported her to the hospital and fetched their emergency nevirapine supplies, which had just arrived from the United States and were being stored in a locker in the hospital pharmacy. The mother and her newborn received the first doses of nevirapine from the American shipment. When she proceeded to deliver twins, the staff went back to the locker and got more nevirapine to treat the second baby. Both girls were born healthy.

In the first two months of the program, the Kamuzu clinic saw 300 women. All but six of them accepted HIV testing, and all of those who tested positive accepted the single-dose nevirapine regimen. At a follow up visit eighteen months later, both of the twins who had launched the clinic were thriving and remained free from HIV infection.

* * *

In Uganda, one of the first countries to implement an aggressive educational campaign and coordinated AIDS healthcare services, HIV infections had dropped from fifteen percent of the population in 1991 to five percent in 2001.[64] Leaders in many other African countries, after nearly two decades of silence and denial, had also begun to acknowledge AIDS and were taking steps to address the epidemic.[65] But not in South Africa, where President Thabo Mbeki, along with many in his government, dodged the issue. South Africa had the highest AIDS caseload in the world, with about 4.7 million people affected and an estimated 70,000 babies born with HIV every year.[66] Although South Africa was the richest country on the subcontinent, treating its entire HIV-infected population with AZT would cost the government ten times what it was currently spending on healthcare, and healthcare already consumed nine percent of the country's gross national product.[67]

Month after month, while the AIDS epidemic ravaged the nation, especially an increasing number of infants, many South Africans felt their government's sluggish response was unnecessary and misguided.[68] The world's leading AIDS experts and healthcare organizations agreed and repeatedly urged South Africa's leaders to take action, but the gap between the government and its ailing citizens only widened. "There was no common ground."[69] For the next three years, Boehringer Ingelheim and nevirapine would be caught in the middle of an emotionally charged, litigious debate between patient advocacy groups, healthcare workers, elected officials, international health agencies, and the courts, all struggling with what to do about South Africa's growing population of HIV-infected children. Each day of that debate, 1500 South African babies were born with HIV.

21

Justice Delayed

History was repeating itself. After nearly a decade, a little boy in Africa followed in Ryan White's footsteps so closely that it defied mere coincidence, two boys leading comparable lives, shifted only in space and time. Xolani Nkosi was born on February 4, 1989, to Nonthlanthla Daphne Nkosi in a township east of Johannesburg, South Africa. Whereas Ryan's HIV infection was typical of hemophilia patients in the United States, ninety percent of whom contracted AIDS, Xolani's HIV infection was typical of the 70,000 HIV-positive babies born each year to women in South Africa. Xolani was among the fortunate few who survived his second birthday. But Daphne's HIV-related illness weakened her too much to care for her son, and she reluctantly placed him in an AIDS care center in Johannesburg. The newly admitted two-year-old was again fortunate, because he captured the affection of Gail Johnson, a volunteer worker at the crowded center. Realizing that Daphne was dying, Gail offered to become Xolani's foster mother. The two women collaborated on an arrangement that guaranteed proper care for Xolani while also maintaining his family ties. Xolani became Nkosi Johnson and moved into Gail's home in Melville, a neat suburb of Johannesburg, where he attracted a wide circle of friends. But frequently, Nkosi also visited Daphne. A lucky lad with two loving mothers. Then, in 1997, Daphne died in her sleep while on a holiday in Newcastle, 185 miles away. Nkosi mourned the loss of his mother with a maturity and poise far beyond his eight years. "She is on my shoulder watching over me and in my heart."[1]

That same year, Gail tried to enroll Nkosi at Melpark Primary School, disclosing on the application form that her foster son had AIDS. At a meeting reminiscent of what Ryan had faced at his Indiana school, half of the parents and teachers at Melpark School opposed Nkosi's admission. "No one seemed to know what to do with me because I am infected."[2] The media soon picked up the story, and like Ryan's situation a decade earlier, the controversy made Nkosi a national figure in the campaign to destigmatize AIDS. Like Ryan's school in Cicero, Indiana, Nkosi's school sponsored AIDS workshops for the parents and teachers. They overcame their fear of a child with AIDS, and the school reversed its decision, allowing him to attend. The difficulties that Nkosi faced also prompted the South African Parliament to pass legislation requiring provincial education departments to establish non-discrimination policies.

Ryan had reached his largest audience at the New Orleans Superdome. Nkosi's reach was global. On July 9, 2000, the eleven-year-old delivered the keynote speech on the opening day of the 13th International AIDS Conference in Durban, South Africa. A tiny figure in a shiny dark suit and sneakers, Nkosi, whose name in Zulu means "King," bravely faced 10,000 delegates and spoke frankly about his birth, life, experiences with HIV, and the issues surrounding AIDS in South Africa. He called on the delegates to destigmatize the disease and on the South African government to introduce programs to prevent HIV transmission from mother to child. In addition to the Conference delegates, who sat in rapt and tearful silence, the Zulu boy with soulful eyes and full-blown AIDS melted the hearts of millions of television viewers. His simple, sincere words resonated around the world. "You can't get AIDS if you touch, hug, kiss, hold hands with someone who is infected.... We are all human beings. We are normal.... We can walk, we can talk, we have needs just like everyone else ... we are all the same."[3]

But there was one big difference between the worlds where Ryan and Nkosi had been born: the availability of drugs that could keep people with AIDS alive. Nkosi's speech capped a day-long set of events that had begun with a march through the streets of Durban and established the unofficial but resounding theme of the International AIDS Conference: equal access to HIV/AIDS treatment. Zachie Achmat, the charismatic leader of the Treatment Action Campaign, South Africa's largest and most influential AIDS advocacy group, had organized the march and wanted to call attention to President Thabo Mbeki's reluctance to make AIDS drugs available to South Africans.[4]

* * *

Thabo Mbeki became politically active as a teenager and along with others who forcefully resisted apartheid had spent his early adult life in exile. While based in London, he rapidly rose through the ranks of the African National Congress party, groomed his diplomatic skills, and established an extensive network of decision makers and power brokers. By the time he returned to South Africa in the late 1980s, he was recognized by businessmen and mainstream journalists as the best known and most receptive black South African politician.[5]

During South Africa's transition from apartheid to democracy, Mbeki was an influential member of the African National Congress party's top leadership and negotiated many post-apartheid legal reforms. A leader blessed with a magnetic personality and imposing intellect, Mbeki was among those who advocated broad legal equality and ensured that the country's new constitution guaranteed equal rights for all groups who had experienced discrimination under apartheid, including gays and lesbians.[6]

In January 1997, Mbeki was serving as Nelson Mandela's Deputy President when Minister of Health Nkosazana Zuma brought him some exciting news. A South African scientist, Olga Visser, had found a drug that represented a breakthrough in the treatment AIDS, perhaps even a cure.[7] As chairman of the Inter-Ministerial Committee on HIV/AIDS, Mbeki was keenly aware of the growing AIDS epidemic in South Africa and actively promoted AIDS prevention measures.[8] He shared Zuma's enthusiasm for the new drug and invited Visser to present her results to the Cabinet.

The ministers in Mandela's cabinet carried a tremendous burden of responsibility, the first government democratically elected by South Africa's black majority. They were anxious to show the world that they were capable, responsible leaders. But decades of colonial and apartheid rule had also sensitized them to the motives of foreign governments and corporations, which had denied them justice, exploited their resources, and impoverished their nation. The new government sought to establish a stable democracy, respect human rights, end violent conflicts, and deliver a better life for all Africans. Mbeki called it the African Renaissance, and he championed African solutions to the country's problems.[9]

On January 22, 1997, Visser introduced the Cabinet to her new discovery, a drug she called Virodene.[10] She claimed that the drug was safe and destroyed the AIDS virus. Two

HIV/AIDS patients, whom she had treated in a preliminary experiment in Pretoria, were also present and attested to their remarkable recovery. At the end of the presentation, the cabinet ministers broke into spontaneous applause. They immediately saw Virodene's value, medically and politically — a drug discovered in South Africa by South Africans to eliminate South Africa's devastating AIDS epidemic.

The cabinet ministers also saw the financial attractiveness of Virodene, which Visser estimated would cost one-tenth the price of the triple-drug regimens that had become the standard treatment for AIDS. With government ownership and sponsorship, Virodene could be developed and distributed to state hospitals cheaper and faster than relying on a foreign drug company, which would develop it overseas and then charge a high price. Better still, if Visser's initial research was confirmed, the cure for AIDS would be worth billions of dollars to South Africa. Visser and her husband, Zigi, had established a company to develop Virodene, but they needed money to secure the worldwide patent rights and to conduct a proper clinical trial. The cabinet authorized, on the spot and without debate, millions of dollars to support the Vissers' work.[11]

Within days, Virodene came to the attention of the Medicines Control Council, the government agency responsible for regulating drugs in South Africa. Olga Visser had conducted minimal laboratory tests. Her claims of the drug's antiviral effects were based entirely on a few reports published by other investigators, and none of them mentioned HIV. The main ingredient in Virodene is dimethylformamide, an industrial solvent known to cause irreversible liver toxicity, but Visser had not conducted any preclinical safety tests. And she had not obtained permission from either the hospital's human ethics committee or the Medicines Control Council prior to giving Virodene to eleven patients in Pretoria.[12] In short, Visser had broken all of the ethical and scientific rules for human experimentation. At the Council's request, Visser and her colleagues stopped treating patients.

For the next two years, the Vissers submitted revision after revision of the protocol for their clinical trial, and each time the Medicines Control Council rejected it. To address some of the Council's questions, the investigators contracted a commercial laboratory in Germany to test Virodene. Unfortunately, the German technicians saw no anti-HIV activity in their cell-based assays.[13] The Vissers also failed to address the Council's concerns about Virodene's safety or to answer questions about the drug's dosage, stability, and purity.[14] Yet, Mbeki and Zuma continued to champion the drug and worked behind the scenes to negotiate a resolution between the Vissers and the Council. When those attempts failed, representatives from Mbeki's political party, the African National Congress, accused the Medicines Control Council of conspiring with western drug companies and denying work that "is on the brink of a major breakthrough on the scourge of AIDS."[15] The government's suspicions and frustration reached a peak in March 1998, when Zuma accepted the recommendations of a special review committee, which she had established in January to investigate the Council's lack of cooperation.[16] Zuma dismissed the chairman and two senior officials of the Medicines Control Council and replaced them with political allies, hoping they would be more sympathetic toward Virodene. Instead, the incoming Council chairman sided with her medical reviewers and like her predecessor, denied clinical testing of the drug.

Also in March 1998, news reached South Africa of the results of the short term AZT regimen in the Thailand clinical trial. The government's AIDS health director began a South African pilot program to assess the new AZT regimen in preventing HIV transmission from mothers to newborns. If the pilot program, which was running in three provinces, proved successful, the director planned to expand AZT access. Nationwide use of the shortened

AZT regimen would cost less than one percent of the national health budget, a cost-effective solution to South Africa's growing problem of pediatric AIDS.[17]

Well known for his "quiet diplomacy" and personal charm, Mbeki often tapped his vast network of lawyers, businessmen, academics, political consultants, and bureaucrats to broker agreements and advance the government's agenda.[18] Over the next six months, he introduced the Vissers to political consultants and party officials, who channeled hundreds of thousands of dollars to secure international patents for Virodene. In September 1998, the Vissers launched a small clinical trial at Guy's Drug Research Unit in London, a necessary first step to determine the clinical safety of Virodene and hopefully alleviate some of the Medicines Control Council's concerns. This trial was financed by funds linked to senior leaders of the African National Congress.[19]

A few weeks later, Mbeki and Zuma cancelled the AZT pilot program for preventing mother-to-child HIV transmission, explaining that it would put "a further strain on an already limited health budget."[20] Instead, Mbeki announced an anti-AIDS advertising campaign in a televised broadcast to the nation.[21] His speech highlighted the well-established scientific facts that AIDS is a sexually transmitted disease caused by HIV and that nothing could prevent infection except protection during sex. In a veiled reference to Virodene, he assured his audience that "we shall work together to support medical institutions to search for a vaccine and a cure."[22] Unaware of the government's involvement and support of Virodene, South Africans criticized the AZT program cancellation. To them, the financial argument made no sense. Investment in the AZT regimen, which represented a tiny portion of the country's healthcare budget, could eliminate HIV infections and the huge, long-term costs of caring for terminally ill AIDS patients. Angered by this lack of drug access, a small group headed by Zackie Achmat launched their advocacy organization, the Treatment Action Campaign, in December 1998. Newspaper editorials became increasingly critical of the Health Ministry, citing among other things the government's unwillingness to embrace Glaxo-Wellcome's substantially reduced pricing of AZT.[23]

Although the clinical safety study at the Guy's Unit ran smoothly, the Vissers had difficulty finding a location for their controlled clinical trial, the one that could prove Virodene reversed AIDS. They had given up trying to obtain permission from the Medicines Control Council to conduct the trial in South Africa. As alternatives, they considered Botswana and Tanzania, but the regulatory authorities in those countries also rejected the trial protocol. Through the first half of 1999, the Vissers frequently sent Zuma updates on the Virodene trial at Guy's, patent documents, and status reports of their holding company's activities. The investigators' glowing reports kept senior African National Congress leaders emotionally and financially invested in the development of Virodene as an African cure for AIDS.[24] Funds continued to flow to the Vissers as they struggled to find a site for their pivotal clinical trial.

In June 1999, Thabo Mbeki was elected President of South Africa by a wide margin. Politically, the election marked a shift from the Mandela era of reconciliation to an era preoccupied by social realities: the widening inequalities of health, wealth, and opportunity.[25] After decades of struggle and years in exile, Mbeki had earned the right to celebrate his job as the leader of the young democracy. Instead, he faced massive social issues and a growing number of people dying from AIDS. De-racialization of the state and civil service permitted rapid growth of the black middle class, but the apartheid legacy of social prejudices, particularly accusations of African promiscuity, were not easily erased. Still fresh in the minds of Mbeki's followers was South Africa's long practice of racially-biased public health, including a chemical and biological warfare program aimed at eliminating black leaders and creating infertility among black people.[26] Regarding AIDS, Mbeki and his government viewed the pharmaceutical industry, medical researchers, and Westerners in general with suspicion, at best, and accused them of conspiracy, at worst.

A few months after taking office, President Mbeki received another packet of documents from Zigi Visser, including an article entitled "Debating AZT" written by Anthony Brink, a leading South African AIDS dissident who claimed that the evidence for the AIDS virus was flawed.[27] Brink's article asserted that AZT was useless as a medicine and was exceptionally toxic. Like other dissidents, Brink had selectively culled statements from Ellen Cooper's official medical review, which had formed the basis of AZT's approval by the Food and Drug Administration, to support his views. He neglected to mention that investigators subsequently found that lower doses reduced the likelihood and severity of AZT's side effects, and that in Cooper's mind, "there is no question that the drug worked."[28]

Brink accused the established scientific community of what amounted to a racial conspiracy meant to demean Africans by berating their sexual dignity and to exploit them by selling them useless and toxic drugs.[29] Brink's AZT article offered an alternative viewpoint, one that, like the Vissers, challenged the established truths of AIDS. For two years, Mbeki had witnessed firsthand the resistance of the official scientific community to Virodene and the Vissers' attempts to treat patients with it. Now, Brink's article bolstered his confidence in both Virodene and the Vissers.

The AIDS dissidents' explanations made sense to Mbeki, based on what he knew about Virodene. The Vissers had tried but failed to find any evidence that Virodene suppressed HIV in laboratory assays. But Mbeki, leaders in his political party, and the Vissers clung to their unforgettable, eyewitness observations of the first AIDS patients who had made a miraculous recovery after Virodene treatment. Clearly, here was evidence that a drug could improve, if not cure, AIDS, even though it had no effect on the virus called HIV. Best of all, South Africans had made this important discovery — a perfect example of Mbeki's African Renaissance.

Mbeki immediately adopted the dissidents' view and told his assembled parliament that "a large volume of scientific evidence" exists on the toxicity of AZT and suggested that it caused some forms of cancer and "is in fact a danger to health."[30] He directed his new Minister of Health, Manto Tshabalala-Msimang, to investigate the drug's safety further.[31] Convinced that industrial conspirators were out to poison and kill Africans, Mbeki shifted his reasons for stopping the AZT distribution program from concerns about the drug's cost to claims that it was toxic.

* * *

Like many bright, young Africans in the then-outlawed African National Congress party, Manto Tshabalala-Msimang had been sent into exile to complete her education. She received her medical training in Leningrad, completed her residency in obstetrics and gynecology in Tanzania, and earned a master's degree in public health from the University of Antwerp in Belgium. While providing healthcare services in Tanzania and Botswana, she also assumed positions of increasing responsibility within the exiled African National Congress party, accumulating considerable political savvy. Prior to her appointment as Mbeki's Minister of Health, she had served as Deputy Minister of Justice in President Mandela's administration.

In the spring of 2000, Tshabalala-Msimang followed up and expanded the scope of

Mbeki's request to investigate AZT by forming a Presidential AIDS Panel.[32] She asked the thirty-member international panel, nearly half of whom were AIDS dissidents, to assess the science of HIV/AIDS. Increasingly swayed by the dissidents' views, Tshabalala-Msimang also directed the Medicines Control Council to review the use of AZT, made a series of public statements questioning the drug's safety, and declared that the government would "never use AZT" to prevent mother-to-child HIV transmission.[33] Privately, Mbeki and Tshabalala-Msimang were encouraged by the Vissers' progress. The investigators had finally arranged to conduct their controlled clinical trial at two military hospitals in Tanzania. To finance this Virodene trial, millions of dollars meandered their way from the African National Congress through a series of accounts to the Vissers' company.[34]

Meanwhile, Mbeki's statements about AZT's toxicity and his actions to limit its use were causing a furor among physicians and AIDS patients.[35] Only a fraction of the millions of Africans living with AIDS were receiving treatment. The rest, knowing that they would likely die within three years, wandered from clinic to clinic in a futile search for help from the government. Some resorted to drinking bleach, a last-ditch attempt to kill the virus that was destroying their bodies.[36] In a principled act of solidarity, Zackie Achmat refused to take antiviral drugs to treat his AIDS symptoms until the government made those drugs available to all South African AIDS patients through the public health system.[37] He could afford treatment, but he refused because the $500 monthly cost was outside the reach of most South Africans.[38]

When news of the HIVNET 012 trial reached Health Minister Tshabalala-Msimang, she used it to diffuse growing pressure from the Treatment Action Campaign. She indicated that nevirapine was the government's probable medicine of choice for preventing mother-to-child HIV transmission, rather than the AZT regimen the government opposed.[39] But to be certain, she wanted to wait for the outcome of SAINT, the clinical trial that was examining single-dose nevirapine in South Africa.[40] Unfortunately, when the SAINT results were delivered in June 2000 and showed that nevirapine worked as well as a short-term AZT/3TC regimen, the Health Minister issued "a new catalogue of excuses" opposing AIDS drugs.[41] That prompted Achmat to organize a rally at Durban City Hall on the eve of the 13th International AIDS Conference in July.

The rally attracted thousands of supporters, representing a wide cross-section of South Africans and Conference delegates: nuns, doctors, nurses, traditional native healers, unionists, gay activists, and dudes on skateboards.[42] From City Hall, Achmat, Winnie Mandela, Catholic Archbishop Denis Hurley, Anglican Archbishop Njongonkulu Ndungane, and Muslim theologian Farid Essack led a peaceful and orderly procession through the streets of central Durban to Kingsmead Stadium, the site of the Conference's opening ceremonies. There, they presented their demands in the form of a memorandum to Conference Chair Hoosen "Jerry" Coovadia, UNAIDS Executive Director Peter Piot, and Health Minister Manto Tshabalala-Msimang. The memorandum asked the Mbeki government to ease restrictions and make life-saving AIDS drugs available to all South Africans who needed them, and to provide nevirapine, AZT, or both to pregnant women and their newborn babies. Coovadia and Piot wholeheartedly expressed their support. Tshabalala-Msimang assured the demonstrators that the government was working on these issues, but evidence of that was hard to see.[43]

President Mbeki's address, officially opening the Durban AIDS Conference that same evening, was widely criticized as a missed opportunity. Instead of engaging his international audience and inviting drug companies to help address South Africa's AIDS epidemic, he presented AIDS as an African problem that would be tackled by Africans. He acknowledged that AIDS was a disease characterized by a collapse of the immune system, but the real causes of AIDS in Africa, he said, were the widespread conditions that collectively weakened immunity, such as malaria, tuberculosis, diarrhea, respiratory infections, and malnutrition. In short, poverty caused AIDS.[44] He avoided any references to HIV and casually dismissed the Durban Declaration, a statement signed by more than 5000 Conference delegates affirming that AIDS was caused by HIV.[45]

At breakfast the next morning, Edwin Cameron scribbled a last minute addition to his prepared speech. In front of 14,000 delegates on that balmy morning of Durban's southern hemisphere winter, Cameron declared, "I cannot believe that President Mbeki's speech at the official opening of this conference last night has done enough."[46] Like most of those in the audience, Cameron had expected an unequivocal statement from his president that HIV caused AIDS, primarily by sexual transmission, and that effective and affordable drugs were available to treat it. "To my grief, his speech was bereft of this."[47]

* * *

Following the Durban Conference, Tshabalala-Msimang called a meeting with South Africa's nine provincial health department heads to discuss AZT and nevirapine.[48] They agreed to continue the policy of not using AZT for treating mother-to-child HIV transmission. After nevirapine's registration in South Africa, which they anticipated would soon happen, they agreed to test the drug at two pilot sites in each of the country's nine provinces. If the two-year pilot exercise demonstrated that the single-dose regimen was feasible and if they could set up the necessary operational procedures, the Health Ministry would proceed with stepwise, nationwide implementation.[49]

In November 2000, Mbeki's new, politically appointed Medicines Control Council leaders granted conditional approval of nevirapine to treat mother-to-child HIV transmission, and clinicians at the pilot sites made preparations to launch the long-delayed nevirapine pilot program.[50] Boehringer Ingelheim officials were hopeful that distribution of nevirapine, which the company was donating for free, would begin shortly.[51] Instead, negotiations over the final wording of the product's label, a detail that is usually resolved between the regulatory agency and manufacturer in a few days, dragged on for months.[52]

* * *

All year, the Treatment Action Campaign had been lobbying the government to address AIDS-related opportunistic infections that inflicted so much misery in South Africa. Thrush, a yeast infection, attacked the esophagus and digestive tract, which made swallowing painful, caused severe weight loss, and accounted for the deaths of nearly half of AIDS patients in Africa. One in ten suffered cryptococcal meningitis, a brain inflammation.[53] Fluconazole, an antifungal drug, treated both conditions, but few patients could afford the $12 per tablet price.[54] Frustrated by the government's inaction to make fluconazole more widely available, Achmat made a highly publicized trip to Thailand in October 2000. He returned with a suitcase full of generic fluconazole that he had bought for a fraction of the price charged to South Africans.[55] The police investigated Achmat for drug smuggling, and the publicity stunt accelerated discussions about drug pricing.[56] Finally in December 2000, the South African government announced that it had accepted a $50 million donation of fluconazole from Pfizer.[57] That agreement triggered a series of negotiated price reductions of AIDS drugs made by other manufacturers.

* * *

After his speech at the Durban AIDS Conference, Nkosi Johnson leveraged his celebrity status to inspire creation of centers where women and children with AIDS received shelter, medical care, and emotional support. Unlike many South African children with AIDS, he had been accepted and was loved, and he wanted to do the same for other children. "When I grow up, I want to lecture to more and more people about AIDS."[58] Nkosi spent a quiet Christmas and then on December 29, 2000, he collapsed while visiting one of the AIDS care centers that he had inspired. Doctors found that AIDS had damaged his brain, and he subsequently suffered several seizures. He slipped into a semi-coma but hung on, month after month, fighting until his diminutive body was drained of all its reserves. Nkosi Johnson died on June 1, 2001, at the age of twelve.

Among those who called at his home to pay their respects were school friends whose parents once warned them not to get close to Nkosi. They missed their friend, a little boy who organized cops-and-robbers games and always wanted to be the top cop. Like Ryan White's death, the news of Nkosi's death galvanized AIDS-awareness campaigners. The editors of South Africa's largest newspaper noted that for people around the world, but most especially in South Africa, a wide-eyed child in sneakers had "made us confront our frail humanity and our own deepest fears.... We South Africans and all others on this continent and in the world have to learn to acknowledge and treat with humanity those who are living with AIDS."[59]

* * *

The fits and starts of single-dose nevirapine continued. In January 2001, after a meeting with representatives of sub–Saharan African countries, the World Health Organization added single-dose nevirapine to its Model List of Essential Drugs. On April 18, 2001, after months of assurances — some said foot-dragging — by government officials, the South African Medicines Control Council granted full approval of nevirapine.[60] Over the next few months, the country's nine provinces finally launched their pilot sites for distributing nevirapine to pregnant women. But the program created more problems than it solved. Doctors and nurses who practiced at locations outside the program faced an ethical dilemma when confronted with women who knew they were HIV-positive and requested nevirapine. Because nevirapine was now approved, anyone who could afford private healthcare could get a prescription for it. But that excluded three-fourths of South Africans, who relied on cost-free public hospitals for their medical care. Most of those hospitals were not part of the nevirapine pilot program. Doctors at Bethesda Hospital in Ubombo, a rural area in KwaZulu-Natal province, bought nevirapine with their own money to give to their patients.[61]

Vivienne Matebula worked as a nurse and counselor in the outpatient unit at Kopanong Hospital in Gauteng province.[62] The hospital provided prenatal and maternity services to women from the surrounding district and delivered about one hundred babies each month. Vivienne counseled ten to fifteen patients every day, many of whom tested positive for HIV. Her responsibilities included referring patients with HIV and other illnesses to the appropriate hospital clinic, but unfortunately, the hospital was not authorized to dispense nevirapine. For pregnant women who were HIV-positive, she could only refer them to another hospital to obtain nevirapine.

In May 2001, Vivienne counseled a woman she identified as "S," who was pregnant and knew she was infected with HIV. Vivienne referred "S" to Chris Hani Baragwanath Hospital in Soweto, the nearest clinic in the nevirapine pilot program. The Baragwanath

Hospital staff assessed each patient's situation individually. In "S's" case, they were helpful and friendly but instructed her to return to the hospital when she went into labor. She would receive the nevirapine regimen during childbirth.

At the end of June, "S" went into labor and came to Kopanong Hospital. She told the nurses that she needed to go to Baragwanath Hospital, 37 miles away. She asked for an ambulance but was told to go there herself by taxi. Although "S" was already two centimeters dilated, she set out for Baragwanath Hospital. From Kopanong, "S" needed to take three taxis, waiting for each one to fill up before it departed on the next leg of the journey. After the last taxi ride, "S" had to climb the bridge over a road to reach the hospital, all of this while she was in labor. But she arrived in time to take her special pill of nevirapine and ensure that her baby got the drops of nevirapine syrup.

In the pediatric ward at Kopanong Hospital, Vivienne saw "a lot of HIV and mothers losing their children. For me this is very sad."[63] The women were poor, and making the trip to a pilot site during labor was challenging in the extreme. Vivienne and her hospital coworkers wanted to help these women and give them nevirapine, but the drug was simply not available to them.

Not far away in Thokoza, Sarah Hlalele was facing similar challenges.[64] She knew she was HIV-positive when she became pregnant with her second child, and she knew about nevirapine from attending an HIV support group. Sarah wanted to take the drug to protect her baby and was evaluated by the staff at Chris Hani Baragwanath Hospital. They gave her a tablet of nevirapine and written instructions for taking it when she went into labor. But they explained that the amount of the syrup for her baby depended on the baby's weight. So they told her to bring her baby for treatment within three days after birth.

In her sixth month of pregnancy, Sarah became very sick and the doctors told her she had hepatitis B. They gave her medicine for the pain and sent her home. The next month, she again had severe pain. In the ambulance on the way to Sebokeng Hospital, the nurse told her that he thought she was in labor. But because she was only in her seventh month and did not think she was in labor when she boarded the ambulance, she had not brought along her nevirapine tablet. When she arrived at Sebokeng Hospital, Sarah was already eight centimeters dilated. She told the doctors that she was HIV-positive, but they could not give her nevirapine. They did not have it. She delivered a baby boy on July 18, 2001, and still wanted him to get the nevirapine syrup. She asked for an ambulance to take him to Baragwanath Hospital for treatment, 35 miles away. Instead, the hospital arranged for a bus to transport him. Sarah thought this was unsafe for her tiny, premature son. Instead, he remained at Sebokeng Hospital for the first month of his life. "It worries me to think that my baby didn't get the drops. I feel very angry."[65] Because of the difficulties in diagnosing HIV in babies at that time, Sarah would need to wait 18 months to have her son, Kgotso, tested for HIV. Unfortunately, she never found out his status. Although she was undergoing treatment for AIDS, she was often too weak to make the two-hour journey to keep her appointments at the hospital. On April 14, 2002, Sarah died.[66]

* * *

South Africa was one of 69 countries where BI had obtained approval, or conditional approval, of single-dose nevirapine to prevent mother-to-child transmission of HIV.[67] But in the United States, BI had only obtained FDA approval to use nevirapine in combination with other AIDS drugs to treat HIV-infected children and adults. The company could not advertise or market the drug for other uses, such as preventing mother-to-child HIV transmission. To support this new claim, BI needed to submit the findings from all of the single-dose nevirapine clinical trials, including the Ugandan HIVNET 012 trial, for FDA review.[68] Brooks Jackson had not originally designed HIVNET 012 with the specific intent of meeting FDA's documentation requirements for regulatory approval, and the BI team had not been actively involved in conducting it. Even so, the FDA would accept the data from the Ugandan trial as evidence for the new indication, if FDA inspectors audited Mulago Hospital in Uganda (where the study had been conducted) and confirmed that the trial met FDA's standards.[69]

BI informed Jackson that the company was considering a label change in the United States to permit nevirapine's use in preventing mother-to-child HIV transmission and asked Jackson for permission to submit his data, as well as his cooperation with the audits. Jackson agreed, and in June 2001, BI began the process of obtaining FDA's approval of single-dose nevirapine for this new indication, following the same procedure that the company had used for nevirapine's pediatric use (a supplement to its original New Drug Application).[70]

* * *

Meanwhile, the South African pilot program was only reaching one-tenth of the women and babies who could have benefited from single-dose nevirapine treatment.[71] Patients, physicians, and advocacy groups soon grew frustrated with the slow pace of Mbeki's government to address the growing epidemic. On August 21, 2001, the Treatment Action Campaign, along with a coalition of patients and pediatricians, filed a lawsuit against Health Minister Tshabalala-Msimang and the heads of the nine provincial health departments.[72] The patient advocates wanted the government to distribute single-dose nevirapine for use in the public health sector and to produce a clear timeframe for implementing a national program to prevent mother-to-child transmission of HIV.

Under increasing pressure, both from the publicity surrounding the Treatment Action Campaign's lawsuit and from Mbeki's cabinet ministers, whose departmental budgets were being decimated by AIDS-related costs, the South African finance minister announced in October 2001 that the government would increase spending four-fold on AIDS-related programs over the next three years.[73] Activists hoped that the money would be used to expand prevention programs, such as single-dose nevirapine to pregnant women and their newborns, but the Treatment Action Campaign still pressed forward with its lawsuit.

On November 25, 2001, the Treatment Action Campaign had its day in court.[74] While 600 demonstrators marched outside, the Pretoria High Court heard arguments from both sides in a room packed with health professionals, journalists, and people wearing "HIV Positive" T-shirts.[75] The Health Ministry had submitted affidavits from the heads of the provincial health departments, meant to represent independent statements of support. Unfortunately, the affidavits showed signs of being drawn from a common template. They resembled each other so closely that they repeated typographical errors. The same error of "pubic hospitals" occurred at the same point in each of the affidavits from four of the provinces.[76] The government's lawyers assured the court that nevirapine distribution would be expanded, but the Health Ministry needed time to monitor hospital experiences during the pilot program. They wanted to resolve problems such as lack of adequate space and staff to handle the surge of women coming for HIV testing and counseling, even though this contradicted the well-known capabilities of hospitals in South Africa's major urban areas and port cities. They were also concerned about nevirapine-induced viral resistance and possible side effects. In short, they were "trying to be responsible."[77]

The Treatment Action Campaign's lawyers argued that the government's pilot program was arbitrary, unnecessary, and irrational. Women in rural areas were denied access to nevirapine, resulting in the predictable but avoidable deaths of many children. Geography was determining which children lived and which died. The lawyers presented affidavits from pregnant women, including Sarah Hlalele, who sought nevirapine treatment and from physicians who were eager to begin dispensing it. One doctor declared, "It is an easy drug to administer and we have seen no side effects on this regime except extreme gratefulness."[78]

Due to the legal action and mounting public pressure, South Africa's national and provincial health departments found it increasingly difficult to enforce the government's restrictive policy. Gauteng province had large teaching hospitals with the capacity to implement the nevirapine program, but they were initially excluded as pilot sites. With the backing of the hospital's administration, Johannesburg Hospital was added as a pilot site in October, and by December 2001, with the support of the province's premier, Gauteng had twelve pilot sites covering many of the major hospitals in the province.[79] Once the "two pilot sites per province rule" had been broken, it became unenforceable, and health officials in other provinces soon followed Gauteng's lead.

The Western Cape Province creatively ramped up its treatment program. Provincial health officials agreed with Tshabalala-Msimang that the Mbeki government should take responsibility for managing health policy. They worried that putting this decision solely in the hands of physicians, as the Treatment Action Campaign advocated, would strain the health department's budget. But the province implemented the nevirapine distribution policy on a rapid timetable, with a goal of reaching ninety percent of pregnancies in the province by mid–2002 and covering everyone by the following year. The Western Cape's program for preventing mother-to-child transmission ignored Mbeki's Health Ministry limitations and offered both the nevirapine and AZT regimens, as well as voluntary counseling and HIV testing services.[80]

* * *

In parallel with the court proceedings in South Africa, representatives from Boehringer Ingelheim traveled to Uganda to assess Mulago Hospital's readiness for an audit by the FDA's inspectors, who were expected to arrive at the site in March 2002.[81] Laura Guay had returned to the United States after the HIVNET 012 trial had completed the 18-month follow up assessment of the babies born during the trial.[82] She returned to Uganda to host the BI visitors during their two-day review of the trial's records. Because Brooks Jackson and his team had conducted the trial independently and had not intended to submit their results to regulatory authorities, their documents in some ways did not comply with FDA standards. The BI visitors identified potential issues requiring follow up, mostly questions about recordkeeping, but were satisfied that Guay and her colleagues had followed good clinical practices.[83] The BI inspectors submitted copies of their preliminary findings to officials at the National Institutes of Health, which had funded the trial, the trial's investigators at the Johns Hopkins and Makerere universities, and others involved in conducting the trial, encouraging them to correct the observed procedural and recordkeeping deficiencies prior to the planned FDA audit.[84] After reviewing the BI report, officials at the National Institutes of Health's Division of AIDS contracted Westat Corporation, an independent auditing firm, to visit Mulago Hospital and help the Ugandan clinical team prepare for the FDA audit.[85]

* * *

On December 14, 2001, the Pretoria High Court, after only two weeks of deliberations, ruled in favor of the Treatment Action Campaign, saying that every HIV-positive woman in South Africa had a constitutional right to healthcare.[86] The court ordered the South African government to provide single-dose nevirapine to all pregnant women and babies when it was medically indicated and, within three months, to develop a comprehensive national program to prevent or reduce mother-to-child transmission of HIV.[87] The following week, Health Minister Tshabalala-Msimang announced that the government would appeal the court's ruling. While confirming that the nevirapine pilot program would continue and that the government was "making every effort possible" to reduce mother-to-child transmission of HIV, Tshabalala-Msimang said the court had overstepped its authority by interfering with the government's right to set policy and ordering the government to supply a specific medicine, namely nevirapine.[88]

The appeal bought Tshabalala-Msimang time until the results of the government-sponsored Virodene clinical trial could be announced. A few months earlier, she had visited the clinical sites in Tanzania and assured Mbeki and Parliament that things were going well. The clinical trial concluded in March 2001, and throughout the remainder of the year the Vissers confidently predicted that the unblinded results would be overwhelmingly positive.[89] While awaiting the outcome of the data analysis, which took an unusually long time, Mbeki issued a document entitled *Castro Hlongwane, Caravans, Cats, Geese, Foot & Mouth and Statistics: HIV/AIDS and the Struggle for the Humanisation of the African* to the National Executive Committee of the African National Congress. Although authorship of this manifesto remains uncertain, it clearly stated Mbeki's ideology and was intended to persuade his colleagues during an executive meeting on HIV/AIDS. The document declared as illogical the notion that AIDS is a single disease caused by a single virus and instead argued that "there are many conditions that cause acquired immune deficiency, including malnutrition and disease."[90] Whether they agreed with Mbeki's ideology or not, the party leaders were reluctant to oppose a president who put a high value on political loyalty.[91] The National Executive Committee supported Mbeki's opposition to AIDS drugs such as AZT, affirmed the government's policy limiting nevirapine, and blocked the use of AIDS drugs in public hospitals for rape victims and needle-stick injuries.[92]

* * *

By 2002, the Elizabeth Glaser Pediatric AIDS Foundation's Call to Action had implemented large-scale programs to distribute single-dose nevirapine in Cameroon, Uganda, and Zimbabwe.[93] But in South Africa, those programs were constrained. In January 2002, Health Minister Tshabalala-Msimang met with the provincial health officials to discuss a progress report on the nevirapine pilot program. The report said that the eighteen pilot sites had generated "a lot of useful and important lessons that can now be put to use."[94] It recommended phased expansion of services for preventing HIV transmission and concluded that "nevirapine can and should be provided immediately to all pregnant women who are already known to be HIV-positive."[95] Tensions escalated within the ministry, as government leaders mulled over how to reconcile the report's recommendations with their political ideology. Increasingly, the provincial health officials and even officials within the Health Ministry were breaking ranks, saying they could no longer defend the indefensible. Tshabalala-Msimang publicly criticized the actions of Gauteng province, which had made nevirapine widely available, and one of the nation's largest newspapers reacted by labeling her "Dr. No."[96]

How to address South Africa's growing number of HIV-infected babies had become one of the country's most emotionally charged issues. The legal appeals process threatened to take many months, and in the meantime the Health Ministry slogged along with its limited pilot program for distributing single-dose nevirapine. The Treatment Action Campaign and other patient advocacy groups were quick to criticize the government's failure to comply with the Pretoria High Court's ruling, and they were joined by doctors, trade unions, religious leaders, and members of South Africa's provincial and local governments, all strongly opposing the Health Ministry's stance.

In late January 2002, Lionel Mtshali, premier of South Africa's KwaZulu-Natal province, became the first elected official to publicly challenge the national government's nevirapine policy.[97] A soft-spoken, retired school teacher, Mtshali was a most unlikely person to defy the Mbeki government, but KwaZulu-Natal had more HIV-infected adults than anywhere else in South Africa, which had more HIV-infected people than anywhere else in the world. When the head of his provincial health department explained that the single-dose nevirapine program was limited to two hospitals in the province, Mtshali consulted doctors, colleagues, AIDS advocates, his relatives, and friends at church. The province had 61 hospitals and 390 clinics. Some hospitals outside the pilot program freely acknowledged that they had the capacity to implement the nevirapine regimen, and Mtshali commended "the courageous decision of doctors who have committed themselves to supply antiretroviral drugs to pregnant mothers" on their own.[98] KwaZulu-Natal faced "a desperate situation," and he decided to act.[99] At the opening of the provincial legislature on February 25, 2002, Mtshali announced his decision to distribute nevirapine to every HIV-infected pregnant woman in his province, and he implemented the program immediately.[100]

The actions taken by Gauteng, the Western Cape, and KwaZulu-Natal provinces emboldened individuals and organizations to follow their lead nationwide. Doctors and nurses began quietly distributing single-dose nevirapine to pregnant women in other provinces without government permission.[101] Public, private, professional, and parochial groups all put unprecedented pressure on the government to change its policy and expand access to single-dose nevirapine. The Colleges of Medicine of South Africa, representing thousands of physicians, officially declared it was "unethical and against medical principles" to withhold nevirapine treatment for HIV transmission from mother to child.[102] Prominent clinicians from university medical centers across South Africa, including Jerry Coovadia at the University of KwaZulu-Natal, echoed that view in a published commentary, saying it was "ethically and morally unacceptable" to delay the national program of single-dose nevirapine.[103]

Premier Mtshali's bold action prompted Health Minister Tshabalala-Msimang to call a meeting of the nine provincial health department heads. She struck a deal allowing individual provinces to expand the single-dose nevirapine program, if they wished. Western Cape Province, Gauteng, and KwaZulu-Natal immediately forged ahead, but the other provinces had more limited resources and were unable to act without federal assistance. That financial assistance would come from the court-ordered nationwide distribution plan, which Tshabalala-Msimang still had not produced.[104]

* * *

Meanwhile, the team of Westat auditors arrived at Mulago Hospital in Uganda in February 2002 to inspect documents associated with the HIVNET 012 trial, as requested by the National Institutes of Health.[105] Laura Guay again traveled to Kampala to host their four-day audit.[106] The lead auditor, a former FDA employee, examined the records according to FDA's guidelines as if the trial had been conducted in the United States. His assessment made no allowance for the situation and standard of medical care in Uganda.[107] In the United States, unplanned hospitalization of a patient during a clinical trial always causes concern and extensive investigation. But in Uganda, where malaria and other tropical diseases were widespread, such hospitalizations were handled routinely and not automatically assumed to result from trial participation.

The auditors found inconsistencies in study procedures such as gaps and irregularities in the assigned patient identification numbers. Each woman who enrolled in the HIVNET 012 trial had been assigned a sequential study ID number. After the trial was temporarily stopped and the placebo treatment was dropped from the protocol, the trial was restarted with new patient ID numbers, creating a gap in the number sequence.[108]

For women who required hospitalization or visited a hospital clinic during the trial, Mulago Hospital assigned a new hospital ID number for each visit, unlike the United States, where all of a patient's hospitalizations and hospital clinic visits are recorded under the same ID number. Consequently, when the Westat auditor wanted to verify all hospitalizations of the study participants, the Mulago Hospital staff could not easily retrieve the records. Instead, the study investigators were granted permission by the hospital to perform the time-consuming task of sorting through stacks of files and locating the relevant medical records in the hospital's storage room.[109]

The auditors also faulted how the investigators defined, graded, and reported serious adverse events, including deaths. Westat had requested trial data for a fixed time interval, which HIVNET's Seattle-based data management team provided. In Uganda, the Westat auditors compared those database entries with the site's original patient records, which included clinical observations outside the requested database timeframe. Noting the mismatch but not the reason for it, the auditors incorrectly concluded that the site had underreported the number of adverse events and deaths.[110]

On March 8, 2002, Westat submitted its preliminary report to the Division of AIDS at the National Institutes of Health. As is customary in such audits, the investigators were given an opportunity to respond. Guay wrote responses to all of the auditors' findings, many of which were resolved by straightforward clarifications or explanations.[111] The recordkeeping errors and omissions cited by the auditors were, for the most part, "fixable" but resolving those problems took time.[112] Boehringer Ingelheim wanted all of the recordkeeping deficiencies corrected prior to the planned FDA audit, and the FDA inspectors were due to visit Mulago Hospital very soon.[113] Based on the Westat audit, Guay's responses, and BI's desire to have FDA-quality documentation, officials at the Division of AIDS decided that they needed to comprehensively review all of the study documents, a process called monitoring.[114] (All of the documents had been monitored during the trial but not according to the standards that the FDA and BI now required.) In addition, the Division shut down Mulago Hospital as a site for new HIVNET clinical trials and prevented further enrollment in the site's ongoing trials, pending the outcome of the re-monitoring exercise.[115] But Guay's colleagues in Kampala continued to evaluate the mothers and babies in the HIVNET 012 trial, which was now in the midst of the trial's five-year follow up period.[116]

Realizing that the National Institutes of Health and the site staff would not be able to complete the re-monitoring process before the scheduled FDA audit, BI withdrew its supplemental New Drug Application, and the FDA cancelled its audit.[117] On March 22, 2002, the National Institutes of Health issued a public statement about the HIVNET 012 trial on behalf of its Division of AIDS, acknowledging that "certain aspects of the collection of the primary data may not conform to FDA regulatory requirements."[118] But the National Institutes of Health's statement and a companion statement issued simultaneously by the World Health Organization both cited other trials that had confirmed the results of the HIVNET 012 trial and concluded that "there is no reason for programs implementing this life-saving regimen to change."[119]

* * *

On March 1, 2002, the Treatment Action Campaign's lawyers returned to the Pretoria High Court. They claimed that the delay imposed by the government's appeal was causing irreparable harm to women and children by denying them access to the court-ordered single-dose nevirapine regimen. The Pretoria High Court agreed and again ordered the government to comply with its ruling to make nevirapine available to HIV-infected pregnant women. The Mbeki government refused, saying it would appeal this latest court ruling, as well as the original court order.[120] The Treatment Action Campaign's legal team reacted by accusing the government of using delaying tactics to avoid the court's rulings.

In its original appeal, the government sought to overturn the court's decision based on the right of elected officials to set policy, but now the government's lawyers also cited recent news reports of the data irregularities in the Ugandan clinical trial. Despite statements from the National Institutes of Health and the World Health Organization that the problems with the HIVNET 012 trial were technical and did not affect nevirapine's safety or value as a prevention regimen, the government's lawyers argued that nevirapine had been approved in South Africa partly based on data from the Ugandan trial. The Health Ministry did not want to expand the nevirapine program until they reviewed that drug license. The Pretoria High Court judge dismissed this argument, saying, "Right now, the drug is legal in South Africa."[121] On March 25, 2002, the Pretoria High Court, for the third time, ordered the Health Ministry to begin distributing single-dose nevirapine immediately, in parallel with the appeals process.

By April, the court case had become a public relations nightmare for the Mbeki government. Powerful religious organizations and trade unions that had formerly been strong allies of the ruling African National Congress party now marched in the streets alongside the Treatment Action Campaign. Nelson Mandela, still a member of the African National Congress's Executive Committee, and Archbishop Desmond Tutu both urged the government to offer universal access to nevirapine.[122] Visiting United States Congressman Jim Kolbe (R-AZ), who chaired the House Appropriations Subcommittee on Foreign Operations, told reporters in Cape Town the situation was "tragic" and warned that United States aid to South Africa might be "reconsidered."[123] Dissatisfaction with President Mbeki's policy was also spreading within the African National Congress, some of whose leaders were secretly taking the AIDS drugs his party opposed.[124] Nearly everyone in South Africa knew a family member who had died from AIDS, and Mandela, always in the lead, had been the first party official to acknowledge he had lost family members — a niece and two sons of a nephew — to AIDS.[125]

The Constitutional Court, South Africa's highest court, had not yet ruled on the government's appeal, but the justices made it clear that the government, at least temporarily, must distribute nevirapine to HIV-infected pregnant women, as ordered by the Pretoria High Court.[126] The next day, the newspaper's headline was, "Yes, you will, Dr. No."[127] But

Mbeki, now firmly embracing the dissidents' views, defied the courts. "We will not be intimidated, terrorized, bludgeoned, manipulated, stampeded, or in any other way forced to adopt policies and programs inimical to the health of our people."[128] Unfortunately, Mbeki and his cabinet ministers had just received some very bad news. The final results of the clinical trial in Tanzania revealed that Virodene had no effect on HIV and was no cure for AIDS.[129] Some of the patients developed abdominal swelling, pain, and other symptoms associated with liver toxicity.[130]

On April 17, 2002, with Virodene's failure, public pressure mounting, provincial health departments already defying the government's policy, and no options remaining, Mbeki's Cabinet announced that the government would comply with the Pretoria High Court's order and offer single-dose nevirapine to all pregnant women infected with HIV.[131] Despite public bravado and chest-thumping by Tshabalala-Msimang, who threatened to ignore the court, the Cabinet, led by Justice Minister Penuell Maduna, reassured the nation that the government would follow the rule of law. In addition, the Cabinet admitted, for the first time, that AIDS drugs "can improve the quality of life of people living with AIDS, if administered at certain stages in the progression of the condition and in accordance with international guidelines."[132] The Cabinet also tripled the budget for AIDS prevention and treatment programs, including, for the first time, rape victims treated in public hospitals.[133] A week later, Mbeki publicly promised to lead the fight against AIDS, a major shift from his previous official policy.[134] But when the government made its case before the Constitutional Court on May 2, 2002, supplies of nevirapine had still not arrived at many of the country's hospitals and clinics.[135] And the controversy surrounding nevirapine continued.

22

Am-Bushed

On June 19, 2002, President George W. Bush stepped to microphones in the White House Rose Garden and announced a major foreign aid initiative. He had already pledged $500 million to the United Nations' newly created Global Fund to Fight AIDS, Tuberculosis, and Malaria. Now, on this sunny Wednesday morning, Bush was budgeting another $500 million specifically to prevent mother-to-child transmission of HIV in the countries hit hardest by the AIDS epidemic, including Uganda and South Africa. Bush's prevention strategy consisted of three parts, one of which would "support programs that administer a single dose of nevirapine," the only drug he mentioned by name.[1]

Within weeks, the Elizabeth Glaser Pediatric AIDS Foundation announced that it had received a $100 million federal funding agreement, in conjunction with the President's new prevention initiative.[2] The Foundation's ongoing Call to Action was already operating programs at 231 clinics in seventeen developing countries. Those programs had proven that the Foundation could establish services to prevent babies from becoming infected with HIV, and many of the prevention clinics had started with the single-dose nevirapine regimen. With the infusion of government funds, the Call to Action campaign hoped to reach three million women and prevent thousands of new HIV infections throughout the developing world. The new funds also permitted the Foundation to broaden the scope of its existing programs beyond pediatric AIDS and provide AIDS care and treatment for mothers, families, and entire communities.[3] But while the Foundation was preparing to ramp up its Call to Action, the single-dose nevirapine regimen was still under the microscope.

*   *   *

In July 2002, the National Institutes of Health, responding to the observations cited in Boehringer Ingelheim's inspection report and the Westat audit, sent an internal team from its Division of AIDS to Uganda to re-monitor the HIVNET 012 study documents and hospital records. The clinical site had no director at the time, so Laura Guay once again returned to Kampala to assist the monitors and ensure that they were given access to all the documents and information they requested during their comprehensive six-month assessment.[4] They first inspected the laboratory and pharmacy facilities and documents. Then, they reviewed all the study procedures to confirm that the study team had followed the trial's protocol. Next, they systematically compared the patients' medical charts with the recorded entries in the study files, confirming that each of 25,000 data points correctly documented the babies' delivery and birth, the HIV-RNA assay measurements, and adverse events. Finally, they reviewed all of the patient charts — more than 600 mother/infant pairs — for completeness in reporting drug side effects and patient safety issues.[5] The work was tedious for both the monitors and Guay's Ugandan team, but they systematically worked through and addressed the list of problems originally identified by the Westat auditors.[6]

* * *

Meanwhile, in South Africa, Zackie Achmat's "drug strike" was taking its toll. He entered the hospital in July 2002 with a severe lung infection. His relatives, friends, and colleagues were worried about his health and begged him to begin treatment for his AIDS symptoms, but he steadfastly refused. He would lead the Treatment Action Campaign's demonstrations and court appeals until his demand of AIDS treatment for all South Africans was met. Or he would die trying. "I don't want to live in a world where people die every day simply because they are poor."[7] His declining health rallied even stronger support for his cause, not only from the rank and file but also from Nelson Mandela, the country's most respected statesman.[8] When Mandela emerged from his visit to Achmat's home wearing one of the activists' distinctive T-shirts emblazoned with "HIV Positive," Edwin Cameron said it "marked a turning point in our national struggle about the meaning of AIDS."[9] While Achmat was still resting at home, he learned that his persistence had paid off and his campaign was one step closer to reaching its goal.

On July 5, 2002, the South African Constitutional Court issued its decision regarding the government's appeal of the Treatment Action Campaign's lawsuit. In their precedent-setting decision, the justices unanimously agreed with the lower court's original ruling: restricting the supply of nevirapine infringed on the constitutional rights of both HIV-infected mothers and their babies. The justices cited explicit provisions in South Africa's constitution, which guarantees everyone the right to access healthcare and protects the "best interests" of children.[10] Consequently, they ordered the government to remove all restrictions on single-dose nevirapine and, with its available resources, to implement a comprehensive program to combat mother-to-child transmission of HIV.[11]

Having already shifted policy in reaction to mounting public pressure and the lower court's ruling, the Mbeki government, through a spokesman, said the Constitutional Court's order was "workable" and promised to facilitate the nevirapine mother-to-child HIV prevention program.[12] The Treatment Action Campaign and its many supporters celebrated the Constitutional Court's decision, confident that they had finally overcome the last hurdle to distribution of single-dose nevirapine. But their elation did not last long.

Within a month, officials at South Africa's Medicines Control Council said that they had serious concerns about nevirapine, citing the National Institutes of Health's disclosure of problems with the HIVNET 012 trial.[13] The Medicines Control Council's original approval of single-dose nevirapine to treat pregnant women and their infants was largely based on that study. If the Ugandan clinical trial was not good enough for the FDA, then it was not good enough for South Africa, either. The Council's Registrar declared, "We are not going to promote bad science."[14]

The Medicines Control Council was also concerned about nevirapine-induced resistance. Nevirapine was widely used in triple-drug regimens to treat HIV-infected people in South Africa, and regardless of its decision about single-dose nevirapine, the Council intended to support continued use of nevirapine in the triple-drug regimens. The Council worried that pregnant women who took a single tablet of nevirapine during labor to protect their infants might become resistant and not benefit in the future from triple-drug therapy that contained nevirapine.[15] Resistance was a legitimate concern. Several clinical teams had reported that viral resistance could develop after only a single dose of nevirapine, but by this time the scientific community had already addressed this problem. Investigators found that resistance to single-dose nevirapine fades over time, and nevirapine-containing triple-drug regimens were effective if women waited to begin their triple-drug therapy at least one year after taking the single-dose nevirapine regimen.[16]

Once again, AIDS advocates in South Africa reacted angrily to the possibility of another government restriction. By withdrawing its approval, the Medicines Control Council could prevent doctors from prescribing single-dose nevirapine to pregnant women and effectively render the Constitutional Court's decision moot, just as the single-dose regimen was beginning to make a significant impact.[17] In Gauteng, one of the provinces that had defied the government's restrictions, doctors reported a 75 percent drop in the number of HIV-infected babies, one year after launching the single-dose nevirapine program throughout the province.[18]

More determined than ever, Zackie Achmat continued his drug strike. The fight was not over. The government was still threatening barriers to prevent AIDS drugs from reaching South Africans who needed them. In December 2002, doctors warned Achmat that unless he started drug treatment, he had a fifty-fifty chance of surviving another year.[19] But he remained true to his pledge.

* * *

Meanwhile, the United States, which was already providing 45 percent of all international HIV/AIDS assistance, increased its support even further.[20] In December 2002, the

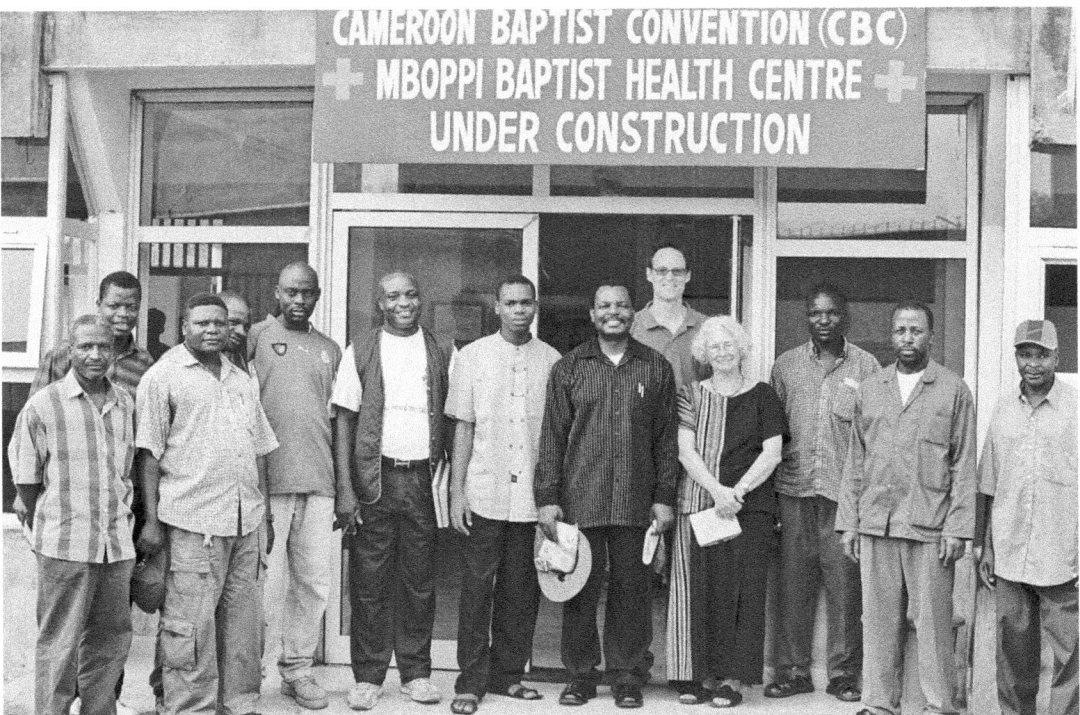

Catherine Wilfert meeting with representatives of the Cameroon Baptist Convention to establish an HIV prevention program at the new Mboppi Baptist Health Center (courtesy Elizabeth Glaser Pediatric AIDS Foundation).

United States Trade Office announced it would permit African countries to override patents on drugs produced outside their countries.[21] International trade agreements, meant to protect intellectual property rights, had actually prevented poor countries from importing life-saving drugs. The Trade Office's move provided a practical solution to this barrier, allowing African and other developing countries greater access to AIDS drugs, and the United States called on other World Trade Organization members to follow its lead.

In parallel, former President Bill Clinton launched the Clinton HIV/AIDS Initiative to create comprehensive AIDS care and treatment plans in Rwanda, Mozambique, Tanzania, Haiti, the Organization of Eastern Caribbean States, and the Dominican Republic. Clinton's foundation also took advantage of the Trade Office's newly announced policies, struck deals with drug companies to secure major price reductions for AIDS drugs, and facilitated drug delivery to more than seventy developing countries.[22]

In January 2003, President Bush asked Congress in his State of the Union address for a five-year, $15 billion initiative called the President's Emergency Plan for AIDS Relief. The PEPFAR funds would expand the program Bush had announced in the Rose Garden the previous summer. While continuing to support programs to prevent mother-to-child HIV transmission, PEPFAR would also pay for AIDS drugs to treat two million people already infected with HIV and general medical care for ten million HIV-infected people and AIDS orphans in Africa.[23]

The PEPFAR announcement was welcomed at the Elizabeth Glaser Pediatric AIDS Foundation, where Elizabeth had begun her uphill campaign fifteen years earlier. Using privately donated funds and the previously awarded government grant, the Foundation had already been doing what the President proposed to do. For three years under the Foundation's Call to Action initiative, Cathy Wilfert had been visiting clinics and helping hundreds of them set up HIV prevention programs—each one adapted to local conditions and the clinic's existing resources.[24] Wilfert had a soft touch, infinite patience, and a quiet expertise that earned her the respect and admiration of policy makers and patients alike. She built constructive relationships with the Health Ministers of each country, worked within their regulatory framework, and welcomed them as full partners, not just participants, in the Call to Action programs.

Wilfert also applied her laboratory management expertise to set up a patient evaluation and monitoring system, which was not easy with limited technology and resources. At the time, there was no rapid HIV test. Women needed to return weeks after their blood draw to learn their test results. Wilfert helped the clinics devise creative

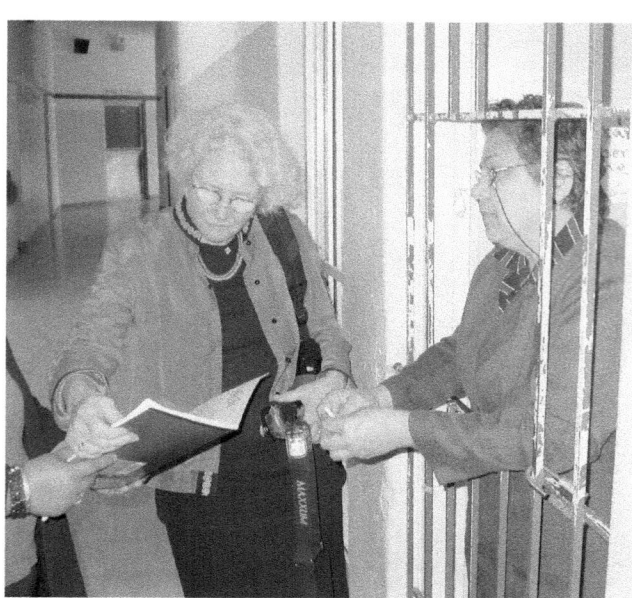

Catherine Wilfert reviewing pharmacy records at an HIV prevention clinic in the Dominican Republic in 2004 (courtesy Catherine Wilfert, photographer Arthur Ammann).

and culturally acceptable ways to follow up with infected women and to address the concerns of those who opted out of testing.[25] She and her staff also kept detailed records on the status and progress of the clinics that received Call to Action funds.

To jump-start the PEPFAR program, the American government limited the initial round of funding to organizations that could demonstrate a proven record of success.[26] The Elizabeth Glaser Pediatric AIDS Foundation's accumulated statistics on patient treatment and clinic performance confirmed its skill in managing a multinational HIV prevention and treatment program, and it was one of four organizations to receive PEPFAR Track 1.0 funds.[27] The grant allowed the Foundation to rapidly scale up its HIV prevention, care, and treatment programs in Côte d'Ivoire, Zambia, Tanzania, South Africa, and Mozambique.[28]

The Foundation was now supported more by government funds than by private donations and now spent more of its resources on service delivery than on research. Single-dose nevirapine continued to be a key component of those service delivery programs. It allowed clinics in a number of countries to initiate mother-to-child HIV prevention programs and laid the groundwork for more elaborate AIDS drug regimens and more comprehensive healthcare for both children and their parents. Under Wilfert's leadership and with PEPFAR support, the Foundation had opened 532 HIV clinics in 20 countries. And the Foundation had grown from three mothers sitting around a kitchen table in Los Angeles to 84 employees, most of whom were citizens and residents of the developing countries where the Call to Action programs were implemented.[29]

* * *

In March 2003, a full year after the audits by Boehringer Ingelheim and Westat, the Division of AIDS at the National Institutes of Health finally issued the report of its re-monitoring efforts on the HIVNET 012 trial. After an intensive, six-month review of trial procedures and documents, Division officials concluded that the trial's original findings were valid. Single-dose nevirapine was safe and effective when given to women during labor and infants right after birth, a conclusion that the World Health Organization also reconfirmed in an independently issued statement.[30]

For Brooks Jackson, Laura Guay, and their Kampala-based colleagues, the past two years had been a difficult time, as they constantly revisited the trial and responded to critics who kept raising new concerns. But more than anyone, they wanted to make sure that the trial's conclusions were true. Children's lives were at stake. With guidance from the regulatory group at the National Institutes of Health, they corrected the trial's documentation deficiencies and made substantial improvements in the site's operational procedures.[31] In resolving the issues raised by the auditors, inspectors, and monitors, they realized that they all could have done their jobs better.[32] And they would avoid those problems on future clinical trials. Impressed with the investigators' responsiveness, officials at the Division of AIDS concluded that now "the site is the best in Africa run by black Africans."[33] In June 2003, they reopened the Ugandan site, allowing the investigators to conduct new clinical trials with HIVNET funding. Unfortunately, the controversy surrounding the HIVNET 012 trial and the use of single-dose nevirapine continued.

* * *

In South Africa, the Treatment Action Campaign saw its victories undermined at every turn by its own government. Despite orders from the country's highest appellate court, distribution of single-dose nevirapine had stalled because the Medicines Control Council questioned the validity of the HIVNET 012 trial. President Mbeki distanced himself from the controversy and made no further public statements.[34] He had never emphatically stated that AIDS is not caused by HIV, instead viewing the virus as a contributing factor and blaming poverty as the underlying cause. Privately, he still clung to the views of the AIDS dissidents, asserting that AIDS drugs were toxic.[35] Publicly, his loyal lieutenant, Health Minister Manto Tshabalala-Msimang, who had been politically aligned with Mbeki since their departure together in 1962 from South Africa into exile, stepped up to carry the banner of the AIDS dissident movement and defend the government's position.[36] Her latest tactic to impede progress was arguing that the AIDS drug regimens, which required swallowing multiple pills at specific times throughout the day, were too complicated for people in inaccessible villages to follow. They "do not understand the importance of completing a course of drug therapy. People don't have watches."[37] Instead, she urged AIDS patients to take home remedies such as garlic, lemon juice, olive oil, and beets to boost their immune system because "these things are affordable for South Africans."[38] The Global Fund to Fight AIDS, Tuberculosis, and Malaria had awarded a $72 million grant to the province of KwaZulu-Natal, but Tshabalala-Msimang blocked distribution of the funds, claiming that the grant had been improperly filed.[39]

Zackie Achmat reluctantly had to admit that the target of his protests needed to focus squarely on his own political party, the African National Congress. Achmat considered himself a loyal party member and had won the support of Nelson Mandela. But President Mbeki and Health Minister Tshabalala-Msimang had thwarted every AIDS health initiative in South Africa, and he now had no choice but to confront them. Throughout the spring of 2003, Achmat organized a nationwide campaign of civil disobedience, the biggest and most organized protests and sit-in demonstrations in South Africa since the days of apartheid.[40] South Africans willingly went to jail, pressing their demand for universal access to nevirapine.

Achmat had now been on his drug strike for four years and he looked worn out. He suffered from bronchitis and his CD4 count hovered around 200, a sign that his immune system was failing. Privately, he began reassessing whether he should abandon his pledge and start drug treatment.[41] But publicly, he continued the marches, sit-ins, and demonstrations, leading by example in defiance of his poor health.

On July 28, 2003, the Medicines Control Council proceeded to revoke its provisional approval of single-dose nevirapine. Prompted by the documentation irregularities in the HIVNET 012 trial, which were first announced by the National Institutes of Health's officials, and then BI's withdrawal of its application to the FDA, the Medicines Control Council expressed doubts about authorizing permanent approval of the drug. The Council found faults with both the Ugandan HIVNET 012 trial and the SAINT trial, which had subsequently been conducted by John Sullivan, Jerry Coovadia, and other investigators in South Africa.[42] The Medicines Control Council gave BI ninety days to provide further evidence that single-dose nevirapine prevented mother-to-child transmission of HIV. Otherwise, the Council would de-register the drug. But BI had already submitted all of its data to the Medicines Control Council, in compliance with regulatory requirements, and replied that it had nothing more to offer.[43]

Coincidently, the following week, South Africa held its first national conference on AIDS, a conference that should have signaled another step in the country's willingness to address its most pressing health problem. Instead, the topic that dominated the conference from beginning to end was nevirapine. Health Minister Tshabalala-Msimang was heckled when she opened the conference.[44] Speaker after speaker urged the government to announce its long-promised AIDS drug plan and to end the threatened withdrawal of nevirapine. Scientists and physicians attending the conference could not fathom why regulators would take away one of the few medical options for fighting HIV in infants. Conference Chairman Jerry Coovadia called the Council's pending decision a "dreadful mistake."[45] Fearing the nevirapine withdrawal, health workers and patient advocates signed petitions and protested in the streets, criticizing the Medicines Control Council's "confusing and seemingly unjustified decision."[46]

President Mbeki, as always, diplomatically crafted his words and avoided public comments on this latest controversy. His Cabinet also distanced itself from the Medicines Control Council, explaining that the Council was an independent body charged with making decisions "on scientific grounds."[47] But Cabinet members assured the public that they were preparing a contingency plan to cope with HIV-infected mothers and babies, if nevirapine was de-registered. The chief director of the Health Ministry's HIV/AIDS program admitted she had been "spending sleepless nights asking what we are to do with mother-to-child transmission if we can't have nevirapine."[48]

The conference organizers hastily arranged an emergency plenary session before the closing ceremonies to discuss the nevirapine issue. Precious Matsoso, the Registrar of the Medicines Control Council, presented the regulators' perspective, confirming that the Council would revoke nevirapine's approval unless BI provided further safety and efficacy data and pointing out that effective combination drug regimens were available as alternatives.[49] Although the conference delegates agreed that there were alternatives to nevirapine, they found it hard to imagine how those regimens could be implemented in a country that had no national AIDS treatment plan. Cathy Wilfert, who was leading the Elizabeth Glaser Pediatric AIDS Foundation's efforts to roll out HIV prevention programs throughout Africa, and James McIntyre, an investigator on the SAINT trial, presented data defending the use of nevirapine for preventing mother-to-child HIV transmission. They explained that the single-dose nevirapine regimen "has been the building block of programs" that rapidly expanded to include other treatment regimens and comprehensive medical care for pregnant women.[50] Prudence Mabale, director of the Positive Women Network, agreed and made an impassioned plea for access to AIDS drugs. Nevirapine had given women hope and overcame their fears to seek counseling and other AIDS services. "It is not just the drug — these programs have changed women's lives."[51]

By the end of the conference, scientists, practitioners, and the Medicines Control Council came to a common understanding and agreed to collaborate on a workable solution to the nevirapine crisis.[52] For Zackie Achmat and his Treatment Action Campaign, it was another victory in a string of successes since his drug strike began. Religious leaders, trade unions, and many other groups had aligned with his cause. Now, widespread distribution of nevirapine was within reach and, for Achmat, not a moment too soon. He had been plagued all year by a recurring lung infection and was constantly exhausted. Only President Mbeki's pragmatic views now stood in their way, and many thought that Achmat was the only person who could punch through that one remaining barrier and ensure that Mbeki's government followed through on its pledge. More than ever, Achmat's friends and followers needed him alive and healthy. On August 4, 2003, Achmat announced that he intended to end his drug strike and begin treatment, explaining, "I don't want to kill myself for Thabo. I want to make sure that people get medicines."[53]

In November 2003, the South African government finally unveiled its national AIDS treatment plan and vastly increased the Health Ministry's budget for AIDS healthcare.[54] Among those who benefited from the government's new initiatives was Vuyiseka Dubula. Like many South Africans, she had joined the Treatment Action Campaign and participated in the organization's efforts to broaden access to single-dose nevirapine. Vuyiseka was twenty-two years old when she learned she was HIV-positive in 2001. She was healthy, enjoying life, and not feeling sick, but she went for testing because she was "just curious to know."[55] She lived with her family in Philippi, a township in Cape Town, and like many South Africans, her family was poor. Gender inequality and gender-based violence were huge problems in the country, and the poor economic and social status of women made them especially vulnerable to HIV. "I realized that it was not coincidence when I found myself amongst those living with HIV."[56] Fortunately, she did not suffer the fate of many women in South Africa who were coerced into sterilization because of their HIV status. Before the Constitutional Court ruling and the introduction of nationwide HIV/AIDS treatment programs, such sterilization practices were commonly forced on HIV-infected women (but not on their male partners).

When Vuyiseka and her husband decided to start a family in 2004, she went to her doctor for advice and to discuss her options. Her CD4 count was 269.[57] Vuyiseka and her doctor agreed that her best option was to begin treatment to reduce her viral load and increase her CD4 count prior to becoming pregnant. She took a regimen of nevirapine, AZT, and 3TC for two years before giving birth to her first child. Her daughter was given a single dose of nevirapine after delivery and AZT for a week. After her baby's birth, Vuyiseka continued taking her triple-drug regimen, her CD4 count rose to 460, and her viral load fell below detection and stayed there. Best of all, her daughter has remained free of HIV.[58]

* * *

Nevirapine had prevailed in the courts of law and public opinion, but it was also facing another hurdle. At the same time that the Medicines Control Council was grappling with whether to de-register nevirapine, the South African Competition Commission was investigating accusations that the manufacturers of AIDS drugs were employing unfair pricing and licensing policies.[59] The Treatment Action Campaign, along with a collection of AIDS support groups, trade unions, healthcare workers, and people with HIV/AIDS, filed the complaint using the experiences of Hazel Tau to make their point.[60]

Hazel, who lived in Soweto, was diagnosed with HIV in 1991. Two years later, she began treatment with AZT, which was covered by her husband's medical insurance.[61] After six months, Hazel decided to stop taking the drug, because she felt better. At the same time, she began working as a volunteer counselor at an AIDS information center. One day, she returned home from her counseling job to discover that her husband had locked her out and proceeded to divorce her because of her HIV status. Through a miscarriage of justice during the divorce proceedings, she lost all of her possessions — her house, her clothes, and furniture — and over the next eight years, Hazel was forced to rebuild her life from scratch. She worked at a series of HIV counseling and support centers and managed to maintain her health. Then in April 2002, her health began to decline. She developed several opportunistic infections including thrush and a lung infection. By September, her CD4 count had dropped to 168 and she had lost 55 pounds. She knew that she should begin treatment with a triple-drug regimen, but on her meager salary, "I cannot afford to pay the prices the drug companies charge for antiretroviral treatment."[62]

The Treatment Action Campaign and its sister organizations claimed that Glaxo-SmithKline and Boehringer Ingelheim were unlawfully charging patients like Hazel excessive prices.⁶³ GSK made AZT and 3TC, which along with BI's nevirapine comprised the most widely used triple-drug regimen for treating AIDS patients in South Africa. In October 2003, after an extensive investigation of the pricing complaint, the Competition Commission found sufficient justification to refer the matter to the courts.

BI denied the charges. Since July 2000, the company had been distributing nevirapine free of charge to prevent mother-to-child HIV transmission — a program that was running successfully in more than fifty developing countries — and had recently announced it would extend the program beyond its original five-year commitment.⁶⁴ In addition, BI had collaborated with five other drug companies, several United Nations agencies, and the World Bank to make triple-drug AIDS therapy affordable and available to large numbers of HIV-infected people in Africa.⁶⁵ As part of that commitment, BI had granted a license in October 2002 to Aspen Pharmacare, a generic drug manufacturer in South Africa. The license allowed Aspen to make and distribute generic nevirapine for use in combination-drug regimens in South Africa and thirteen other sub–Saharan countries and put its generic product in direct competition with BI's branded Viramune.⁶⁶

Both sides — the Treatment Action Campaign accusers and the drug companies — wanted to avoid a prolonged court battle, because "the enormity of the HIV/AIDS problem facing South Africa ... demands unity of resolve."⁶⁷ On December 10, 2003, BI reached an agreement with the Competition Commission and the AIDS advocacy groups representing Hazel. BI agreed to grant licenses to two additional generic companies to make nevirapine. Although the agreement with the Commission allowed BI to charge the generic companies up to a five percent royalty, BI's licenses were royalty-free, making generic nevirapine even less expensive to private insurers and the South African government.⁶⁸ In return, the Treatment Action Campaign withdrew its complaint. GSK struck a similar agreement, and consequently, the South African government's cost of supplying the generic triple-drug regimen to AIDS patients dropped to $25 per month.⁶⁹

The United States government also took steps to facilitate distribution of low-cost generic AIDS drugs to African and other developing countries. In May 2004, the FDA, in association with the President's Emergency Plan for AIDS Relief, launched a new "tentative approval" procedure, which allowed generic manufacturers to submit generic versions of AIDS drugs for FDA consideration, while the original drug was still protected by a patent.⁷⁰ FDA would review and approve these generic drugs according to its usual standards but issue a "tentative" rather than "full" approval. Tentative approval allowed the PEPFAR program to purchase and distribute generic drugs of the same, FDA-approved quality as the patented products but at a substantial cost savings. Nevirapine, manufactured by Aspen Pharmacare in South Africa, was the second generic drug to receive tentative approval through this procedure. Subsequently, BI granted voluntary licenses to other generic manufacturers in South Africa, Nigeria, Egypt, and Kenya. After obtaining FDA's tentative approval, those manufacturers also distributed generic nevirapine through the PEPFAR program to HIV/AIDS patients throughout Africa.⁷¹

* * *

By 2004, investigators had learned a lot about HIV transmission to newborns and how to prevent it. The Ariel Project and other studies had pointed to the mother's viral load as a major factor responsible for infant infections.⁷² When pregnant women took a triple-drug regimen and their viral load fell below detection, their babies did not become infected with HIV. Without drug treatment during pregnancy, women had a one-in-three chance of transmitting their HIV infection to their babies, and in most cases, the baby became infected during childbirth. Single-dose nevirapine to the mother during labor and to the baby after birth reduced the chances of HIV transmission to about one in ten. Unfortunately, as Jackson and Guay soon discovered, the single-dose nevirapine regimen also triggered viral resistance in the mothers, as well as in the one-in-ten babies who became infected despite nevirapine treatment.[73] This was a significant concern because nevirapine was also widely used in developing countries as a component various triple-drug regimens to treat HIV/AIDS in both adults and children. If those patients were resistant to nevirapine, the drug regimen was more likely to fail, and alternative drug regimens were often unavailable.

For those reasons, clinical investigators continued to search for drug regimens that worked better than single-dose nevirapine to prevent mother-to-child HIV transmission but that were feasible in resource-limited settings. They found that combining a single dose of nevirapine with a short course of treatment with AZT, 3TC, or both, made HIV transmission to babies less likely.[74] And in addition to preventing infant HIV infections, the short-term regimen of AZT and 3TC, along with a dose of nevirapine during labor, reduced the likelihood that mothers would develop resistance to nevirapine.[75] Clinics in metropolitan areas of Africa soon adopted these improved regimens. But unfortunately, the new regimens were still not convenient enough to impact HIV transmission to infants in the tiny, remote villages of Africa where the single-dose nevirapine regimen remained the only feasible choice.

* * *

In May 2004, shortly after his reelection, President Mbeki addressed the South African Parliament and announced that one of his government's goals was to treat 53,000 AIDS patients within a year.[76] By July 2004, single-dose nevirapine to prevent mother-to-child HIV transmission had been implemented nationwide in South Africa. Then, the Medicines Control Council, reacting to the new clinical findings about the advantages of adding AZT and 3TC, ruled that single-dose nevirapine should only be given in combination with other AIDS drugs to prevent mother-to-child HIV transmission.[77]

Speaking at the 15th International AIDS Conference in Bangkok, Health Minister Tshabalala-Msimang implied that the Treatment Action Campaign's court case had forced the South African government to implement an unsafe treatment (namely, single-dose nevirapine) and used the concerns about nevirapine-induced resistance to justify the Medicines Control Council's revised policy. Scientists, physicians, and patient advocates strongly criticized the Medicines Control Council's decision.[78] Although everyone acknowledged that the combination regimens (which added multiple doses of AZT and 3TC to single-dose nevirapine) were more effective in preventing mother-to-child HIV transmission, those regimens were also more complicated to administer and more expensive. Conference delegates worried that many mothers and newborns who currently benefited from the single-dose nevirapine program would not have access to the more complicated regimens. Joep Lange, co-chairman of the Bangkok conference and president of the International AIDS Society, had been among the most vocal and concerned scientists warning about nevirapine-induced resistance, but he agreed that "in many settings the single dose of nevirapine is the only option."[79] Zackie Achmat, having regained his strength after a year of AIDS therapy, told reporters in Bangkok that limiting the use of nevirapine was another sign of how the South African government had sowed confusion over AIDS.[80] The World Health Organization also issued a statement supporting the use of single-dose nevirapine, which it said should not be limited while health organizations worked toward implementing more complex drug regimens.[81]

* * *

Meanwhile, questions about the Ugandan HIVNET 012 trial continued to bounce around the Division of AIDS offices at the National Institutes of Health. Three separate inspections had confirmed the validity of the trial and its conclusions, but those inspections also raised suspicions that some of the trial's problems stemmed from poor grant management by the Division. So, the National Institutes of Health conducted an internal investigation to determine whether the Division was properly overseeing the AIDS clinical trials that it funded through its HIVNET network. The investigation cleared officials and staff in the Division of AIDS of any wrongdoing, but the Institute's leaders acknowledged that important lessons had come from the intensive reviews of the Ugandan trial. Those lessons would "help us do our clinical research, both domestically and internationally, much better" in the future.[82]

All of the inspections and reviews of the HIVNET 012 trial, although extensive and thorough, had been conducted by individuals or organizations with a vested interest the trial: Boehringer Ingelheim (the drug's manufacturer), Westat Corporation (paid by the National Institutes of Health under contract), and Division of AIDS auditors (employees of the National Institutes of Health). In addition, the reports of those inspections were internal documents that would not be made public. Consequently, lingering concerns and uncertainty about the use of single-dose nevirapine for preventing mother-to-child HIV transmission persisted among the media, politicians, and the general public.[83] Those concerns compelled officials at the National Institutes of Health to seek yet another assessment of the HIVNET 012 trial. In August 2004, they asked the Institute of Medicine, an independent professional organization with no ties to the trial, to convene a committee and evaluate the HIVNET 012 trial's design, conduct, results, and validity.[84] For the next seven months, the prestigious nine-member committee reviewed the investigators' files, previous auditors' reports, information from the trial's database, and primary source documents from Uganda. They also conducted an independent statistical analysis of key parts of the trial.

Once again, Jackson and Guay fully cooperated, testifying before the committee in both open and closed sessions.[85] Jackson transferred an extensive collection of data files and study-related documents for the committee's review, and Guay responded in a series of emails to numerous questions, explaining trial procedures, study staff activities, and patient management. The committee also asked experts to comment on aspects of the trial's procedures and conduct. David Feigal, who had been Director of FDA's Antiviral Drug Products Division at the time of nevirapine's approval, reviewed the Westat audit report. Although the auditor cited presumed regulatory deficiencies in the trial's investigator training and monitoring practices, Feigal said the investigators' activities met FDA's standards.[86]

The committee's review proceeded smoothly and inconspicuously until December, 13, 2004, when the first of a series of wire service articles put nevirapine back in the headlines. Referencing leaked documents from within the National Institutes of Health, the wire service reporter challenged the validity of the HIVNET 012 trial. Among the harshest criticisms in his articles were that the Ugandan study was flawed and "riddled with sloppy record keeping," the investigators "underreported thousands of severe reactions including deaths" and were slow to report those safety concerns to the FDA, and the National Institutes of Health, which funded the study, failed to enforce the clinical standards required by regulators in the United States.[87]

Newspapers and radio stations around the world carried the wire service stories, and those stories generated an emphatic rebuttal from scientists, patient advocacy groups, government officials, and Boehringer Ingelheim. Within twenty-four hours, the National Institutes of Health and BI issued press releases, recounting their actions over the previous four years, correcting the inaccuracies in the wire service articles, and repeating their conclusions that the HIVNET 012 trial's procedural flaws and recordkeeping deficiencies did not negate its key findings.[88] Other organizations were concerned that the wire service articles' inaccuracies might provide ammunition to dissident groups who had long denied HIV, opposed using AIDS drugs, and interfered with efforts to address the growing AIDS epidemic in developing countries. The Elizabeth Glaser Pediatric AIDS Foundation, Doctors Without Borders, and Global Strategies for HIV Prevention issued statements reaffirming their confidence in the safety and efficacy of single-dose nevirapine.[89] While they urged continued efforts to find more effective drug regimens, they said it was premature and inappropriate to withdraw single-dose nevirapine as an option for preventing mother-to-child HIV transmission and continued to support its use in resource-limited settings where alternatives were not yet available. Many prominent investigators and patient advocacy groups around the world agreed with them.[90]

But the South African government used the ammunition. The African National Congress, through its official journal, *ANC Today*, cited the wire service articles as evidence that the National Institutes of Health and BI had conspired to treat Africans as "guinea pigs, given a drug [that they] knew very well should not be prescribed."[91] Jerry Coovadia, a prominent and outspoken South African investigator, countered by saying that the controversy was "more manufactured rather than being real" and pointed out that no new data had emerged to change the established conclusions that nevirapine was safe, well tolerated in mothers and babies, and highly effective in preventing mother-to-child transmission of HIV.[92] Zackie Achmat's Treatment Action Campaign added, "There is not a single reported life threatening adverse event associated with this regimen, which is widely used in the developing world."[93]

On January 4, 2005, three weeks after the initial wire service article appeared, the Institute of Medicine committee heard testimony from the Director of Policy in Research Operations, who represented a newly created unit within the Division of AIDS.[94] The Director read an 18-page statement criticizing the Division of AIDS's re-monitoring report and echoed the concerns that had been widely reported in the wire service articles.[95] But all of criticisms raised in the articles and repeated by the Director had already been addressed by Jackson, Guay, Feigal, and other experts. Some were auditor misinterpretations that had been successfully explained. Some were documentation errors that had been subsequently corrected or annotated. And some were procedural deficiencies that, although they were unfortunate mistakes, did not affect the study's outcome. The Director's testimony did not present any new issues for the committee to consider.

On April 7, 2005, the Institute of Medicine published its report on the HIVNET 012 trial.[96] The committee found that the study's design met all relevant ethical requirements. The data on adverse outcomes, including hospitalizations and deaths, was accurate, complete, and permitted a reliable assessment of drug safety. The extent and significance of missing documents was quite limited and had no bearing on the integrity of the trial. And the data and original findings of the trial's investigators were sound and presented in a balanced manner. The committee therefore concluded that the trial "can be relied upon for scientific and policy-making purposes."[97]

The Ugandan trial, HIVNET 012, stands as the most thoroughly reviewed of all AIDS clinical trials. Auditors, inspectors, and statisticians had repeatedly combed through every aspect of this clinical trial — its design, enrollment procedures, patient care, data handling, and analysis — and consistently concluded that the investigators' original findings could be trusted. Despite this proof of the trial's value, BI did not resubmit the HIVNET 012 data to the FDA or request approval of the single-dose nevirapine regimen in the United States. Regulatory approval to use single-dose nevirapine for preventing mother-to-child HIV transmission had already been granted in the developing countries where this regimen was most urgently needed.[98] In the United States, the Public Health Service Task Force still recommended single-dose nevirapine as an option for preventing mother-to-child HIV transmission, regardless of the drug's regulatory approval status, in cases where HIV-infected women had not received AIDS drugs during pregnancy.[99] But in general, BI acknowledged, better drug regimens had emerged for protecting infants from HIV infection.[100] In the United States, most HIV-infected women received HAART triple-drug therapy, a treatment regimen that preserved their health and prevented HIV transmission whether they were pregnant or not.

* * *

In the early years of the twenty-first century, Uganda and South Africa both faced a devastating AIDS crisis. Uganda's swift and aggressive response won praise from the international community, and by 2005, its nationwide programs had dramatically reduced HIV infection rates and AIDS-related deaths.[101] On the other hand, the South African government's resistance, restrictions, and delays not only provoked worldwide condemnation but also caused widespread and unnecessary suffering. From 2000 to 2005, more than 330,000 South Africans lost their lives, because their government denied them feasible AIDS treatment. In addition, an estimated 35,000 South African babies were born with HIV infections that could have been prevented by implementing the single-dose nevirapine regimen.[102]

For years, Florence Ngobeni-Allen had worked as a counselor at Chris Hani Baragwanath Hospital in Soweto, South Africa, and she had listened to thousands of HIV-infected pregnant women and new mothers.[103] Their faces were sad and hopeless as they told their stories and hesitantly admitted their fears. At first, Florence had little to offer them except sympathy and understanding. She was also HIV-positive, and she had lost a daughter to AIDS. Florence knew she was providing essential moral support, but it was depressing work. After these stressful sessions, she would often retire to a quiet corner and cry.

She knew as well as anyone the struggles that they faced at home and in their communities. As a young child, her parents were unemployed and the family was homeless. When Florence was fourteen, her mother remarried and she was sent to live with her grandmother, whose full-time domestic work kept her away from home except on Fridays and Saturdays. The rest of the time, Florence was under the care of an abusive, drug-using uncle who frequently beat her, sometimes in the middle of the night. When she grew old enough and strong enough, the feisty teenager fought back, physically able to hold her own against any man. She wanted a better life and was determined to finish high school. Despite living with different family members and transfers to different schools each year, Florence, at the age of twenty-one, became the only person in her family to earn her high school qualification.

Unfortunately, her plans for a better life with her new fiancé changed sharply when her baby daughter died and Florence learned she was infected with HIV. Like legions of other South Africans, Florence joined the crusade against AIDS, demanding the Mbeki government to show leadership and make AIDS drugs available to everyone who needed them.[104] When investigators at Chris Hani Baragwanath Hospital began conducting clinical

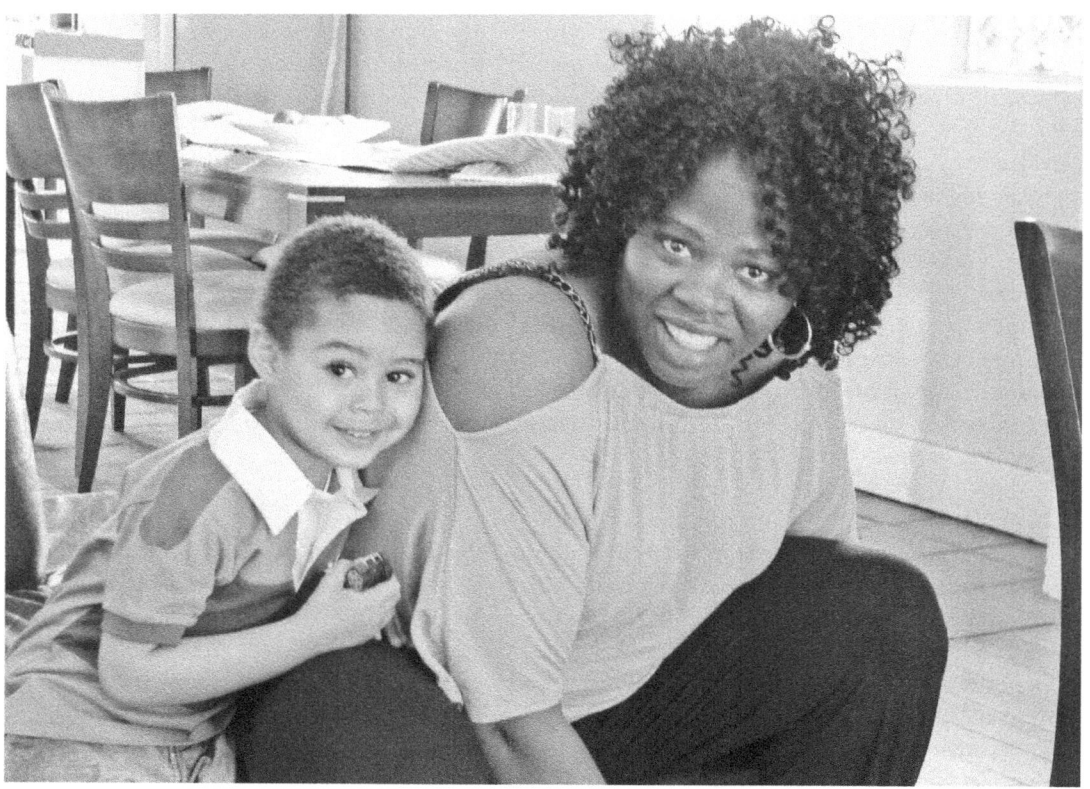

Florence Ngobeni-Allen and her son, Alexander (courtesy Elizabeth Glaser Pediatric AIDS Foundation).

trials, she served on the Community Advisory Board, drafted informed consent forms, and recruited women to participate. Pregnant women readily signed up for the trials, even though they knew they might be assigned to a placebo group or that the experimental drug might not work. At least, the clinical trials offered them a chance to save their children. Otherwise, they had nothing.

Then, after years of struggle and controversy, South Africa began distributing drugs to treat AIDS and the single-dose nevirapine regimen to prevent mother-to-child HIV transmission. Despite fears of retaliation, pregnant women mustered the strength to fight the social stigma that AIDS had imposed on them. "There is nothing a mother wouldn't do to protect her baby."[105] They bravely stepped forward to be tested. And at Chris Hani Baragwanath Hospital, Florence introduced HIV-positive women to programs that would protect their babies from infection.

Florence spent less time crying in her quiet corner. Instead, she brought smiles to mothers' faces when she gave them the test results, informing them that their infants were HIV-negative. After watching so many other HIV-positive mothers give birth to healthy babies, she began to wonder, "What am I waiting for?"[106] She had remarried and had been taking AIDS drugs as a participant in clinical trials. For the first time in almost a decade, she thought it might be possible to have a family—a healthy family. In 2006, her son, Alexander, was born, and Florence was overjoyed that he was HIV-negative. But for months, she could not bring herself to get close to her son, unwilling to risk infecting him. Over time, her fears faded away, and the Ngobeni-Allens adjusted to a normal family life. In 2011, her second son, Kulani, was born, also HIV-negative.

The prevention programs emboldened HIV-infected women like Florence across Africa. Losing a child to AIDS was heartbreaking, but the experience also made them strong. And seeing children playing in the neighborhoods — healthy children, thanks to the HIV prevention programs — gave them hope. Their determination extended beyond protecting their own children. They wanted to help others and sought opportunities to work as counselors, advocates, or, after additional training, as healthcare workers. To the physicians, foreign aid workers, and agency officials who witnessed this phenomenon, the brigades of women like Florence were the true heroes: mothers who had suffered so much and lost so much but were still willing to talk about what they had gone through and were determined to "keep going until we end pediatric AIDS once and for all."[107]

President Mbeki resigned in 2008, reacting to charges of government corruption and a loss of his party's confidence in his ability to lead. Health Minister Tshabalala-Msimang left her post at the same time. The following year, after a short interim government, Jacob Zuma was elected as South Africa's new president. The new leaders in Zuma's Health Ministry tackled the country's HIV/AIDS epidemic as a top priority and made rapid progress. In 2010, the South African government partnered with the Clinton Health Access Initiative and other organizations to implement HIV testing, treatment, and consulting services throughout all nine of the country's provinces. That year, more than 2200 nurses were trained to deliver AIDS therapies and deployed to work in newly established healthcare centers in all 250 South African municipalities. At those centers, AIDS drugs, including nevirapine, were distributed free of charge to millions of HIV-infected South Africans.[108] Most significantly, comprehensive programs to prevent mother-to-child transmission of HIV were established in 98 percent of the country's health facilities, and the rate of HIV infections in newborns was cut in half.[109] South Africa now manages the largest AIDS treatment program in the world and is well on its way to eliminating mother-to-child HIV transmission.

As foreign aid programs found cost-effective ways to provide developing countries with newer AIDS drugs, nevirapine became more widely used in combination-drug regimens than as a single-dose treatment. But investigators were still discovering ways that nevirapine could be used to prevent HIV transmission to newborns.

23

If Nothing Else ...

"If you had told me in 1984 that there would be twenty-plus drugs and about twelve co-formulated combos that decreased HIV below the level of detection, I would have said, No way."[1] Martin Hirsch, like so many of his fellow researchers, had embarked on his quest to study the new clinical syndrome called AIDS because it fascinated him. AIDS tickled his scientific curiosity and presented a puzzle, which scientists cannot resist. As investigators, Hirsch and his colleagues wanted to know what was killing their patients. As physicians, they wanted to ease their patients' suffering. But even when their suspicions were confirmed and the culprit turned out to be a virus, they knew a cure was unlikely. No one had ever found a drug that could knock out any virus the way that antibiotics knocked out bacteria, and they doubted that they could make a vaccine. They would try, of course. But they all knew the odds were against them.

For the first ten years, despite the efforts of some of the world's best scientific minds and a string of technological breakthroughs, this shifty virus always kept one step ahead. It found ways to resist the most promising drugs. Experimental vaccines failed. To make matters worse, public health officials faced political, cultural, social, and religious barriers to their HIV prevention campaigns: gay men did not want to curb their sexual freedom, many parents and church leaders did not want condoms distributed in schools, law enforcement officials often opposed distribution of clean needles to injection drug users, and elected officials avoided discussion of AIDS altogether. Still, teams of dedicated researchers persisted — urged on by desperate patients and their advocates — and learned from their failures. When they reached a dead end, they simply redirected their efforts. Slowly but surely, their path became smoother, their pace became faster, and their prize came within reach. In three short years, from 1993 to 1996, AIDS went from a raging epidemic that provoked only despair to a manageable disease that gave people hope — if not for a cure, at least for a second chance. HAART regimens brought people who were already infected back from the brink of death and restored their health. Other drug regimens — starting with multi-dose AZT, then single-dose nevirapine, and finally combined drug regimens — prevented babies from becoming infected.

* * *

Katherine Luzuriaga witnessed the impact of HAART on pediatric AIDS from a unique and personal perspective. While she was planning the first pediatric AIDS clinical trials of nevirapine in 1990, she was also pregnant with her first son.[2] Mothers of the children in those early pediatric trials identified with Luzuriaga, an instant rapport between mothers sharing common experiences and expectations: informal, intimate, and apprehensive feelings that trial subjects rarely disclose to clinical investigators. Luzuriaga's baby bump made her one of them, an expectant mother who understood their hopes and fears. Unfortunately, in the early 1990s, Luzuriaga and the project team at Boehringer Ingelheim were still learning how to optimize nevirapine, and no one had yet figured out how to use drug combinations to change the course of the disease. The youngsters who participated in those early pediatric AIDS trials died within a few years, and their HIV-infected mothers did, too.[3]

In 1995, Luzuriaga was still conducting pediatric clinical trials with nevirapine when she became pregnant with her second son. In the intervening five years, she and the BI team had refined the conditions for effective nevirapine treatment and were now conducting the first nevirapine-containing triple-drug clinical trials in children and infants. Again, Luzuriaga found herself building a rapport with the mothers of the children in her clinical trial. But this time, the outcome was different. Clinicians had more choices. The new triple-drug regimens suppressed HIV below detection and kept the virus bottled up indefinitely. Consequently, most of the children that Luzuriaga treated in those later clinical trials, as well as their HIV-infected mothers, are still alive and healthy — including Jason and Jane, the fraternal twins who were among the first infants that Luzuriaga treated with nevirapine, AZT, and ddI.[4] Over the years, Luzuriaga adjusted the twins' triple-drug regimen, substituting the AZT/ddI backbone with third-generation compounds (emtricitabine and tenofovir) and replacing nevirapine with an HIV protease inhibitor.[5] Jason and Jane are now approaching adulthood, having remained free of detectable HIV replication and other signs of immune deficiency longer than any other babies infected at birth.[6]

The widespread use of HAART regimens and the success of HIV prevention programs have virtually eliminated pediatric AIDS in the United States. Pediatric AIDS wards, which were once overflowing with sick children, are now empty. The babies and children who became infected prior to 1994 and survived are now teenagers or young adults, and HAART regimens have kept them healthy. Despite the number of HIV-infected women, which has changed little in the past decade, American mothers no longer infect their babies. Their HAART regimens and other prevention procedures have eliminated HIV infections in newborns. Most American pediatricians who began practicing medicine in the twenty-first century have never seen HIV-related opportunistic infections or other AIDS symptoms in children.[7] In fact, they rarely see HIV-infected children, and perhaps in the future they never will.

In 2012, Luzuriaga and Doug Richman consulted on a case that reinforced the notion that aggressively treating HIV-infected babies with a HAART regimen within days after birth might be able to prevent the virus from becoming infectious. A baby born in Mississippi with HIV was given nevirapine, AZT, and 3TC, starting just thirty hours after birth and continued a triple-drug regimen for about 18 months.[8] At two years of age, despite having stopped drug treatment for at least six months, the baby had no detectable HIV when assessed by conventional assays, and the minute traces of virus, measured in the baby's body by the most sophisticated assays, appeared to be unable to replicate. Luzuriaga and her colleagues think that early and aggressive drug treatment markedly curtailed the amount of virus and the extent of the "viral reservoirs" that otherwise would have colonized in the baby's body. They guardedly called it a "functional cure."[9] Investigators like Luzuriaga think that Jason, Jane, and other HIV-infected teenagers who began HAART treatment as newborns might also be candidates for stopping drug treatment, having reduced the virus in their bodies to a residual and apparently harmless microbe.[10] "It may be as close as we can come to a cure before a vaccine."[11]

* * *

After the introduction of HAART, the dreaded hallmarks of AIDS, such as pneumocystis pneumonia and Kaposi's sarcoma, disappeared. People are now living with HIV, not dying from AIDS. But the longer life expectancy that they now enjoy has uncovered new problems: side effects that result from long-term exposure to these powerful drug combinations. Both the virus and certain AIDS drugs produce changes in insulin sensitivity that put HIV-infected people at an increased, long-term risk of developing diabetes.[12] People who take HIV protease inhibitors or the AZT-like drugs are three to four times more likely to develop type 2 diabetes than uninfected people.[13] Investigators think these AIDS drugs either interfere directly with insulin's ability to regulate blood sugar or contribute indirectly to diabetes through changes in body fat distribution.

The redistribution of body fat also leads to a cluster of cosmetic changes, which many patients consider the most disturbing side effects of long term HAART treatment. The AZT-like drugs and HIV protease inhibitors account for the most frequently occurring and severe cases.[14] People lose superficial fat in their face, arms, and legs, and accumulate deeper fat deposits in their breasts and abdomen. They also develop a fat pad at the back of the neck called a buffalo hump. These physical changes can affect a person's self-image and present profound social and psychological challenges. The sunken cheeks, hollow eyes, and belly fat can be so disfiguring and stigmatizing that people stop taking their drug regimens, or worse, take their drugs intermittently.

In addition to cosmetic changes, the alterations in fat metabolism after long term HAART treatment can lead to an increased risk of cardiovascular disease.[15] Some of the AZT-like drugs and HIV protease inhibitors, especially when coupled with booster doses of ritonavir, decrease HDL-cholesterol (the "good" cholesterol) and increase triglycerides and LDL-cholesterol (the "bad" cholesterol).[16] Drugs in the nevirapine class (the non-nucleoside reverse transcriptase inhibitors) cause more modest increases and a favorable shift in the cholesterol balance. Specifically, nevirapine causes a large, selective increase in HDL-cholesterol and improvement in the ratio of good-to-bad cholesterol.[17] Because of this "protease inhibitor-sparing" effect, nevirapine is a preferred alternative for patients who have high blood lipids and are at risk of coronary heart disease.[18]

* * *

In addition to its relatively favorable side effect profile, nevirapine's proven value in preventing HIV transmission to newborns led many physicians to choose nevirapine when treating healthy people who were accidentally exposed to HIV through needle sticks or other mishaps. In 2000, Wanda, a 43-year-old healthcare worker in Chicago, was accidentally injured by a needle stick while drawing blood from a patient who suffered from HIV and hepatitis C viral infections.[19] Based on the patient's advanced disease, his treatment history with AIDS drugs, and the severity of her exposure, Wanda's doctors, as a precaution, decided to give her the triple-drug regimen of nevirapine, AZT, and 3TC. When she started the drug regimen, Wanda's blood contained no HIV or hepatitis C virus, and her liver function was normal.

After fourteen days of drug treatment, Wanda developed malaise, fatigue, fever, and chills. Six days later, her doctors noticed the first signs of liver damage, and they stopped her drug treatment. Unfortunately, Wanda's condition continued to worsen over the following week. Although her blood remained free of HIV infection, she developed acute liver failure and slipped into a coma. Eight days later, Wanda received a liver transplant. After the doctors removed her liver, they examined it more closely and saw a pattern of dead and damaged tissue. Wanda recovered from the transplant operation without complications. At a checkup six months later, her new liver continued to function normally, and her blood still showed no signs of infection with either HIV or the hepatitis C virus.

From the beginning of the nevirapine clinical trials, investigators had consistently noted some patients who had changes in liver function, but this side effect occurred infrequently and had been overshadowed by the problems associated with nevirapine-induced skin rash and Stevens-Johnson Syndrome, the most severe form of skin rash. The observed liver problems did not cause physicians to favor one HAART regimen over another. All of the AIDS drugs could cause liver damage, and many HIV-infected patients had damaged livers due to the stage of their disease or as a consequence of their lifestyle (such as alcoholism, injection drug use, or concurrent hepatitis C viral infection).[20] Aware of this potential risk, physicians always paid close attention to each patient's liver function, but they balanced the possibility of causing liver damage against the clear value of HAART regimens, which could suppress HIV indefinitely.

The situation was different for healthy people, like Wanda, who were accidentally exposed to HIV. In these cases, aggressive drug treatment offered fewer benefits and posed greater risks. The likelihood of becoming infected with HIV from a needle stick was relatively low, and preventative treatment with the powerful AIDS drugs could cause serious side effects, perhaps permanent damage. With little experience to guide them, officials at the United States Public Health Service recommended a conservative approach when treating accidental HIV exposures: a four-week course of treatment with AZT and 3TC.[21] But based on the theoretical advantages of nevirapine, which worked faster than other AIDS drugs and had other attractive pharmaceutical properties, some physicians — like Wanda's — added nevirapine to the treatment regimen for accidentally exposed people.[22]

By 2000, the Food and Drug Administration had received a dozen reports of liver toxicity in people who had taken nevirapine after accidental HIV exposure. Although Wanda was the only person who required a liver transplant, the Centers for Disease Control and Prevention warned physicians that nevirapine could cause serious liver toxicity when given to healthy people.[23] As the reports accumulated from widespread use of nevirapine, both as a treatment regimen in HIV-infected patients and as a preventative measure for healthy people after accidental HIV exposure, clinicians at BI saw more clearly the conditions under which nevirapine would likely cause liver damage. Women appeared to be more sensitive to nevirapine's side effects than men, and people with a healthy immune system appeared to be more sensitive than those with lower CD4 cell counts.[24] Unfortunately, the early clinical trials of nevirapine had included mostly people with low CD4 cell counts and only a small number of women, delaying awareness of possible liver damage. But with the new information gleaned from wider nevirapine use, BI revised the drug's label to include warnings about liver toxicity, instructions for minimizing the risk to vulnerable patients, and a directive to avoid its use in healthy people.[25]

* * *

Despite the restrictions on using nevirapine, the success of various drug regimens in preventing infection after accidental HIV exposure and preventing HIV transmission to newborns led investigators to systematically examine whether HAART regimens could prevent the spread of HIV. From the beginning of the AIDS epidemic, investigators and funding agencies had followed two parallel, and largely unrelated, research strategies. One pursued programs for treating people already infected with HIV. The other directed efforts toward preventing HIV infection (primarily, vaccine research and public health initiatives). But investigators later established that the HAART regimens can both treat and prevent HIV infections, a finding that has eliminated the distinction between treatment and prevention programs. HAART keeps the viral load of HIV-infected people below detection, preserving their own health and significantly reducing their ability to transmit HIV to others.[26] In addition, regimens of appropriately chosen AIDS drugs given to healthy people protect them from infection by their HIV-positive partners.[27] These successes have led health officials to conclude that "treatment itself can serve as a major form of prevention."[28]

Until an effective AIDS vaccine is developed, transmission of HIV to healthy people of any age, whether to newborns or adults, can be prevented by a HAART regimen, especially when combined with other proven prevention strategies (such as condom use, male circumcision, and clean needle use by injection drug users). According to Anthony Fauci, "We are now on solid scientific ground that even without a cure we [can] turn around the trajectory of the pandemic."[29] In devising their treatment-as-prevention strategies, clinicians now have many drugs to choose from.

* * *

Following the first wave of AIDS drugs, researchers soon found better compounds, some more potent, others less toxic, and still others with superior pharmaceutical properties. GlaxoSmithKline continued HIV/AIDS research to find better AZT-like drugs, including 3TC and abacavir. Gilead Sciences emerged as a major developer of AIDS drugs and introduced several third-generation, AZT-like drugs, including emtricitabine and tenofovir, which are used together as a popular and convenient backbone of many HAART regimens.

On the other hand, of the three original drugs in the nevirapine class of non-nucleoside reverse transcriptase inhibitors, only nevirapine survived. Merck discontinued development of its "L" drugs, preferring to concentrate its research efforts on HIV protease inhibitors. Merck's indinavir was among the first HIV protease inhibitors approved by the FDA, and Merck also led research efforts to introduce the first drug in the new class of HIV integrase inhibitors, launching raltegravir in 2007. Janssen also stopped development of its original drug candidates, the TIBO compounds, but has continued an active HIV/AIDS research program. The company developed etravirine and rilpivirine as alternatives to nevirapine and also received approval for its HIV protease inhibitor, darunavir.

But of all the non-nucleoside reverse transcriptase inhibitors, Bristol-Myers Squibb's efavirenz emerged as the best-in-class agent and replaced nevirapine as the first-line choice for treating HIV-infected children and adults. Efavirenz and nevirapine have many properties in common.[30] But efavirenz is less prone to cause liver toxicity, and overall, patients tolerate it better than nevirapine. When combined with a backbone of tenofovir and emtricitabine, efavirenz has become a popular once-daily HAART regimen because of its convenience, effectiveness, and long-term tolerability.

Unfortunately, efavirenz has two drawbacks that limit its value in preventing mother-to-child HIV transmission. The drug does not easily cross biological barriers, making it difficult to protect against HIV infection in relatively inaccessible parts of the body such as the brain and a fetus. Also, efavirenz is known to cause birth defects in animals, and for that reason, physicians advise women wishing to become pregnant or who are pregnant not to take it, especially in the first trimester. Instead, they recommend switching to a nevirapine-containing regimen.

* * *

In addition to the new drug regimens that minimize HIV transmission from mother to child, public health authorities also advocate Cesarean delivery and formula feeding.[31] Newborns are most likely to become infected as they slide through the birth canal, making delivery by Cesarean section safer than natural childbirth. Even with Cesarean delivery, one-third to one-half of infants who are breastfed can still become infected through their mother's milk.[32] For this reason, public health authorities in regions with robust sanitation and healthcare systems advise HIV-infected mothers to give their babies infant formula instead.[33]

Tatu works as a counselor at Kilimanjaro Christian Medical Center in Tanzania and has held the hands of many clients who feared AIDS.[34] In 2004, she became pregnant and went to the medical center's clinic for prenatal care. Like many women in sub–Saharan Africa, Tatu was not sure when she contracted HIV, but a routine blood test during her pregnancy checkups confirmed that she was HIV-positive. "I was very shocked ... and I felt scared for my health and the health of my baby."[35] Fortunately, the Elizabeth Glaser Pediatric AIDS Foundation had established an HIV prevention clinic at the medical center, and the clinic's counselors gave Tatu hope. They explained the things that she could do to prevent her baby from becoming infected with HIV, and she followed their advice.

She began taking a drug regimen, which reduced her viral load and also reduced the chance that she would infect others, including her baby. When she went into labor, she was given a dose of nevirapine. Doctors delivered Tatu's baby by Cesarean section, and her new daughter, whom she named Faith, received a dose of nevirapine shortly after birth. Fortunately,

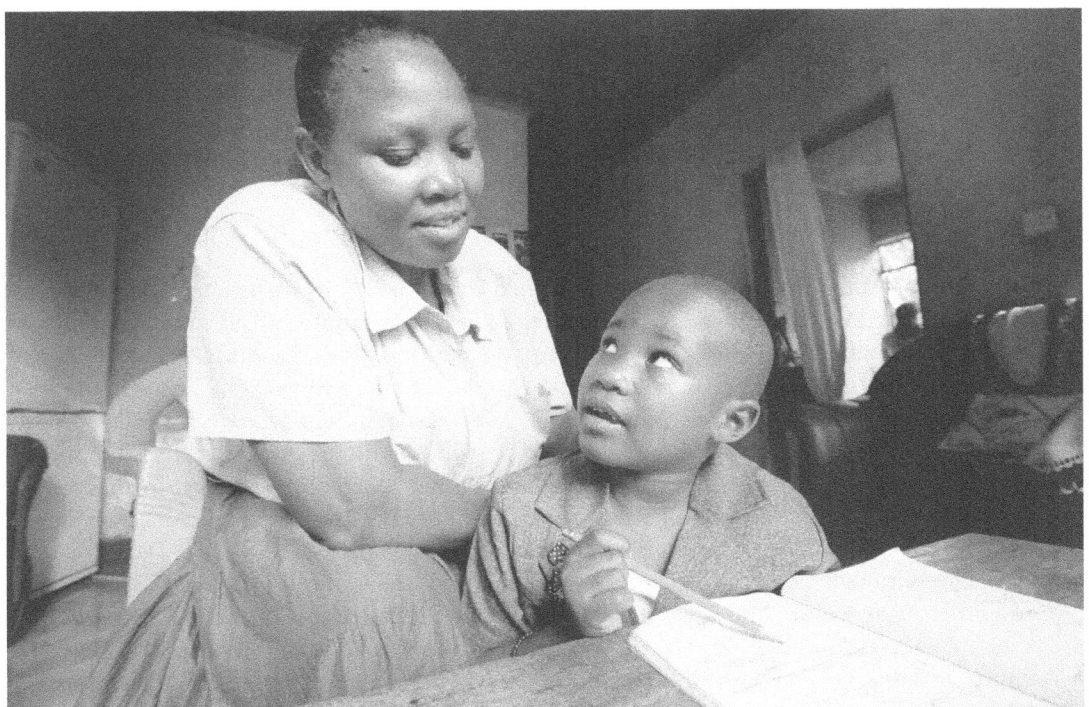

Tatu and Faith at home in Tanzania (Elizabeth Glaser Pediatric AIDS Foundation, photographer James Pursey).

Tatu could access clean water, and she fed Faith with infant formula rather than breastfeeding. As a result, Faith has remained HIV-negative. Under Tatu's watchful eye, Faith goes to school and studies hard. In the evenings, after she finishes her homework, she plays with her kitten or goes outside to join in games with her friends in the neighborhood. Thanks to the advice and care they received, Tatu and Faith "have a bright future ahead of us."[36]

Although using infant formula reduces the risk of HIV transmission, not everyone in developing countries can follow the advice that kept Faith healthy. Often, nutritional, economic, and social factors make breastfeeding preferable. Breast milk contains a powerful mixture of natural substances that protect babies from diarrhea and pneumonia, which are major killers of malnourished infants in developing countries. In some regions, breastfeeding is an essential part of the culture, and women who do not breastfeed may be ostracized.[37] In addition, women may not have access to sterile equipment and clean water to prepare infant formula safely. So, deciding between breastfeeding and formula feeding posed the ultimate dilemma for HIV-infected mothers. Breastfeeding was relatively simple, inexpensive, and widely available but increased the risk of HIV infection in babies. Formula feeding reduced the risk of HIV but made other life-threatening infections more likely, especially if clean water was not available to mix the formula.

Joep Lange was among the first investigators to address the breastfeeding issue. In the PETRA trial, one of the first clinical trials aimed at finding a feasible, short-term drug regimen to prevent HIV transmission, he could protect babies from HIV at birth, but they subsequently became infected by their mothers through breast milk.[38] Lange and his colleagues quickly followed up with another trial called SIMBA.[39] In 2003, they reported that giving a daily dose of either nevirapine or 3TC to breastfed infants prevented HIV infection. A series of clinical trials by other investigators followed, all of which confirmed that HIV transmission to infants during breastfeeding could be prevented by a variety of drug regimens given to the mother, infant, or both.[40] The most convenient drug was nevirapine.[41] Consequently, the World Health Organization revised its guidelines in 2010, recommending that babies who are breastfed by an HIV-infected mother should receive a daily dose of the nevirapine syrup until after they are weaned.[42]

* * *

Although programs to treat pregnant women and their infants are beneficial, preventing the spread of HIV and pediatric AIDS requires additional measures. In sub–Saharan Africa, HIV/AIDS is a family disease, and men are often the family's decision maker. Mobilizing them is essential. During her counseling sessions at the clinic in Kilimanjaro, Tatu encourages the women, as girlfriends, wives, and mothers, to bring along their partners for HIV counseling, testing, and treatment. "Once a man gets involved with his partner in the prevention of mother-to-child transmission process, it makes a big difference — not just to that man but to the men around him. Men will listen to another HIV-positive man more than they will a woman. That's our culture."[43]

The Elizabeth Glaser Pediatric AIDS Foundation, the Clinton HIV/AIDS Initiative, and other organizations and agencies that have tackled pediatric AIDS in developing countries are now family-focused.[44] They seek to keep the whole family in treatment, which improves the survival of both children and adults and helps prevent future HIV infections.[45] Many are structured like the Child Centered Family Care Clinic in Tanzania. The Elizabeth Glaser Pediatric AIDS Foundation awarded a grant to build the Clinic and provide comprehensive HIV/AIDS services and treatment under one roof. The trained clinic staff coordinates the mother-to-child HIV prevention programs, primary and specialty medical care, home-based care, and social services to families affected by HIV/AIDS — all centered around children in need. The Child Centered Family Care Clinic sits next door to the Kilimanjaro Christian Medical Center, and the integrated services of the two units provide medical care for malaria, tuberculosis, and other common diseases, as well as HIV/AIDS.

* * *

In 2009, Cathy Wilfert retired after fourteen years as Scientific Director at the Elizabeth Glaser Pediatric AIDS Foundation, capping a remarkable career. She had conducted the first pediatric clinical trial of the first AIDS drug, AZT. She had served as the first chairman of the Pediatric Core Committee of the AIDS Clinical Trials Group, which sponsored early pediatric testing of the newly emerging AIDS drugs. She championed, against strong opposition, the landmark ACTG 076 trial, proving that AZT could prevent mother-to-child HIV transmission. And when single-dose nevirapine was recognized as a feasible alternative to AZT in developing countries, Wilfert led the Foundation's Call to Action initiative.

Blessed with a brilliant mind and gentle nature and guided by her experiences in the pediatric AIDS wards and virology laboratory at Duke University, Wilfert crisscrossed Africa, Asia, and the Caribbean, schmoozing health ministers, placating politicians, advising clinic administrators, inspiring healthcare workers, and playing games with children on dusty, barren playgrounds. She kept a demanding schedule, at a time when the virus was spreading faster than the Foundation could set up programs. Even so, during her tenure, 2800 service sites were established in seventeen countries to prevent mother-to-child HIV transmission, and those services reached nearly five million women.[46] Through the Foundation's programs, which followed years of pediatric AIDS research, Wilfert, along with the in-country staff and teams of dedicated local country workers, could easily claim to have spared more children from HIV infection and AIDS than any other group in the world. She carved a path that made it easier for others to follow, and as Emerita Scientific Director, Wilfert continues to advise the Foundation's staff.

By 2012, the Foundation had supported 9000 clinics, reached nearly 16 million pregnant women with services to prevent mother-to-child HIV transmission, and provided treatment and care to more than 1.9 million HIV-infected children and their families.[47] As mandated by the President's Emergency Program for AIDS Relief, the Foundation worked with national governments and local institutions to shift responsibilities and transition ownership of its treatment and prevention programs to existing organizations in the host countries. In Tanzania, Mozambique, and Côte d'Ivoire, where no organizations already existed to pick up these new responsibilities, the Foundation helped local officials create new national organizations. In each country, officials chose to name their new national organizations the Ariel Glaser Foundation, in tribute to the little girl who painted colorful pictures of flower gardens more than twenty-five years before.[48] Although they maintain a voluntary affiliation with the Elizabeth Glaser Pediatric AIDS Foundation, the country-specific organizations now operate independently, with their own governance boards led by citizens of the country. They take responsibility for managing clinic operations, setting strategy, and raising funds, and they continue marching ever closer to Elizabeth Glaser's goal of eliminating pediatric AIDS.

* * *

On Laura Guay's desk sits a photograph of a dozen Ugandan children, a class reunion of sorts because they are all the same age.[49] But the bond between them has less to do with school or friendships than with a decision their mothers made before they were born, a decision that saved their lives. They were among the hundreds of babies born during the HIVNET 012 clinical trial. Now, they are ready to enter high school, still healthy, thanks to the single dose of nevirapine they received at birth and the follow up medical care they received at Mulago Hospital during the five-year trial.

The children in Guay's photo also have one other thing in common. They are all orphans. While the single-dose nevirapine regimen prevented them from becoming infected with HIV and allowed them to get a disease-free start in life, it did nothing to improve the health of their mothers. The women's HIV infections led to AIDS symptoms at a time when Mulago Hospital was unable to provide anything but supportive care. Within a few years, they all died, and their babies joined the ranks of the nearly two million children who become orphans each year in Africa and Asia due to AIDS. In some countries, including Botswana and South Africa, all pregnant women who are HIV-positive now receive highly effective drug regimens, and HIV transmission from mother to child is increasingly rare. In other countries, women and children are less fortunate, and overall, the number of "AIDS orphans" continues to rise.[50] Globally, only half of HIV-infected pregnant women receive adequate drug treatment for their own health and to protect their babies.[51]

Those who benefit from HIV/AIDS healthcare are often the easiest for the international network of agencies and non-profit organizations to reach. Many of them live in urban areas of countries with governments that put a priority on their citizens' health and have the resources to implement nationwide programs. Hitting that fifty percent milestone is certainly a remarkable accomplishment — one that Martin Hirsch and his fellow scientists could not imagine twenty years ago. Unfortunately, the international network of HIV/AIDS clinics has not reached millions of women who should be tested, could benefit from counseling, and need treatment. Consequently, 300,000 babies in the world still become infected with HIV each year, and only one-quarter of the children who subsequently need treatment for HIV are receiving it.[52] Elizabeth Glaser's quest to eliminate pediatric AIDS remains a quest.

In an effort to find a regimen that would be effective and convenient enough to prevent HIV infection in all babies everywhere, investigators built on the early successes with AZT and nevirapine, tweaking the combination of drugs, treatment schedules, and dosing conditions before, during, and after a child's birth. But the findings of these follow up trials varied little and always reached the same conclusion. All of the current drug regimens work.[53] Success in preventing mother-to-child HIV transmission now depends less on what treatment regimen is used and more on getting the drugs to all of the women and babies who need them. Public health officials urged investigators to end the "debate about which intervention is optimal and most effective" and concentrate on eliminating the barriers that have restricted universal access to AIDS drugs.[54]

In 2008, Laura Guay, the investigator who had spent most of her early career in Africa, joined the Elizabeth Glaser Pediatric AIDS Foundation. Her mission is to reach that final fifty percent.[55] And that is a formidable mission. People in developing countries still struggle with stigma, denial, and discrimination. Even in countries with supportive governments, emotional, psychological, social, and cultural barriers hinder efforts to deliver HIV/AIDS treatment and prevention services. In many infected individuals, HIV initially causes few if any symptoms. They may carry out their normal activities for years, not knowing they are infected and not taking precautions to prevent spreading HIV to others. Some of those who think they may be infected prefer not knowing. And because they do not feel sick, they do not seek medical care. Many women, like Tatu, only discover they are HIV-positive when they become pregnant and undergo routine blood testing as part of their prenatal care.

Those who discover they are infected after taking an early HIV test, but are still healthy, face other challenges. Their physician will want to monitor their HIV status and, when their immune system begins to fail, start treatment. But the routine monitoring without drug treatment (as outlined by current World Health Organization guidelines) may go on for years, and many people — feeling healthy — fail to report for their scheduled checkups. Emotionally, they go through denial, fear social stigma, and, in some cases, suffer discrimination. They struggle with how the news of their infection will affect their relationships with family members, friends, and coworkers. Consequently, many people avoid HIV testing, checkups, and treatment until they have developed late-stage AIDS symptoms, which decreases the ability of any treatment to control their disease and restore their health — even if they stick to their drug regimen. Worldwide, one-third of those who begin drug treatment discontinue therapy within five years.[56]

* * *

In sub–Saharan Africa, HIV is spread primarily by heterosexual transmission, and more women are infected than men.[57] To facilitate reaching the final fifty percent, Guay and the leaders of other international organizations now rely on a sisterhood of dedicated women who have bravely stepped forward and become the strongest advocates for improved HIV/AIDS healthcare in their countries. Women like Vuyiseka in South Africa and Tatu in Tanzania have taken control of their lives, turned their misfortune into a mission, and become influential role models in their communities.

Vuyiseka and many other HIV-positive women joined the Treatment Action Campaign and supported its lawsuit (demanding universal access to single-dose nevirapine), because they wanted their sexual reproductive rights protected, as guaranteed by the South African Constitution. They knew that the benefits of single-dose nevirapine and combination drug regimens went far beyond prevention of HIV transmission to babies. "Prevention of mother-to-child transmission was an entry point to addressing the sexual reproductive health and the rights of women living with HIV."[58] The Constitutional Court's ruling affirmed their right to be treated with dignity, their right to sexual reproductive health, and their right to have a healthy child. After the birth of her daughter, Vuyiseka went back to school, earning a bachelor's degree in health sciences and social work from the University of South Africa and a master's degree in HIV/AIDS management from the University of Stellenbosch. She has continued her affiliation with the Treatment Action Campaign, where she started as a receptionist and now serves as General Secretary. She remains a committed advocate for people living with HIV, ensuring that women and girls have access to health services and pushing for a society that is free of gender-based and sexual violence.

In Tanzania, Tatu also wanted to do more. After Faith started school, Tatu, at the age of thirty-seven, enhanced her counseling skills by earning a bachelor's degree in science and nursing. Every day at the Kilimanjaro Christian Medical Center, she sees frightened women, but she knows what they are going through, and as an HIV-infected mother with a healthy child, she speaks from her heart. She tells them her own story and reassures them that they, too, can give birth to HIV-negative children. "That's a fact — Faith and I are proof."[59] Tatu and her colleagues at the clinic show pregnant women how to live a normal, healthy life despite their HIV infection and how to protect their babies during pregnancy, childbirth, and infant nursing. When a baby is born and Tatu informs the mother that the baby's HIV test is negative, she sees "relief and joy on the mother's face. That's when you know that you have been part of something worthwhile."[60]

* * *

Nevirapine continues to be an integral part of AIDS treatment worldwide. More than half of the HIV-infected adults and children being treated in developing countries receive a triple-drug regimen containing nevirapine, usually in combination with the AZT/3TC backbone, a regimen that is less expensive than the comparable HAART regimens without nevirapine.[61] For preventing mother-to-child HIV transmission, the World Health Organization currently recommends multi-dose, multi-drug regimens and advises against using single-dose nevirapine. Drug combinations are more effective and less prone to induce viral resistance than single-dose nevirapine, and in general, longer drug exposure is more effective in protecting babies than short term treatment. Consequently, many health ministries and local clinics have replaced single-dose nevirapine with multi-drug regimens that often include nevirapine as a component.[62] Implementing the most effective regimens requires not only drug availability but also a healthcare infrastructure that encourages people to be tested for HIV, provides counseling services, conscientiously monitors their health status, prescribes an appropriate drug regimen, and oversees its use — a system of comprehensive medical care that is increasingly common in developing countries.

Many of those comprehensive medical centers can be traced back to the courageous actions of a single person, like Hauwa, who established a tiny HIV prevention clinic in her remote village of Bakin Kogi in 2004. Hauwa's success in using single-dose nevirapine to prevent HIV infections in newborns was a cause for celebration, and when a group of Americans visited, the grateful village elders presented them with a photograph of the first village child saved by nevirapine. That was just the beginning. Hauwa's newly learned skills inspired other volunteers in Bakin Kogi to seek training in home-based care, and they became influential in raising public health and HIV awareness throughout that remote region of Nigeria. Their commitment convinced the staff at Faith Alive Hospital in Jos to set up a satellite HIV testing and counseling center. Within two years, the Faith Alive Foundation broke ground for an affiliated clinic to serve the impoverished rural communities of Bakin Kogi and nearby Kafanchan.[63] A critical component of the new clinic was construction of a borehole to provide clean, drinkable well water for the patients and residents in the community. Now, instead of traveling three hours to Jos, Bakin Kogi patients have their own doctor, trained healthcare staff, and medical facilities, which provide comprehensive 24-hour HIV/AIDS care and other medical treatment. And it all started with Hauwa, who bravely packed her bags one day, journeyed to Jos, and attended the Faith Alive Hospital's first workshop on the use of single-dose nevirapine.

Healthcare professionals agree that in a perfect world, everyone should get the best drugs and the best medical care. But in developing countries, not all communities have achieved the healthcare success that Hauwa inspired in Bakin Kogi. Even at the neighborhood clinics that provide services to prevent mother-to-child HIV transmission, only half of the HIV-exposed infants receive the minimal regimen of single-dose nevirapine.[64] Treatment with the more elaborate drug combinations and dosing schedules recommended by the World Health Organization reaches even fewer people. Healthcare professionals who have extensive experience working in developing countries echo Voltaire's warning that "the great is the enemy of the good" and argue it is better to give a less-than-perfect regimen that reaches patients in need than to insist on a perfect regimen that reaches no one.[65]

Simple, inexpensive, and convenient HIV drug regimens — though less than perfect — still save lives.

The search for better and safer drugs continues, and the hope for an AIDS vaccine remains promising. But until a practical cure is found, healthcare practitioners must rely on multi-drug regimens surrounded by a robust healthcare infrastructure to prevent HIV transmission. Unfortunately, preventing the spread of HIV will remain a challenge until those drugs and services reach everyone who needs them. As long as AIDS persists, unchecked and unyielding, in the most remote corners of the world — where people have limited access to healthcare and their governments cannot afford the newest drugs — one drug remains the simplest, least expensive, and most convenient choice in the toolkit to prevent HIV transmission from mother to child. At the very least, and if nothing else, they have nevirapine.

Epilogue

For want of a nail the shoe was lost,
For want of a shoe the horse was lost,
For want of a horse the rider was lost,
For want of a rider the battle was lost,
For want of a battle the kingdom was lost,
And all for the want of a nail.
— English proverb

Some call it the butterfly effect: the notion that small actions can result in large consequences. Many scientific breakthroughs can be traced back to a seemingly trivial event that just happened to trigger other events, all of which aligned at a time and in a sequence that amplified their individual importance. In studying the facts and piecing together such events, one quickly realizes how remarkable, and unlikely, those scientific breakthroughs were. In a similar manner, the nevirapine duck's flight was buffeted and blown toward its final destination by a series of events, many of which were not anticipated or the result of conscious planning. If even one element in that chain of events had played out differently, nevirapine might not have happened at all.

When Catherine Wilfert took early retirement from Duke University, she could have steered her leisure activities in almost any direction. Her reputation as a pediatrician was secure, and she had already made major contributions to the treatment of pediatric AIDS and preventing HIV transmission to infants in the United States. Her immediate goals did not include extending her professional reach internationally.

If Elizabeth Glaser had received one less pint of blood in 1981, she might have led a long and healthy life. Undoubtedly, she would have expended her considerable energy devising educational programs to enrich the lives of children. She would have proudly watched her own children grow to adulthood, doted over her grandchildren, and engaged her wide circle of friends in tennis and a range of social activities.

If John Sullivan had been accepted for admission to the United States Air Force Academy, he likely would have served in Vietnam. From there, his uncertain path would have led, one way or another, to active research in virology and infectious diseases. But he probably would not have been working at the University of Massachusetts Medical Center, down the hall from Robert Eckner's laboratory, in 1986.

If Maureen Myers had chosen to accept the offer of a position at Roche, she would have guided that company's portfolio of AIDS drugs, including ddC and several first-generation HIV protease inhibitors. Roche would have benefited from her twenty-plus years at the National Institutes of Health, where she had established the framework for AIDS clinical trials and fostered strong professional relationships with the world's HIV/AIDS experts.

If Albert Boehringer had not decided to expand his company's market position in opiates, Karl Thomae would have remained an independent pharmaceutical firm, and the series of pirenzapine analogs would still be sitting on a dusty shelf in the Thomae archives.

If Alan Rosenthal had chosen to stay at Merck, he would have orchestrated the ongoing efforts to develop Merck's impressive roster of AIDS drugs, and the scientists at Boehringer Ingelheim would have continued their narrowly defined search for new allergy drugs.

Instead, Alan Rosenthal chose to move to Connecticut and head BI's research and development division, where he inspired expansion of the company's drug discovery efforts to include viral diseases — AIDS, in particular. The BI chemists then took pirenzepine off a dusty shelf and transformed it into nevirapine. John Sullivan did set up his laboratory in nearby Worcester, Massachusetts, where he confirmed the activity of nevirapine as an AIDS drug and relentlessly championed its use in pediatric clinical trials. Maureen Myers opted to move to BI instead of Roche and applied her accumulated knowledge of AIDS clinical trials and her network of the world's top HIV investigators to nevirapine. And Elizabeth Glaser's Pediatric AIDS Foundation leveraged nevirapine's value in preventing mother-to-child HIV transmission as a call to action, setting up thousands of prevention programs throughout the world, under Cathy Wilfert's able leadership. One nail hammered into a shoe that sustained the horse that bore its rider through many battles and saved a kingdom of children from AIDS.

In the twenty years between Alan Rosenthal's arrival at Boehringer Ingelheim and Hauwa's roundtrip to Jos and back to set up her tiny clinic, thousands of people contributed to nevirapine's development. Some came to BI specifically to work on the nevirapine project. Others volunteered their time in addition to their assigned duties. And some just assayed samples, dosed animals, or punched numbers into a computer database. A few were generals, others were work horses, some forged the horseshoes, and others hammered the nails. Whether their job was large or small, they were all guided by a moral compass, which they turned into a moral imperative — for the patients, young and old, who were waiting. For most of those researchers, the nevirapine experience was the highlight of their career.

After nevirapine's approval, Jay Merluzzi and, later, Maureen Myers left BI. For Merluzzi, nevirapine's successful development capped a distinguished research career that he felt he could not top. Along with his success, the all-consuming nevirapine project had deprived him of valuable time with his family, and he resolved to change that. At the age of 49, he retired and moved his family to his newly built home in Vermont. Myers held executive positions at Idenix (originally named Novirio) Pharmaceuticals and remained active in clinical drug development until her retirement in 2004.

Other key contributors to nevirapine's development also moved to new companies. In 1993, Rosenthal joined Abbott Laboratories where he guided research efforts including the development of ritonavir, an early HIV protease inhibitor that is still widely used as a booster of other protease inhibitors. After launching two start-up companies, he now serves on several corporate and scientific advisory boards and still enjoys fine wine, frozen yoghurt, and soft-shell crabs. In 1994, Julian Adams, who steered BI's chemistry efforts and collected the first evidence of nevirapine's ability to prevent HIV transmission, left BI to lead research and development efforts at Proscript, LeukoSite, and Millennium Pharmaceuticals. He is now president of research and development at Infinity Pharmaceuticals and serves on the boards of directors and scientific advisory boards of several other pharmaceutical firms. Jim Wright, who oversaw the nevirapine formulations and served the team in many other ways, left BI in 1994 to head drug development at Alkermes Pharmaceuticals. He is currently Chief Scientific Officer at BIND Biosciences.

Mark Labadia, the first scientist to observe the HIV activity of BI's compounds, completed his Ph.D. in immunology in 1994 and returned to BI, where he now heads his own research laboratory. Other members of the nevirapine project team remained at BI to work on other drug development projects. Chemists Karl Hargrave and Karl Grozinger retired from BI after 31 and 41 years of service, respectively.

John Sullivan and Doug Richman, the investigators who led both the early laboratory and clinical testing of nevirapine, continued to make significant contributions in HIV/AIDS research at the University of Massachusetts and the University of California, San Diego, and their protégés followed in their footsteps. Katherine Luzuriaga is now Director of the University of Massachusetts Center for Clinical and Translational Science. As Associate Provost of Global Health at the University of Massachusetts Medical School, she works to translate advances in HIV prevention and treatment to limited-resource settings, where most pediatric infections now occur. Diane Havlir became chief of the HIV/AIDS division and Positive Health Program at San Francisco General Hospital, is professor of medicine at the University of California, San Francisco, and is spearheading research in East Africa to evaluate whether universal HIV testing and antiretroviral therapy offered to all infected individuals can "break the back" of the epidemic. Havlir co-chaired the 19th International AIDS Conference, in Washington, DC, in 2012, the first time that the conference had been held in the United States since the travel ban on HIV-infected individuals was lifted by President Obama.

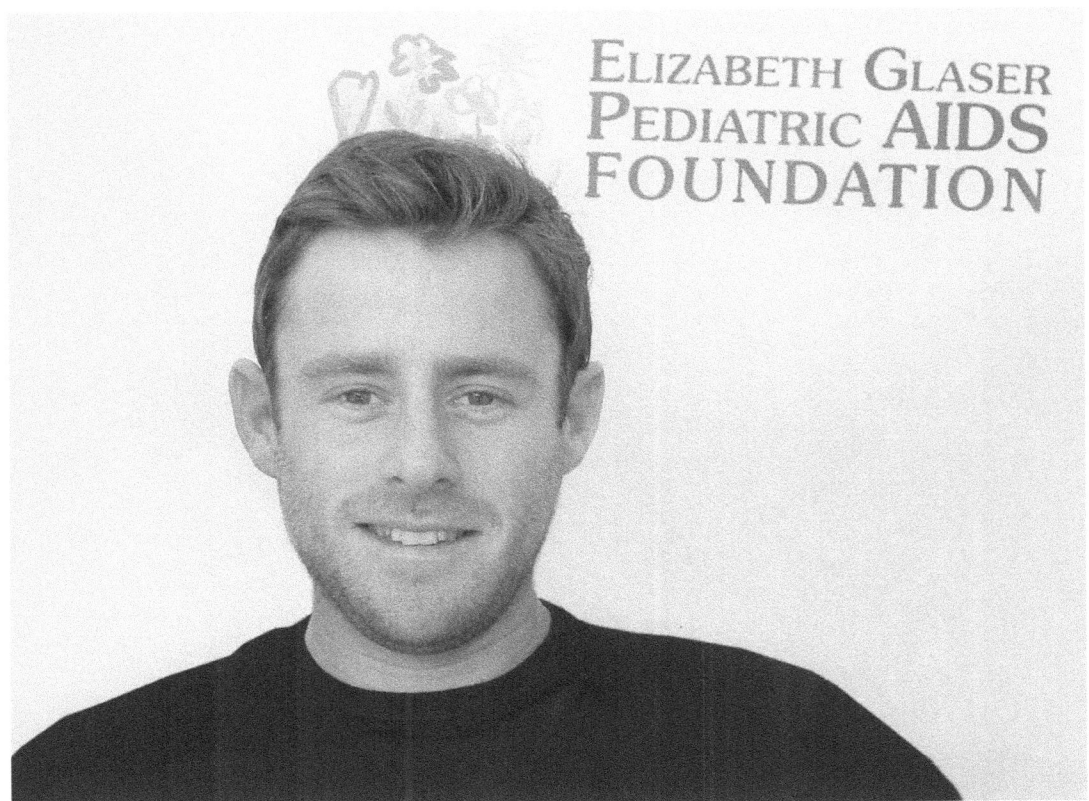

Jake Glaser (courtesy Elizabeth Glaser Pediatric AIDS Foundation).

Joep Lange (the Netherlands), David Cooper (Australia), Stefano Vella (Italy), and Julio Montaner (Canada), the lead investigators on nevirapine's international clinical trials, also continued to be influential leaders in HIV/AIDS research. Each of them has been active in the International AIDS Society, the sponsoring organization of the International AIDS Conferences, and has served a term as the Society's president.

ACT UP, Treatment Action Campaign, Project Inform, and many other organizations continue their mission, advocating medical research, treatment, and social services for people living with HIV. As a result of their efforts, new drugs for life-threatening diseases are now developed with input from patients and patient advocates, and those drugs are now approved more quickly. Bill Snow transitioned from his work at ACT UP to champion AIDS vaccines. He has served on numerous private and government advisory boards that oversee HIV vaccine research and currently is Director of the Global HIV Vaccine Enterprise's Secretariat.

Zackie Achmat, a co-founder of the Treatment Action Campaign, continues to be a strong voice advocating for the legal rights of disadvantaged South Africans. He currently serves as co-director of Ndifuna Ukawzi, an organization devoted to building and supporting social justice organizations and leaders in South Africa. Edwin Cameron was appointed a justice on South Africa's Constitutional Court (the country's highest court) in 2009 and continues to make scholarly contributions to the understanding of gay issues. He remains the only senior government official in South Africa to publicly state his HIV status.

Jeanne White continued to champion healthcare services for HIV-infected people after her son's death. The Ryan White Care Act has been reauthorized every few years since 1990 and is now the largest federally funded program to assist people living with HIV/AIDS in the United States.

Jamie Gentille (courtesy Elizabeth Glaser Pediatric AIDS Foundation).

Jake Glaser and Jamie Gentille are now healthy and thriving adults. Jake supports and is an occasional blogger for his mother's foundation. Jamie continued taking research medications and was lucky that most of them were very successful. She was instrumental in lobbying efforts that led to creating a longitudinal study at the National Institutes of Health to medically monitor adults, like herself, who had participated in pediatric AIDS clinical trials.

For a while, scientists at BI continued HIV research but never found a drug superior to nevirapine. Their research efforts then shifted to develop drugs to treat hepatitis C viral infections. In 2012, Boehringer Ingelheim announced that it was closing its virology research laboratories. Although the company remains committed to improving access to medicines and healthcare in developing countries, including for the treatment of HIV/AIDS, BI's senior executives realized that medical innovation to treat viruses is now focused on prevention through vaccines, a field in which BI is not active.

The ugly lucky duck that served as the BI project team's unofficial mascot still sits on a shelf in Pam Strode's office.

Chapter Notes

Introduction

1. By permission of Global Strategies for HIV Prevention.
2. *Faith Alive Foundation Annual Report*, 2006.
3. Global Strategies for HIV Prevention, "Pennies from heaven," *Global Strategies for HIV Prevention Newsletter*, December 2004.
4. Ryan White and Ann Marie Cunningham, *Ryan White: My own story* (New York: Signet, 1992), 5–6.
5. White and Cunningham, *My own story*, 18.
6. White and Cunningham, *My own story*, 22–23.
7. White and Cunningham, *My own story*, 48–49.
8. White and Cunningham, *My own story*, 50.
9. James R. Stringer et al., "A new name (*Pneumocystis jiroveci*) for Pneumocystis from humans," *Emerging Infectious Diseases* 8 (2002): 891–896. The pneumonia seen in early AIDS patients was commonly attributed to *Pneumocystis carinii*, which is actually found only in rats. In 2002, the causative organism of pneumonia in immune-suppressed patients was renamed *Pneumocystis jiroveci*, with a recommendation that the widely used acronym, PCP, be retained and refer to the opportunistic infection, *Pneumocystis p*neumonia, without specifying the responsible species.
10. White and Cunningham, *My own story*, 52.
11. White and Cunningham, *My own story*, 127–128.
12. White and Cunningham, *My own story*, 72–73.
13. White and Cunningham, *My own story*, 81–82.
14. White and Cunningham, *My own story*, 102.
15. White and Cunningham, *My own story*, 189.
16. White and Cunningham, *My own story*, 224.
17. White and Cunningham, *My own story*, 244.
18. White and Cunningham, *My own story*, 245–247.
19. White and Cunningham, *My own story*, 252.
20. White and Cunningham, *My own story*, 261.
21. Andrew Orkin, "Sixth international AIDS conference featured some notable absentees," *Canadian Medical Association Journal* 143 (1990): 407–410; Elizabeth Glaser and Laura Palmer, *In the absence of angels: A Hollywood family's courageous story* (New York: Putnam, 1991), 292.
22. John S. James, "San Francisco AIDS Conference, related events: Issues and update," *AIDS Treatment News*, May 4, 1990; Rex Wockner, "AIDS conference closes in chaos," *Outweek*, July 11, 1990. The travel ban that barred anyone with HIV infection from entering the United States was finally lifted in 2009 by President Barack Obama.
23. John Lauritsen, "They left their HIV in San Francisco: A report on the sixth International Conference on AIDS," *New York Native*, June 24, 1990.
24. Associated Press, "Officials fear hemophiliac will spread disease: School in Indiana bars boy with AIDS," *Los Angeles Times*, July 31, 1985.
25. William H. Danforth et al., *The AIDS research program of the National Institutes of Health* (Washington, DC: National Academy Press, 1991), 24–25.
26. John Sullivan, interview, December 6, 2011.
27. Danforth et al., *AIDS research program*, 25.
28. Samuel Grubman and James Oleske, "Primary care for the HIV-infected child," *PAACNOTES* (January 1993); Philip A. Pizzo, quoted in FDA Antiviral Drugs Advisory Committee meeting, July 18, 1991, 119.
29. White and Cunningham, *My own story*, 219.
30. Ellen Cooper et al., "Development of new drugs for the treatment of pediatric AIDS: Scientific and regulatory issues," in *Pediatric AIDS: Challenge of HIV infection in infants, children and adolescents*, eds. Philip A. Pizzo and Catherine M. Wilfert (Baltimore: Williams and Wilkins, 1991), 605–618.
31. Jean L. Marx, "Drug-resistant strains of AIDS virus found," *Science* 243 (1989): 1551–1552.
32. Marcus Conant, "Sixth International Conference overview from Marcus Conant," *AIDS Treatment News*, July 6, 1990.
33. White and Cunningham, *My own story*, 274.
34. Mark Harrington, interview, April 4, 2012.
35. Ellen Cooper, interview, December 20, 2011.
36. Ellen Cooper, interviews, December 20, 2011 and March 7, 2013.
37. Ellen Cooper, interview, December 20, 2011.
38. Gina Kolata, "Citing stress, FDA aide wants out," *New York Times*, December 22, 1990; David A. Kessler, *A question of intent: A great American battle with a deadly industry* (New York: PublicAffairs, 2001), 38–39.
39. The Antiviral Drug Products Division reviewed Investigational New Drug applications from sponsors seeking permission to test new drugs in humans and to review New Drug Applications from sponsors of drugs with completed clinical trials, seeking marketing approval.
40. Glaser and Palmer, *Absence of angels*, 221.
41. White and Cunningham, *My own story*, 174.
42. Glaser and Palmer, *Absence of angels*, 221.
43. Ellen Cooper, interview, December 20, 2011.

Chapter 1

1. Elizabeth Glaser and Laura Palmer, *In the absence of angels: A Hollywood family's courageous story* (New York: Putnam, 1991), 36.
2. Glaser and Palmer, *Absence of angels*, 38.
3. Glaser and Palmer, *Absence of angels*, 39.
4. Glaser and Palmer, *Absence of angels*, 33.
5. Glaser and Palmer, *Absence of angels*, 40.
6. Glaser and Palmer, *Absence of angels*, 44.
7. Glaser and Palmer, *Absence of angels*, 44–45.
8. Glaser and Palmer, *Absence of angels*, 48, 85.

9. Glaser and Palmer, *Absence of angels*, 48, 51.
10. Margaret A. Fischl et al., "The efficacy of azidothymidine (AZT) in the treatment of patients with AIDS and AIDS-related complex," *New England Journal of Medicine* 317 (1987): 185–191.
11. Jessica Roseberry, Catherine Wilfert interview, *Women in Duke medicine: An oral history exhibit*, August 25, 2006.
12. Ross E. McKinney Jr., "Dr. Catherine Wilfert's indomitable will," in *Duke magic: A history*, June 2009.
13. Frank M. Balis et al., "Pharmacokinetics of zidovudine administered intravenously and orally in children with human immunodeficiency virus infection," *Journal of Pediatrics* 114 (1989): 880–884; Ross E. McKinney Jr. et al., "Safety and tolerance of intermittent intravenous and oral zidovudine therapy in human immunodeficient virus-infected pediatric patients," *Journal of Pediatrics* 116 (1990): 640–647.
14. Glaser and Palmer, *Absence of angels*, 80, 85.
15. Glaser and Palmer, *Absence of angels*, 87–88.
16. Glaser and Palmer, *Absence of angels*, 89.
17. Glaser and Palmer, *Absence of angels*, 92.
18. Glaser and Palmer, *Absence of angels*, 98–101.
19. Glaser and Palmer, *Absence of angels*, 101. A broviac catheter was implanted for administration of Total Parenteral Nutrition (TPN).
20. Glaser and Palmer, *Absence of angels*, 101–107.
21. Glaser and Palmer, *Absence of angels*, 109. Lasix was administered as the diuretic.
22. Glaser and Palmer, *Absence of angels*, 110.
23. Glaser and Palmer, *Absence of angels*, 121.
24. Glaser and Palmer, *Absence of angels*, 113.
25. Glaser and Palmer, *Absence of angels*, 135.
26. Glaser and Palmer, *Absence of angels*, 137–138.
27. *Elizabeth Glaser Pediatric AIDS Foundation Annual Report*, 1999; Susan DeLaurentis, interview, May 14, 2013. This painting now serves as the logo of the Elizabeth Glaser Pediatric AIDS Foundation.
28. Glaser and Palmer, *Absence of angels*, 130–131.
29. Glaser and Palmer, *Absence of angels*, 139.
30. Glaser and Palmer, *Absence of angels*, 155–156.
31. Glaser and Palmer, *Absence of angels*, 157. GM-CSF is granulocyte macrophage colony stimulating factor.
32. Jake Glaser, "What I want you to know about AIDS," *Glamour Magazine*, May 2011.
33. Glaser and Palmer, *Absence of angels*, 158–159.
34. Joep Lange, interview, February 28, 2012.
35. Vincent Merluzzi, interview, July 5, 2011.
36. Vincent Merluzzi, interview, July 5, 2011.
37. Mark Labadia, interview, August 5, 2011.
38. Julian Adams and Vincent J. Merluzzi, "Discovery of nevirapine, a nonnucleoside inhibitor of HIV-1 reverse transcriptase," in *The search for antiviral drugs: Case histories from concept to clinic*, eds. Julian Adams and Vincent J. Merluzzi (Boston, Birkhäuser, 1993), 45–70; Mark Labadia, interview, August 5, 2011.
39. The genetic material in retroviruses is RNA, rather than DNA. In order to reproduce, the virus must first produce DNA from its RNA genome (a process called reverse transcription, which is facilitated by the enzyme, reverse transcriptase). The newly formed DNA is then incorporated into the host's genome (human cells, in the case of HIV), and the virus replicates using the host cell's DNA.
40. Vincent Merluzzi, interview, December 9, 2011.
41. Robert Eckner, interview, July 18, 2011.
42. Robert Eckner, interview, July 18, 2011.
43. Adams and Merluzzi, "Discovery of nevirapine," 45–70.
44. Karl Hargrave, interview, August 11, 2011.

45. Adams and Merluzzi, "Discovery of nevirapine"; Karl Hargrave, interview, August 11, 2011.
46. Ronald Swanstrom, letter to Robert Eckner, March 8, 1988; Robert Eckner, interview, July 18, 2011. Swanstrom's clones expressed HIV reverse transcriptase from *E. coli*. The RT product was an auto-cleaved product from the full length pol precursor polyprotein.
47. Adams and Merluzzi, "Discovery of nevirapine."
48. Robert Eckner, interview, July 18, 2011; John Sullivan, interview, December 6, 2011.
49. John Sullivan, interview, February 16, 2012.
50. John Sullivan, interview, December 6, 2011.
51. Adams and Merluzzi, "Discovery of nevirapine."
52. Adams and Merluzzi, "Discovery of nevirapine."
53. Robert Eckner, interview, July 18, 2011; Mark Labadia, interview, August 5, 2011.
54. Mark Labadia, interview, August 5, 2011.
55. Adams and Merluzzi, "Discovery of nevirapine."
56. Adams and Merluzzi, "Discovery of nevirapine." Mark Labadia repeated the assay and then produced a dose-response curve to obtain an IC50 of 6 μM.
57. Mark Labadia, interview, January 6, 2012. The compound was UD-PM 0147BS, which was chemically related to pirenzepine.
58. Robert Eckner, interview, July 18, 2011.
59. Mark Labadia, interview, January 6, 2012.
60. Karl Hargrave, interview, August 11, 2011.
61. Robert Eckner, interview, July 18, 2011; Mark Labadia, interview, August 5, 2011.
62. Robert Eckner, interview, July 18, 2011; Mark Labadia, interview, January 6, 2012.

Chapter 2

1. Julian Adams and Vincent J. Merluzzi, "Discovery of nevirapine, a nonnucleoside inhibitor of HIV-1 reverse transcriptase," in *The search for antiviral drugs: Case histories from concept to clinic*, eds. Julian Adams and Vincent J. Merluzzi (Boston, Birkhäuser, 1993), 45–70; Karl Grozinger et al., "Discovery and development of nevirapine," in *Drug Discovery and Development*, ed. Mukund S. Chorghade, (Hoboken, NJ: Wiley, 2006), 353–363.
2. Adams and Merluzzi, "Discovery of nevirapine."
3. James Keirns, interview, September 19, 2011.
4. Karl Hargrave, interview, August 11, 2011; Karl Grozinger, interview, October 12, 2011.
5. Julian Adams, interview, December 9, 2011.
6. Margaret I. Johnston and Daniel F. Hoth, "Present status and future prospects for HIV therapies," *Science* 260 (1993): 1286–1293.
7. Johnston and Hoth, "Prospects for HIV therapies."
8. Adams and Merluzzi, "Discovery of nevirapine."
9. Julian Adams, interview, December 9, 2011.
10. Karl Hargrave, interview, August 11, 2011.
11. Karl Hargrave, interview, August 11, 2011.
12. Adams and Merluzzi, "Discovery of nevirapine."
13. Robert Eckner, interview, July 18, 2011.
14. Robert Eckner, interview, July 18, 2011; Mark Labadia, interview, August 5, 2011.
15. Mark Labadia, interview, August 5, 2011.
16. Adams and Merluzzi, "Discovery of nevirapine."
17. Vincent Merluzzi, interview, July 5, 2011.
18. Vincent Merluzzi, interview, July 5, 2011.
19. Vincent Merluzzi, interview, December 15, 2011.
20. Karl Grozinger, interview, October 12, 2011.
21. Adams and Merluzzi, "Discovery of nevirapine."
22. Karl Hargrave, interview, August 11, 2011.
23. Karl Hargrave, interview, August 11, 2011.

24. Vincent Merluzzi, interview, July 5, 2011.
25. Vincent Merluzzi, interview, July 5, 2011.
26. Adams and Merluzzi, "Discovery of nevirapine."
27. Vincent Merluzzi, interview, July 5, 2011.
28. Adams and Merluzzi, "Discovery of nevirapine." The L-S 1170 characterization included its solubility, metabolism, virus specificity, toxicity, pharmacology, and preliminary formulation/stability.
29. Karl Grozinger, interview, October 12, 2011.
30. Robert Eckner, interview, July 18, 2011.
31. Julian Adams, interview, December 9, 2011.
32. Karl Hargrave, interview, August 11, 2011; Julian Adams, interview, December 9, 2011.
33. Julian Adams, interview, December 9, 2011.
34. Julian Adams, interview, December 9, 2011; Karl Hargrave, interview, August 11, 2011.
35. Karl Hargrave, interview, August 11, 2011.
36. Karl D. Hargrave et al., "5,11-dihydro-6H-dipyrido(3,2-B:2',3'-E)(1,4)diazepines and their use in the prevention or treatment of HIV infection," United States Patent 5,366,972, issued November 22, 1994.
37. Mark Labadia, interview, August 5, 2011.
38. Brendan A. Larder et al., "HIV with reduced sensitivity to zidovudine (AZT) isolated during prolonged therapy," *Science* 243 (1989): 1731–1734.
39. Robert Eckner, interview, July 18, 2011.
40. Douglas Richman, interview, December 8, 2011.
41. Robert Eckner, interview, July 18, 2011. Richman used a plaque reduction assay to screen the compounds.
42. Douglas D. Richman et al., "Human immunodeficiency virus type 1 mutants resistant to nonnucleoside inhibitors of reverse transcriptase arise in tissue culture," *Proceedings of the National Academy of Sciences* 88 (1991): 11241–11245; Douglas D. Richman et al., "BI-RG-587 is active against zidovudine-resistant human immunodeficiency virus type 1 and synergistic with zidovudine," *Antimicrobial Agents and Chemotherapy* 35 (1991): 305–308.
43. Cheng-Kon Shih et al., "Chimeric human immunodeficiency virus type 1/type 2 reverse transcriptases display reversed sensitivity to non-nucleoside analog inhibitors," *Proceedings of the National Academy of Sciences* 88 (1991): 9878–9882.
44. Mark Labadia, interview, January 6, 2012.

Chapter 3

1. Elizabeth Glaser and Laura Palmer, *In the absence of angels: A Hollywood family's courageous story* (New York: Putnam, 1991), 8.
2. Glaser and Palmer, *Absence of angels*, 9–10.
3. Michael S. Gottlieb et al., "Pneumocystis Pneumonia — Los Angeles," *Morbidity and Mortality Weekly Report* 30 (1981): 1–3.
4. Glaser and Palmer, *Absence of angels*, 55.
5. Glaser and Palmer, *Absence of angels*, 69–70.
6. Glaser and Palmer, *Absence of angels*, 69–70.
7. "A failure led to drug against AIDS," *New York Times*, September 19, 1986; "Jerome P. Horwitz: AZT, the anticancer drug he developed 22 years ago, is now our best hope in the battle against AIDS," *People Magazine*, December 22, 1986; Kathryn Pattishall, "Discovery and development of zidovudine as the cornerstone of therapy to control human immunodeficiency virus infection," in *The search for antiviral drugs: Case histories from concept to clinic*, eds. Julian Adams and Vincent J. Merluzzi, 23–43 (Boston: Birkhäuser, 1993).
8. AZT, or azidothymidine, is a nucleoside analog of thymidine and ddC, or dideoxycytidine, is a nucleoside analog of cytidine.
9. Jerome P. Horwitz, quoted in "AZT, the anticancer drug," *People Magazine*, December 22, 1986.
10. Jerome P. Horwitz et al., "The monomesylates of 1-(2'-Deoxy-β-D-lysofuranosyl) thymine," *Journal of Organic Chemistry* 29 (1964): 2076–2078.
11. Pattishall, "Discovery of zidovudine."
12. Burroughs Wellcome used a plaque reduction assay, infecting FG-10 cells with the murine retroviruses, Friend leukemia virus and Harvey sarcoma virus.
13. Pattishall, "Discovery of zidovudine."
14. Pattishall, "Discovery of zidovudine"; "Failure led to AIDS," *New York Times*.
15. Pattishall, "Discovery of zidovudine."
16. Brendan A. Larder et al., "HIV with reduced sensitivity to zidovudine (AZT) isolated during prolonged therapy," *Science* 243 (1989): 1731–1734.
17. ddI, or dideoxyinosine, is a nucleoside analog of guanosine.
18. FDA Antiviral Drugs Advisory Committee meeting, July 18, 1991, 20.
19. "Drugs for HIV infection," *Medical Letter* 31 (1990): 11–13.
20. "Drugs for HIV infection," *Medical Letter*.
21. Gina Kolata, "Citing stress, FDA aide wants out," *New York Times*, December 22, 1990; ACT UP, "Treatment Agenda, 1990: VI International AIDS Conference," June 1990; FDA Antiviral Drugs Advisory Committee meeting, July 18, 1991, 18. A treatment IND for ddI was approved in September 1989 and the expanded access program began in October 1989.
22. "Drugs for HIV infection, *Medical Letter*."
23. Julian Adams and Vincent J. Merluzzi, "Discovery of nevirapine, a nonnucleoside inhibitor of HIV-1 reverse transcriptase," in *The search for antiviral drugs: Case histories from concept to clinic*, eds. Julian Adams and Vincent J. Merluzzi (Birkhäuser, 1993), 45–70; Karl Grozinger et al., "Discovery and development of nevirapine," in *Drug Discovery and Development*, ed. Mukund S. Chorghade (Hoboken, NJ: Wiley, 2006), 353–263. The selection criteria included acceptable potency, metabolism, solubility, pharmacokinetics, synthesis, and pharmacology.
24. Adams and Merluzzi, "Discovery of nevirapine."
25. James Keirns, interview, September 9, 2011.
26. Karl Hargrave, interview, August 11, 2011.
27. Karl Hargrave, interview, August 11, 2011.
28. In mid-1989, the HIV assay was transferred to Eckner's laboratory, where Janice Rose assumed responsibility for testing BIRH-414, BIRG-587, and other analogs in the series.
29. Adams and Merluzzi, "Discovery of nevirapine."
30. Adams and Merluzzi, "Discovery of nevirapine."
31. Adams and Merluzzi, "Discovery of nevirapine."
32. Karl Grozinger, interview, October 12, 2011.
33. Karl Hargrave, interview, August 11, 2011.
34. Karl D. Hargrave et al., "5,11-dihydro-6H-dipyrido(3,2-B:2',3'-E)(1,4)diazepines and their use in the prevention or treatment of HIV infection," United States patent 5,366,972, issued November 22, 1994.
35. John Tiso, interview, December 1, 2011; Julian Adams, interview, December 9, 2011.
36. Julian Adams, interview, December 9, 2011.
37. Hargrave et al., U.S. Patent No. 5,366,972.
38. Hargrave et al., U.S. Patent No. 5,366,972. The other co-inventors were Gunther Schmidt, Wolfhard Engel, Gunther Trummlitz, and Wolfgang Eberlein.
39. Adams and Merluzzi, "Discovery of nevirapine."
40. Vincent Merluzzi, interview, July 5, 2011.

41. Adams and Merluzzi, "Discovery of nevirapine" ; Grozinger et al., "Development of nevirapine."
42. Tommy Cheng, Yale University, provided several cellular DNA pol assays to test the selectivity of the BI compounds.
43. Vincent Merluzzi, interview, July 5, 2011.
44. Adams and Merluzzi, "Discovery of nevirapine," 45–70; Grozinger et al., "Development of nevirapine," 353–363; NDA 20-636 Pharmacologist's Review (1996): 73–74.
45. Joann S. Lublin, "Scientists report discovering compounds that could lead to powerful AIDS drug," *Wall Street Journal*, February 1, 1990; Rudi Pauweis et al., "Potent and selective inhibition of HIV-1 replication in vitro by a novel series of TIBO derivatives," *Nature* 343 (1990): 470–474.
46. The active series of BI compounds are dipyridodiazepinones.
47. Pauweis et al., "TIBO derivatives."
48. Ron Dagani, "New anti–HIV-1 agents most potent ever," *Chemical & Engineering News*, February 5, 1990.
49. Alfons Raeymaekers et al., "Preparation and formulation of antiviral tetrahydroimidazo (1,4) benzodiazepine-2-ones," European Patent 336466, A1, issued October 11, 1989.
50. Adams and Merluzzi, "Discovery of nevirapine"; Grozinger et al., "Development of nevirapine."
51. James Keirns, interview, September 19, 2011.
52. Mark Labadia, interview, August 5, 2011.

Chapter 4

1. James Wright, interview, October 20, 2011.
2. James Wright, interview, October, 20, 2011.
3. Vincent Merluzzi, email, March 5, 2013.
4. Vincent Merluzzi, interview, July 5, 2011.
5. James Wright, interview, October 20, 2011.
6. James Wright, interview, October 20, 2011.
7. James Wright, interview, October 20, 2011. This formulation also was quite similar to the final tablets produced commercially.
8. Vincent Merluzzi, interview, March 5, 2013.
9. James Wright, interview, October 20, 2011.
10. Vincent Merluzzi, interview, July 5, 2011.
11. Vincent Merluzzi, interview, July 5, 2011.
12. Laura Andrews, interview, October 12–13, 2011.
13. Vincent Merluzzi, interview, July 5, 2011.
14. Laura Andrews, interview, October 12–13, 2011.
15. Laura Andrews, interview, October 12–13, 2011. Conducted at Bio-Research Laboratories in Montreal.
16. Laura Andrews, interview, October 12–13, 2011.
17. Karl Grozinger, interview, October 12, 2011.
18. Karl Grozinger, interview, October 12, 2011.
19. Karl Grozinger, interview, October 12, 2011.
20. James Wright, interview, October 20, 2011.
21. William H. Danforth et al., *The AIDS research program of the National Institutes of Health*, (Washington, DC: National Academy Press, (1991), 21.
22. Danforth et al., *AIDS research program*, 22.
23. James Hill, interview by Victoria A. Harden, October 4, 1988, *In their own words*, NIH Historical Office; Maureen Myers, email, May 11, 2012.
24. Maureen Myers, interview, November 17, 2011.
25. Maureen Myers, email, May 11, 2012.
26. Maureen Myers, interview, March 19, 2012.
27. Maureen Myers, interview, March 19, 2012.
28. Maureen Myers, email, May 11, 2012.
29. Martin Hirsch, interview, February 3, 2012.
30. Maureen Myers, interview, March 19, 2012.

31. Martin Hirsch, interview, February 3, 2012.
32. James Hill, interview by Victoria A. Harden, October 4, 1988, *In their own words*, NIH Historical Office; Greg Folkers, "NIAID funds adult AIDS clinical trials group," NIAID news release, November 30, 1995.
33. Folkers, "NIAID funds clinical trials."
34. Vincent Merluzzi, interview, July 5, 2011.
35. The group was the AIDS Clinical Drug Development Committee, the ACTG's steering committee.
36. Vincent Merluzzi, interview, July 5, 2011.
37. C. Everett Koop, "Foreword," in *Pediatric AIDS: Challenge of HIV infection in infants, children and adolescents*, eds. Philip A. Pizzo and Catherin M. Wilfert (Baltimore: Williams and Wilkins, 1991), vii.
38. UNAIDS, "Report on the global AIDS epidemic 2008," WHO Library.
39. Elizabeth Glaser and Laura Palmer, *In the absence of angels: A Hollywood family's courageous story* (New York: Putnam, 1991), 115.
40. Elizabeth Glaser quoted in Glaser and Palmer, *Absence of angels*, 115.
41. Glaser and Palmer, *Absence of angels*, 173, 198.
42. Glaser and Palmer, *Absence of angels*, 199.
43. Glaser and Palmer, *Absence of angels*, 199.
44. Glaser and Palmer, *Absence of angels*, 152, 198.
45. Glaser and Palmer, *Absence of angels*, 228.
46. Glaser and Palmer, *Absence of angels*, 221.
47. Glaser and Palmer, *Absence of angels*, 217.
48. Glaser and Palmer, *Absence of angels*, 221.
49. FDA, "Points to consider in preparation of IND applications for new drugs intended for the treatment of HIV-infected individuals," February 1990.
50. Vincent Merluzzi, interview, July 5, 2011; Kathryn Jason, interview, October 3, 2011.
51. Ellen Cooper, interview, March 7, 2013.
52. Ellen Cooper, interview, December 20, 2011.
53. Vincent Merluzzi, interview, July 5, 2011.
54. James Keirns, interview, September 19, 2011.
55. Vincent Merluzzi, interview, July 5, 2011.
56. In addition to Jane Kinsel and Carla Pettinelli from NIH and John Sullivan from UMass, the BI contingent consisted of Kathryn Jason, Jack Weet, Jay Merluzzi, James Keirns, Laura Andrews, Ross Rocklin, Peggy McLaughlin, Julian Adams, John Tiso, and Alan Rosenthal. The FDA reviewers present were Ellen Cooper, Eileen Leonard, Larry Rosenstein, Chi-Wan Chen, Manfred Ruthsatz, Jim Ramsey, Mike Ussery, Cynthia Cunard, and Toni Anthony.
57. Ellen Cooper, interview, December 20, 2011.
58. Vincent Merluzzi, interview, July 5, 2011; James Keirns interview, September 19, 2011; Laura Andrews, interview, October 3, 2011.
59. Julian Adams, interview, December 9, 2011.
60. Ellen Cooper et al., "Development of new drugs for the treatment of pediatric AIDS: Scientific and regulatory issues," in *Pediatric AIDS: Challenge of HIV infection in infants, children and adolescents*, eds. Philip A. Pizzo and Catherine M. Wilfert (Baltimore: Williams and Wilkins, 1991), 605–618.
61. Ellen Cooper, interview, December 20, 2011.
62. Philip A. Pizzo and Catherine M. Wilfert, "Treatment considerations for children with HIV infection," in *Pediatric AIDS: Challenge of HIV infection in infants, children and adolescents*, eds. Philip A. Pizzo and Catherine M. Wilfert (Baltimore: Williams and Wilkins, 1991), 487–488; David Kessler, interview, December 12, 2011.
63. Laura Andrews, interview, October 12–13, 2011.
64. ACT UP, "Treatment Agenda."
65. ACT UP, "Treatment Agenda."

Chapter 5

1. Digby Barrios, quoted by Judee Schuler, "Executive Profile: Digby Barrios," *Pharmaceutical Executive*, June 1985.
2. Elizabeth Glaser and Laura Palmer, *In the absence of angels: A Hollywood family's courageous story* (New York: Putnam, 1991), 59–61; Doug Nelson, personal communication.
3. Janet Huck, "Breaking a silence: Starsky star, wife share their family's painful battle against AIDS," *Los Angeles Times*, August 25, 1989.
4. Glaser and Palmer, *Absence of angels*, 290, 292.
5. Glaser and Palmer, *Absence of angels*, 301.
6. Glaser and Palmer, *Absence of angels*, 302.
7. David Feigal, interview, May 24, 2012.
8. David Feigal, interview, May 24, 2012.
9. David Feigal, interview, May 24, 2012.
10. David Feigal, interview, May 24, 2012.
11. Terri Pascarelli, interview, December 19, 2011.
12. Terri Pascarelli, interview, December 19, 2011.
13. Julian Adams, interview, December 9, 2011.
14. Julian Adams, interview, December 9, 2011.
15. Gina Kolata, "Medical data: who should hear it first?" *New York Times*, May 22, 1990.
16. Vincent Merluzzi, interview, July 5, 2011.
17. Vincent Merluzzi, interview, July 5, 2011.
18. The Pharmaceutical Research and Manufacturers of America (PhRMA.org) estimates that one new drug is approved for every 250 that enter preclinical development.
19. Vincent Merluzzi, interview, July 5, 2011; Julian Adams, interview, December 9, 2011.
20. John Sullivan, interview, December 6, 2011.
21. Julian Adams, interview, December 9, 2011; Kathryn Pattishall, "Discovery and development of zidovudine as the cornerstone of therapy to control human immunodeficiency virus infection," in *The search for antiviral drugs: Case histories from concept to clinic*, eds. Julian Adams and Vincent J. Merluzzi (Boston: Birkhäuser, 1993), 23–43.
22. Vincent Merluzzi, interview, July 5, 2011.
23. Paul P. Heldman, "AIDS drug called promising," *Worcester Telegram & Gazette*, October 23, 1990.
24. Meg Angus-Smith, "Boehringer develops new AIDS drug," *Danbury News-Times*, October 25, 1990; Meg Angus-Smith, "Boehringer optimistic about new AIDS drug," *Danbury News-Times*, October 28, 1990.
25. Terri Pascarelli, interview, December 19, 2011.
26. Vincent J. Merluzzi et al., "Inhibition of HIV-1 replication by a nonnucleoside reverse transcriptase inhibitor," *Science* 250 (1990): 1411–1413.
27. The other authors were Mark Labadia, Mark Skoog, Joe Wu, C-K Shih, Susan Hattox, and Ron Faanes.
28. "This week in science: Novel HIV-1 inhibitor," *Science* 250 (1990): 1315.
29. Paul Recer, "New compound blocks AIDS spread in test tube experiments, study says," Associated Press, December 6, 1990; Rebecca Kolberg, "New AIDS drug may be less toxic, reach brain," United Press International, December 6, 1990.
30. Vincent Merluzzi, interview, July 5, 2011.
31. Vincent Merluzzi, interview, July 5, 2011.
32. Vincent Merluzzi, interview, July 5, 2011.
33. Michael Waldholz, "Merck develops drug to combat virus causing AIDS: Human tests begun," *Wall Street Journal*, December 21, 1990.

Chapter 6

1. James Keirns, interview, September 19, 2011.
2. James Wright, interview, October 20, 2011.
3. Julian Adams, interview, December 9, 2011.
4. Julian Adams, interview, December 9, 2011.
5. John Sullivan, interview, December 6, 2011; Douglas Richman, interview, December 8, 2011.
6. John Sullivan, interview, December 6, 2011
7. John Sullivan, interview, December 6, 2011
8. Douglas D. Richman et al., "BI-RG-587 is active against zidovudine-resistant human immunodeficiency virus type 1 and synergistic with zidovudine," *Antimicrobial Agents and Chemotherapy* 35 (1991): 305–308.
9. James Keirns, interview, September 19, 2011.
10. FDA, "Points to consider in the preparation of IND applications for new drugs intended for the treatment of HIV-infected individuals," February 1990.
11. NDA 20-636 Pharmacologist's Review (1996) 73, 76.
12. The first and second branches of the Christmas tree trial became studies BI 744 (ACTG 164) and BI 834 (ACTG 168), respectively.
13. Kathryn Jason, interview, October 3, 2011.
14. Douglas Richman, interview, December 8, 2011.
15. Martin Delaney, Project Inform, comments at ACTG Core Committee, November 14, 1990.
16. Laura Andrews, interview, October 12–13, 2011.
17. Laura Andrews, interview, October 12–13, 2011.
18. Vincent Merluzzi, interview, July 5, 2011.
19. IND No. 36,026.
20. Gina Kolata, "Citing stress, FDA aide wants out," *New York Times*, December 22, 1990.
21. Michael L. Millenson, "Cancer institute: AIDS drug unduly delayed," *Chicago Tribune*, January 5, 1989.
22. David Kessler, *A question of intent: A great American battle with a deadly industry* (New York: PublicAffairs, 2001), 38–39; Kolata, "FDA aide wants out"; Ellen Cooper, interview, December 20, 2011.
23. Vincent Merluzzi, interview, July 5, 2011.
24. Vincent Merluzzi, interview, July 5, 2011.
25. John Tiso, interview, November 8, 2011.
26. John Tiso, interview, November 8, 2011.
27. CDC, "HIV/AIDS Surveillance Report," January 1991.
28. ACT UP New York (Treatment and Data Committee) issued a treatment agenda for 1990 in conjunction with the 6th International Conference on AIDS in San Francisco, June 1990.
29. Kathryn Jason, interview, October 3, 2011.

Chapter 7

1. Phil is a fictitious name to protect the patient's identity, but he represents a documented clinical case.
2. This profile is a composite of the patients who enrolled in the first clinical trial of BIRG-587, along with accounts from the following sources: Marcus Conant, quoted by Dennis L. Breo, "Tired of taking the blame, AIDS drug regulator Ellen Cooper quits," *JAMA* 265 (1991): 1027–1028; Randy Shilts, *And the band played on: Politics, people, and the AIDS epidemic* (New York: St. Martin's Griffin, 1987), 356–357; and Diane Havlir, interview, February 17, 2012.
3. James Keirns, interview, September 19, 2011.
4. Michael J. Lamson et al., "Single dose pharmacokinetics and bioavailability of nevirapine in healthy volunteers," *Biopharmaceutics & Drug Disposition* 20 (1999):

285–291; Thomas MacGregor, interview, January 23, 2012. Bioavailability of BIRG-587 is > 90 percent, mean residence time is 80 hr.
5. Kathryn Jason, interview, October 3, 2011.
6. James Keirns, interview, September 19, 2011.
7. John Tiso, interview, November 8, 2011.
8. Karl Grozinger, interview, October 12, 2011.
9. The dose levels were 12.5, 50, and 200 mg, given once daily.
10. Sarah H. Cheeseman et al., "Phase I/II evaluation of nevirapine alone and in combination with zidovudine for infection with human immunodeficiency virus," *Journal of Acquired Immune Deficiency Syndrome and Human Retrovirology* 8 (1995): 141–151.
11. Patients in a BIRG-587-only dosing group started treatment two months before the corresponding group who received the same dose of BIRG-587 plus AZT.
12. Maureen Myers, interview, November 17, 2011; Joep Lange, interview, February 28, 2012.
13. Vincent Merluzzi, interview, July 5, 2011; Maureen Myers, interview, March 19, 2012.
14. Vincent Merluzzi, interview, July 5, 2011; Kathryn Jason, interview, October 3, 2011.
15. Bristol-Myers Squibb's U.S.–Canada clinical trials of ddI were described at the FDA Antiviral Drugs Advisory Committee meeting, July 18–19, 1991.
16. Vincent Merluzzi, interview, July 5, 2011; Maureen Myers, interview, November 17, 2011.
17. Julio Montaner, interview, January 31, 2012.
18. Julio Montaner, interview, January 31, 2012.
19. Julio Montaner, interview, January 31, 2012.
20. Julio Montaner, interview, January 31, 2012.
21. Amale Hawi, interview, November 17, 2011.
22. Amale Hawi, interview, November 17, 2011.
23. Katherine Luzuriaga, interview, December 21, 2011.
24. Katherine Luzuriaga, interview, December 21, 2011.
25. Katherine Luzuriaga, interview, January 24, 2012; Thomas MacGregor, interview, January 23, 2011.
26. Amale Hawi, interview, November 17, 2011.
27. Katherine Luzuriaga, interview, December 21, 2011.
28. Karl Grozinger, interview, October 12, 2011.
29. James Wright, interview, October 20, 2011; Amale Hawi, interview, November 17, 2011.
30. Karl Grozinger and Amale Hawi, "Pharmaceutical suspension comprising nevirapine hemihydrate," United States Patent 6,255,481, issued July 3, 2001; Karl Grozinger, interview, October 12, 2011; James Wright, interview, October 20, 2011; Amale Hawi, interview, November 17, 2011. The nevirapine hemihydrate contains about 0.5 mole of water.
31. The pediatric study was designated ACTG 165.
32. Age ranged from 2 months to 15 years and weight ranged from 9 to 140 pounds.
33. Many companies make generic versions of acetaminophen but only Johnson & Johnson makes the Tylenol® brand of acetaminophen.
34. Janice M. Klunder et al., "Synthesis of a series of dipyrido[3,2-b:2',3'-e]diazepinones: potent and selective non-nucleoside inhibitors of HIV-1 reverse transcriptase," 7th International AIDS Conference, Florence, 1991.
35. Joe C. Wu et al., "A novel dipyridodiazepinone inhibitor of HIV-1 reverse transcriptase acts through a non-substrate binding site," 7th International AIDS Conference, Florence, 1991.
36. Julian Adams and Vincent J. Merluzzi, "Discovery of nevirapine, a nonnucleoside inhibitor of HIV-1 reverse transcriptase," in *The search for antiviral drugs: Case histories from concept to clinic*, eds. Julian Adams and Vincent J. Merluzzi (Boston: Birkhäuser, 1993), 45–70; John Proudfoot, interview, February 7, 2012.

37. Joe Wu, interview, January 26, 2012.
38. Joe Wu, interview, January 26, 2012.
39. Joe Wu, interview, January 26, 2012.
40. Mike Tsianco, interview, January 27, 2012.
41. James Keirns, interview, September 19, 2011.
42. F-D-C Reports, "Janssen's TIBO/benzodiazepine AIDS drugs," *Pink Sheet*, October 15, 1990; G. Pialoux et al., "Pharmacokinetics of R 82913 in patients with AIDS or AIDS-related complex," *Lancet* 338 (1991): 140–143; Stephan DeWit et al., "Pharmacokinetics of R 82913 in AIDS patients: A phase I dose-finding study of oral administration compared with intravenous infusion," *Antimicrobial Agents and Chemotherapy* 36 (1992): 2661–2663.
43. Merck's "L" drugs were L-679,539 and L-679,661.
44. Garance Franke-Ruta, "A new tide in antiviral research," *GMHC Treatment Issues*, May 15, 1991; Michael S. Saag et al., "A short-term clinical evaluation of L-679,661, a non-nucleoside inhibitor of HIV-1 reverse transcriptase," *New England Journal of Medicine* 329 (1993): 1065–1072.
45. Maureen Myers, interview, November 17, 2011.
46. John Tiso, interview, November 16, 2011.
47. John Tiso, interview, November 16, 2011; David Hall, interview, December 9, 2011.

Chapter 8

1. Gifford S. Leoung et al., "Aerosolized pentamidine for prophylaxis against *Pneumocystis carinii* pneumonia," *New England Journal of Medicine* 323 (1990): 769–775.
2. David Feigal, interview, May 24, 2012.
3. David Feigal, interview, May 24, 2012.
4. Leoung et al., "Aerosolized pentamidine prophylaxis."
5. Beverly Merz, "Aerosolized pentamidine promising in *Phenmocystis* therapy, prophylaxis," *JAMA* 259 (1988): 3223–3224.
6. John Mills, "Ganciclovir for cytomegalovirus retinitis," *Western Journal of Medicine* 151 (1989): 543–544.
7. Gina Kolata, "FDA gives quick approval to two drugs to treat AIDS," *New York Times*, June 27, 1989; Mark Harrington, interview, April 3, 2012.
8. Victoria A. Harden, *AIDS at 30: A history* (Washington, DC: Potomac Books, 2012), 144; Jim Eigo, "ACT UP crashes the gates," *Global Forum* 5 (2013): 13–20.
9. United Press International, "Police arrest AIDS protesters blocking access to FDA offices," *Los Angeles Times*, October 11, 1988; Paul Duggan, "1,000 Swarm FDA's Rockville office to demand approval of AIDS drugs," *Washington Post*, October 12, 1988.
10. Eigo, "ACT UP crashes the gates"; Mark Harrington, interview, April 3, 2012.
11. *How to Survive a Plague*, DVD, MPI Media Group, 2013.
12. United Press International, "Police arrest protesters."
13. Ellen Cooper, interview, December 20, 2011.
14. Subpart E 21 CFR 312.80; 53 Federal Register 41523, October 21, 1988.
15. Kolata, "FDA gives quick approval"; ACT UP, "Treatment Agenda, 1990: VI International AIDS Conference," June 1990. The trial was ACTG 071 (ClinicalTrials.gov ID: NCT00000688).
16. Eigo, "ACT UP crashes the gates"; Louis Lasagna et al., "Final report of the national committee to review current procedures for approval of new drugs for cancer and AIDS," National Cancer Institute, August 15, 1990.
17. Steven Morris, "AIDS-related drug wins limited ok," *Chicago Tribune*, February 7, 1989.

18. Associated Press, "Panel backs drug to fight eye danger," *New York Times*, May 4, 1989; Harden, *AIDS at 30*, 143.
19. Ellen Cooper, interview, March 7, 2013.
20. Ellen Cooper, interview, March 7, 2013.
21. John S. James, "Aerosol pentamidine, ganciclovir recommended for approval," *AIDS Treatment News*, May 5, 1989.
22. Robert Steinbrook, "FDA approves sale of AIDS pneumonia drug," *Los Angeles Times*, June 16, 1989.
23. ACT UP, "Treatment Agenda."
24. Jeffrey Levi, "Unproven AIDS therapies: The Food and Drug Administration and ddI," in *Biomedical Politics*, ed. Kathi E. Hanna (Washington, DC: National Academy Press, 1991), 9–42; Eigo, "ACT UP crashes the gates."
25. Levi, "Unproven AIDS therapies."
26. Tim McCaskell, "Taking our place," *The Positive Side*, Summer 2011.
27. David Barr, "Enemies at the gate: Storming Montreal's Palais de Congrès, and makeshift battle stations in fortress San Francisco," *The Body*, December 2002; McCaskell, "Taking our place."
28. Barr, "Enemies at the gate"; James Hale, "After Montreal, international AIDS conferences will never be the same," *Canadian Medical Association Journal* 141 (1999): 144–146.
29. Ellen Cooper, "Clinical trials in AIDS: the regulatory perspective," Abstract No. W.B.O.47, 5th International AIDS Conference, Montreal, 1989.
30. Eigo, "ACT UP crashes the gates"; David Kirschenbaum, interviewed by Sarah Schulman, October 19, 2003, ACT UP oral history project No. 031.
31. John Bowen, quoted by David Kirschenbaum in interview by Sarah Shulman, October 19, 2003.
32. Harden, *AIDS at 30*, 145; Eigo, "ACT UP crashes the gates"; Levi, "Unproven AIDS therapies."
33. Anthony Fauci, quoted by Victor F. Zonana and Marlene Cimons, "Ease AIDS drug rules, health chief urges," *Los Angeles Times*, June 24, 1989.
34. Barr, "Enemies at the gate"; Harden, *AIDS at 30*, 145; Levi, "Unproven AIDS therapies."
35. Gina Kolata, "AIDS researcher seeks wider access to drugs in tests," *New York Times*, June 26, 1989; Eigo, "ACT UP crashes the gates"; ACT UP, "Treatment Agenda"; Levi, "Unproven AIDS therapies."
36. ACT UP, "Treatment Agenda"; Levi, "Unproven AIDS therapies."
37. Milt Freudenheim, "Sick get experimental drugs free," *New York Times*, October 21, 1989; Gina Kolata, "Innovative AIDS drug plan may be undermining testing," *New York Times*, November 21, 1989.
38. Ellen Cooper, interview, December 20, 2011.
39. Mark Harrington, interview, April 3, 2012.
40. Philip M. Boffey, "Food and Drug Administration: At fulcrum of conflict, regulator of AIDS drugs," *New York Times*, August 19, 1988.
41. Ellen Cooper, interview, March 7, 2013.
42. Gina Kolata, "Citing stress, FDA aide wants out," *New York Times*, December 22, 1990.
43. David Kessler, *A question of intent: A great American battle with a deadly industry* (New York: PublicAffairs, 2001), 38–39; Kolata, "FDA aide wants out"; Victor F. Zonana, "Top AIDS drug regulator to step down," *Los Angeles Times*, December 22, 1990; Ellen Cooper, interview, December 20, 2011.
44. Michael L. Millenson, "Cancer institute: AIDS drugs unduly delayed," *Chicago Tribune*, January 5, 1989; Zonana, "Top AIDS drug regulator steps down"; Kolata, "FDA aide wants out."
45. Dennis L. Breo, "Tired of taking the blame, AIDS drug regulator Ellen Cooper quits," *JAMA* 265 (1991): 1027–1028; Ellen Cooper, interview, December 20, 2011.
46. Breo, "Ellen Cooper quits."
47. Mark Harrington, interview, April 3, 2012.
48. Philip J. Hilts, "82 held in protest on pace of AIDS research," *New York Times*, May 22, 1990.
49. Mark Harrington, interview, April 3, 2012.
50. Mark Harrington, interview, April 3, 2012; Gregg Gonsalves and Mark Harrington, "AIDS research at NIH: A critical review," 8th International AIDS Conference, Amsterdam, July 20, 1992.
51. Hilts, "Protest on AIDS research"; Eigo, "ACT UP crashes the gates."
52. A 1987 amendment by Sen. Jesse Helms (R-NC) required the Public Health Service to classify HIV infection as a contagious disease that barred foreigners from entering the United States. In April 1990, the Immigration and Naturalization Service issued a temporary waiver granting a 10-day visa that allowed people to enter the U.S. for professional or scientific conferences without declaring that they were infected with HIV.
53. Avert, "History of AIDS: 1987–1992," Avert International AIDS & HIV Charity.
54. Michael Vinikoor, "Celebrating the end of the HIV/AIDS travel ban," *Health Affairs* blog, July 20, 2012.
55. Bruce Lambert, "Jay C. Lipner, 46, a lawyer-lobbyist for victims of AIDS," *New York Times*, November 7, 1991; David Barr, "Marking time: Commune of shell shocked soldiers springs up then quickly crumbles inexplicably," *The Body*, November 2002.
56. Barr, "Enemies at the gate."
57. Harden, *AIDS at 30*, 144; Kolata, "FDA gives quick approval."
58. Lambert, "Jay Lipner."
59. John Lauritsen, "They left their HIV in San Francisco: A report on the sixth International Conference on AIDS," *New York Native*, June 24, 1990; Barr, "Enemies at the gate."
60. Robert Pear, "Faster approval of AIDS drugs is urged," *New York Times*, August 15, 1990. The panel of the National Committee to Review Current Procedures for Approval of New Drugs for Cancer and AIDS consisted of Louis Lasagna (chair), Theodore Cooper, Gertrude Elion, Emil Frei, Samuel Hellman, Peter Barton Hutt, Charles Leighton, Thomas C. Merigan, Jr., and Henry C. Pitot.
61. Lasagna et al., "Approval of new drugs."
62. Lasagna et al., "Approval of new drugs."
63. Mark Harrington, interview, April 3, 2012.
64. Gonsalves and Harrington, "AIDS research at NIH"; Eigo, "ACT UP crashes the gates."
65. Elizabeth Glaser and Laura Palmer, *In the absence of angels: A Hollywood family's courageous story* (New York: Putnam, 1991), 74.
66. Glaser and Palmer, *Absence of angels*, 48.
67. Michael S. Gottlieb et al., "Pneumocystis Pneumonia—Los Angeles," *Morbidity and Mortality Weekly Report* 30 (1981): 1–3; Glaser and Palmer, *Absence of angels*, 55; Elizabeth's initial CD4 cell count was 210.
68. Glaser and Palmer, *Absence of angels*, 235.
69. Glaser and Palmer, *Absence of angels*, 234.
70. Glaser and Palmer, *Absence of angels*, 215. Routine blood work included a CBC and blood chemistry screen.
71. Glaser and Palmer, *Absence of angels*, 55, 215.
72. Glaser and Palmer, *Absence of angels*, 246. Elizabeth's CD4 count was 140.
73. Glaser and Palmer, *Absence of angels*, 287.
74. Glaser and Palmer, *Absence of angels*, 288. Elizabeth had a highly elevated level of creatinine phosphokinase.

75. Glaser and Palmer, *Absence of angels*, 289.
76. Glaser and Palmer, *Absence of angels*, 289.
77. Glaser and Palmer, *Absence of angels*, 290.
78. Glaser and Palmer, *Absence of angels*, 298.
79. Ann Moravick, "Toward a common ground for activists and innovators," *Pharmaceutical Executive*, April 1991; Lew Sibert, "Partnering with community — Could the past hold more promise than the future?" *Global Forum* 5 (2013): 31–40.
80. Mark Harrington, quoted by Moravick, "Toward a common ground."
81. Maureen Myers, interview, November 17, 2011.
82. Direct-to-consumer drug advertising was many years in the future.
83. Mark Harrington, interview, April 3, 2012.
84. Moravick, "Toward a common ground."
85. John Tiso, interview, October 6, 2011; Vincent Merluzzi, interview, December 15, 2011.
86. James Keirns, interview, September 19, 2011.
87. Terri Pascarelli, interview, December 19, 2011.
88. Vincent Merluzzi, interview, July 5, 2011.
89. Vincent Merluzzi, interview, July 5, 2011; Maureen Myers, interview, November 17, 2011.
90. Mike Barr, "Pressing hard for change at Boehringer," *ACT UP Treatment and Data Digest*, June 10, 1991.
91. Garance Franke-Ruta, "A new tide in antiviral research," *GMHC Treatment Issues*, May 15, 1991.
92. Barr, "Pressing Boehringer."
93. Sibert, "Partnering with Community," 31–40.
94. John S. James, "Convergent combination therapy," *AIDS Treatment News*, March 5, 1993.
95. Kathryn Jason, interview, October 3, 2011; Vincent Merluzzi, interview, July 5, 2011; Maureen Myers, interview, November 17, 2011; Terri Pascarelli, interview, December 19, 2011.
96. Maureen Myers, interview, November 17, 2011.
97. Kathryn Jason, interview, October 3, 2011.
98. Vincent Merluzzi, interview, July 5, 2011; Kathryn Jason, interview, October 3, 2011; Maureen Myers, interview, November 17, 2011.
99. Terri Pascarelli, interview, December 19, 2011.
100. William Snow, email, April 30, 2012.
101. Barr, "Pressing Boehringer."
102. Barr, "Pressing Boehringer."
103. Terri Pascarelli, interview, December 19, 2011; William Snow email, April 30, 2012.
104. William Snow, letter to Digby Barrios, August 15, 1991.
105. William Snow, letter to Digby Barrios, August 15, 1991.
106. William Snow, email, April 30, 2012.
107. Maureen Myers, interview, November 17, 2011.
108. Patrick Robinson, interview, December 22, 2011.

Chapter 9

1. Sarah H. Cheeseman et al., "Pharmacokinetics of nevirapine: Initial single-rising-dose study in humans," *Antimicrobial Agents and Chemotherapy* 37 (1993): 178–182.
2. Sarah H. Cheeseman et al., "Phase I/II evaluation of nevirapine alone and in combination with zidovudine for infection with human immunodeficiency virus," *Journal of Acquired Immune Deficiency Syndrome and Human Retrovirology* 8 (1995): 141–151.
3. Overall, p24 is detected in 30–50 percent of HIV-infected individuals. Detectable levels of p24 are most easily found 2–8 weeks after HIV exposure, but then anti-p24 antibodies develop and make detection of p24 more difficult.
4. Maureen Myers, interview, November 17, 2011; John Tiso, interview, November 16, 2011; Douglas Richman, interview, December 8, 2011.
5. Douglas Richman, interview, December 8, 2011.
6. Brendan A. Larder et al., "HIV with reduced sensitivity to zidovudine (AZT) isolated during prolonged therapy," *Science* 243 (1989): 1731–1734.
7. Douglas D. Richman et al., "BI-RG-587 is active against zidovudine-resistant human immunodeficiency virus type 1 and synergistic with zidovudine," *Antimicrobial Agents and Chemotherapy* 35 (1991): 305–308.
8. Douglas D. Richman et al., "Human immunodeficiency virus type 1 mutants resistant to nonnucleoside inhibitors of reverse transcriptase arise in tissue culture," *Proceedings of the National Academy of Sciences* 88 (1991): 11241–11245.
9. Dennis L. Kasper et al., *Harrison's Principles of Internal Medicine*, 16th ed. (New York: McGraw-Hill, 2005), 961; Douglas Richman, interview, December 8, 2011; Julian Adams, interview, December 9, 2011.
10. Martin Hirsch, interview, February 3, 2012.
11. Richman et al., "BIRG-587 synergistic with zidovudine."
12. Douglas Richman, interview, December 8, 2011.
13. Robert Eckner, interview, July 18, 2011; Peter Grob, interview, October 20, 2011.
14. Peter Grob, interview, October 20, 2011.
15. Julian Adams, interview, December 9, 2011.
16. Peter Grob, interview, October 20, 2011; Johanna Griffin, interview, November 9, 2011.
17. Johanna Griffin, interview, November 9, 2011; Julian Adams, interview, December 9, 2011.
18. Julian Adams, interview, December 9, 2011.
19. Joe C. Wu et al., "A novel dipyridodiazepinone inhibitor of HIV-1 reverse transcriptase acts through a non-substrate binding site," *Biochemistry* 30 (1991): 2022–2026.
20. BI scientists included C-K Shih, Janice Rose, Ken Cohen, Johanna Griffin, Racheline Schwartz, and Mark Skoog.
21. Lori A. Kohlsteadt et al., "Reverse transcriptase of human immunodeficiency virus can use either human tRNA^{Lys3} or *Escherichia coli* tRNA^{Gln2} as a primer in an *in vitro* primer-utilization assay," *Proceedings of the National Academy of Sciences* 89 (1992): 9652–9656; Lori A. Kohlsteadt et al., "Crystal structure at 3.5 Å resolution of HIV-1 reverse transcriptase complexed with an inhibitor," *Science* 256 (1992): 1783–1790.
22. Kohlsteadt et al., "Crystal structure of HIV-1 RT." Following the successful crystallization efforts of BI biochemist Tom Warren, Steitz's laboratory co-crystallized nevirapine and HIV-1 reverse transcriptase to demonstrate that nevirapine was a non-competitive inhibitor in a binding pocket on the 66 kD subunit of RT, separate from the enzyme's active site. This work confirmed Joe Wu's results using the photoaffinity probe, which had predicted the Y181C point mutation of reverse transcriptase that was responsible for nevirapine-induced resistance.
23. Richman et al., "HIV-1 mutants to RT."
24. Marilyn Chase, "Merck setback shows problems of AIDS drugs," *Wall Street Journal*, November 16, 1991; Vera W. Byrnes et al., "Comprehensive mutant enzyme and viral variant assessment of human immunodeficiency virus type 1 reverse transcriptase resistance to nonnucleoside inhibitors," *Antimicrobial Agents and Chemotherapy* 37 (1993): 1576–1579.
25. Boehringer Ingelheim, "BIPI announced today its plans to halt the single agent testing of nevirapine (BIRG-

587) in HIV-positive patients," press release, November 27, 1991.

26. Douglas D. Richman et al., "Nevirapine resistance mutations of human immunodeficiency virus type 1 selected during therapy," *Journal of Virology* 68 (1994): 1660–1666.

27. Cheeseman et al., "Phase I/II nevirapine and zidovudine."

28. Maureen Myers, interview, November 17, 2011.

29. Maureen Myers, interview, November 17, 2011.

30. Maureen Myers, interview, November 17, 2011.

31. Cheeseman et al., "Phase I/II nevirapine and zidovudine."

32. Boehringer Ingelheim, "BIPI announced today."

33. "Boehringer Ingelheim Corp. said it would curtail development of an AIDS drug," *New York Times*, November 28, 1991; "Boehringer Ingelheim halts AIDS drug human tests," *Reuters News Service*, November 27, 1991; "Pharmaceutical company plans to end testing of AIDS drug," *Associated Press*, November 27, 1991; Marilyn Chase, "Boehringer Ingelheim Corp. is expected to announce today that it is curtailing development of an AIDS drug because it encountered a problem with viral resistance," Dow Jones News Service, November 27, 1991; Douglas Richman, quoted by Marilyn Chase, "Boehringer is seen scaling back testing on AIDS drug facing viral resistance," *Wall Street Journal*, November 27, 1991.

34. Michael Becker, quoted by Marilyn Chase, "Merck setback."

35. Janssen statement quoted by Reuters, "Johnson/Johnson unit stays with AIDS drugs," November 27, 1991.

36. John Tiso, interview, November 16, 2011.

37. Kathryn Jason, interview, October 3, 2011; John Tiso, interview, November 8, 2011.

38. Julian Adams, interview, December 9, 2011.

39. Peter Grob, interview, October 20, 2011; Peter Farina, personal communication.

40. David Hall, interview, December 9, 2011.

41. Vincent Merluzzi, interview, December 15, 2011.

42. Julian Adams, March 30, 2013.

43. Douglas Richman, interview, December 8, 2011; Martin Hirsch, interview, February 3, 2012.

44. Peter Grob, interview, October 20, 2011.

45. Peter Grob, interview, October 20, 2011.

46. Johanna Griffin, interview, November 9, 2011.

47. Kohlsteadt et al., "Crystal structure of HIV-1 RT"; Scott Hammer, quoted in FDA Antiviral Drugs Advisory Committee meeting, June 7, 1996, 177.

48. Richman et al., "Nevirapine resistance mutations." Nevirapine in vitro induces a single mutation in the p66 subunit of HIV-1 reverse transcriptase changing the 181 residue from tyrosine to cysteine, which was 100-fold less susceptible to nevirapine — an observation that was later confirmed in clinical isolates from nevirapine-resistant patients. Clinical isolates showed additional mutations, primarily at residues 103, 108, and 188, which fluctuated (appearing and disappearing) over the first 12 weeks of therapy.

49. Peter Grob, interview, October 20, 2011.

50. Susan E. Hattox, "Pharmacokinetics of nevirapine alone and in combination with zidovudine," Abstract No. PoB 3591, 8th International AIDS Conference, Amsterdam, 1992; T. C. Greenough, "Quantitative virology: The experience during the nevirapine phase I/II trials," Abstract No. PoB 3610, 8th International AIDS Conference, Amsterdam, 1992; Sarah H. Cheeseman, "Nevirapine (NVP) alone and in combination with zidovudine (ZDV): Safety and activity," Abstract No. MoB 0053, 8th International AIDS Conference, Amsterdam, 1992; Douglas D. Richman, "Loss of nevirapine activity associated with the emergence of resistance in clinical trials," Abstract No. PoB 3576, 8th International AIDS Conference, Amsterdam, 1992.

51. Boehringer Ingelheim, "Nevirapine, a new approach to the treatment of AIDS under development at Boehringer Ingelheim," press release, August 18, 1992.

52. Diane Havlir, quoted by Chris Vaughn, "Diane Havlir: AIDS doctor," *UCSF Magazine*, June 2003.

53. Diane Havlir, interview, February 17, 2012.

54. Menno D. De Jong et al., "Alternating nevirapine and zidovudine treatment of human immunodeficiency virus type 1-infected persons does not prolong nevirapine activity," *Journal of Infectious Diseases* 169 (1994): 1346–1350.

55. Richman et al., "Nevirapine resistance mutations."

56. James Keirns, interview, September 19, 2011.

57. Cheeseman et al., "Phase I/II nevirapine and zidovudine."

58. They had safely given 200 mg daily, and they increased the daily dose to 400 mg.

59. Dianne Havlir et al., "High-dose nevirapine: Safety, pharmacokinetics, and antiviral effect in patients with human immunodeficiency virus infection," *Journal of Infectious Diseases* 171 (1995): 537–545. Viral load measured by ICD-p24 antigen and HIV-RNA.

60. Havlir et al., "High-dose nevirapine safety."

61. Diane Havlir et al., "Nevirapine: Further dose escalation of monotherapy (600 mg/daily) and combination therapy with zidovudine," Conference on Human Retrovirus Related Infections, Washington, DC, December 1993.

62. Maureen Myers, interview, November 17, 2011.

63. Menno D. De Jong et al., "High-dose nevirapine in previously untreated human immunodeficiency virus type 1-infected persons does not result in sustained suppression of viral replication," *Journal of Infectious Diseases* 175 (1997): 966–970. HIV-RNA, a more reliable marker for viral load, returned to baseline levels within 12 weeks of dosing at 400 mg per day.

Chapter 10

1. Kelly J. Warren et al., "Nevirapine-associated Stevens-Johnson syndrome," *Lancet* 351 (1998): 567. Stuart is a fictitious name to protect the patient's identity, but this is a documented clinical case. The regimen was AZT 300 mg bid, lamivudine 150 mg bid, and nevirapine 200 mg qd.

2. Diane Havlir et al., "High-dose nevirapine: Safety, pharmacokinetics, and antiviral effect in patients with human immunodeficiency virus infection," *Journal of Infectious Diseases* 171 (1995): 537–545.

3. Havlir et al., "High-dose nevirapine safety."

4. Havlir et al., "High-dose nevirapine safety."

5. Maureen Myers, interview, November 17, 2011.

6. Maureen Myers, interview, November 17, 2011.

7. Havlir et al., "High-dose nevirapine safety"; NDA 20-636 Medical Review (1996) 17.

8. Havlir et al., "High-dose nevirapine safety."

9. Havlir et al., "Nevirapine: Further dose escalation of monotherapy (600 mg/daily) and combination therapy with zidovudine," Conference on Human Retrovirus Related Infections, Washington, DC, December 1993; Joel Gibson, "Update on the use of nevirapine in clinical trials," *STEP Perspective*, July 1993.

10. Diane Havlir, interview, February 17, 2012.

11. James Wright, interview, October 20, 2011. The PK curves suggested that the 400 mg dose was creating a saturated suspension of nevirapine in the gI tract, making absorption slower and less efficient.

12. The two-week lead-in dose of nevirapine is 200 mg per day, followed by a standard dose of 400 mg per day.

13. Sarah H. Cheeseman et al., "Pharmacokinetics of nevirapine: Initial single-rising-dose study in humans," *Antimicrobial Agents and Chemotherapy* 37 (1993): 178–182; Andreas Barner and Maureen Myers, "Nevirapine and rashes," *Lancet* 351 (1998): 1133–1134. About 16 percent of patients experience a skin rash, which usually resolves with continued drug administration. About 7 percent of patients discontinue nevirapine treatment due to skin rash. Stevens-Johnson syndrome, a life-threatening skin rash condition, is rare but occurs in 0.3 percent of nevirapine treated patients.

14. Anna Maria Cattelan et al., "Severe hepatic failure related to nevirapine treatment," *Clinical Infectious Diseases* 29 (1999): 455–456. Stefano is a fictitious name to protect the patient's identity, but this is a documented clinical case.

15. The regimen was stavudine 40 mg bid, lamivudine 150 mg bid, and nevirapine 200 qd.

16. The new regimen was stavudine, lamivudine, and saquinavir.

17. Sarah H. Cheeseman et al., "Phase I/II evaluation of nevirapine alone and in combination with zidovudine for infection with human immunodeficiency virus," *Journal of Acquired Immune Deficiency Syndrome and Human Retrovirology* 8 (1995): 141–151. Six of 62 patients exhibited an increase in gamma-glutamyl transferase greater than 5 times the upper limit of normal. Three of these had baseline GGT levels greater than 3 times the upper limit of normal; the other three were within the normal range at baseline.

18. Havlir et al., "High-dose nevirapine safety." Six of 21 patients exhibited an increase in GGT greater than 5 times the upper limit of normal. Three of these also had a less pronounced elevation in aspartate aminotransaminase and alanine aminotransaminase. One patient had a history of IV drug use but no evidence of hepatitis, one had chronic active hepatitis B, and another developed abnormal liver function tests in conjunction with fever and intolerable rash.

19. Diane Havlir, interview, February 17, 2012.

20. Dennis L. Kasper et al., *Harrison's Principles of Internal Medicine*, 16th ed. (New York: McGraw-Hill, 2005), 1111.

21. David B. Hall and Thomas R. MacGregor, "Case-control exploration of relationships between early rash or liver toxicity and plasma concentrations of nevirapine and primary metabolites," *HIV Clinical Trials* 8 (2007): 381–399.

22. Maureen Myers, interview, November 17, 2011.

23. Robert L. Murphy, "Defining the toxicity profile of nevirapine and other antiretroviral drugs," *Journal of Acquired Immune Deficiency Syndrome* 34 (2003): S15–S20.

Chapter 11

1. Randy Shilts, *And the band played on: Politics, people, and the AIDS epidemic* (New York: St. Martin's Griffin, 1987), 194.

2. R. O'Reilly et al., "Unexplained immunodeficiency and opportunistic infections in infants — New York, New Jersey, California," *Morbidity and Mortality Weekly Report* 31 (1982): 665–667.

3. Arthur Ammann, interview, February 24, 2012.

4. O'Reilly et al., "Unexplained immunodeficiency."

5. Arthur Ammann, interview, February 24, 2012.

6. Elizabeth Glaser and Laura Palmer, *In the absence of angels: A Hollywood family's courageous story* (New York: Putnam, 1991), 123, 126, 127.

7. Glaser and Palmer, *Absence of angels*, 199.

8. Jake Glaser, interview, September 19, 2012.

9. Susan DeLaurentis, email, May 2, 2013.

10. Glaser and Palmer, *Absence of angels*, 143; Jacob W. Stahl, "A history of accelerated approval: Overcoming the FDA's bureaucratic barriers in order to expedite desperately needed drugs to critically ill patients," *Harvard Law School Third Year Paper*, March 31, 2005; The Watkins Commission reported to President Reagan in 1988 and the Lasagna Commission reported to President Bush in 1990.

11. Elizabeth Glaser, Address to the Democratic National Convention, New York, July 14, 1992.

12. Glaser and her doctors assumed that she had passed the virus to Jake in utero, but confirmatory tests were not available at the time; subsequent research has demonstrated that in cases with a medical history similar to the Glasers', HIV transmission most likely occurs during childbirth.

13. Glaser, Address to the Democratic National Convention, July 14, 1992.

14. Glaser and Palmer, *Absence of angels*, 115–116, 119.

15. Stéphanie Blanche et al., "A prospective study of infants born to women seropositive for human immunodeficiency virus type 1," *New England Journal of Medicine* 320 (1989): 1643–1648; Margaret J. Oxtoby, "Perinatally acquired human immunodeficiency virus infection," *Pediatric Infectious Disease Journal* 9 (1990): 609–619; Glaser and Palmer, *Absence of angels*, 197.

16. Arthur Ammann, interview, February 24, 2012.

17. Elizabeth Glaser, quoted in *Elizabeth Glaser Pediatric AIDS Foundation Annual Report*, 2003.

18. Russell B. Van Dyke et al., "The Ariel Project: A prospective cohort study of maternal-child transmission of human immunodeficiency virus type 1 in the era of maternal antiretroviral therapy," *Journal of Infectious Diseases* 179 (1999): 319–328.

19. Julian Adams, interview, December 9, 2011.

20. Julian Adams, interview, December 9, 2011.

21. Julian Adams, interview, December 9, 2011.

22. Bruce K. Johnson et al., "Long-term observations of human immunodeficiency virus-infected chimpanzees," *AIDS Research and Human Retroviruses* 9 (1993): 375–378; Francis J. Novembre et al., "Development of AIDS in a chimpanzee infected with human immunodeficiency virus type 1," *Journal of Virology* 71 (1997): 4086–4091. HIV-1 infection in chimpanzees leads to seroconversion, viremia in peripheral blood mononuclear cells, and plasma viral PCR-RNA.

23. Peter Grob et al., "Prophylaxis against HIV-1 infection in chimpanzees by nevirapine, a nonnucleoside inhibitor of reverse transcriptase," *Nature Medicine* 3 (1997): 665–670.

24. Joep Lange, interview, February 28, 2012.

25. "HIV/AIDS Update — International conference paints bleak picture of pandemic with severe socioeconomic consequences," *MedPRO Month*, August 1992.

26. "HIV/AIDS Update," MedPRO Month.

27. John Sullivan, interview, December 6, 2011.

28. John Sullivan, interview, December 6, 2011.

29. A. Ehrnst et al., "HIV in pregnant women and their offspring: Evidence for late transmission," *Lancet* 338 (1991): 203–207; A. Krivine et al., "HIV replication during the first weeks of life," *Lancet* 339 (1992): 1187–1189; Paolo Rossi et al., "Maternal factors involved in mother-to-child transmission of HIV-1: Report of a consensus workshop, Siena, Italy, January 17–18, 1992," *Journal of Acquired Immune Deficiency Syndrome* 5 (1992): 1019–1029; John Sullivan, interview, December 6, 2011.

30. David Feigal, interview, May 24, 2012.

31. Philip A. Rea et al., "Ivermectin and river blindness," *American Scientist* 98 (2010): 294–303.

32. Rea et al., "Ivermectin and river blindness."

33. NDA 20-636 Pharmacologist's Review (1996) 50-59.
34. Grob et al., "Prophylaxis in chimpanzees by nevirapine."
35. Peter Farina, personal communication.
36. Julian Adams, interview, December 9, 2011.
37. Douglas Richman, interview, December 8, 2011.
38. Arthur Ammann, interview, February 24, 2012; Ross E. McKinney, Jr., "Dr. Catherine Wilfert's indomitable will," *Duke magic: A history*, June 2009.
39. Jessica Roseberry, Catherine Wilfert interview, *Women in Duke medicine: An oral history exhibit*, August 25, 2006.
40. Roseberry, Catherine Wilfert interview.
41. McKinney, "Catherine Wilfert's will."
42. A. H. Sharpe et al., "Retroviruses and mouse embryos: a rapid model for neurovirulence and transplacental antiviral therapy," *Science* 236 (1987): 1671–1674.
43. Catherine Wilfert, interview, January 18, 2012; Arthur Ammann, interview, February 24, 2012.
44. McKinney, "Catherine Wilfert's will."
45. Catherine Wilfert, interview, January 18, 2012.
46. Van Dyke et al., "Ariel Project."
47. David Feigal, interview, May 24, 2012.
48. Catherine Wilfert, interview, January 18, 2012.
49. Arthur Ammann, interview, March 2, 2012.
50. Edward M. Connor et al., "Reduction of maternal-infant transmission of human immunodeficiency virus type 1 with zidovudine treatment," *New England Journal of Medicine* 331 (1994): 1173–1180.
51. Katherine Luzuriaga, interview, December 21, 2011.
52. Connor et al., "Maternal-infant transmission with zidovudine"; Rhoda S. Sperling et al., "Maternal viral load, zidovudine treatment, and the risk of transmission of human immunodeficiency virus type 1 from mother to infant," *New England Journal of Medicine* 335 (1996): 1621–1629.
53. Centers for Disease Control and Prevention, "Zidovudine for the prevention of HIV transmission from mother to infant," *Morbidity and Mortality Weekly Report* 43 (1994): 285–287; Lynne M. Mofenson et al., "Recommendations of the U.S. Public Health Service Task Force on the use of zidovudine to reduce perinatal transmission of human immunodeficiency virus," *Morbidity and Mortality Weekly Report* 43, no. RR-11 (1994): 1–20.
54. Greg Folkers, "New ACTG 076 analysis emphasizes importance of offering AZT therapy to all HIV-infected pregnant women," *NIH News*, November 27, 1996; John L. Sullivan, "Prevention of mother-to-child transmission of HIV—What next?" *Journal of Acquired Immune Deficiency Syndrome* 34 (2003): S67–S72.
55. Maria, Jason, and Jane are fictitious names to protect the identity of these patients, but this is a documented clinical case.
56. Katherine Luzuriaga, interview, January 24, 2012; John Sullivan, interview, December 6, 2011.
57. Katherine Luzuriaga et al., "Combination treatment with zidovudine, didanosine, and nevirapine in infants with human immunodeficiency virus type 1 infection," *New England Journal of Medicine* 336 (1997): 1343–1349.
58. Sullivan, "Prevention of mother-to-child transmission," S67–S72.
59. Elliot Marseille et al., "Cost effectiveness of single-dose nevirapine regimen for mothers and babies to decrease vertical HIV-1 transmission in sub–Saharan Africa," *Lancet* 354 (1999): 803–809.
60. Maureen Myers, interview, November 29, 2011.
61. Ehrnst et al., "HIV in pregnant women"; Arlette Simonon et al., "An assessment of the timing of mother-to-child transmission of human immunodeficiency virus type 1 by means of polymerase chain reaction," *Journal of Acquired Immune Deficiency Syndrome* 7 (1994): 952–957; Philip A. Mock et al., "Maternal viral load and timing of mother-to-child HIV transmission, Bangkok, Thailand," *AIDS* 13 (1999): 407–414.
62. Nathan Shaffer et al., "Short-course zidovudine for perinatal HIV-1 transmission in Bangkok, Thailand: A randomized controlled trial," *Lancet* 353 (1999): 773–380. The short term regimen consisted of 300 mg of AZT twice a day to pregnant mothers from 36 weeks gestation and every 3 hrs from onset of labor until delivery; mothers did not breastfeed and infants received no AZT.
63. Centers for Disease Control and Prevention, "Administration of zidovudine during late pregnancy and delivery to prevent perinatal HIV transmission—Thailand, 1996–1998," *Mortality and Morbidity Weekly Report* 47 (1998): 151–154.
64. The three treatment arms were: A—AZT plus 3TC starting at 36 weeks gestation, followed by 7 days dosing to mothers and infants; B—AZT plus 3TC starting at onset of labor through delivery, followed by 7 days dosing to mothers and infants; C—AZT plus 3TC at onset of labor through delivery.
65. PETRA study team, "Efficacy of three short-course regimens of zidovudine and lamivudine in preventing early and late transmission of HIV-1 from mother to child in Tanzania, South Africa, and Uganda (Petra study): A randomized, double-blind, placebo-controlled trial," *Lancet* 359 (2002): 1178–1186.

Chapter 12

1. Lawrence K. Altman, "Drug mixture halts HIV in lab, doctors say in a cautious report," *New York Times*, February 18, 1993.
2. Yung-Kang Chow et al., "Use of evolutionary limitations of HIV-1 multidrug resistance to optimize therapy," *Nature* 361 (1993): 650–645.
3. Max Finland Award, Martin Hirsch biography, National Foundation for Infectious Diseases, 2008.
4. Victoria A. Johnson et al., "Three-drug synergistic inhibition of HIV-1 replication in vitro by zidovudine, recombinant soluble CD4, and recombinant interferon-alpha A," *Journal of Infectious Diseases* 161 (1990): 1059–1067; Martin Hirsch, interview, February 3, 2012.
5. Martin Hirsch, interview, February 3, 2012. Hirsch's dinner colleagues were Tom Merigan and Steve Lagakos.
6. Scott M. Hammer et al., "A trial comparing nucleoside monotherapy with combination therapy in HIV-infected adults with CD4 cell counts from 200 to 500 per cubic millimeter," *New England Journal of Medicine* 335 (1996): 1081–1090. The trial was ACTG 175.
7. John S. James, "Convergent combination therapy," *AIDS Treatment News*, March 5, 1993.
8. Peter Farina, personal communication.
9. Peter Grob, interview, October 20, 2011.
10. Maureen Myers, interview, November 17, 2011; David Hall, interview, December 9, 2011; Patrick Robinson, interview, December 22, 2011.
11. Altman, "Drug halts HIV in lab"; Joel Gibson, "Update on the use of nevirapine in clinical trials," *STEP Perspective*, July 1993. Patients received either nevirapine and ddI together, alternating doses of nevirapine and ddI, a combination of nevirapine, AZT and ddI, or a combination of nevirapine, AZT and ddC.
12. "Recent news about ddI," *The Body*, September 1999. Bristol-Myers Squibb subsequently reformulated ddI to eliminate the antacid co-medication and simplify dosing with other AIDS drugs.

13. James Wright, interview, October 20, 2011.
14. James Wright, interview, October 20, 2011.
15. Maureen Myers, interview, November 17, 2011; Johanna Griffin, interview, November 9, 2011.
16. Victor Hartmann quoted by Barbara Loecher, "AIDS drug given another shot," *Danbury News-Times*, May 12, 1993.
17. Chow et al., "Limitations of multidrug resistance."
18. Maureen Myers, interview, November 17, 2011.
19. Altman, "Drug halts HIV in lab"; John Rennie, "Triple whammy: Will an AIDS therapy live up to its advance billing?" *Scientific American*, May 1993, 18–19.
20. James, "Convergent combination therapy."
21. George E. Curry, "AIDS conference ends with optimism," *philly.com*, August 1, 2010.
22. John Lauritsen, "Looking back on Berlin," *HEAL Newsletter*, Fall/Winter 1993.
23. Curry, "AIDS conference ends with optimism"; Maureen Myers, interview, November 17, 2011.
24. Lauritsen, "Looking back on Berlin."
25. The other designated clinical sites were Albert Einstein University, Cornell University, Indiana University, Mt. Sinai Medical Center, Northwestern University, University of Alabama at Birmingham, University of California San Diego, University of California San Francisco, University of Colorado, University of Cincinnati, University of Colorado, University of Miami Florida, University of Minnesota, University of North Carolina, University of Pennsylvania Philadelphia, and University of Southern California.
26. Hammer et al., "Comparing monotherapy with combination therapy."
27. Mark Harrington, "The crisis in clinical AIDS research," *The Body*, December 1993.
28. Maureen Myers, interview, November 17, 2011; Patrick Robinson, interview, December 22, 2011.
29. Gibson, "Update on nevirapine trials."
30. Harrington, "Crisis in AIDS research"; Gibson, "Update on nevirapine trials."
31. "Pitt researchers to investigate new drug combination for treatment of AIDS," PR Newswire, February 24, 1993.
32. The designated clinical sites were University of Pennsylvania in Philadelphia, Pitt Treatment Evaluation unit in Pittsburg, and Miriam Hospital/Brown University in Providence, Rhode Island.
33. Harrington, "Crisis in AIDS research"; Maureen Myers, interview, November 17, 2011.
34. Case details provided by John Sullivan, interview, December 6, 2011, and Katherine Luzuriaga, interview, December 21, 2011.
35. David is a fictitious name to protect the patient's identity, but this is a documented clinical case.
36. John Sullivan, interview, December 6, 2011; Katherine Luzuriaga, interview, December 21, 2011.
37. Katherine Luzuriaga, interview, December 21, 2011.
38. Rennie, "Triple whammy."
39. Harrington, "Crisis in AIDS research."
40. Loecher, "AIDS drug given another shot."
41. Roy Vagelos, quoted in *Wall Street Journal*, "Top firms plan joint testing of AIDS drugs," April 20, 1993.
42. David W. Barry and Linda M. Distlerath, "History and accomplishments of inter-company collaboration for AIDS drug development," *Drug Information Journal* 34 (2000): 741–752.
43. Barry and Distlerath, "History of inter-company collaboration," 741–752. ICC member companies were AB Astra, Boehringer Ingelheim, Bristol-Myers Squibb, Burroughs Wellcome, DuPont Merck, Glaxo, Hoechst AG, Hoffmann-La Roche, Eli Lilly, Merck, Pfizer, Miles, Sigma-Tau, SmithKlein Beecham, and Syntex.
44. Barry and Distlerath, "History of inter-company collaboration."
45. Johanna Griffin, interview, November 9, 2011.
46. Barry and Distlerath, "History of inter-company collaboration"; Maureen Myers, interview, November 17, 2011; Johanna Griffin, interview, November 9, 2011.
47. Johanna Griffin, interview, November 9, 2011; Maureen Myers, interview, November 17, 2011; Barry and Distlerath, "History of inter-company collaboration."
48. Brendan A. Larder et al., "Convergent combination therapy can select viable multidrug-resistant HIV-1 in vitro," *Nature* 365 (1993): 451–453; Emillo A. Emini et al., "HIV and multidrug resistance," *Nature* 364 (1993): 679.
49. Henry E. Chang, "Triple-drug therapy still worth testing, despite laboratory error," *AIDS Treatment News*, August 20, 1993.
50. Yung-Kang Chow et al., "HIV-1 error revealed," *Nature* 364 (1993): 679.
51. Yung-Kang Chow et al., "In vitro selection of multidrug resistant HIV-1," Abstract No. WS-A19-6, 9th International AIDS Conference, Berlin, 1993; Maureen Myers, interview, November 17, 2011.
52. Margaret A. Fischl et al., "The safety and efficacy of zidovudine (ZDV) and zalcitabine (ddC) or ddC alone versus ZVD," Abstract No. WS-B25-1, 9th International AIDS Conference, Berlin, 1993; Margaret A. Fischl et al., "Combination and monotherapy with zidovudine and zalcitabine in patients with advanced HIV disease, ACTG 155," *Annals of Internal Medicine* 122 (1995): 24–32. The AZT-ddC combination trial was ACTG 155.
53. Chang, "Triple-drug therapy despite laboratory error."
54. NDA 20–636 Medical Review (1996) 8.
55. James, "Convergent combination therapy."

Chapter 13

1. Kenneth H. Bacon, "Plan to speed availability of drugs for AIDS backed by US officials," *Wall Street Journal*, June 22, 1989; Kenneth H. Bacon, "US moves to help critically ill get new AIDS drugs," *Wall Street Journal*, May 21, 1990; 55 Federal Register 20856, May 21, 1990.
2. ACT UP, "Treatment Agenda, 1990: VI International AIDS Conference," June 1990; Joanna E. Siegel and Marc J. Roberts, "Reforming FDA policy lessons from the AIDS experience," *Regulation* 14 (1991): 71–77.
3. ACT UP, "Treatment Agenda"; FDA Antiviral Drugs Advisory Committee meeting, July 18, 1991, 18; The existing FDA regulations allowed enrollment of patients under a Treatment IND and in an open label safety study, in cases where they did not meet clinical trial enrollment criteria.
4. Ann M. Moravick, "Toward a common ground for activists and innovators," *Pharmaceutical Executive*, April 1991.
5. FDA, "HIV specific resources, expanded access and expedited approval of new therapies related to HIV/AIDS, August 13, 2009."
6. David Kessler, interview, December 12, 2011.
7. FDA Antiviral Drugs Advisory Committee meeting, July 18, 1991, 80, 118; Gina Kolata, "Innovative AIDS drug plan may be undermining testing," *New York Times*, November 21, 1989; Jeffrey Levi, "Unproven AIDS therapies: The Food and Drug Administration and ddI," in *Biomedical Politics*, ed. Kathi E. Hanna (Washington. DC: National Academy Press, 1991), 9–42.
8. Moravick, "Toward a common ground."

9. Mike Barr, "Pressing hard for change at Boehringer," *Treatment and Data Digest*, June 10, 1991.
10. ACT UP, "Treatment agenda"; Gina Kolata, "FDA debate on speedy access to AIDS drugs is reopening," *New York Times*, September 12, 1994.
11. ACT UP, "Treatment agenda"; Barr, "Pressing Boehringer."
12. James Wright, interview, October 20, 2011.
13. James Wright, interview, October 20, 2011.
14. Karl Grozinger et al., "Discovery and development of nevirapine," in *Drug Discovery and Development*, ed. Mukund S. Chorghade (Hoboken, NJ: Wiley, 2006), 353–363.
15. Grozinger et al., "Drug development." The chemical reaction was an exothermic nitration step.
16. Grozinger et al., "Drug development."
17. CAPIC is 3-amino-2-chloro-4-methylpyridine.
18. Robert L. Murphy and Julio Montaner, "Drug evaluations anti-infectives: Nevirapine: A review of its development, pharmacological profile and potential for clinical use," *Expert Opinion on Investigational Drugs* 5 (1996): 1183–1199.
19. Julian Adams, interview, December 9, 2011.
20. Julian Adams, interview, December 9, 2011.
21. Julian Adams, interview, December 9, 2011.
22. Laura Andrews, interview, October 12–13, 2011.
23. James Wright, interview, October 20, 2011.
24. James Wright, interview, October 20, 2011; Julian Adams, interview, December 9, 2011.
25. Karl Grozinger, interview, October 12, 2011; Julian Adams, interview, December 9, 2011.
26. Julian Adams, interview, December 9, 2011.
27. John Tiso, interview, October 6, 2011.
28. James Wright, interview, October 20, 2011.
29. Karl Grozinger, interview, October 12, 2011; James Wright, interview, October 20, 2011; Julian Adams, interview, December 9, 2011.
30. Karl Grozinger, interview, October 12, 2011.
31. Karl Grozinger, interview, October 12, 2011.
32. NDA 20-636 Environmental Assessment (1996) 1.
33. Karl Grozinger, interview, October 12, 2011; Julian Adams, interview, December 9, 2011.
34. The tablets were used for bioequivalence studies and NDA batches.
35. James Wright, interview, October 20, 2011.
36. James Wright, interview, October 20, 2011.

Chapter 14

1. John A. Bartlett, "Management and counseling for persons with HIV infection," in *Cecil Textbook of Medicine*, eds. J. Claude Bennett and Fred Plum (Philadelphia: Saunders, 1996), 1888–1892.
2. Maureen Myers, interview, November 17, 2011.
3. Maureen Myers, interview, November 17, 2011.
4. CD4 cell counts are expressed as the number of cells per microliter (or per cubic millimeter).
5. Elizabeth Glaser and Laura Palmer, *In the absence of angels: A Hollywood family's courageous story* (New York: Putnam, 1991), 55.
6. John Modlin and Anne Gershon in FDA Antiviral Drugs Advisory Committee meeting, July 18, 1991, 335.
7. Ryan White and Ann Marie Cunningham, *Ryan White: My own story* (New York: Signet, 1992).
8. Glaser and Palmer, *Absence of angels*, 46.
9. Margaret A. Fischl et al., "The efficacy of azidothymidine (AZT) in the treatment of patients with AIDS and AIDS-related complex," *New England Journal of Medicine* 317 (1987): 181–191.

10. Ellen Cooper, quoted in F-D-C, "Surrogate endpoints for AIDS drugs: long-term studies needed," *Pink Sheet*, October 11, 1989.
11. Louis Lasagna et al., "Final report of the national committee to review current procedures for approval of new drugs for cancer and AIDS," National Cancer Institute, August 15, 1990. National Committee to Review Current Procedures for Approval of New Drugs for Cancer and AIDS members were Louis Lasagna, Theodore Cooper, Gertrude Elion, Emil Frei, Samuel Hellman, Peter Barton Hutt, Charles Leighton, Thomas C. Merigan, and Henry C. Pitot.
12. Robert Pear, "Faster approval of AIDS drugs is urged," *New York Times*, August 16, 1990.
13. David A. Kessler, *A question of intent: A great American battle with a deadly industry* (New York: PublicAffairs, 2001), 38.
14. Kessler, *A question of intent*, 40.
15. Kessler, *A question of intent*, 41.
16. John S. James, "ddI and ddC approval effort—interview with Martin Delaney," *AIDS Treatment News*, December 7, 1990; John S. James, "ddC/ddI approval update," *AIDS Treatment News*, January 4, 1991.
17. Gina Kolata, "Interest grows in licensing shortcut for 2 AIDS drugs," *New York Times*, September 25, 1990.
18. The controlled trials were ACTG 116A/B, ACTG 117, and ACTG 118.
19. James, "Interview with Martin Delaney," December 7, 1990.
20. James, "Interview with Martin Delaney," December 7, 1990.
21. James Bilstad, quoted in FDA Antiviral Drugs Advisory Committee meeting, July 18, 1991, 201. The Advisory Committee meeting to consider CD4 as a surrogate marker was held on February 13–14, 1991.
22. FDA, "HHS Secretary Lewis W. Sullivan announces FDA's approval of ddI," news release, October 9, 1991.
23. Kessler, *A question of intent*, 41; David Feigal, interview, May 24, 2012; FDA Antiviral Drugs Advisory Committee meeting, July 18, 1991, 37.
24. FDA Antiviral Drugs Advisory Committee meeting, July 18, 1991.
25. Kessler, *A question of intent*, 42.
26. The ACTG trials were 116A, 116B, 117, and 118, each testing two doses of ddI versus AZT in double blind, placebo-controlled trials.
27. In the first 12 weeks, CD4 counts increased by 15 cells in the ddI groups versus a decrease of about 10 cells in the AZT group.
28. Kessler, *A question of intent*, 42.
29. Jacob W. Stahl, "A history of accelerated approval: Overcoming the FDA's bureaucratic barriers in order to expedite desperately needed drugs to critically ill patients," *Harvard Law School Third Year Paper*, March 31, 2005.
30. David W. Barry and Linda M. Distlerath, "History and accomplishments of inter-company collaboration for AIDS drug development," *Drug Information Journal* 34 (2000): 741–752.
31. James O. Kahn et al., "A controlled trial comparing continued zidovudine with didanosine in human immunodeficiency virus infection," *New England Journal of Medicine* 327 (1992): 581–587; R. W. Coombs et al., "Association of plasma human immunodeficiency virus type 1 RNA level with risk of clinical progression in patients with advanced infection," *Journal of Infectious Diseases* 174 (1996): 704–712.
32. David Kessler, quoted in FDA, "HHS Secretary Lewis W. Sullivan announces FDA's approval of ddI," news release, October 9, 1991.

33. David Feigal, interview, May 24, 2012.
34. Stahl, "History of accelerated approval"; 57 FR 13234; 57 FR 58942; 21 CFR 314.500 to 314.550 (Subpart H).
35. Accelerated approval of ddC was for use in combination with AZT, rather than as a standalone treatment.
36. Richard T. D'Aquila et al., "Nevirapine, zidovudine, and didanosine compared with zidovudine and didanosine in patients with HIV-1 infection," *Annals of Internal Medicine* 124 (1996): 1019–1030.
37. The trials were BI 1037 and BI 1038.
38. Maureen Myers, interview, November 17, 2011.
39. Johanna Griffin, interview, November 9, 2011.
40. Peter Grob, interview, October 20, 2011; James Wright, interview, October 20, 2011.
41. Julian Adams, interview, December 9, 2011.
42. Maureen Myers, interview, November 17, 2011.
43. Johanna Griffin, interview, November 9, 2011; Barry and Distlerath, "History of inter-company collaboration," 741–752.
44. James Wright, interview, October 20, 2011.
45. James Wright, interview, October 20, 2011.
46. Peter Grob, interview, October 20, 2011; James Wright, interview, October 20, 2011.
47. James Wright, interview, October 20, 2011.
48. Maureen Myers, interview, November 17, 2011.
49. James Wright, interview, October 20, 2011.
50. James Wright, interview, October 20, 2011.
51. A. Carr et al., "A controlled trial of nevirapine plus zidovudine versus zidovudine alone in p24 antigenaemic HIV-infected patients," *AIDS* 10 (1996): 635–641.

Chapter 15

1. Arthur Ammann, interview, February, 24, 2012.
2. Arthur Ammann et al., "Epidemiologic notes and reports possible transfusion-associated acquired immune deficiency syndrome (AIDS) — California," *Morbidity and Mortality Weekly Report* 31 (1982): 652–654; Arthur Ammann et al., "Acquired immunodeficiency in an infant: Possible transmission by means of blood products," *Lancet* 1 (1983): 956–958.
3. Arthur Ammann quoted by Randy Shilts, *And the band played on: Politics, people, and the AIDS epidemic* (New York: St. Martin's Griffin, 1987), 179; Arthur Ammann, interview, February 24, 2012.
4. Ammann et al., "Possible transmission by blood products."
5. Shilts, *And the band played on*, 178.
6. Shilts, *And the band played on*, 57.
7. Ammann et al., "Possible transfusion-associated AIDS"; Shilts, *And the band played on*, 178.
8. John Sullivan, interview, February 16, 2012.
9. Catherine Wilfert, interview, January 18, 2012.
10. Ross E. McKinney, Jr., "Dr. Catherine Wilfert's indomitable will," in *Duke magic: A history*.
11. Jessica Roseberry, "Catherine Wilfert Interview," *Women in Duke medicine: An oral history exhibit*, August 25, 2006.
12. Roseberry, Catherine Wilfert "Interview."
13. McKinney, "Wilfert's indomitable will"; Catherine Wilfert, interview, January 18, 2012.
14. Frank M. Balis and David G. Poplack, "Drug development and clinical pharmacology," in *Pediatric AIDS: Challenge of HIV infection in infants, children and adolescents*, eds. Philip A. Pizzo and Catherine M. Wilfert (Baltimore: Williams and Wilkins, 1991); 457–477; Charles G. Prober and Anne A. Gershon, "Medical management of newborns and infants born to seropositive mothers," in *Pediatric AIDS: Challenge of HIV infection in infants, children and adolescents*, eds. Philip A. Pizzo and Catherine M. Wilfert (Baltimore: Williams and Wilkins, 1991); 516–530; Wilfert, interview, January 18, 2012.
15. Elizabeth Glaser and Laura Palmer, *In the absence of angels: A Hollywood family's courageous story* (New York: Putnam, 1991), 32, 49.
16. Glaser and Palmer, *Absence of angels*, 233.
17. Jake Glaser, interview, September 19, 2012.
18. Glaser and Palmer, *Absence of angels*, 234.
19. Glaser and Palmer, *Absence of angels*, 290, 301.
20. Jake Glaser, interview, September 19, 2012
21. Jake Glaser, interview, September 19, 2012.
22. Elizabeth Glaser, quoted by Jake Glaser, interview, September 19, 2012.
23. 21 CFR 201.57 (f)(9).
24. Cooper et al., "Development of new drugs for the treatment of pediatric AIDS: Scientific and regulatory issues," in *Pediatric AIDS: Challenge of HIV infection in infants, children and adolescents*, eds. Philip A. Pizzo and Catherine M. Wilfert (Baltimore: Williams and Wilkins, 1991); 605–618.
25. Maureen Myers, interview, November 29, 2011; James Keirns, interview, September 19, 2011.
26. Cooper et al., "New drugs for pediatric AIDS."
27. Glaser and Palmer, *Absence of angels*, 218.
28. Catherine Wilfert, interview, January 18, 2012.
29. Philip A. Pizzo and Catherine M. Wilfert, "Treatment considerations for children with HIV infection," in *Pediatric AIDS: Challenge of HIV infection in infants, children and adolescents*, eds. Philip A, Pizzo and Catherine M. Wilfert, (Baltimore; Williams and Wilkins,1991): 478–494.
30. Katherine Luzuriaga et al., "Pharmacokinetics, safety, and activity of nevirapine in human immunodeficiency virus type 1-infected children," *Journal of Infectious Diseases* 174 (1996): 713–721.
31. Katherine Luzuriaga, interview, December 21, 2011.
32. John Tiso, interview, December 1, 2011.
33. John Sullivan, interview, December 6, 2011; Maureen Myers, interview, November 29, 2011; John Tiso, interview, December 1, 2011.
34. The three dose levels were 7.5, 30, and 120 mg/m^2.
35. Amale Hawi, interview, November 17, 2011.
36. NDA No. 20–636/SE1–009 and 20–933 Medical Review (1998) 5.
37. The pediatric dose level was 120 mg/m^2 and was equivalent to the 200 mg adult dose.
38. Amale Hawi, interview, November 17, 2011.
39. NDA No. 20–636/SE1–009 and 20–933 Medical Review (1998) 5–6. The new pediatric dose level was 240 mg/m^2.
40. NDA No. 20–636/SE1–009 and 20–933 Medical Review (1998) 15–16.
41. Children older than 9 years received 120 mg/m^2 for four weeks followed by 240 mg/m^2; children younger than 9 years received 120 mg/m^2 for four weeks followed by 400 mg/m^2.
42. Luzuriaga et al., "Safety and activity of nevirapine in children."
43. NDA No. 20–636/SE1–009 and 20–933 Medical Review (1998) 6.
44. NDA No. 20–636/SE1–009 and 20–933 Medical Review (1998) 7.
45. Luzuriaga et al., "Safety and activity of nevirapine in children"; NDA No. 20–636/SE1–009 and 20–933 Medical Review (1998) 5–18. Children younger than 9 years received 120 mg/m^2 for four weeks followed by 400 mg/m^2.

46. Katherine Luzuriaga, interview, January 24, 2012.
47. Cooper et al., "New drugs for pediatric AIDS."
48. The study was ACTG 245.
49. ClinicalTrials.gov, NCT00000814.
50. Amale Hawi, interview, November 17, 2011.
51. NDA 20-636/009 and NDA 20-933 Medical Review (1998) 26.
52. Amale Hawi, interview, November 17, 2011.
53. Amale Hawi, interview, November 17, 2011.
54. James Curran, CDC, quoted at 10th Annual AMA Science Writers' Conference, September 30–October 1, 1991.
55. Jamie Gentille, interview, August 28, 2012.
56. Jamie Gentille, interview, August 28, 2012.
57. Jamie Gentille, interview, August 28, 2012.
58. Karina M. Butler et al., "Dideoxyinosine in children with symptomatic human immunodeficiency virus infection," *New England Journal of Medicine* 324 (1991): 137–144.
59. Jamie Gentille, interview, August 28, 2012.
60. Jamie Gentille, interview, August 28, 2012.
61. Jamie Gentille, interview, August 28, 2012; Butler et al., "Dideoxyinosine in children."
62. Jamie Gentille, interview, August 28, 2012.
63. Jamie Gentille, interview, August 28, 2012.
64. She enrolled in clinical trials to assess 3TC and IL2.
65. Sandra K. Burchett et al., "Virologic activity of didanosine (ddI), zidovudine (ZDV), and nevirapine, (NVP) combinations in pediatric subjects with advanced HIV disease (ACTG 245)," Abstract No. 271, Conference on Retroviruses and Opportunistic Infections, 1998.
66. Sandra K. Burchett and Katherine Luzuriaga, cochairs, ClinicalTrials.gov, 1999, NCT00000814. The final protocol consisted of three placebo-controlled treatment groups of 130 patients each: nevirapine/AZT/ddI, nevirapine/ddI, and AZT/ddI.
67. James Keirns, interview, September 19, 2011.

Chapter 16

1. Maureen Myers, interview, November 17, 2011.
2. Richard T. D'Aquila et al., "Nevirapine, zidovudine, and didanosine compared with zidovudine and didanosine in patients with HIV-1 infection," *Annals of Internal Medicine* 124 (1996): 1019–1030.
3. From NDA 20-636 Medical Review (1996): change in $\log_{10}$ HIV-RNA (copies/ml) was 0.11; change in absolute CD4 count (cells/mm^2) was -15.60 at weeks 40–48.
4. From NDA 20-636 Medical Review (1996): change in $\log_{10}$ HIV-RNA (copies/ml) was -0.14; change in absolute CD4 count (cells/mm^2) was 5.81 at weeks 40–48.
5. John S. James, "Nevirapine triple combination: preliminary results," *AIDS Treatment News*, November 18, 1994; "Nevirapine triple combination shows efficacy for treatment of HIV-infection," *Antiviral Agents Bulletin*, December 1994.
6. Maureen Myers, quoted by Robert Miller, "Boehringer HIV fighter drug looks promising," *Danbury News-Times*, December 16, 1994.
7. Maureen Myers, interview, November 17, 2011.
8. A. Carr et al., "A controlled trial of nevirapine plus zidovudine versus zidovudine alone in p24 antigenaemic HIV-infected patients," *AIDS* (1996): 635–641; BI studies 1011, 1037, and 1038.
9. Julio Montaner, interview, January 31, 2012.
10. Julio Montaner, interview, January 31, 2012.
11. Julio Montaner, interview, January 31, 2012; Joep Lange, interview, February 28, 2012.
12. Julio Montaner et al., "A randomized, double-blind trial comparing combinations of nevirapine, didanosine, and zidovudine for HIV-infected patients," *JAMA* 279 (1998): 930–937; NDA 20-636 Medical Review (1996) 28–29.
13. David W. Barry and Linda M. Distlerath, "History and accomplishments of inter-company collaboration for AIDS drug development," *Drug Information Journal* 34 (2000): 741–752.
14. M. Thompson et al., "A master protocol to evaluate the safety and efficacy of multidrug combination antiretroviral therapy with zidovudine and zalcitabine with or without saquinavir or nevirapine for the treatment of HIV infection," Abstract No. 242, Conference on Retroviruses and Opportunistic Infections, 1997. The drug combinations were nevirapine+AZT+ddC vs. AZT+ddC+saquinavir vs. AZT+ddC.
15. The drug combinations were nevirapine+AZT+ddI vs AZT+ddI+3TC.
16. Patrick Robinson, interview, December 22, 2011.
17. Randy Kennedy, "Elizabeth Glaser dies at 47: Crusader for pediatric AIDS," *New York Times*, December 4, 1994.
18. Arthur Ammann, interview, March 2, 2012; Trish Karlin, interview, March 8, 2012.
19. Kennedy, "Elizabeth Glaser dies"; Jake Glaser, interview, September 19, 2012.
20. Josh Baran, quoted by David Ellis, "The defiant one," *People Magazine*, December 19, 1994.
21. Ellis, "The defiant one."
22. Jake Glaser, interview, September 19, 2012.
23. Arthur Ammann, interview, March 2, 2012.
24. Elizabeth Glaser, Address to the Democratic National Convention, July 14, 1992.
25. Elizabeth Glaser and Laura Palmer, *In the absence of angels: A Hollywood family's courageous story* (New York: Putnam, 1991), 306.

Chapter 17

1. Gina Kolata, "FDA debate on speedy access to AIDS drugs is reopening," *New York Times*, September 12, 1994.
2. Pamela Strode, interview, February 8, 2012.
3. Pamela Strode, interview, February 8, 2012.
4. Maureen Myers, interview, November 29, 2011.
5. Pamela Strode, interview, February 8, 2012.
6. Pamela Strode, interview, February 8, 2012.
7. Pamela Strode, interview, February 8, 2012.
8. Strode and Watson developed a coordinated division of regulatory responsibilities, in which Strode focused on the preclinical/clinical sections and Watson on the chemistry/manufacturing/controls sections. This model was soon adopted by the company's regulatory departments as the model for preparing BI's future regulatory submissions worldwide.
9. John Tiso, interview, November 16, 2011.
10. Peter Grob, interview, October 20, 2011. Grob coordinated preparation of the microbiology/resistance data.
11. Pamela Strode, interview, February 8, 2012.
12. Keith Henry et al., "A randomized, controlled, double-blind study comparing the survival benefit of four different reverse transcriptase inhibitor therapies (three-drug, two-drug, and alternating drug) for the treatment of advanced AIDS," *Journal of Acquired Immune Deficiency Syndrome and Human Retrovirology* 19 (1998): 339–349. The study was ACTG 193a. The four groups received AZT alternating monthly with ddI, AZT plus ddC, AZT plus ddI, or AZT plus ddI plus nevirapine.

13. Henry et al., "Survival benefit for advanced AIDS."
14. The goal of this survival study was observing a total of 525 deaths. Patients were randomized between June 24, 1993, and November 7, 1995. Close out was between April 15 and June 14, 1996.
15. Maureen Myers, interview, November 29, 2011; Joep Lange, interview, February 28, 2012.
16. Joep Lange, "Efficacy and durability of nevirapine in antiretroviral drug naïve patients," *Journal of Acquired Immune Deficiency Syndromes* 34 (2003): S40–S52. The study was BI 1090. All patients received 3TC, but could opt to substitute AZT for another antiretroviral agent and many chose to take an HIV protease inhibitor.
17. Pamela Strode, interview, February 24, 2012.
18. FDA Antiviral Drugs Advisory Committee meeting, June 7, 1996, 13, 18.
19. Vincent Merluzzi, interview, July 5, 2011.
20. Elsa Scott, "Marinol: The little synthetic that couldn't," *High Times*, July 1994; Boehringer Ingelheim, "Viramune® receives accelerated approval to treat AIDS: Represents first drug in class to receive designation," press release, June 24, 1996.
21. Pamela Strode, interview, February 8, 2012.
22. NDA 20–636.
23. Pamela Strode, interview, February 8, 2012.
24. UNAIDS, "AIDS epidemic update," December 2009, 7.
25. Pamela Strode, interview, February 8, 2012; Maureen Myers, interview, November 29, 2011; Mike Tsianco, interview, January 27, 2012.
26. Mike Tsianco, interview, January 27, 2012.
27. FDA Antiviral Drugs Advisory Committee meeting, June 7, 1996, 15.
28. Patrick Robinson, interview, December 22, 2011.
29. David Hall, interview, December 9, 2011; Pamela Strode, interview, February 8, 2012.
30. Pamela Strode, interview, February 8, 2012; Maureen Myers, interview, November 29, 2011.
31. Pamela Strode, interview, February 8, 2012.
32. Pamela Strode, interview, February 8, 2012.
33. Maureen Myers, interview, November 29, 2011.
34. Pamela Strode, interview, February 8, 2012.
35. Pamela Strode, interview, February 8, 2012.
36. Pamela Strode, interview, February 8, 2012.
37. NDA 20–636 Medical Review (1996) 4.
38. Pamela Strode, email, April 22, 2013.
39. Pamela Strode, interview, February 8, 2012.
40. Maureen Myers, interview, November 29, 2011.
41. Pamela Strode, interview, February 8, 2012.
42. NDA 20–636, FDA approval letter, June 21, 1996.
43. NDA 20–636 Medical Review (1996) 5.
44. NDA 20–636 Medical Review (1996) 13.
45. Mark Wainberg, interview, February 28, 2012.
46. Julio Montaner, interview, January 31, 2012.
47. Julio Montaner, interview, January 31, 2012; Mark Wainberg, interview, February 28, 2012.
48. Julio Montaner, interview, January 31, 2012.
49. Julio Montaner et al., "Rebound of plasma HIV viral load following prolonged suppression with combination therapy," *AIDS* 12 (1998): 1398–1399.
50. Colin is a fictitious name to protect the patient's identity, but this is a documented clinical case.
51. Montaner et al., "Rebound of viral load." The patient's pre-treatment viral load was 2142 copies/ml.
52. Douglas Richman, interview, December 8, 2011.
53. Diane Havlir, interview, February 17, 2012.
54. Maureen Myers, interview, November 29, 2011.
55. Maureen W. Myers and Julio G. Montaner, "A randomized, double-blinded comparative trial of the effects of zidovudine, didanosine and nevirapine combinations in antiviral naïve, AIDS-free, HIV-infected patients with CD4 counts 200–600/mm^3," Abstract No. Mo.B.294, 11th International AIDS Conference, Vancouver, 1996; NDA 20–636 Medical Review (1996) 28.
56. Myers and Montaner, "Nevirapine combinations in AIDS-free patients."
57. Julio Montaner, interview, January 31, 2012; Maureen Myers, interview, November 29, 2011.
58. NDA 20–636 Medical Review (1996) 28; Pamela Strode, interview, February 8, 2012; Myers, interview, November 29, 2011.
59. NDA 20–636 Medical Review (1996) 28.
60. Pamela Strode, interview, February 8, 2012.
61. David Hall, interview, December 9, 2011; Pamela Strode, interview, February 8, 2012.
62. NDA 20–636 Medical Review (1996) 28; David Hall, interview, December 9, 2011; Myers, interview, November 29, 3011.
63. NDA 20–636 Chemistry Review (1996) 2; NDA 20–636, FDA approval letter, June 21, 1996.
64. Pamela Strode, interview, February 8, 2012.
65. FDA Antiviral Drugs Advisory Committee meeting, June 7, 1996, 13–18.
66. FDA Antiviral Drugs Advisory Committee meeting, June 7, 1996, 18–61.
67. Pamela Strode, interview, February 8, 2012.
68. Spokespersons were Jules Levin, National AIDS Treatment Advocacy Project in New York, Spencer Cox, Treatment Action Group in New York, and Martin Delaney, Project Inform in San Francisco.
69. Jules Levin quoted at FDA Antiviral Drugs Advisory Committee meeting, June 7, 1996, 141.
70. Martin Delaney quoted at FDA Antiviral Drugs Advisory Committee meeting, June 7, 1996, 145–146.
71. Martin Delaney quoted at FDA Antiviral Drugs Advisory Committee meeting, June 7, 1996, 150–151.
72. James Keirns, interview, September 19, 2011; Thomas MacGregor, interview, January 23, 2012.
73. NDA 20–636 Medical Review (1996) 41.
74. Julio Montaner et al., "A randomized, double-blind trial comparing combinations of nevirapine, didanosine, and zidovudine for HIV-infected patients," *JAMA* 279 (1998): 930–937.
75. Montaner et al., "Combinations of nevirapine, didanosine and zidovudine."
76. Maureen Myers, interview, November 17, 2011; FDA Antiviral Drugs Advisory Committee meeting, June 7, 1996, 13–14.
77. FDA Antiviral Drugs Advisory Committee meeting, June 7, 1996, 185–206.
78. Mark Harrington, "Once we were warriors: Activist corpses born in protest, furtive legislative coups, and the devastation that was Berlin," *The Body*, March 2002; Joep Lange, interview, February 28, 2012.
79. Scott Hammer, quoted in FDA Antiviral Drugs Advisory Committee meeting, June 7, 1996, 177.
80. Scott Hammer, quoted in FDA Antiviral Drugs Advisory Committee meeting, June 7, 1996, 177.
81. Patrick Robinson, interview, December 22, 2011; Fred Valentine, quoted in FDA Antiviral Drugs Advisory Committee meeting, June 7, 1996, 179–180.
82. Maureen Myers, interview, November 17, 2011.
83. Patrick Robinson, interview, December 22, 2011.
84. NDA 20–636, BI letter to FDA, June 20, 1996.
85. Pamela Strode, interview, February 8, 2012.
86. NDA 20–636, FDA letter to BI, June 21, 1996.
87. NDA 20–636 Medical Review (1996) 41. The actual FDA-approved indication for Viramune® (nevirapine) was

for use "in combination with nucleoside analogues for the treatment of HIV-1 infected adults who have experienced clinical and/or immunologic deterioration."
88. Pamela Strode, interview, February 8, 2012.
89. NDA 20-636, 3.0 Chemistry, Manufacturing and Controls, Environmental Assessment Amendment, March 29, 1996, 12; Boehringer Ingelheim, "Viramune® receives accelerated approval," press release, June 24, 1996.
90. Boehringer Ingelheim, "Viramune® receives accelerated approval." BI launched an expanded access program in March 1996 and transitioned patients after FDA approval in June.
91. Boehringer Ingelheim, "Viramune® receives accelerated approval."
92. Pamela Strode, interview, February 8, 2012.
93. EPAR: Viramune Background Information. The marketing application was submitted through the centralized procedure, Prof. M. Forte was the designated Rapporteur and Pharm. G. De Greff was the Co-Rapporteur.
94. Pamela Strode, interview, February 8, 2012.
95. Pamela Strode, interview, February 8, 2012.
96. Boehringer Ingelheim, "Potent new HIV/AIDS drug focus of European Conference," press release, March 12, 1998.
97. Julio Montaner, interview, January 31, 2012.
98. Thomas Maugh, "Studies of combined HIV drugs promising," *Los Angeles Times*, July 12, 1996.
99. John W. Mellors et al., "Prognosis in HIV-1 infection predicted by the quantity of virus in plasma," *Science* 272 (1996): 1167–1170; John W. Mellors et al., "Plasma viral load and CD4+ lymphocytes as prognostic markers of HIV-1 infection," *Annals of Internal Medicine* 126 (1997): 946–954; William A. O'Brien et al., "Changes in plasma HIV-1 RNA and CD4+ lymphocyte counts and the risk of progression to AIDS," *New England Journal of Medicine* 334 (1996): 426–431; R. W. Coombs et al., "Association of plasma human immunodeficiency virus type 1 RNA level with risk of clinical progression in patients with advanced infection," *Journal of Infectious Diseases* 174 (1996): 704–712.
100. Roche's Amplicor HIV-1 Monitor Test was approved by FDA on June 3, 1996.
101. David Feigal, interview, May 24, 2012.
102. David Feigal, interview, May 24, 2012.
103. David Feigal, interview, May 24, 2012; NDA 20-636 Medical Review (1996) 41.
104. 3TC was approved on November 17, 1995, saquinavir on December 6, 1995, ritonavir on March 1, 1996, and indinavir on March 13, 1996.
105. Roy M. Gulick et al., "Treatment with indinavir, zidovudine, and lamivudine in adults with human immunodeficiency virus infection and prior antiretroviral therapy," *New England Journal of Medicine* 337 (1997): 734–739; Scott M. Hammer et al., "A controlled trial of two nucleoside analogues plus indinavir in persons with human immunodeficiency virus infection and CD4 cell counts of 200 per cubic millimeter or less," *New England Journal of Medicine* 337 (1997): 725–733.
106. Warren E. Leary, "Scientists optimistic on use of new therapies for AIDS," *New York Times*, June 15, 1996; Hammer et al., "Two nucleoside analogues plus indinavir," 725–733.
107. Lawrence K. Altman, "Scientists display substantial gains in AIDS treatment," *New York Times*, July 12, 1996.
108. John A. Bartlett, "Management and counseling for persons with HIV infection," in *Cecil Textbook of Medicine*, eds. J. Claude Bennett and Fred Plum (Philadelphia: Saunders, 1996), 1888.
109. Centers for Disease Control and Prevention, "HIV/AIDS surveillance report," December 1999, 31.
110. David D. Ho, "Time to hit HIV, early and hard," *New England Journal of Medicine* 333 (1995): 450–451.
111. David D. Ho, "Dynamics of HIV-1 replication in vivo," *Journal of Clinical Investigation* 99 (1997): 2565–2567.
112. Montaner et al., "Rebound of viral load."
113. In June 1996, Montaner replaced ddI with 3TC, because Colin experienced stomach and gut irritation from ddI treatment.
114. Montaner et al., "Rebound of viral load."
115. David Barr, "Yin and Yang: Yokohama, Vancouver, Twin Pacific Ports, serve as polar opposites for scientific advances," *The Body*, March 2003.
116. Julio Montaner, interview, January 31, 2012.
117. John Bowersox, "NIAID's clinical trial ACTG 241 was central to nevirapine FDA approval," press release, September 1996.
118. Steven M Schnittman, quoted by John Bowersox, "Nevirapine FDA approval," September 1996.

Chapter 18

1. Mark Mirochnick et al., "Pharmacokinetics of nevirapine in human immunodeficiency virus type 1-infected pregnant women and their neonates," *Journal of Infectious Diseases* 178 (1998): 368–374. The study was ACTG 250.
2. Mirochnick et al., "Nevirapine in pregnant women and neonates."
3. FDA Antiviral Drugs Advisory Committee meeting, June 7, 1996, 158.
4. FDA Antiviral Drugs Advisory Committee meeting, June 7, 1996, 158.
5. FDA Antiviral Drugs Advisory Committee meeting, June 7, 1996, 160.
6. Mark Wainberg, interview, February 28, 2012.
7. Thomas Maugh, "Studies of combined HIV drugs promising," *Los Angeles Times*, July 12, 1996.
8. Abigail Zuger, "XI international AIDS conference: Two worlds, two hopes," *Journal Watch*, September 1, 1996.
9. Connie Osborne, quoted by Abigail Zugar, "Two worlds, two hopes," September 1, 1996.
10. Florence Ngobeni-Allen, interview, October 30, 2012.
11. Florence Ngobeni-Allen, interview, October 30, 2012.
12. Florence Ngobeni-Allen, interview, October 30, 2012.
13. Florence Ngobeni-Allen, "AIDS@30," December 2, 2011.
14. Florence Ngobeni-Allen, interview, October 30, 2012.
15. Florence Ngobeni-Allen, "AIDS@30," December 2, 2011.
16. Florence Ngobeni-Allen, interview, October 30, 2012
17. Florence Ngobeni-Allen, AIDS@30, December 2, 2011.
18. John Sullivan, interview, December 6, 2011.
19. John Sullivan, interview, December 6, 2011.
20. Laura Guay, interview, March 14, 2012. Zaire is now the Democratic Republic of the Congo.
21. Susan A. Cohen, "Beyond slogans: Lessons from Uganda's experience with ABC and HIV/AIDS," *Guttmacher Report* 6 (2003): 1–3; Annie Kelly, "Background: HIV/AIDS in Uganda," *The Guardian*, December 1, 2008.
22. Laura Guay, interview, February 29, 2012.
23. Laura Guay, interview, March 14, 2012.

24. Alejandro Dorenbaum et al., "Two-dose intrapartum/newborn nevirapine and standard antiretroviral therapy to reduce perinatal HIV transmission," *JAMA* 288 (2002): 189–198. The study was PACTG 316.
25. Dorenbaum et al., "Two-dose nevirapine to reduce HIV transmission."
26. John Sullivan, interview, December 6, 2011.
27. J. Brooks Jackson, interview, February 29, 2012.
28. Maureen Myers, interview, November 17, 2011.
29. Douglas Wilson, letter to J. Brooks Jackson, August 25, 1997.
30. Maureen Myers, interview, March 19, 2012; Douglas Wilson, letter to J. Brooks Jackson, August 25, 1997.
31. *Global Strategies for HIV Prevention Newsletter*, June 2002.
32. Arthur Ammann, interview, February 24, 2012.
33. Maureen Myers, interview, November 29, 2011.
34. Arthur Ammann, interview, February 24, 2012.
35. Marcia Angell, "The ethics of clinical research in the third world," *New England Journal of Medicine* 337 (1997): 847–849.
36. Lawrence K. Altman, "AIDS experts leave journal after studies are criticized," *New York Times*, October 15, 1997.
37. Catherine Wilfert, quoted by Lawrence Altman, "AIDS experts leave journal."
38. Harold Varmus and David Satcher, "Ethical complexities of conducting research in developing countries," *New England Journal of Medicine* 337 (1997): 1003–1005.
39. Stephen Lagakos et al., *Review of the HIVNET 012 perinatal HIV prevention study* (Washington, DC: National Academies Press, 2005), 28.
40. Edward K. Mbidde, quoted by Harold Varmus and David Satcher, "Ethical complexities."
41. Laura Guay, interview, March 14, 2012; Lagakos et al., "Review of HIVNET 012," 29.
42. Philippa Musoke et al., "A phase I/II study of the safety and pharmacokinetics of nevirapine in HIV-1-infected pregnant Ugandan women and their neonates (HIVNET 006)," *AIDS* 13 (1999): 479–486. The study was HIVNET 006.
43. Musoke et al., "Safety of nevirapine in Ugandan neonates."
44. The nevirapine regimen consisted of 200 mg at onset of labor to the mother and 2 mg/kg to the infants within 72 hr of birth. The AZT regimen consisted of 600 mg at the onset of labor, followed by 300 mg every 3 hr until delivery to the mothers and 4 mg/kg twice daily for 7 days to the infants.
45. Nathan Shaffer et al., "Short-course zidovudine for perinatal HIV-1 transmission in Bangkok, Thailand: A randomized controlled trial," *Lancet* 353 (1999): 773–780. The Thailand study's abbreviated treatment schedule was twice daily AZT starting at 36 weeks gestation and every 3 hours from onset of labor until delivery; no AZT treatment to the infant.
46. Centers for Disease Control and Prevention, "Administration of zidovudine during late pregnancy and delivery to prevent perinatal HIV transmission — Thailand, 1996–1998," *Morbidity and Mortality Weekly Report* 47 (1998): 151–154.
47. Lagakos et al., "Review of HIVNET 012," 33.
48. Lagakos et al., "Review of HIVNET 012," 30.
49. J. Brooks Jackson, interview, February 29, 2012.
50. HIVNET 012 Proposed Interim Plan, quoted in Lagakos et al., "Review of HIVNET 012," 30.
51. Lagakos et al., "Review of HIVNET 012," 90–91. The requirement to include fathers in the informed consent process was imposed by the Division of AIDS at NIH and the IRBs; it exceeded U.S. regulatory requirements.
52. Lagakos et al., "Review of HIVNET 012," 90.
53. J. Brooks Jackson, interview, February 29, 2012.
54. Laura Guay, interview, March 14, 2012; Lakagos et al., "Review of HIVNET 012," 90.
55. Lagakos et al., "Review of HIVNET 012," 92.
56. Lagakos et al., "Review of HIVNET 012," 51–52.
57. Laura Guay, interview, March 14, 2012.
58. Laura Guay, interview, March 14, 2012.
59. Laura Guay, interview, March 14, 2012.
60. Lagakos et al., "Review of HIVNET 012," 57–58.
61. The statistical center supporting the data management and analysis of HIVNET 012 was SCHARP, Statistical Center for HIV/AIDS Research and Prevention at the Fred Hutchinson Cancer Center in Seattle, Washington.
62. Laura Guay, interview, March 14, 2012.
63. J. Brooks Jackson, interview, February 29, 2012.
64. Lagakos et al., "Review of HIVNET 012," 25. The DSMB met on June 24, 1999.
65. NIAID, "A Phase IIB randomized, controlled trial to evaluate the safety, tolerance, and HIV vertical transmission rates associated with short course nevirapine (NVP) vs. short course zidovudine (ZDV) in HIV infected pregnant women and their infants in Uganda," news release, July 12, 1999.
66. Laura A. Guay, et al., "Intrapartum and neonatal single-dose nevirapine compared with zidovudine for prevention of mother-to-child transmission of HIV-1 in Kampala, Uganda: HIVNET 012 randomized trial," *Lancet* 354 (1999): 795–802.
67. Laura Guay, interview, March 14, 2012.
68. J. Brooks Jackson, interview, February 29, 2012; Laura Guay, interview, March 14, 2012.
69. Laura Guay, interview, March 14, 2012.
70. Lagakos et al., "Review of HIVNET 012," 25.
71. Guay et al., "Nevirapine compared with zidovudine in Uganda," 795–802. At 14–16 weeks, the risk of transmission in the nevirapine group was 13.1 percent compared with 25.1 percent in the AZT group, a 47 percent reduction.
72. NIAID, "Researchers identify a simple, affordable drug regimen that is highly effective in preventing HIV infection in infants of mothers with the disease," news release, July 14, 1999.
73. NIAID, "Researchers identify a simple, affordable regimen."
74. Anthony Fauci, quoted by Lawrence K. Altman, "New means found for reducing HIV passed to child," *New York Times*, July 15, 1999.
75. Altman, "Reducing HIV passed to child."
76. Guay et al., "Nevirapine compared with zidovudine in Uganda."
77. Michael Chung et al., "Breast milk HIV-1 suppression and decreased transmission: A randomized trial comparing HIVNET 012 nevirapine versus short-course zidovudine," *AIDS* 19 (2005): 1415–1422.
78. Boehringer Ingelheim, "Results of landmark studies support use of AIDS drug Viramune® (nevirapine)," press release, October 25, 1999.
79. Guay et al., "Nevirapine compared with zidovudine in Uganda."
80. Guay et al., "Nevirapine compared with zidovudine in Uganda."
81. In the nevirapine group, mothers received one 200 mg dose during labor and another dose 1–2 days after delivery and the infants received one 6 mg dose 1–2 days after delivery. In the other group, mothers received a loading dose of 600 mg AZT and 150 mg 3TC followed by 300 mg of AZT and 150 mg of 3TC every 12 hours until

delivery, followed by twice-daily 300 mg AZT and 150 mg 3TC for one week; infants weighing > 2 kg received twice-daily doses of 12 mg AZT and 6 mg 3TC for one week, starting at 12 hours after birth; infants weighing < 2 kg received 4 mg/kg AZT and 2 mg/kg 3TC.

Chapter 19

1. James Hale, "After Montreal, international AIDS conferences will never be the same," *Canadian Medical Association Journal* 141 (1989): 144–146; Tim McCaskell, "Taking our place," *The Positive Side*, Summer 2011.
2. David Barr, "Enemies at the gate: Storming Montreal's Palais de Congrès, and makeshift battle stations in fortress San Francisco," *The Body*, December, 2002.
3. Zambian President Kenneth Kaunda, quoted by James Hale, "After Montreal."
4. Hale, "After Montreal."
5. Hale, "After Montreal."
6. Hale, "After Montreal."
7. Hale, "After Montreal."
8. Arthur Ammann, interview, February 24, 2012.
9. Arthur Ammann, interview, February 24, 2012.
10. Catherine Wilfert, interview, January 18, 2012.
11. Russell B. Van Dyke et al., "The Ariel Project: A prospective cohort study of maternal-child transmission of human immunodeficiency virus type 1 in the era of maternal antiretroviral therapy," *Journal of Infectious Diseases* 179 (1999): 319–328.
12. *Global Strategies for HIV Prevention Newsletter*, June 2002. By 1999, the incidence of HIV-infected newborns had dropped from 2000 per year to less than 200.
13. Arthur Ammann, Call to Action, Global Strategies for HIV Prevention, 2003.
14. Catherine Wilfert, email to Arthur Ammann, August 25, 1999.
15. David S. MacDougall, "The second conference on global strategies for the prevention of HIV transmission from mothers to infants," *Global Strategies for HIV Prevention*, September 2–5, 1999.
16. Catherine Wilfert, interview, January 18, 2012.
17. Keri Oberg, interview, February 2, 2012.
18. Trish Karlin, interview, March 8, 2012.
19. Trish Karlin, interview, March 8, 2012.
20. Arthur Ammann, personal communication.
21. *Global Strategies for HIV Prevention Newsletter*, January 2000 and June 2002; J. Brooks Jackson, interview, February 29, 2012.
22. Catherine Wilfert, interview, January 18, 2012.
23. Catherine Wilfert, interview, January 18, 2012; David Kessler, interview, December 12, 2011.
24. *Global Strategies for HIV Prevention Newsletter*, June 2002.
25. Trish Karlin, interview, March 8, 2012.
26. Catherine Wilfert, interview, January 18, 2012; Jessica Roseberry, "Catherine Wilfert Interview," *Women in Duke medicine: An oral history exhibit*, August 25, 2006.
27. *Global Strategies for HIV Prevention Newsletter*, June 2002; Boehringer Ingelheim, "Boehringer Ingelheim offers Viramune® (nevirapine) free of charge to developing economies for the prevention of HIV-1 mother-to-child transmission," press release, July 7, 2000; Boehringer Ingelheim, "World AIDS day report: First supplies of Viramune® donation program for developing countries," press release, November 28, 2000.
28. Trish Karlin, interview, March 8, 2012.
29. Catherine Wilfert, interview, January 18, 2012
30. Catherine Wilfert, interview, January 18, 2012.
31. Roseberry, "Catherine Wilfert Interview," August 25, 2006.
32. Laura Guay, interview, March 14, 2012.
33. Catherine Wilfert, interview, January 18, 2012.
34. Roseberry, "Catherine Wilfert Interview."
35. Roseberry, "Catherine Wilfert Interview."
36. Roseberry, "Catherine Wilfert Interview."
37. Catherine Wilfert, interview, January 18, 2012.
38. Mark Wainberg, interview, February 28, 2012.
39. Mark Wainberg, interview, February 28, 2012.
40. Edwin Cameron, "The deafening silence of AIDS," 13th International AIDS Conference, Durban, plenary presentation, July 10, 2000.
41. Edwin Cameron and Nathan Geffen, *Witness to AIDS* (London: I.B. Tauris, 2005), 9, 121.
42. Cameron, "Deafening silence"; Samantha Power, "The AIDS rebel," *The New Yorker*, May 19, 2003.
43. Edwin Cameron, interview, June 13, 2012.
44. Edwin Cameron, interview, June 13, 2012.
45. Cameron, "Deafening silence."
46. Power, "The AIDS rebel."
47. Jonathan Mann, quoted by Edwin Cameron, "Deafening silence."
48. Cameron, "Deafening silence."
49. Boehringer Ingelheim, "Nevirapine free of charge," July 7, 2000; Lawrence K. Altman, "Report dims hope for AIDS therapy to protect babies," *New York Times*, July 8, 2000.
50. Boehringer Ingelheim, "World AIDS day report," November 28, 2000.
51. Jeffery Stringer et al., "Timing of the maternal drug dose and risk of perinatal HIV transmission in the setting of intrapartum and neonatal single-dose nevirapine," *AIDS* 17 (2003): 1659–1665; Dhayendre Moodley et al., "A multicenter randomized controlled trial of nevirapine versus a combination of zidovudine and lamivudine to reduce intrapartum and early postpartum mother-to-child transmission of human immunodeficiency virus type 1," *Journal of Infectious Diseases* 187 (2003): 725–735; Taha E. Taha et al., "Nevirapine and zidovudine at birth to reduce perinatal transmission of HIV in an African setting: A randomized controlled trial," *JAMA* 292 (2004): 202–209; Benjamin H. Chi et al., "Timing of maternal and neonatal dosing of nevirapine and the risk of mother-to-child transmission of HIV-1: HIVNET 024," *AIDS* 19 (2005): 1857–1864; Michael H. Chung et al., "Breast milk HIV-1 suppression and decreased transmission: A randomized trial comparing HIVNET 012 nevirapine versus short-course zidovudine," *AIDS* 19 (2005): 1415–1422; Paul Thistle et al., "A randomized, double-blind, placebo-controlled trial of combined nevirapine and zidovudine compared with nevirapine alone in the prevention of perinatal transmission of HIV in Zimbabwe," *Clinical Infectious Diseases* 44 (2007): 111–119.
52. Haroon Saloojee, "The real value of nevirapine," in *Nevirapine—godsend or drug from hell?* May 29, 2002; Boehringer Ingelheim, "World AIDS day report," November 28, 2000.

Chapter 20

1. Jason, Jane, and Maria are fictitious names to protect the patients' identity, but they represent a documented clinical case.
2. Katherine Luzuriaga et al., "Combination treatment with zidovudine, didanosine, and nevirapine in infants with human immunodeficiency virus type 1 infection," *New England Journal of Medicine* 336 (1997): 1343–1349.

3. The standard assay at this time measured HIV-1 RNA by PCR after reverse transcription (Amplicor HIV-1 Monitor Test, Roche), and the limit of detection was 400 copies per milliliter of plasma.

4. Luzuriaga et al., "Combination treatment in infants"; Luzuriaga et al., "Absent HIV-specific immune responses and replication-competent HIV reservoirs in perinatally infected youth treated from infancy: Toward cure," Abstract No. 171LB, Atlanta, March 3–6, 2013.

5. David Feigal, quoted at FDA Antiviral Drugs Advisory Committee meeting, June 7, 1996, 211.

6. David Feigal, quoted at FDA Antiviral Drugs Advisory Committee meeting, June 7, 1996, 211.

7. John Sullivan, quoted at FDA Antiviral Drugs Advisory Committee meeting, June 7, 1996, 160.

8. David Feigal, quoted at FDA Antiviral Drugs Advisory Committee meeting, June 7, 1996, 211.

9. Sandra K. Burchett et al., "Virologic activity of didanosine (ddI), zidovudine (ZDV), and nevirapine, (NVP) combinations in pediatric subjects with advanced HIV disease (ACTG 245)," Abstract No. 271, Conference on Retrovirology and Opportunistic Infections, 1998; Sandra K. Burchett et al., "Combinations of didanosine (ddI), zidovudine (ZDV) and nevirapine (NVP) can reduce CSF HIV-1 viral load in pediatric patients with advanced HIV disease," Abstract No. 12253, 12th International AIDS Conference, Geneva, 1998; ClinicalTrials.gov No. NCT00000814. The three groups in the ACTG 245 trial were nevirapine/AZT/ddI vs. nevirapine/ddI vs. AZT/ddI.

10. NDA 20–636/SE1–009 and 20–933 Administrative Documents/Correspondence (1998) Record of FDA/Industry [Pre-NDA] Meeting, June 25, 1997.

11. NDA 20–636/SE1–009 and 20–933 Medical Review (1998) 19.

12. NDA 20–636/SE1–009 and 20–933 Administrative Documents/Correspondence (1998) Record of FDA/Industry [Pre-NDA] Meeting, June 25, 1997.

13. NDA 20–636/SE1–009 (1998).

14. Both children had switched to a regimen of 3TC, d4T, and nelfinavir. Viral load was determined by HIV-RNA assay.

15. NDA 20–933 (1998).

16. ACTG 250, HIVNET 012, PACTG 316, cited in NDA 20–636/SE1–009 and 20–933 Medical Review (1998) 4, 5, 27.

17. Heidi Jolson, FDA Approval Letter for NDA 20–636/SE1–009 and 20–933, September 11, 1998; NDA 20–636/SE1–009 and 20–933 Administrative Documents/Correspondence (1998).

18. Heidi Jolson, FDA Approval Letter for NDA 20–636/SE1–009 and 20–933, September 11, 1998.

19. EPAR: Viramune Steps Taken after Granting Marketing Authorization.

20. NDA 20–636/SE1–009 and 20–933 Medical Review (1998) 30.

21. John Sullivan, quoted in Boehringer Ingelheim, "First NNRTI suspension, Viramune®, now available for use in HIV-positive children: European Commission approval advances fight against pediatric HIV/AIDS," press release, July 7, 1999.

22. WHO statistics, quoted in Boehringer Ingelheim, "First NNRTI available," July 7, 1999.

23. Jake Glaser, interview, September 19, 2012.
24. Jake Glaser, interview, September 19, 2012.
25. Jake Glaser, interview, September 19, 2012.
26. Jake Glaser, interview, September 19, 2012.
27. Jake Glaser, interview, September, 19, 2012.
28. Jake Glaser, interview, September 19, 2012.
29. Jake Glaser, interview, September 19, 2012.
30. Jake Glaser, interview, September 19, 2012.
31. Jamie Gentille, interview, August 28, 2012.
32. Jamie Gentille, interview, August 28, 2012.
33. Jamie Gentille, interview, August 28, 2012.
34. The trials were ACTG 193a and BI 1090, respectively.

35. NDA 20–636/017 and 20–933/007 Medical Review (2002) 5.

36. David Hall, interview, December 9, 2011; Pamela Strode, interview, February 8, 2012.

37. FDA Guidance for Industry: Antiretroviral drugs using plasma HIV RNA measurements, October 2002.

38. NDA 20–636/017 and 20–933/007, FDA letter to Kevin Dransfield, March 27, 2002.

39. NDA 20–636/017 and 20–933/007 Group Leader's Memorandum (2002) 2. A person-year is the number of years times the number of people who have been treated.

40. NDA 20–636/017 and 20–933/007 Medical Review (2002) 4. Clinical trials were BI-1090, Atlantic/BI-1229, INCAS/BI-1046, BI-1037, and BI-1038.

41. David Hall, interview, December 9, 2011.

42. Joep Lange et al., "Efficacy and durability of nevirapine in antiretroviral drug naïve patients," *Journal of Acquired Immune Deficiency Syndromes* 34 (2003): S40–S52. FDA approval was based on the 48 week data, and the label was later updated to include the 96 week data.

43. FDA letter to Kevin Dransfield, March 27, 2002.
44. Pamela Strode, interview, February 8, 2012.
45. Boehringer Ingelheim, "Viramune® receives full marketing approval," press release, July 9, 2002.

46. P. Krogstad et al., "Nucleoside-analogue reverse-transcriptase inhibitors plus nevirapine, nelfinavir, or ritonavir for pretreated children infected with human immunodeficiency virus type 1," *Clinical Infectious Diseases* 34 (2002): 991–1001; Gwenda Verweel et al., "Nevirapine use in HIV-1-infected children," *AIDS* 17 (2003): 1639–1647; Katherine Luzuriaga et al., "A trial of three antiretroviral regimens in HIV-1-infected children," *New England Journal of Medicine* 350 (2004): 2471–2480; Tripti Pensi, "Fixed-dose combination of lamivudine, stavudine and nevirapine in the treatment of pediatric HIV-infection: a preliminary report," *Indian Pediatrics* 44 (2007): 519–521.

47. Burchett et al., "Combinations of ddI, ZDV, and nevirapine reduce CSF viral load"; Sandra Burchett, presentation at FDA Antiviral Drugs Advisory Committee meeting, June 7, 1996, 165–166.

48. NDA 20–636/009 and 20–933 Medical Review (1998) 29–30.

49. Glenda Gray, "The PETRA study: Early and late efficacy of three short ZDV/3TC combination regimens to prevent mother-to-child transmission of HIV-1," Abstract No. LbOr5 2000, 13th International AIDS Conference, Durban, 2000.

50. Joep Lange, quoted by Lawrence K. Altman, "Report dims hope for AIDS therapy to protect babies," *New York Times*, July 8, 2000; PETRA Study Team, "Efficacy of three short-course regimens of zidovudine and lamivudine in preventing early and late transmission of HIV-1 from mother to child in Tanzania, South Africa, and Uganda (Petra study): A randomized, double-blind, placebo-controlled trial," *Lancet* 359 (2002): 1178–1186.

51. Maxensia Owor, "The one year safety and efficacy data of the HIVNET 012 trial," Abstract No. LbOr1 2000, 13th International AIDS Conference, Durban, 2000; Lawrence K. Altman, "AIDS studies on infants appear to conflict," *New York Times*, July 13, 2000; J. Brooks Jackson et al., "Intrapartum and neonatal single-dose nevirapine compared with zidovudine for prevention of mother-to-

child transmission of HIV-1 in Kampala, Uganda: 18-month follow-up of the HIVNET 012 randomised trial," *Lancet* 362 (2003): 859–868.

52. National Institutes of Health statement quoted by Lawrence Altman, "AIDS studies conflict," July 13, 2000.

53. Joep Lange, quoted by Bob Huff, "Let nevirapine do what it does best," *GMHC Treatment Issues*, March 10–11, 2002.

54. Stephen Lagakos et al., *Review of the HIVNET 012 perinatal HIV prevention study*, (Washington, DC: National Academies Press, 2005), 20.

55. Susan H. Eshleman et al., "Selection and fading of resistance mutations in women and infants receiving nevirapine to prevent HIV-1 vertical transmission (HIVNET 012)," *AIDS* 15 (2001): 1951–1957; Susan H. Eshleman and J. Brooks Jackson, "Nevirapine resistance after single dose prophylaxis," *AIDS Reviews* 4 (2002): 59–63.

56. Shayne Loubser et al., "Decay of K103N mutants in cellular DNA and plasma RNA after single-dose nevirapine to reduce mother-to-child HIV transmission," *AIDS* 20 (2006): 995–1002; Susan H. Eshleman et al., "Resistance after single-dose nevirapine prophylaxis emerges in a high proportion of Malawian newborns," *AIDS* 19 (2005): 2167–2175; Roger L. Shapiro et al., "Maternal single-dose nevirapine versus placebo as part of an antiretroviral strategy to prevent mother-to-child HIV transmission in Botswana," *AIDS* 20 (2006): 1281–1288.

57. Neil A. Martinson et al., "Transmission rates in consecutive pregnancies exposed to single-dose nevirapine in Soweto, South Africa and Abidjoan, Côte d'Ivoire," *Journal of Acquired Immune Deficiency Syndromes* 45 (2007): 206–209; Michelle S. McConnell et al., "Effectiveness of repeat single-dose nevirapine for prevention of mother-to-child transmission of HIV-1 in repeat pregnancies in Uganda," *Journal of Acquired Immune Deficiency Syndromes* 46 (2007): 291–296.

58. Shahin Lockman et al., "Response to antiviral therapy after a single, peripartum dose of nevirapine," *New England Journal of Medicine* 356 (2007): 135–147.

59. Lawrence K. Altman, "Infant drugs for HIV put mothers at risk," *New York Times*, February 10, 2004.

60. Alejandro Dorenbaum, et al., "Two-dose intrapartum/newborn nevirapine and standard antiretroviral therapy to reduce perinatal HIV transmission," *JAMA* 288 (2002): 189–198.

61. *Elizabeth Glaser Pediatric AIDS Foundation Annual Report*, 2001.

62. Boehringer Ingelheim, "World AIDS day 2001—Progress in the battle against AIDS," press release, November 30, 2001. The African countries were Burundi, Benin, Cameroon, Congo, Ghana, Ivory Coast, Kenya, Malawi, Namibia, Nigeria, Rwanda, Senegal, Sierra Leone, Uganda, Zambia, and Zimbabwe.

63. By permission, Arthur Ammann, Global Strategies for HIV Prevention.

64. Susan A. Cohen, "Beyond slogans: Lessons from Uganda's experience with ABC and HIV/AIDS," *Guttmacher Report on Public Policy* 6 (2003): 1–3.

65. Lawrence K. Altman, "A new regimen to fight AIDS in newborns," *New York Times*, July 18, 1999.

66. Adele Baleta, "South African government threatens to ban nevirapine," *Lancet* 362 (2003): 451; Rachel Swarns, "A move to force South Africa to give AIDS drug for newborns," *New York Times*, November 27, 2001.

67. George J. Annas, "Reply: The right to health and the nevirapine case in South Africa," *New England Journal of Medicine* 348 (2003): 2470; Sharon LaFraniere, "South Africa rejects use of AIDS drug for women," *New York Times*, July 14, 2004; Swarns, "Safety of common AIDS drug questioned in South Africa," *New York Times*, November 25, 1999.

68. Kerry Cullinan, "Court orders South Africa to treat pregnant HIV-positive women with nevirapine," *Bulletin of the World Health Organization* 80 (2002): 335.

69. Mark Wainberg, interview, February 28, 2012.

Chapter 21

1. Nkosi Johnson, 13th International AIDS Conference, Durban, keynote speech, July 9, 2000.

2. Nkosi Johnson, 13th International AIDS Conference, Durban, keynote speech, July 9, 2000.

3. Nkosi Johnson, 13th International AIDS Conference, Durban, keynote speech, July 9, 2000.

4. Richard Pithouse, "Report on global march for treatment access," *Treatment Action Campaign*, July 9, 2000; Janet Howse, "Treatment Access March," *South African Medical Journal*, July 9, 2000.

5. Tom Lodge, *Politics in South Africa: From Mandela to Mbeki* (Cape Town: David Philip, 2002), 241–243.

6. Edwin Cameron and Nathan Geffen, *Witness to AIDS* (London: I. B. Tauris, 2005), 125–126.

7. James Myburgh, "The Virodene affair (I): The secret history of the ANC's response to the HIV/AIDS epidemic," *Politicsweb*, September 17, 2007.

8. Lodge, *Politics in South Africa*, 256.

9. Lodge, *Politics in South Africa*, 227.

10. Myburgh, "Virodene affair (I)."

11. James Myburgh, "Virodene, transformation and the constitution," *Politicsweb*, March 19, 2012.

12. Myburgh, "Virodene affair (I)."

13. James Myburgh, "The Virodene affair (III): How the MCC was eventually taken out, and why Virodene was nonetheless still banned in SA," *Politicsweb*, September 18, 2007.

14. James Myburgh, "The Virodene affair (II): How Mbeki and Nkosazana Zuma allied with the Vissers against the MCC," *Politicsweb*, September 18, 2007.

15. ANC Secretary General Kgalema Mothanthe, quoted by James Myburgh, "Virodene affair (III)"; Lodge, *Politics in South Africa*, 256.

16. Myburgh, "Virodene affair (III)." The Commission consisted of two university-based experts, four Health Ministry employees, and a health advisor to Zuma.

17. James Myburgh, "The Virodene affair (IV): How the involvement in Virodene led to Thabo Mbeki's AIDS denialism," *Politicsweb*, September 20, 2007.

18. Cameron and Geffen, *Witness to AIDS*, 125.

19. Myburgh, "The Virodene affair (IV)."

20. Department of Health press release, quoted by James Myburgh, "The Virodene affair (IV)."

21. Lodge, *Politics in South Africa*, 257.

22. Thabo Mbeki, quoted by James Myburgh, "The Virodene affair (IV)."

23. Myburgh, "The Virodene affair (IV)"; Lodge, *Politics in South Africa*, 257.

24. Myburgh, "The Virodene affair (IV)."

25. Helen Schneider and Didier Fassin, "Denial and defiance: a socio-political analysis of AIDS in South Africa," *AIDS* 16 (2002): S45–S51.

26. Schneider and Fassin, "Denial and defiance."

27. Myburgh, "The Virodene affair (IV)"; Brink, "Debating AZT."

28. Ellen Cooper, interview, March 7, 2013.

29. Cameron and Geffen, *Witness to AIDS*, 135.

30. Thabo Mbeki, quoted by Rachel L. Swarns, "Safety

of AIDS drug questioned," November 25, 1999, and by Cameron and Geffen, *Witness to AIDS*, 104.

31. Swarns, "Safety of AIDS drug questioned"; Cameron and Geffen, *Witness to AIDS*, 106.

32. Lodge, *Politics in South Africa*, 257.

33. Manto Tshabalala-Msimang, quoted by Mark Heywood, "Preventing mother-to-child HIV transmission in South Africa," *South African Journal on Human Rights* 19 (2003): 278–315.

34. James Myburgh, "The Virodene affair (V): How the efficacy of Virodene was finally put to the test, and why the war on antiretrovirals ended," *Politicsweb* September 21, 2007.

35. Swarns, "Safety of AIDS drug questioned."

36. Pithouse, "Global march for treatment access."

37. Tony Karon, "South African AIDS activist Zackie Achmat," *Time*, April 19, 2001.

38. Pithouse, "Global march for treatment access"; African Success Biography, "Biography of Zackie Achmat," November 7, 2008.

39. Heywood, "Preventing HIV transmission in South Africa"; Swarns, "Safety of AIDS drug questioned."

40. Nevirapine treatment in the SAINT trial was 200 mg during labor and 200 mg 1–2 days after delivery to the mother and 6 mg within 3 days of birth to infants. In the AZT/3TC group, mothers received a loading dose of 600 mg AZT and 150 mg 3TC followed by 300 mg AZT every 3 hr and 150 mg 3TC every 12 hr until delivery and twice-daily 300 mg AZT and 150 mg 3TC for one week after delivery; infants received twice-daily 12 mg AZT and 6 mg 3TC for one week after birth.

41. Dhayendre Moodley, "The SAINT trial: nevirapine (NVP) versus zidovudine (ZDV) + lamivudine (3TC) in prevention of peripartum HIV transmission," Abstract No. LbOr2 2000, 13th International AIDS Conference, Durban, 2000; Heywood, "Preventing HIV transmission in South Africa."

42. Pithouse, "Global march for treatment access."

43. Howse, "Treatment Access March."

44. David Barr, "Tipping Point: MSF, Oxfam redefine the possible, and Y2K activist trek to Durban marks a watershed," *The Body*, April 2003; James Myburgh, "Here is the evidence of Mbeki's denialism: A reply to the Minister in the Presidency, Essop Pahad," *Politicsweb* July 12, 2007.

45. Pithouse, "Global march for treatment access"; Schneider and Fassin, "Denial and defiance"; Jon Cohen, "South African leader declines to join the chorus on HIV and AIDS," *Science* 289 (2000): 222.

46. Cameron and Geffen, *Witness to AIDS*, 113.

47. Cameron and Geffen, *Witness to AIDS*, 113.

48. Heywood, "Preventing HIV transmission in South Africa."

49. Challiss S. McDonough, "S. African group urges nationwide distribution of AIDS drug," *Voice of America News*, August 21, 2001; Chris Bateman, "Nevirapine all set to succeed in Gauteng," *South African Medical Journal* 92 (2002): 932–933.

50. Heywood, "Preventing HIV transmission in South Africa."

51. Rachel L. Swarns, "South Africa to distribute $50 million in donated AIDS drugs," *New York Times*, December 2, 2000.

52. Heywood, "Preventing HIV transmission in South Africa."

53. Swarns, "South Africa distributes donated AIDS drugs."

54. Cameron and Geffen, *Witness to AIDS*, 158–159; Marcus Low et al., *Fighting for our lives: The history of the Treatment Action Campaign 1998–2010* (Cape Town: Treatment Action Campaign, 2010), 43.

55. Karon, "South African activist Zackie Achmat"; Samantha Power, "The AIDS rebel," *The New Yorker*, May 19, 2003; Cameron and Geffen, *Witness to AIDS*, 163–164.

56. Chris McGreal, "Zackie Achmat: Profile," *The Guardian*, September 12, 2008; Power, "The AIDS rebel"; Cameron and Geffen, *Witness to AIDS*, 164–165.

57. Swarns, "South Africa distributes donated AIDS drugs."

58. Nkosi Johnson, 13th International AIDS Conference, Durban, keynote speech, July 9, 2000.

59. Editorial, *National Sunday Times*, 2001.

60. George J. Annas, "The right to health and the nevirapine case in South Africa," *New England Journal of Medicine* 348 (2003): 750–754.

61. Dr. Andrew James Grant quoted in Replying Affidavit TAC v Minister of Health TPD 21182/2001, Annexure X 2095–98.

62. Personal Affidavit of Vivienne Nokuzola Matebula, Treatment Action Campaign and others v. Minister of Health and others [2001] Pretoria High Court (S. Afr.).

63. Personal Affidavit of Vivienne Nokuzola Matebula, Treatment Action Campaign and others v. Minister of Health and others [2001] Pretoria High Court (S. Afr.).

64. Personal Affidavit of "SH," Treatment Action Campaign and others v. Minister of Health and others [2001] Pretoria High Court (S. Afr.).

65. Personal Affidavit of "SH," Treatment Action Campaign and others v. Minister of Health and others [2001] Pretoria High Court (S. Afr.).

66. Cameron and Geffen, *Witness to AIDS*, 203; Heywood,"Preventing HIV transmission in South Africa."

67. Boehringer Ingelheim, "Viramune® receives full marketing approval," press release, July 9, 2002.

68. Boehringer Ingelheim, "Boehringer Ingelheim provides key background on nevirapine," press release, December 16, 2004; Stephen Lagakos et al., *Review of the HIVNET 012 perinatal HIV prevention study*, (Washington, DC: National Academies Press, 2005), 25.

69. Lagakos et al., "Review of HIVNET 012," 12–13.

70. J. Brooks Jackson, interview, February 29, 2012; Boehringer Ingelheim, "Key background on nevirapine"; Lagakos et al., "Review of HIVNET 012."

71. Rachel L. Swarns, "A move to force South Africa to give AIDS drug for newborns," *New York Times*, November 27, 2001.

72. McDonough, "Nationwide distribution of AIDS drug"; Heywood, "Preventing HIV transmission in South Africa."

73. Voice of America, "S. Africa AIDS activists welcome spending increase, *VOA News*, October 31, 2001.

74. Challiss S. McDonough, "African activists sue for AIDS drug access," *VOA News*, November 26, 2001; Swarns, "AIDS drug for newborns."

75. Heywood, "Preventing HIV transmission in South Africa."

76. Heywood, "Preventing HIV transmission in South Africa."

77. Marumo Moerane, quoted by Rachel Swarns, "AIDS drug for newborns."

78. Dr. Andrew James Grant in Replying Affidavit TAC v Minister of Health TPD 21182/2001, Annexure X 2095–98.

79. Heywood, "Preventing HIV transmission in South Africa"; Lodge, *Politics in South Africa*, 262.

80. Heywood, "Preventing HIV transmission in South Africa."

81. Boehringer Ingelheim, "Key background on nevirapine"; Lakagos et al., "Review of HIVNET 012," 12–13.
82. Laura Guay, interview, March 14, 2012.
83. Patrick Robinson, interview, December 22, 2011; Laura Guay, interview, March 14, 2012.
84. Boehringer Ingelheim, "Key background on nevirapine," December 16, 2004.
85. Lakagos et al., "Review of HIVNET 012," 13.
86. Annas, "Nevirapine case in South Africa"; Heywood, "Preventing HIV transmission in South Africa."
87. Delia Robertson, "South Africa agency to appeal ruling on AIDS drug," *VOA News*, December 19, 2001; Heywood, "Preventing HIV transmission in South Africa."
88. Manto Tshabalala-Msimang quoted by Delia Robertson, "Agency to appeal ruling"; Henri E. Cauvin, "South Africa to appeal ruling ordering access to AIDS drug," *New York Times*, December 20, 2001; Heywood, "Preventing HIV transmission in South Africa."
89. Myburgh, "The Virodene affair (V)."
90. *Castro Hlongwane, Caravans, Cats, Geese, Foot & Mouth and Statistics: HIV?AIDS and the Struggle for the Humanisation of the African*, quoted by James Myburgh, "Mbeki's denialism."
91. Lodge, *Politics in South Africa*, 262, 266.
92. Myburgh, "The Virodene affair (V)"; Lodge, *Politics in South Africa*, 258.
93. Elizabeth Glaser Pediatric AIDS Foundation, "Elizabeth Glaser Pediatric AIDS Foundation awarded $100 million by United States Agency for International Development," press release, July 31, 2002.
94. Jillian Nicholson et al., "Interim findings of the national PMTCT pilot sites: Summary of lessons and recommendations," *Health Systems Trust*, February 2002.
95. Nicholson et al., "Interim Findings on PMTCT Pilot Sites."
96. Heywood, "Preventing HIV transmission in South Africa."
97. Rachel L. Swarns, "A bold move on AIDS in South Africa," *New York Times*, February 5, 2002.
98. Office of the Premier KwaZulu-Natal Media Statement, January 21, 2002.
99. Lionel Mtshali, quoted by Rachel Swarns, "Bold move on AIDS."
100. Heywood, "Preventing HIV transmission in South Africa."
101. Swarns, "Bold move on AIDS."
102. Colleges of Medicine of South Africa, quoted by Joe De Capua, "South Africa/Nevirapine," *VOA News*, February 13, 2002.
103. Salim Abdool Karim et al., "Vertical HIV transmission in South Africa: translating research into policy and practice," *Lancet* 359 (2002): 992–993.
104. Baleta, "Nevirapine policy faces pressure."
105. Lagakos et al., "Review of HIVNET 012," 13. The Westat audit included a review of regulatory compliance, laboratory facilities, pharmacy facilities and processes, and trial records.
106. Laura Guay, interview, March 14, 2012.
107. Laura Guay, interview, March 14, 2012.
108. Laura Guay, interview, March 14, 2012.
109. Lagakos et al., "Review of HIVNET 012," 55–56.
110. J. Brooks Jackson, interview, February 29, 2012.
111. Laura Guay, interview, March 14, 2012.
112. John Solomon, "NIH dismissed concerns about AIDS treatment," Associated Press, December 14, 2004.
113. Boehringer Ingelheim, "Key background on nevirapine."
114. Lagakos et al., "Review of HIVNET 012," 13.
115. Jon Cohen, "HIV Transmission: Allegations raise fears of backlash against AIDS prevention strategy," *Science* 306 (2004): 2168–2169.
116. Laura Guay, interview, March 14, 2012; J. Brooks Jackson, interview, February 29, 2012.
117. Boehringer Ingelheim, "Key background on nevirapine."
118. NIAID, "Review of HIVNET 012 (A clinical trial to determine the efficacy of oral AZT and the efficacy of oral nevirapine for prevention of vertical transmission of HIV-1 infection in pregnant Ugandan women and their neonates)," news release, March 22, 2002.
119. NIAID, "Review of HIVNET 012 (in Ugandan women)"; WHO, "WHO and UNAIDS continue to support use of nevirapine for prevention of mother-to-child HIV transmission," press release, March 22, 2002.
120. Challiss S. McDonough, "Africa court orders distribution of anti–AIDS drug," *VOA News*, March 25, 2002; Heywood, "Preventing HIV transmission in South Africa."
121. Judge Chris Botha, quoted by Challiss McDonough, "Court orders distribution of AIDS drug," March 25, 2002.
122. Kerry Cullinan, "Court orders South Africa to treat pregnant HIV-positive women with nevirapine," *Bulletin of the World Health Organization* 80 (2002): 335; Rachel L. Swarns, "In a policy shift, South Africa will make AIDS drugs available to more pregnant women," *New York Times*, April 20, 2002; Myburgh, "Mbeki's denialism," July 12, 2007.
123. Jim Kolbe, quoted by Voice of America, "US congressman slams South Africa's AIDS policies," *VOA News*, April 9, 2002.
124. "South Africa addresses AIDS," *New York Times*, August 18, 2003.
125. Power, "The AIDS rebel."
126. Henri E. Cauvin, "South Africa to appeal ruling ordering access to AIDS drug," *New York Times*, December 20, 2001.
127. *The Star*, quoted by Henri Cauvin, "South Africa to appeal ruling," December 20, 2001.
128. Thabo Mbeki, "Health, human dignity and partners for poverty reduction," *ANC Today*, April 5, 2002.
129. Myburgh, "The Virodene affair (V)."
130. Myburgh, "Virodene transformation."
131. South African Cabinet Statement on HIV/AIDS, April 17, 2002.
132. South African Cabinet Statement on HIV/AIDS, April 17, 2002.
133. Swarns, "Policy shift to make AIDS drugs available"; Cullinan, "Court orders treatment with nevirapine"; Power, "The AIDS rebel."
134. Challiss S. McDonough, "Mbeki: Battle against AIDS 'critically important,'" *World News Site*, April 24, 2002.
135. Cullinan, "Court orders treatment with nevirapine."

Chapter 22

1. George W. Bush, "President promotes new mother and child HIV prevention initiative: Rose Garden," White House Archives, June 19, 2002; George W. Bush, "President Bush's international mother and child HIV prevention initiative," White House press release, June 19, 2002; "Bush proposes $500 million to fight AIDS: Pandemic claims over 5000 lives a day in the targeted regions," *About.com*, June 20, 2002.
2. Elizabeth Glaser Pediatric AIDS Foundation, "Elizabeth Glaser Pediatric AIDS Foundation awarded $100

million by United States Agency for International Development," press release, July 31, 2002.
　3. Elizabeth Glaser Pediatric AIDS Foundation, "Foundation awarded $100 million."
　4. Laura Guay, interview, March 14, 2012.
　5. Stephen Lakagos et al., *Review of the HIVNET 012 perinatal HIV prevention study*, (Washington, DC: National Academies Press, 2005), 13–14.
　6. John Solomon, "NIH dismissed concerns about AIDS treatment," Associated Press, December 14, 2004.
　7. Zackie Achmat, quoted by African Success Biography, "Biography of Zackie Achmat," November 7, 2008.
　8. Samantha Power, "The AIDS rebel," *The New Yorker*, May 19, 2003.
　9. Edwin Cameron and Nathan Geffen, *Witness to AIDS* (London: I. B. Tauris, 2005), 130.
　10. George J. Annas, "The right to health and the nevirapine case in South Africa," *New England Journal of Medicine* 348 (2003): 750–754.
　11. Delia Robertson, "Africa court upholds decision on HIV drugs for pregnant women," *VOA News*, July 5, 2002; Mark Heywood, "Preventing mother-to-child HIV transmission in South Africa," *South African Journal on Human Rights* 19 (2003): 278–315.
　12. Patricia Lambert, quoted by Delia Robertson, "Court upholds decision."
　13. Rachel L. Swarns, "South Africa may bar AIDS drug in childbirth," *New York Times*, August 7, 2002.
　14. Precious Matsoso, quoted by Rachel Swarns, "South Africa may bar AIDS drug."
　15. Swarns, "South Africa may bar AIDS drug."
　16. Shayne Loubser et al., "Decay of K103N mutants in cellular DNA and plasma RNA after single-dose nevirapine to reduce mother-to-child HIV transmission," *AIDS* 20 (2006): 995–1002.
　17. Annas, "Nevirapine case in South Africa."
　18. Chris Bateman, "Nevirapine all set to succeed in Gauteng," *South African Medical Journal* 92 (2002): 932–933.
　19. African Success Biography, "Biography of Zackie Achmat," November 7, 2008.
　20. Richard Mills, "U.S. announces interim plan to help poor countries fight HIV/AIDS and other health crises," Office of the United States Trade Representative press release, December 20, 2002.
　21. Mills, "Interim plan to help poor countries." In November 2001, the World Trade Organization called on member states to implement the Doha Declaration on the TRIPS agreement.
　22. *Clinton Foundation Annual Report*, 2008.
　23. George W. Bush, State of the Union Address, January 28, 2003; "Bush's emergency AIDS relief plan: 10 million infected individuals and AIDS orphans would get care," *About.com*, January 2003.
　24. Jessica Roseberry, "Catherine Wilfert Interview," *Women in Duke medicine: An oral history exhibit*, August 25, 2006.
　25. Trish Karlin, interview, March 8, 2012.
　26. Rose McCullough and Lior Miller, "Surveying the Global HIV/AIDS Landscape," in *From the Ground Up: Building Comprehensive HIV/AIDS Care Programs in Resource-Limited Settings*, eds. R. G. Marlink and S. T. Teitleman (Washington, DC: Elizabeth Glaser Pediatric AIDS Foundation, 2009).
　27. Trish Karlin, interview, March 8, 2012. The other organizations were Catholic Relief Services Consortium, Harvard School of Public Health, and Mailman School of Public Health at Columbia University.
　28. McCullough and Miller, "Surveying the global landscape."

　29. *Elizabeth Glaser Pediatric AIDS Foundation Annual Report*, 2003.
　30. Lakagos et al., *Review of HIVNET 012*, 14; Tim Farley and Isabelle De Zoysa, "Nevirapine for the prevention of mother-to-child transmission of HIV: WHO reconfirms its support for the use of nevirapine to prevent mother-to-child transmission of HIV," WHO press release, July 2003.
　31. J. Brooks Jackson, interview, February 29, 2012.
　32. Laura Guay, interview, March 14, 2012.
　33. Edmond Tramont, quoted by Jon Cohen, "HIV Transmission: Allegations raise fears of backlash against AIDS prevention strategy," *Science* 306 (2004): 2168–2169.
　34. Power, "The AIDS rebel."
　35. Cameron and Geffen, *Witness to AIDS*, 117.
　36. Tom Lodge, *Politics in South Africa: From Mandela to Mbeki* (Cape Town: David Philip, 2002), 263.
　37. Manto Tshabalala-Msimang quoted by Laurie Garrett, "AIDS at 20/Seeking global answer/AIDS fund poses worldwide challenge," *Newsday*, June 16, 2001.
　38. Manto Tshabalala-Msimang quoted by Samantha Power, "The AIDS rebel"; Pride Chigwedere et al., "Estimating the lost benefits of antiretroviral drug use in South Africa," *Journal of Acquired Immune Deficiency Syndromes* 49 (2008): 410–415.
　39. Bernard Rivers, "KwaZulu-Natal—the saga continues," *Global Fund Observer Newsletter*, January 10, 2003; Chigwedere et al., "Estimating lost benefits."
　40. Power, "The AIDS rebel."
　41. Power, "The AIDS rebel."
　42. "South Africa's Medicines Control Council may ban use of nevirapine only for prevention of vertical HIV transmission, official says," *The Body*, August 7, 2003.
　43. Adele Baleta, "South African government threatens to ban nevirapine," *Lancet* 362 (2003): 451.
　44. Baleta, "Government threatens to ban nevirapine."
　45. Hoosen Coovadia, quoted by Adele Baleta, "Government threatens to ban nevirapine."
　46. TAC statement quoted by Adele Baleta, "Government threatens to ban nevirapine."
　47. South African Cabinet statement, reported by the South African Press Association, quoted in "Medicines Control Council may ban nevirapine," *The Body*, August 7, 2003.
　48. Nono Simelela, quoted in "Medicines Control Council may ban nevirapine," *The Body*, August 7, 2003.
　49. Polly Clayden, "Nevirapine and MTCT: The single-dose backlash," *HIV Treatment Bulletin* 4 (2003): 20–23; "Medicines Control Council may ban nevirapine," *The Body*.
　50. James McIntyre, quoted by Polly Clayden, "Nevirapine and MTCT backlash."
　51. Prudence Mabale, quoted by Polly Clayden, "Nevirapine and MTCT backlash."
　52. Delia Robertson, "South African AIDS conference ends with renewed calls for government to provide HIV drugs," *VOA News*, August 6, 2003.
　53. Zackie Achmat, quoted by Samantha Power, "The AIDS rebel."
　54. "Operational plan for comprehensive HIV and AIDS care, management and treatment for SA," *South African Government Information*, November 19, 2003.
　55. Vuyiseka Dubula, quoted by Positive Heroes, "Vuyiseka Dubula."
　56. Vuyiseka Dubula quoted by Marcus Low et al., *Fighting for our lives: The history of the Treatment Action Campaign 1998–2010* (Cape Town: Treatment Action Campaign, 2010), 24.
　57. Vuyiseka Dubula quoted by Marcus Low et al., *Fighting for our lives*, 24.

58. Positive Heroes, "Vuyiseka Dubula."
59. Michael Wines, "Agreement expands generic drugs in South Africa to fight AIDS," *New York Times*, December 11, 2003.
60. Low et al., *Fighting for our lives*, 48; Cameron and Geffen, *Witness to AIDS*, 179–180.
61. Cameron and Geffen, *Witness to AIDS*, 180.
62. Affidavit of Complaint: Hazel Tau, Annexure HT, September 2002.
63. Cameron and Geffen, *Witness to AIDS*, 179.
64. Boehringer Ingelheim, "Boehringer Ingelheim offers Viramune® (nevirapine) free of charge to developing economies for the prevention of HIV-1 mother-to-child transmission," press release, July 7, 2000; Boehringer Ingelheim, "Boehringer Ingelheim grants further voluntary licenses," press release, December 11, 2003.
65. Boehringer Ingelheim, "World AIDS day report: First supplies of Viramune® donation program for developing countries," press release, November 28, 2000. The other drug companies were Abbott Laboratories, Bristol-Myers Squibb, Hoffmann-La Roche, GlaxoSmithKline, and Merck; the UN agencies were WHO, UNICEF, UNFPA, and UNAIDS.
66. Boehringer Ingelheim, "Vietnam first Asian country in the Viramune® Donation Program for the prevention of HIV infection from mother to child," press release, November 6, 2002; Wines, "Agreement expands generic drugs."
67. Boehringer Ingelheim, "Further voluntary licenses," press release, December 11, 2003.
68. Boehringer Ingelheim, "Further voluntary licenses," press release, December 11, 2003; Cameron and Geffen, *Witness to AIDS*, 182.
69. Low et al., *Fighting for our lives,* 48; Wines, "Agreement expands generic drugs."
70. FDA.gov, International Programs, President's Emergency Plan for AIDS Relief, May 2004.
71. Boehringer Ingelheim, "World AIDS day 2004 — Boehringer Ingelheim continues its commitment to the HIV/AIDS community," press release, November, 30, 2004; Boehringer Ingelheim, "World AIDS day 2006 — Boehringer ingelheim's patent rights are no obstacle to access to ARV drugs in developing countries," press release, November 28, 2006.
72. Russell B. Van Dyke et al., "The Ariel Project: A prospective cohort study of maternal-child transmission of human immunodeficiency virus type 1 in the era of maternal antiretroviral therapy," *Journal of Infectious Diseases* 179 (1999): 319–328.
73. Susan H. Eshleman et al., "Selection and fading of resistance mutations in women and infants receiving nevirapine to prevent HIV-1 vertical transmission (HIVNET 012)," *AIDS* 15 (2001): 1951–1957.
74. Marc Lallemant et al., "Single-dose perinatal nevirapine plus standard zidovudine to prevent mother-to-child transmission of HIV-1 in Thailand," *New England Journal of Medicine* 351 (2004): 217–228; J. Vyankandondera et al., "Reducing risk of HIV-1 transmission from mother to infant through breastfeeding using antiretroviral prophylaxis in infants (SIMBA study)," Abstract No. LB07 2003, IAS Conference on HIV Pathogenesis and Treatment, Paris, July 2003.
75. James A. McIntyre et al., "Efficacy of short-course AZT plus 3TC to reduce nevirapine resistance in the prevention of mother-to-child HIV transmission: A randomized clinical trial," *PLoS Medicine* 6 (2009): 1–9.
76. Cameron and Geffen, *Witness to AIDS*, 155.
77. Polly Clayden, "Adding Combivir to single dose nevirapine for reduction of MTCT significantly reduces resistance," *HIV Treatment Bulletin* 5 (2004): 14–16; McIntyre et al., "Short-course reduces nevirapine resistance"; Challiss S. McDonough, "Africa group says use of AIDS drug may harm pregnant women," *VOA News*, July 13, 2004.
78. Jonathan Berger and Natan Geffen, "MTCT programmes in South Africa: nevirapine and the minister," *HIV Treatment Bulletin* 5 (2004): 8–9.
79. Joep Lange quoted by Sharon LaFraniere, "South Africa rejects use of AIDS drug for women," *New York Times*, July 14, 2004; Joep Lange, interview, February 28, 2012.
80. LaFraniere, "South Africa rejects drug for women."
81. Iain Simpson and Samantha Bolton, "WHO publishes new guidelines on preventing mother to child transmission of HIV, WHO news release, July 14, 2004.
82. H. Clifford Lane, quoted by John Solomon, "NIH dismissed concerns"; NIAID Q&As, April 7, 2005; John Solomon, "NIH review substantiates fired expert's concerns," Associated Press, July 4, 2005.
83. Lagakos et al., "Review of HIVNET 012," 14.
84. Lakagos et al., "Review of HIVNET 012," 14. A division of the National Academy of Sciences, the Institute of Medicine is an independent, nonprofit organization that works outside of government to provide unbiased and authoritative advice on health and healthcare.
85. Lakagos et al., "Review of HIVNET 012," 110–111; Laura Guay, interview, March 14, 2012; J. Brooks Jackson, interview, February 29, 2012.
86. David Feigal, interview, May 24, 2012.
87. John Solomon, "Top US officials warned of concerns before AIDS drug sent to Africa," Associated Press, December 13, 2004.
88. NIAID, "The HIVNET 012 study and the safety and effectiveness of nevirapine in preventing mother-to-infant transmission of HIV," news release, December 14, 2004; Boehringer Ingelheim, "Boehringer Ingelheim provides key background on nevirapine," press release, December 16, 2004.
89. Elizabeth Glaser Pediatric AIDS Foundation, "Elizabeth Glaser Pediatric AIDS Foundation on issue of prevention of mother-to-child transmission of HIV/AIDS and single-dose nevirapine," press release, December 14, 2004; Global Strategies for HIV Prevention, "Comments on a recent media article on the HIVNET 012 Uganda study," press release, December 15, 2004; Khabir Ahmad, "Controversy around nevirapine trials continues," *Lancet Infectious Diseases* 5 (2005): 74.
90. Project Inform, "Project Inform statement regarding the use of single-dose nevirapine to prevent mother-to-child transmission of HIV," press release, December 15, 2004; NIAID Q&A, April 7, 2005.
91. Alexandra Zavis, "US accused of using Africans for tests," Associated Press, December 18, 2004.
92. Hoosen Coovadia quoted by Joe De Capua, "South African doctor says benefits of nevirapine outweigh any risks."
93. Treatment Action Campaign quoted by Bob Roehr, "Articles criticising nevirapine trial may endanger babies' lives," *BMJ* 330 (2005): 61.
94. Lakagos et al., "Review of HIVNET 012," 14, 112; Ahmad, "Controversy around nevirapine continues."
95. Ahmad, "Controversy around nevirapine continues."
96. Lakagos et al., "Review of HIVNET 012."
97. Lakagos et al., "Review of HIVNET 012," 10.
98. Boehringer Ingelheim, "Viramune® receives full marketing approval," press release, July 9, 2002.
99. NIAID, "Review of HIVNET 012 (A clinical trial

to determine the efficacy of oral AZT and the efficacy of oral nevirapine for prevention of vertical transmission of HIV-1 infection in pregnant Ugandan women and their neonates)," news release, March 22, 2002.

100. Patrick Robinson quoted by John Solomon, "NIH dismissed concerns"; Robinson, interview, December 22, 2011.

101. Annie Kelly, "HIV/AIDS in Uganda," *The Guardian*, December 1, 2008.

102. Chigwedere et al., "Estimating lost benefits."

103. Florence Ngobeni-Allen, AIDS@30, December 2, 2011.

104. Florence Ngobeni-Allen, interview, October 30, 2012.

105. Florence Ngobeni-Allen, AIDS@30, December 2, 2011.

106. Florence Ngobeni-Allen, AIDS@30, December 2, 2011.

107. Florence Ngobeni-Allen, AIDS@30, December 2, 2011; Laura Guay, interview, March 14, 2012.

108. African Success Biography, Biography of Zackie Achmat, November 7, 2008.

109. South Africa, Global AIDS response progress report, 2012; *Clinton Foundation Annual Report*, 2010.

Chapter 23

1. Martin Hirsch, interview, February 3, 2012.
2. Katherine Luzuriaga, interview, December 21, 2011.
3. Katherine Luzuriaga, interview, January 24, 2012.
4. Katherine Luzuriaga, interviews, December 21, 2011, and January 24, 2012.
5. John Sullivan, email, December 7, 2011.
6. Katherine Luzuriaga et al., "Absent HIV-specific immune responses and replication-competent HIV reservoirs in perinatally infected youth treated from infancy: Toward cure," Abstract No. 171LB, Conference on Retriviruses and Opportunistic Infections, Atlanta, March 3–6, 2013.
7. Katherine Luzuriaga, interview, December 21, 2011.
8. John Sullivan, email, March 4, 2013. The baby was switched from nevirapine to an HIV protease inhibitor after the first week of treatment.
9. Deborah Persaud et al., "Functional HIV cure after very early ART of an infected infant," Abstract No. 48LB, Conference on Retroviruses and Opportunistic Infections, Atlanta, March 3–6, 2013.
10. Katherine Luzuriaga et al., "Absent HIV-specific immune responses."
11. Katherine Luzuriaga, interview, December 21, 2011.
12. Jeroen P. H. Van Wijk and Manuel C. Cabezas, "Hypertriglyceridemia, metabolic syndrome, and cardiovascular disease in HIV-infected patients: Effects of antiretroviral therapy and adipose tissue distribution," *International Journal of Vascular Medicine*, Article ID 201027, 2012; Colleen Hadigan, "Insulin resistance among HIV-infected patients: unraveling the mechanism," *Clinical Infectious Diseases* 41 (2005): 1341–1342; Jordan E. Lake and Judith S. Currier, "Switching antiretroviral therapy to minimize metabolic complications," *HIV Therapy* 4 (2010): 693–711.
13. Van Wijk and Cabezas, "Antiretroviral therapy and adipose tissue distribution"; Hadigan, "Insulin resistance in HIV patients," 1341–1342; W. I. W. Ismail et al., "Insulin resistance induced by antiretroviral drugs: Current understanding of molecular mechanisms," *Journal of Endocrinology, Metabolism and Diabetes of South Africa* 14 (2009): 129–132.
14. Van Wijk and Cabezas, "Antiretroviral therapy and adipose tissue distribution."
15. Alexandra Calmy et al., "A new era of antiretroviral drug toxicity," *Antiviral Therapy* 14 (2009): 165–179; Van Wijk and Cabezas, "Antiretroviral therapy and adipose tissue distribution"; Lake and Currier, "Switching antiretroviral therapy."
16. Calmy et al., "New era of drug toxicity"; Van Wijk and Cabezas, "Antiretroviral therapy and adipose tissue distribution."
17. Marc van der Valk et al., "Nevirapine-containing antiretroviral therapy in HIV-1 infected patients in an anti-atherogenic lipid profile," *AIDS* 15 (2001): 2407–2414; Frank Van Leth et al., "Nevirapine and efavirenz elicit different changes in lipid profiles in antiretroviral-therapy-naïve patients infected with HIV-1," *PLoS Medicine* 1 (2004): e19.
18. Van Wijk and Cabezas, "Antiretroviral therapy and adipose tissue distribution."
19. Beverly E. Sha et al., "Adverse events associated with use of nevirapine in HIV postexposure for 2 health care workers," *JAMA* 284 (2000): 2722–2723. Wanda is a fictitious name to protect patient identity, but this is a documented clinical case.
20. Jerry O. Stern et al., "A comprehensive hepatic safety analysis of nevirapine in different populations of HIV infected patients," *Journal of Acquired Immune Deficiency Syndromes* 34 (2003): S21–S33; Robert L. Murphy, "Defining the toxicity profile of nevirapine and other antiretroviral drugs," *Journal of Acquired Immune Deficiency Syndromes* 34 (2003): S15–S20.
21. Centers for Disease Control and Prevention, "Public Health Service guidelines for the management of healthcare worker exposures to HIV and recommendations for postexposure prophylaxis," *Morbidity and Mortality Weekly Report* 47 (RR-7)(1998): 1–28.
22. D. Boxwell et al., "Serious adverse events attributed to nevirapine regimens for postexposure prophylaxis after HIV exposures—worldwide, 1997–2000," *Morbidity and Mortality Weekly Report* 49 (2001): 1153–1156.
23. Boxwell et al., "Nevirapine for postexposure prophylaxis."
24. Judith S. Currier, "Sex differences in antiretroviral therapy toxicity: Lactic acidosis, stavudine, and women," *Clinical Infectious Diseases* 45 (2007): 261–262; David Hall, interview, December 9, 2012.
25. Viramune® label change, January 13, 2005. The current nevirapine label recommends that nevirapine should be given to women with CD4 cell counts below 250 and to men with CD4 cell counts below 400.
26. Myron S. Cohen et al., "Prevention of HIV-1 infection with early antiretroviral therapy," *New England Journal of Medicine*, 365 (2011): 493–505.
27. Hoosen J. Coovadia et al., "Efficacy and safety of an extended nevirapine regimen in infant children of breastfeeding mothers with HIV-1 infection for prevention of postnatal HIV-1 transmission (HPTN 046): A randomized, double-blind, placebo-controlled trial," *Lancet* 379 (2012): 221–228; Kristen J. Kresge, "Treatment is prevention," *IAVI Report* 15 (2011): 14–16.
28. Anthony Fauci, quoted by amfAR, "New momentum for AIDS research: The amfAR interview with Anthony Fauci, MD interview," October 2011.
29. Anthony Fauci, quoted by Kristen Kresge, "Treatment is prevention."
30. Both efavirenz and nevirapine are potent RT inhibitors, are rapidly absorbed, have a long half-life, rapidly induce viral resistance, and in some patients cause a skin rash.

31. John L. Sullivan, "Prevention of mother-to-child transmission of HIV — What next?" *Journal of Acquired Immune Deficiency Syndromes* 34 (2003): S67–S72.

32. Mary Glenn Fowler and Marie L. Newell, "Breastfeeding and HIV-1 transmission in resource-limited settings," *Journal of Acquired Immune Deficiency Syndromes* 30 (2002): 230–239.

33. Sullivan, "Prevention of mother-to-child transmission"; WHO, Report No. WHO/RHR/01.28, 2001.

34. Tatu Story of Hope, by permission from Elizabeth Glaser Pediatric AIDS Foundation.

35. Tatu, quoted in Story of Hope, December 31, 2009.

36. Tatu, quoted in Story of Hope, May 7, 2010.

37. Sullivan, "Prevention of mother-to-child transmission."

38. PETRA Study Team, "Efficacy of three short-course regimens of zidovudine and lamivudine in preventing early and late transmission of HIV-1 from mother to child in Tanzania, South Africa, and Uganda (Petra study): A randomized, double-blind, placebo-controlled trial," *Lancet* 359 (2002): 1178–1186.

39. J. Vyankandondera et al., "Reducing risk of HIV-1 transmission from mother to infant through breastfeeding using antiretroviral prophylaxis in infants (SIMBA study)," Abstract No. LB07, IAS Conference on HIV Pathogenesis and Treatment, July 13–16, 2003.

40. Charles S. Chasela et al., "Maternal or infant antiretroviral drugs to reduce HIV-1 transmission," *New England Journal of Medicine* 362 (2010): 2271–2281; Roger L. Shapiro et al., "Antiretroviral regimens in pregnancy and breast-feeding in Botswana," *New England Journal of Medicine* 362 (2010): 2282–2294; Kesho Bora Study Group, "Triple antiretroviral compared with zidovudine and single-dose nevirapine prophylaxis during pregnancy and breastfeeding for prevention of mother-to-child transmission of HIV-1 (Kesho Bora study): a randomized controlled study," *Lancet Infectious Diseases* 11 (2011): 171–180; Hoosen M. Coovadia et al., "Efficacy and safety of an extended nevirapine regimen in infant children of breastfeeding mothers with HIV-1 infection for prevention of postnatal HIV-1 transmission (HPTN 046): A randomized, double-blind, placebo-controlled trial," *Lancet* 379 (2012): 221–228.

41. Coovadia et al., "Extended nevirapine in infant breastfeeding."

42. Coovadia et al., "Extended nevirapine in infant breastfeeding"; WHO, "Antiretroviral drugs for treating pregnant women and preventing HIV infection in infants: Recommendations for a public health approach," WHO Library, 2010.

43. Tatu, quoted in Story of Hope, May 7, 2010.

44. *Clinton Foundation Annual Report*, 2008.

45. Nicholas Hellmann, interview, March 13, 2012.

46. *Elizabeth Glaser Pediatric AIDS Foundation Annual Report*, 2007.

47. *Elizabeth Glaser Pediatric AIDS Foundation Annual Report*, 2011.

48. Nicholas Hellmann, interview, March 13, 2012; Trish Karlin, interview, March 8, 2012. The full names of these three foundations are Fundação Ariel Glaser contra o SIDA Pediátrico, Ariel Glaser Pediatric AIDS Healthcare Initiative, and Fondation Ariel Glaser pour la Lutte Contre le SIDA Pediatrique.

49. Laura Guay, interview, March 14, 2012.

50. Kevin M. De Cock et al., "Prevention of mother-to-child HIV transmission in resource-poor countries," *JAMA* 283 (2000): 1175–1182; UNAIDS, "Global report: UNAIDS report on the global AIDS epidemic 2010," WHO Library (2010); WHO, "Global HIV/AIDS Response: Epidemic update and health sector progress towards universal access, Progress Report," WHO Library (2011).

51. WHO Global HIV/AIDS Response Progress Report (2011).

52. WHO Global HIV/AIDS Response Progress Report (2011).

53. WHO, "Antiretroviral therapy for HIV infection in infants and children: Towards universal access: Recommendations for a public health approach," WHO Library (2010).

54. Lynne M. Mofenson, "Protecting the next generation — Eliminating perinatal HIV-1 infection," *New England Journal of Medicine* 362 (2010): 2316–2318.

55. Nicholas Hellmann, interview, March 13, 2012; Laura Guay, interview, March 14, 2012; Trish Karlin, interview, March 8, 2012.

56. WHO Global HIV/AIDS Response Progress Report (2011), 84, 105.

57. UNAIDS Global Report (2010).

58. Vuyiseka Dubula quoted by Marcus Low et al., *Fighting for our lives: The history of the Treatment Action Campaign 1998–2010* (Capr Town: Treatment Action Campaign, 2010), 24.

59. Tatu, quoted in Story of Hope, May 7, 2010.

60. Tatu, quoted in Story of Hope, May 7, 2010.

61. WHO Global HIV/AIDS Response Report (2011).

62. For the complete matrix of recommended treatment options for MTCT, see WHO, "Antiretroviral drugs for treating pregnant women and preventing HIV infection in infants: Recommendations for a public health approach, WHO Library (2010).

63. *Faith Alive Foundation Annual Report*, 2006.

64. Elizabeth M. Stringer et al., "Coverage of nevirapine-based services to prevent mother-to-child HIV transmission in 4 African countries," *JAMA* 304 (2010): 293–302. The four countries were Cameroon Côte d'Ivoire, South Africa, and Zambia.

65. Voltaire, La Bégueule, 1772; J. Brooks Jackson, interview, February 29, 2012; Catherine Wilfert, interview, January 18, 2012; Mark Heywood, "Preventing mother-to-child HIV transmission in South Africa," *South African Journal on Human Rights*, 19 (2003): 307.

List of Author Interviews

Julian Adams, director of medicinal chemistry, Boehringer Ingelheim

Arthur Ammann, director of pediatric immunology and clinical research, University of California, San Francisco; director of research, Pediatric AIDS Foundation

Laura Andrews, senior toxicologist, Boehringer Ingelheim

Edwin Cameron, judge on the High Court, South Africa

Ellen C. Cooper, director, antiviral drug products division, FDA

Susan DeLaurentis, co-founder, Elizabeth Glaser Pediatric AIDS Foundation

Robert Eckner, virologist, HIV research team leader, Boehringer Ingelheim

David Feigal, director, antiviral drug products division, FDA

Jamie Gentille, pediatric AIDS patient; ambassador, Elizabeth Glaser Pediatric AIDS Foundation

Jake Glaser, son of Elizabeth and Paul Michael Glaser

Johanna Griffin, director of molecular biology, Boehringer Ingelheim

Peter Grob, biochemist, HIV research team leader, Boehringer Ingelheim

Karl Grozinger, scale up chemist, Boehringer Ingelheim

Laura Guay, investigator of HIVNET 012 clinical trial; vice president of research, Elizabeth Glaser Pediatric AIDS Foundation

David Hall, biostatistician, Boehringer Ingelheim

Karl Hargrave, lead nevirapine chemist, Boehringer Ingelheim

Mark Harrington, policy director and co-founder, Treatment Action Group

Diane Havlir, nevirapine clinical investigator, University of California, San Diego

Amale Hawi, pharmaceutics scientist, Boehringer Ingelheim

Nicholas Hellmann, executive vice president, scientific and medical affairs, Elizabeth Glaser Pediatric AIDS Foundation

Martin Hirsch, nevirapine clinical investigator, Massachusetts General Hospital and Harvard Medical School

J. Brooks Jackson, principal investigator of HIVNET 012 clinical trial, Johns Hopkins University

Kathryn Jason, regulatory affairs, Boehringer Ingelheim

Trish Devine Karlin, vice president, global business planning, Elizabeth Glaser Pediatric AIDS Foundation

James Keirns, director of drug metabolism and pharmacokinetics, Boehringer Ingelheim

David Kessler, FDA commissioner

Mark Labadia, scientist, Boehringer Ingelheim

Joep Lange, nevirapine clinical investigator, University of Amsterdam; chief of clinical research and drug development, World Health Organization

Katherine Luzuriaga, pediatric clinical trial investigator, University of Massachusetts

Thomas MacGregor, drug metabolism and pharmacokinetics scientist, Boehringer Ingelheim

Vincent J. Merluzzi, nevirapine development team leader, Boehringer Ingelheim

Lynne Mofenson, branch chief, maternal and pediatric infectious diseases, National Institutes of Health

Julio Montaner, nevirapine clinical investigator, University of British Columbia

Maureen Myers, nevirapine clinical team leader, Boehringer Ingelheim

Florence Ngobeni-Allen, counselor, Chris Hani Baragwanath Hospital, South Africa; ambassador, Elizabeth Glaser Pediatric AIDS Foundation

Keri Oberg, patient advocacy and professional relations, Boehringer Ingelheim

Terri Pascarelli, group manager, policy and issues analysis, Boehringer Ingelheim

John Proudfoot, medicinal chemist, Boehringer Ingelheim

Douglas Richman, nevirapine clinical investigator, University of California, San Diego, and San Diego Veterans Affairs Medical Center

Patrick Robinson, clinical director, Boehringer Ingelheim

Alan Rosenthal, vice president, research and development, Boehringer Ingelheim

William Snow, treatment and data committee, ACT UP

Pamela Strode, associate director, regulatory affairs, Boehringer Ingelheim

John Sullivan, pediatric clinical trial investigator, University of Massachusetts

John Tiso, nevirapine project manager, Boehringer Ingelheim

Mike Tsianco, director, data management and biostatistics, Boehringer Ingelheim

Mark Wainberg, director, AIDS Center, McGill University and Jewish General Hospital

Catherine Wilfert, pediatric clinical trial investigator, Duke University; scientific director, Elizabeth Glaser Pediatric AIDS Foundation

James Wright, pharmaceutics scientist, Boehringer Ingelheim

Joe C. Wu, biochemist, Boehringer Ingelheim

Bibliography

ACT UP. Treatment Agenda 1990: VI International Conference on AIDS. San Francisco: ACT-UP / New York Treatment and Data Committee, June 1990.

Adams, J., and V. J. Merluzzi. Discovery of nevirapine, a nonnucleoside inhibitor of HIV-1 reverse transcriptase. In *The search for antiviral drugs: Case histories from concept to clinic*, eds. J. Adams and V. J. Merluzzi, 45–70. Boston: Birkhäuser, 1993.

African Success Biography. Biography of Zackie Achmat. November 7, 2008.

Ahmad, K. Controversy around nevirapine trials continues. *Lancet Inf Dis* 5 (2005): 74.

Aliment, A., K. Luzuriaga, B. Stechenberg, and J. L. Sullivan. Quantitation of human immunodeficiency virus in vertically infected infants and children. *J Ped* 119 (1991): 225–229.

Altman, L. K. AIDS experts leave journal after studies are criticized. *New York Times*, October 15, 1997.

Altman, L. K. AIDS studies on infants appear to conflict. *New York Times*, July 13, 2000.

Altman, L. K. The doctor's world: Faith in multiple-drug AIDS trial shaken by report of error in lab. *New York Times*, July 27, 1993.

Altman, L. K. Drug mixture halts HIV in lab, doctors say in a cautious report. *New York Times*, February 18, 1993.

Altman, L. K. Drug reduces HIV rates in newborns, Thai study shows. *New York Times*, July 7, 2002.

Altman, L. K. Infant drugs for HIV put mothers at risk. *New York Times*, February 10, 2004.

Altman, L. K. New means found for reducing HIV passed to child. *New York Times*, July 15, 1999.

Altman, L. K. A new regimen to fight AIDS in newborns. *New York Times*, July 18, 1999.

Altman, L. K. Report dims hope for AIDS therapy to protect babies. *New York Times*, July 8, 2000.

Altman, L. K. Scientists display substantial gains in AIDS treatment. *New York Times*, July 12, 1996.

amfAR. New momentum for AIDS research: The amFAR interview with Anthony Fauci, MD. amfAR, October 2011.

Ammann, A. Call to action. Global Strategies for HIV Prevention, 2003.

Ammann, A., M. Cowan, D. Wara, H. Goldman, H. Perkins, R. Lanzerotti, J. Gullett, A. Duff, S. Dritz, and J. Chin. Epidemiologic notes and reports possible transfusion-associated acquired immune deficiency syndrome (AIDS)—California. *MMWR* 31 (1982): 652–654.

Ammann, A., M. J. Cowan, D.W. Wara, P. Weintrub, S. Dritz, H. Goldman, and H. A. Perkins. Acquired immunodeficiency in an infant: Possible transmission by means of blood products. *Lancet* 1, no. 8331 (1983): 956–958.

Angell, M. The ethics of clinical research in the third world. *N Engl J Med* 337 (1997): 847–849.

Angus-Smith, M. Boehringer AIDS drug reviewed by *Science*. *Danbury News-Times*, December 7, 1990.

Angus-Smith, M. Boehringer develops new AIDS drug. *Danbury News-Times*, October 25, 1990.

Angus-Smith, M. Boehringer optimistic about new AIDS drug. *Danbury News-Times*, October 28, 1990.

Angus-Smith, M. Drug's target: AIDS. Boehringer has fingers crossed. *Danbury News-Times*, January 20, 1991.

Angus-Smith, M. Testing begins on AIDS drug. *Danbury News-Times*, January 25, 1991.

Annas, G. J. Reply: The right to health and the nevirapine case in South Africa. *N Engl J Med* 348 (2003): 2470.

Annas, G. J. The right to health and the nevirapine case in South Africa. *N Engl J Med* 348 (2003): 750–754.

Nevirapine triple combination shows efficacy for treatment of HIV-infection. *Antiviral Agents Bulletin* 7 (1994): 356–357.

Associated Press. Officials fear hemophiliac will spread disease: School in Indiana bars boy with AIDS. *Los Angeles Times*, July 31, 1985.

Associated Press. Panel backs drug to fight eye danger. *New York Times*, May 4, 1989.

Associated Press. Pharmaceutical company plans to end testing of AIDS drug. November 27, 1991.

Avert, International AIDS & HIV Charity. History of AIDS: 1987–1992. http://www.avert.org/aids-history87-92.htm.

Bacon, K. H. Plan to speed availability of drugs for AIDS backed by U.S. officials. *Wall Street Journal*, July 22, 1989.

Bacon, K. H. U.S. moves to help critically ill get new AIDS drugs. *Wall Street Journal*, May 21, 1990.

Baleta, A. South African government threatens to ban nevirapine. *Lancet* 362, no. 9382 (2003): 451.

Baleta, A. South African nevirapine policy faces growing pressure. *Lancet Inf Dis* 2 (2002): 128.

Balis, F. M., P. A. Pizzo, J. Eddy, C. Wilfert, R. McKinney, G. Scott, R. F. Murphy, P. F. Jarosinski, J. Falloon, and D. G. Poplack. Pharmacokinetics of zidovudine administered intravenously and orally in children with human immunodeficiency virus infection. *J Ped* 114 (1989): 880–884.

Balis, F. M., and D. G. Poplack. Drug development and clinical pharmacology. In *Pediatric AIDS: Challenge of HIV infection in infants, children and adolescents*, eds. P. A. Pizzo and C. M. Wilfert, 457–477. Baltimore: Williams and Wilkins, 1991.

Barner, A., and M. Myers. Nevirapine and rashes. *Lancet* 351, no. 9109 (1998): 1133–1134.

Barr, D. Enemies at the gate: Storming Montreal's Palais de Congrès, and makeshift battle stations in fortress San Francisco. *The Body*, December 2002.

Barr, D. Marking time: Commune of shell shocked soldiers springs up then quickly crumbles, inexplicably. *The Body*, November 2002.

Barr, D. Tipping Point: MSF, Oxfam redefine the possible, and Y2K activist trek to Durban marks a watershed. *The Body*, April 2003.

Barr, D. Yin and Yang: Yokohama, Vancouver, Twin Pacific Ports, serve as polar opposites for scientific advances. *The Body*, March 2003.

Barr, M. Pressing hard for change at Boehringer, *The Treatment and Data Digest, ACT UP*, no. 97, June 10, 1991.

Barry, D. W., and L. M. Distlerath. History and accomplishments of inter-company collaboration for AIDS drug development. *Drug Inf J* 34 (2000): 741–752.

Bartlett, J. A. Management and counseling for persons with HIV infection. In *Cecil Textbook of Medicine*, eds. J. C. Bennett and F. Plum, 1888–1892. Philadelphia: Saunders, 1996.

Bateman, C. Nevirapine all set to succeed in Gauteng. *S African Med J* 92 (2002): 932–933.

Berger, J., and N. Geffen. MTCT programmes in South Africa: nevirapine and the minister. *HIV Treatment Bulletin* 5 (2004): 8–9.

Blanche, S., C. Rouzioux, M-LG. Moscato, F. Veber, M-J. Mayaux, C. Jacomet, J. Tricoire, A. Deville, M. Vial, G. Firtion, A. De Crepy, D. Douard, M. Robin, C. Courpotin, N. Ciraru-Vigneron, F. Le Deist, C. Griscelli, and the HIV infection in Newborns French Collaborative Study Group. A prospective study of infants born to women seropositive for human immunodeficiency virus type 1. *N Eng J Med* 320 (1989): 1643–1648.

Boehringer Ingelheim. BIPI announced today its plans to halt the single agent testing of nevirapine (BIRG-587) in HIV-positive patients. Press Release, November 27, 1991.

Boehringer Ingelheim. Boehringer Ingelheim grants further voluntary licenses. Press Release, December 11, 2003.

Boehringer Ingelheim. Boehringer Ingelheim offers Viramune® (nevirapine) free of charge to developing economies for the prevention of HIV-1 mother-to-child transmission. Press Release, July 7, 2000.

Boehringer Ingelheim. Boehringer Ingelheim provides key background on nevirapine. Press Release, December 16, 2004.

Boehringer Ingelheim. Fact Sheet: The Boehringer Ingelheim Corporation and its companies. April 15, 1985.

Boehringer Ingelheim. First NNRTI suspension, Viramune®, now available for use in HIV-positive children: European Commission approval advances fight against pediatric HIV/AIDS. Press Release, July 7, 1999.

Boehringer Ingelheim. A million doses of hope against AIDS: Viramune® Donation Program for the prevention of mother-to-child transmission: one million doses provided. Press Release, July 2, 2007.

Boehringer Ingelheim. Nevirapine, a new approach to the treatment of AIDS under development at Boehringer Ingelheim. Press Release, August 18, 1992.

Boehringer Ingelheim. PMTCT Donation Program, Guidelines for the administration of Viramune® 200 mg tablets and 50 mg/5 ml oral suspension for use in the prevention of mother to child transmission (pMTCT) of HIV-1 (where single dose prophylaxis with Viramune is indicated). http://corporate responsibility.boehringer-ingelheim.com/corporate_citizenship/combating_hiv_aids.html.

Boehringer Ingelheim. Potent new HIV/AIDS drug focus of European Conference. Press Release, March 12, 1998.

Boehringer Ingelheim. Results of landmark studies support use of AIDS drug Viramune® (nevirapine). Press Release, October 25, 1999.

Boehringer Ingelheim. Vietnam first Asian country in the Viramune® Donation Program for the prevention of HIV infection from mother to child. Press Release, November 6, 2002.

Boehringer Ingelheim. Viramune® receives accelerated approval to treat AIDS: Represents first drug in class to receive designation. Press Release, June 24, 1996.

Boehringer Ingelheim. Viramune® receives full marketing approval. Press Release, July 9, 2002.

Boehringer Ingelheim. World AIDS day report: First supplies of Viramune® donation program for developing countries. Press Release, November 28, 2000.

Boehringer Ingelheim. World AIDS day 2001— Progress in the battle against AIDS. Press Release, November 30, 2001.

Boehringer Ingelheim. World AIDS day 2004— Boehringer Ingelheim continues its commitment to the HIV/AIDS community. Press Release, November 30, 2004.

Boehringer Ingelheim. World AIDS day 2005— Boehringer Ingelheim is committed to its fight against AIDS. Press Release, November 28, 2005.

Boehringer Ingelheim. World AIDS day 2006— Boehringer Ingelheim's patent rights are no obstacle to access to ARV drugs in developing countries. Press Release, November 28, 2006.

Boehringer Ingelheim Corp. said it would curtail development of an AIDS drug. *New York Times*, November 28, 1991.

Boehringer Ingelheim halts AIDS drug human tests. Reuters News Service, November 27, 1991.

Boffey, P. M. Food and Drug Administration: At fulcrum of conflict, regulator of AIDS drugs. *New York Times*, August 19, 1988.

Bowersox, J. NIAID's clinical trial ACTG 241 was central to nevirapine FDA approval. NIAID Press Release, September 1996.

Bowersox, J., and A. Blank. Studies shed new light on mother-to-infant HIV transmission. *NIH News*, June 19, 1996.

Boxwell, D., H. Haverkos, S. Kukich, K. Struble, and H. Jolson. Serious adverse events attributed to nevirapine regimens for postexposure prophylaxis after HIV exposures—worldwide, 1997-2000. *MMWR* 49 (2001): 1153–1156.

Breo, D. L. Tired of taking the blame, AIDS drug regulator Ellen Cooper quits. *JAMA* 265 (1991): 1027–1028.

Brink, A. *Debating AZT: Mbeki and the AIDS drug controversy.* Pietermaritzburg: Kendall and Strachan, 2000.

Bryson, Y. J., K. Luzuriaga, and J. L. Sullivan. Proposed definitions for in utero versus intrapartum transmission of HIV-1. *N Engl J Med* 327 (1992): 1246–1247.

Burchett, S. K, V. Carey, F. Yong, J. Sullivan, S. Sutzbacher, L. Civitello, M. Culnane, L. Mofenson, S. Siminski, P. Robinson, and K. Luzuriaga. Virologic activity of didanosine (ddI), zidovudine (ZDV), and nevirapine, (NVP) combinations in pediatric subjects with advanced HIV disease (ACTG 245). *Conf Retrovir Oppor Infect* 5: 130 (abstract no. 271), February 1–5, 1998.

Burchett, S. K., and K. Luzuriaga. A comparative study of combination antiretroviral therapy in children and adolescents with advanced HIV disease, ACTG 245 ClinicalTrials.gov, NCT00000814, 1999.

Burchett, S. K., J. Sullivan, K. Luzuriaga, V. Carey, F. Yong, M. Culnane, L. Mofenson, and P. Robinson. Combinations of didanosine (ddI), zidovudine (ZDV) and nevirapine (NVP) can reduce CSF HIV-1 viral load in pediatric patients with advanced HIV disease. *Int Conf AIDS* 12: 62 (abstract no. 12253), June 28 – July 3, 1998.

Bush proposes $500 million to fight AIDS: Pandemic claims over 5000 lives a day in the targeted regions. *About.com*, June 20, 2002.

Bush, G. W. President Bush's international mother and child HIV prevention initiative. Press Release, June 19, 2002.

Bush, G. W. President promotes new mother and child HIV prevention initiative: The Rose Garden. White House Archives, June 19, 2002.

Bush, G. W. State of the Union Address. January 28, 2003.

Bush's emergency AIDS relief plan: 10 million infected individuals and AIDS orphans would get care. *About.com*, January 2003.

Butler, K. M., R. N. Husson, F. M. Balis, P. Brouwers, J. Eddy, D. El-Amin, J. Gress, M. Hawkins, P. Jarosinski, H. Moss, D. Poplack, S. Santacroce, D. Venzon, L. Wiener, P. Wolters, and P. A. Pizzo. Dideoxyinosine in children with symptomatic human immunodeficiency virus infection. *N Engl J Med* 324 (1991): 137–144.

Byrnes, V. W., V. V. Sardana, W. A. Schleif, J. H. Condra, J. A. Waterbury, J. A. Wolfgang, W. J. Long, C. L. Schneider, J. A. J Schlabach, B. S. Wolanski, D. J. Graham, L. Gotlib, A. Rhodes, D. L. Titus, E. Roth, O. M. Blahy, J. C. Quintero, S. Staszewski, and E. A. Emini. Comprehensive mutant enzyme and viral variant assessment of human immunodeficiency virus type 1 reverse transcriptase resistance to nonnucleoside inhibitors. *Antimicrob Agents Chemother* 37 (1993): 1576–1579.

Calmy, A., B. Hirschel, D. A. Cooper, and A. Carr. Review: A new era of antiretroviral drug toxicity. *Antiviral Therapy* 14 (2009): 165–179.

Cameron, E. The deafening silence of AIDS. 13th International AIDS Conference, Durban, Plenary Presentation, July 10, 2000.

Cameron, E., and N. Geffen. *Witness to AIDS.* London: I.B. Tauris, 2005.

Carr, A., S. Vella, M. D. de Jong, F. Sorice, A. Imrie, C. A. Boucher, and D. A. Cooper. A controlled trial of nevirapine plus zidovudine versus zidovudine alone in p24 antigenaemic HIV-infected patients. The Dutch-Italian-Australian nevirapine study group. *AIDS* 10 (1996): 635–641.

Cattelan, A. M., E. Erne, A. Salatino, M. Trevenzoli, G. Carretta, F. Meneghetti, and P. Cadrobbi. Severe hepatic failure related to nevirapine treatment. *Clin Infect Dis* 29 (1999): 455–456.

Cauvin, H. E. South Africa to appeal ruling ordering access to AIDS drug. *New York Times*, December 20, 2001.

Cauvin, H. E. World Briefing: Africa: South Africa: Provide AIDS drug, court says. *New York Times*, April 5, 2002.

Centers for Disease Control and Prevention. Administration of zidovudine during late pregnancy and delivery to prevent perinatal HIV transmission — Thailand, 1996–1998. *MMWR* 47 (1998): 151–154.

Centers for Disease Control and Prevention. *HIV/AIDS Surveillance Report.* CDC, January 1991. http://www.cdc.gov/hiv/topics/surveillance/resources/reports/pdf/surveillance90.pdf.

Centers for Disease Control and Prevention. *HIV/AIDS Surveillance Report.* CDC, December 1999. http://www.cdc.gov/hiv/pdf/statistics_hasr1102.pdf.

Centers for Disease Control and Prevention. Public Health Service guidelines for the management of health-care worker exposures to HIV and recommendations for postexposure prophylaxis. *MMWR* 47, no. RR-7 (1998): 1–28.

Centers for Disease Control and Prevention. Zidovudine for the prevention of HIV transmission from mother to infant. *MMWR* 43 (1994): 285–287.

Chang, H. E. Triple-drug therapy still worth testing, despite laboratory error. *AIDS Treatment News* no. 181, August 20, 1993.

Chase, M. Boehringer Ingelheim Corp. is expected to announce today that it is curtailing development of an AIDS drug because it encountered a problem with viral resistance. Dow Jones News Service, November 27, 1991.

Chase, M. Boehringer is seen scaling back testing on AIDS drug facing viral resistance. *Wall Street Journal*, November 27, 1991.

Chase, M. Merck setback shows problems of AIDS drugs. *Wall Street Journal*, November 16, 1991.

Chasela, C. S., M. G. Hudgens, D. J. Jamieson, D. Kayira, M. C. Hosseinipour, A. P. Kourtis, F. Martinson, G. Tegha, R. J. Knight, Y. I. Ahmed, D. D. Kamwendo, I. F. Hoffman, S. R. Ellington, Z. Kacheche, A. Soko, J. B. Wiener, S. A. Fiscus, P. Kazembe, I. A. Mofolo, M. Chigwenembe, D. Sichali, and C. M. Van der Horst. Maternal or infant antiretroviral drugs to reduce HIV-1 transmission. *N Eng J Med* 362 (2010): 2271–2281.

Cheeseman, S. H. Nevirapine (NVP) alone and in combination with zidovudine (ZDV): Safety and activity. The ACTG 164/168 Study Team. *Int Conf AIDS* 8: Mo15 (abstract no. MoB 0053), July 19–24, 1992.

Cheeseman, S. H., S. E. Hattox, M. M. McLaughlin, R. A. Koup, C. Andrews, C. A. Bova, J. W. Pav, T. Roy,

J. L. Sullivan, and J. J. Keirns. Pharmacokinetics of nevirapine: Initial single-rising-dose study in humans. *Antimicrob Agents Chemother* 37 (1993): 178–182.

Cheeseman, S. H., D. Havlir, M. M. McLaughlin, T. C. Greenough, J. L. Sullivan, D. Hall, S. E. Hattox, S. A. Spector, D. S. Stein, M. Myers, and D. D. Richman. Phase I/II evaluation of nevirapine alone and in combination with zidovudine for infection with human immunodeficiency virus. *J Acquir Immune Defic Syndr and Human Retrovirology* 8 (1995): 141–151.

Cheeseman, S. H., R. L. Murphy, M. S. Saag, and D. Havlir. Safety of high dose nevirapine (NVP) after 200 mg/d lead-in. ACTG 164/168 Study Team. *Int Conf AIDS* 9: 487 (abstract no. PO-B26-2109), June 6–11, 1993.

Chi, B. H., L. Wang, J. S. Read, M. Sheriff, S. Fiscus, E. R. Brown, T. E. Taha, M. Valentine, and R. Goldenberg. Timing of maternal and neonatal dosing of nevirapine and the risk of mother-to-child transmission of HIV-1: HIVNET 024. *AIDS* 19 (2005): 1857–1864.

Chigwedere, P., G. R. Seage, III, S. Gruskin, T-H. Lee, and M. Essex. Estimating the lost benefits of antiretroviral drug use in South Africa, *J Acquir Immune Defic Syndr* 49 (2008): 410–415.

Chow, Y-K., M. S. Hirsch, J. C. Kaplan, and R. T. D'Aquila. HIV-1 error revealed. *Nature* 364 (1993): 679.

Chow, Y-K., M. S. Hirsch, D. P. Merrill, L. J. Bechtel, J. J. Eron, J. C. Kaplan, and R. T. D'Aquila. Use of evolutionary limitations of HIV-1 multidrug resistance to optimize therapy. *Nature* 361 (1993): 650–654.

Chow, Y-K., D. P. Merrill, J. C. Kaplan, R. T. D'Aquila, and M. S. Hirsch. In vitro selection of multi-drug resistant HIV-1. *Int Conf AIDS* 9: 35 (abstract no. WS-A19-6), June 6–11, 1993.

Chung, M. H., J. N. Kiarie, B. A. Richardson, D. A. Lehman, J. Overbaugh, and G. C. John-Steward. Breast milk HIV-1 suppression and decreased transmission: a randomized trial comparing HIVNET 012 nevirapine versus short-course zidovudine. *AIDS* 19 (2005): 1415–1422.

Clayden, P. Nevirapine and MTCT: The single-dose backlash. *HIV Treatment Bulletin* 4 (2003): 20–23.

Clinton Foundation Annual Report, 2008.

Clinton Foundation Annual Report, 2010.

Cohen, J. HIV Transmission: Allegations raise fears of backlash against AIDS prevention strategy. *Science* 306 (2004): 2168–2169.

Cohen, J. South African leader declines to join the chorus on HIV and AIDS. *Science* 289 (2000): 222.

Cohen, M. S., Y. Q. Chen, M. McCauley, T. Gamble, M. C. Hosseinipour, N. Kumarasamy, J. G. Hakim, J. Kumwenda, B. Grinsztejn, J. H. S. Pilotto, S. V. Godbole, S. Mehendale, S. Chariyalertsak, B. R. Santos, K. H. Mayer, I. F. Hoffman, S. H. Eshleman, E. Piwowar-Manning, L. Wang, J. Makhema, L. A. Mills, G. de Bruyn, I. Sanne, J. Eron, J. Gallant, D. Havlir, S. Swindells, H. Ribaudo, V. Elharrar, D. Burns, T. E. Taha, K. Nielsen-Saines, D. Celentano, M. Essex, and T. R. Fleming for the HPTN 052 Study Team. Prevention of HIV-1 infection with early antiretroviral therapy. *N Engl J Med* 365 (2011): 493–505.

Cohen, S. A. Beyond slogans: Lessons from Uganda's experience with ABC and HIV/AIDS. *The Guttmacher Report on Public Policy* 6 (2003): 1–3.

Conant, M. Sixth International Conference overview from Marcus Conant. *AIDS Treatment News* no. 106, July 6, 1990.

Connor, E. M., R. S. Sperling, R. Gelber, P. Kiselev, G. Scott, M. J. O'Sullivan, R. VanDyke, M. Vey, W. Shearer, R. L. Jacobson, E. Jimenez, E. O'Neill, B. Bazin, J-F. Delfraissy, M. Culnane, R. Coombs, M. Elkins, J. Moye, P. Stratton, and J. Balsley. Reduction of maternal-infant transmission of human immunodeficiency virus type 1 with zidovudine treatment. *N Engl J Med* 331 (1994): 1173–1180.

Coombs, R.W., S. L. Welles, C. Hooper, P. S. Reichelderfer, R. T. D'Aquila, A. J. Japour, V. A. Johnson, D. R. Kuritzkes, D. D. Richman, S. Kwok, J. Todd, J. B. Jackson, V. DeGruttola, C. S. Crumpacker, and J. Kahn for the ACTG 116B/117 Study Team. Association of plasma human immunodeficiency virus type 1 RNA level with risk of clinical progression in patients with advanced infection. *J Infect Dis* 174 (1996): 704–712.

Cooper, E. C. Clinical trials in AIDS: The regulatory perspective. *Int Conf AIDS* 5: 211 (abstract no. W.B.O.47), June 4–9, 1989.

Cooper, E. C., J. E. Knight, and E. M. Leonard. Development of new drugs for the treatment of pediatric AIDS: Scientific and regulatory issues. In *Pediatric AIDS: Challenge of HIV infection in infants, children and adolescents*, eds. P. A. Pizzo and C. M. Wilfert, 605–618. Baltimore: Williams and Wilkins, 1991.

Coovadia, H. M., E. R. Brown, M. G. Fowler, T. Chipato, D. Moodley, K. Manji, P. Musoke, L. Stranix-Chibanda, V. Chetty, W. Fawzi, C. Nankabiito, L. Msweli, R. Kisenge, L. Guay, A. Mwatha, D. J. Lynn, S. H. Eshleman, P. Richardson, K. George, P.Andrew, L. M. Mofenson, S. Zwerski, and Y. Maldanado for the HPTN 046 protocol team. Efficacy and safety of an extended nevirapine regimen in infant children of breastfeeding mothers with HIV-1 infection for prevention of postnatal HIV-1 transmission (HPTN 046): A randomized, double-blind, placebo-controlled trial. *Lancet* 379, no. 9812 (2012): 221–228.

Cullinan, K. Court orders South Africa to treat pregnant HIV-positive women with nevirapine. *Bull WHO* 80 (2002): 335.

Currier, J. S. Sex differences in antiretroviral therapy toxicity: Lactic acidosis, stavudine, and women. *Clin Inf Dis* 45 (2007): 261–262.

Curry, G. E. AIDS conference ends with optimism. *Philly.com*, August 1, 2010.

Dagani, R. New anti–HIV-1 agents most potent ever. *C & E News*, February 5, 1990.

Danforth, W. H., L. H. Aiken, M. H. Becker, V. A. Cargill, J. M. Coffin, R. G. Douglas, Jr., J. Eigo, H. N. Eisen, M. M. Grumbach, D. Hopkins, C. M. Lang, C. Meinert, N. Nathanson, P. S. Schein, and A. Silverstein. *The AIDS research program of the National Institutes of Health*. Washington, DC: National Academy Press, 1991.

D'Aquila, R. T., M. D. Hughes, V. A. Johnson, M. A. Fischl, J-P. Sommadossi, S-H. Liou, J. Timpone, M. Myers, N. Basgoz, M. Niu, M. S. Hirsch, and NIAID

ACTG 241 investigators. Nevirapine, zidovudine, and didanosine compared with zidovudine and didanosine in patients with HIV-1 infection. *Ann Intern Med* 124 (1996): 1019–1030.

De Capua, J. South Africa/Nevirapine. *VOA News*, February 13, 2002.

De Capua, J. South African doctor says benefits of nevirapine outweigh any risks. *VOA News*, December 20, 2004.

De Cock, K. M., M. G. Fowler, E. Mercier, I. De Vincenzi, J. Saba, E. Hoff, D. J. Alnwick, M. Rogers, and N. Shaffer. Prevention of mother-to-child HIV transmission in resource-poor countries. *JAMA* 283 (2000): 1175–1182.

De Jong, M. D., M. Loewenthal, C. A. B. Boucher, I. Van der Ende, D. Hall, P. Schipper, A. Imrie, H. B. Weigel, R. H. Kauffmann, R. Koster, P. Seville, R. Rocklin, D. A. Cooper, and J. M. A. Lange. Alternating nevirapine and zidovudine treatment of human immunodeficiency virus type 1-infected persons does not prolong nevirapine activity. *J Infect Dis* 169 (1994): 1346–1350.

De Jong, M. D., S. Vella, A. Carr, C. A. B. Boucher, A. Imrie, M. French, J. Hoy, S., Sorice, S. Pauluzzi, F., Chiodo, G. J. Weverling, M. E. van der Ende, Ph. J. Frissen, H. M. Weigel, R. H. Kauffmann, J. M. A. Lange, R. Yoon, M. Moroni, E., Hoenderlos, G., Leitz, D. A. Cooper, D. Hall, and P. Reiss. High-dose nevirapine in previously untreated human immunodeficiency virus type 1-infected persons does not result in sustained suppression of viral replication. *J Infect Dis* 175 (1997): 966–970.

DeWit, S., P. Hermans, B. Sommereijns, E. O'Doherty, R. Westenborghs, V. van de Velde, G. F. M. J. Cauwenbergh, and N. Clumeck. Pharmacokinetics of R 82913 in AIDS patients: A phase I dose-finding study of oral administration compared with intravenous infusion. *Antimicrob Agents Chemother* 36 (1992): 2661–2663.

Donnelly, J. The President's Emergency Plan for AIDS Relief: How George W. Bush and aides came to "think big" on battling HIV. *Health Affairs* 31 (2012): 1389–1396.

Dorenbaum, A., C. K. Cunningham, R. D. Gelber, M. Culnane, L. Mofenson, P. Britto, C. Rekacewicz, M-L. Newel, J. F. Delfraissy, B. Cunningham-Schrader, M. Mirochnick, and J. L. Sullivan. Two-dose intrapartum/newborn nevirapine and standard antiretroviral therapy to reduce perinatal HIV transmission. *JAMA* 288 (2002): 189–198.

Drugs for HIV infection. *Medical Letter* 31 (1990): 11–13.

Duggan, P. 1,000 Swarm FDA's Rockville office to demand approval of AIDS drugs. *Washington Post*, October 12, 1988.

Ehrnst, A., B. Johanson, A. Sönnerborg, J. Czajkowski, G. Sundin, S. Lindgren, A-B. Bohlin, and M. Dictor. HIV in pregnant women and their offspring: Evidence for late transmission. *Lancet* 338, no. 8761 (1991): 203–207.

Eigo, J. ACT UP crashes the gates. *Global Forum* 5 (2013): 13–20.

Elizabeth Glaser Pediatric AIDS Foundation. Elizabeth Glaser Pediatric AIDS Foundation awarded $100 million by United States Agency for International Development.Press Release, July 31, 2002.

Elizabeth Glaser Pediatric AIDS Foundation. Elizabeth Glaser Pediatric AIDS Foundation on issue of prevention of mother-to-child transmission of HIV/AIDS and single-dose nevirapine. Press Release, December 14, 2004.

Elizabeth Glaser Pediatric AIDS Foundation Annual Report, 1999.

Elizabeth Glaser Pediatric AIDS Foundation Annual Report, 2001.

Elizabeth Glaser Pediatric AIDS Foundation Annual Report, 2003.

Elizabeth Glaser Pediatric AIDS Foundation Annual Report, 2007.

Elizabeth Glaser Pediatric AIDS Foundation Annual Report, 2011.

Ellis, D. The defiant one. *People Magazine*, December 19, 1994.

Eshleman, S. H., D. R. Hoover, S. Chen, S. E. Hudelson, L. A. Guay, A. Mwatha, S. A. Fiscus, F. Mmiro, P. Musoke, J. B. Jackson, N. Kumwenda, and T. Taha. Resistance after single-dose nevirapine prophylaxis emerges in a high proportion of Malawian newborns. *AIDS* 19 (2005): 2167–2175.

Eshleman, S. H., and J. B. Jackson. Nevirapine resistance after single dose prophylaxis. *AIDS Rev* 4 (2002): 59–63.

Eshleman, S. H., M. Mracna, L. A. Guay, M. Deseyve, S. Cunningham, M. Mirochnick, P. Musoke, T. Fleming, M. G. Fowler, L. M. Mofenson, F. Mmiro, and J. B. Jackson. Selection and fading of resistance mutations in women and infants receiving nevirapine to prevent HIV-1 vertical transmission (HIVNET 012). *AIDS* 15 (2001): 1951–1957.

A failure led to drug against AIDS. *New York Times*, September 19, 1986.

Faith Alive Foundation Annual Report, 2006.

Farley, T., and I. De Zoysa. Nevirapine for the prevention of mother-to-child transmission of HIV: WHO reconfirms its support for the use of nevirapine to prevent mother-to-child transmission of HIV. WHO Press Release, July 2003.

F-D-C Reports. Surrogate endpoints for AIDS drugs: Long-term studies needed. *Pink Sheet*, October 11, 1989.

F-D-C Reports. Janssen's TIBO/benzodiazepine AIDS drugs. *Pink Sheet*, October 15, 1990.

Food and Drug Administration. Points to consider in the preparation of IND applications for new drugs intended for the treatment of HIV-infected individuals. Division of Antiviral Drug Products, CDER, issued February 1990.

Food and Drug Administration. HHS Secretary Lewis W. Sullivan announces FDA's approval of ddI. News Release, October 9, 1991.

Fischl, M. A., D. D. Richman, M. H. Grieco, M. S. Gottlieb, P. A. Volberding, O. L. Laskin, J. M. Leedom, J. E. Groopman, D. Mildvan, R. T. Schooley, G. G. Jackson, D. T. Durack, D. King, and the AZT Collaborative Working Group. The efficacy of azidothymidine (AZT) in the treatment of patients with AIDS and AIDS-related complex. *N Engl J Med* 317 (1987): 185–191.

Fischl, M. A., K. Stanley, J. M. Ardunio, K. Kazial, and D. Stein. The safety and efficacy of zidovudine (ZDV) and zalcitabine (ddC) or ddC alone versus ZDV.

ACTG 155 Team of the NIAID. *Int Conf AIDS* 9: 68 (abstract no. WS-B25–1), June 6–11, 1993.

Fischl, M. A., K. Stanley, A. C. Collier, J. M. Arduino, D. S. Stein, J. E. Feinberg, D. J. Allan, J. C. Goldsmith, W. G. Powderly, and the NIAID AIDS Clinical Trials Group. Combination and monotherapy with zidovudine and zalcitabine in patients with advanced HIV disease (ACTG 155). *Ann Intern Med* 122 (1995): 24–32.

Folkers, G. NIAID funds adult AIDS clinical trials group. NIAID News Release, November 30, 1995.

Fowler, J. Jake Glaser alive and thriving. *People Magazine*, April 7, 2008.

Fowler, M. G., and M. L. Newell. Breast-feeding and HIV-1 transmission in resource-limited settings. *J Acquir Immune Defic Syndr* 30 (2002): 230–239.

Franke-Ruta, G. A new tide in antiviral research. *GMHC Newsletter Treatment Issues*, May 15, 1991.

Freudenheim, M. Sick get experimental drugs free. *New York Times*, October 21, 1989.

Garrett, L. AIDS at 20/Seeking global answer/AIDS fund poses worldwide challenge. *Newsday*, June 16, 2011.

Gebbie, K. M. The president's commission on AIDS: What did it do? *AJPH* 79 (1989): 868–870.

Gibson, J. Update on the use of nevirapine in clinical trials. *STEP Perspective*, July 1993.

Glaser, E. Address to the Democratic National Convention. New York, July 14, 1992.

Glaser, E., and L. Palmer. *In the absence of angels: A Hollywood family's courageous story*. New York: Putnam, 1991.

Glaser, J. What I want you to know about AIDS. *Glamour Magazine*, May 2011.

Global Strategies for HIV Prevention. Comments on a recent media article on the HIVNET 012 Uganda study. Press Release, December 15, 2004.

Global Strategies for HIV Prevention. Pennies from heaven. *Global Strategies for HIV Prevention Newsletter*, December 2004.

Global Strategies for HIV Prevention. Second international conference on global strategies for the prevention of HIV transmission from mothers to infants, Montreal, September 1–6, 1999. *Global Strategies for HIV Prevention Newsletter*, January 2000.

Global Strategies for HIV Prevention. A trilogy of international conferences — moving the HIV prevention agenda forward. *Global Strategies for HIV Prevention Newsletter*, June 2002.

Goldman, M. E. Discovery and development of 2-pyridinone HIV-1 reverse transcriptase inhibitors. In *The search for antiviral drugs: Case histories from concept to clinic*, eds. J. Adams and V. J. Merluzzi, 105–127. Boston: Birkhäuser, 1993.

Gonsalves, G., and M. Harrington. AIDS research at NIH: A critical review, 8th International Conference on AIDS. Amsterdam, July 20, 1992.

Gottlieb, M. S., H. M. Schanker, P. T. Fan, A. Saxon, and J. D. Weisman. Pneumocystis Pneumonia — Los Angeles. *MMWR* 30 (1981): 1–3.

Gottlieb, M. S., R. Schroff, H. M. Schanker, J. D. Weisman, P. T. Fan, R. A. Wolf, and A. Saxon, *Pneumocystis carinii* pneumonia and mucosal candidiasis in previously healthy homosexual men. *N Engl J Med* 305 (1981): 1425–1431.

Gray, G. The PETRA study: early and late efficacy of three short ZDV/3TC combination regimens to prevent mother-to-child transmission of HIV-1. *Int Conf AIDS* 13: 17 (abstract no. LbOr5), July 9–14, 2000.

Greenough, T. C. Quantitative virology: The experience during the nevirapine phase I/II trials, ACTG 164/168 Study Team. *Int Conf AIDS* 8: B192 (abstract no. PoB 3610), July 19–24, 1992.

Grob, P. M., Y. Cao, E. Muchmore, D. D. Ho, S. Norris, J. W. Pav, and J. Adams. Prophylaxis against HIV-1 infection in chimpanzees by nevirapine, a nonnucleoside inhibitor of reverse transcriptase. *Nature Med* 3 (1997): 665–670.

Grozinger, K. G., and A. A. Hawi. Pharmaceutical suspension comprising nevirapine hemihydrate. U.S. Patent 6,255,481, issued July 3, 2001.

Grozinger, K., J. Proudfoot, and K. Hargrave. Discovery and development of nevirapine. In *Drug Discovery and Development*, ed. M. S. Chorghade, 353–363. Hoboken, NJ: Wiley, 2006.

Grubman, S., and J. Oleske. Primary care for the HIV-infected child. *PAACNOTES*, January 1993.

Guay, L. A., P. Musoke, T. Fleming, D. Bagenda, M. Allen, C. Nakabiito, J. Sherman, P. Bakaki, C. Ducar, M. Deseyve, L. Emel, M. Mirochnick, M. G. Fowler, L. Mofenson, P. Miotti, K. Dransfield, D. Bray, R. Mmiro, and J. B. Jackson. Intrapartum and neonatal single-dose nevirapine compared with zidovudine for prevention of mother-to-child transmission of HIV-1 in Kampala, Uganda: HIVNET 012 randomized trial. *Lancet* 354, no. 9181 (1999): 795–802.

Gulick, R. M., J. W. Mellors, D. Havlir, J. J. Eron, C. Gonzalez, D. McMahon, D. D. Richman, F. T. Valentine, L. Jonas, A. Meibohm, E. A. Emini, J. A. Chodakewitz, P. Deutsch, D. Holder, W. A. Schleif, and J. H. Condra. Treatment with indinavir, zidovudine, and lamivudine in adults with human immunodeficiency virus infection and prior antiretroviral therapy. *N Engl J Med* 337 (1997): 734–739.

Gulick, R. M., J. W. Mellors, D. Havlir, J. J. Eron, C. Gonzalez, D. McMahon, D. D. Richman, F. T. Valentine, J. Rooney, L. Jonas, A., Meibohm, E. A. Emini, and J. Chodakewitz. Potent and sustained antiretroviral activity of indinavir AZT and 3TC, Merck 035, *Int Conf AIDS* 11: 19 (abstract no. Th.B. 931), July 7–12, 1996.

Hadigan, C. Insulin resistance among HIV-infected patients: unraveling the mechanism. *Clin Infect Dis* 41 (2005): 1341–1342.

Hale, J. After Montreal, international AIDS conferences will never be the same. *Can Med Assoc J* 141 (1989): 144–146.

Hall, D. B., and T. R. MacGregor. Case-control exploration of relationships between early rash or liver toxicity and plasma concentrations of nevirapine and primary metabolites. *HIV Clin Trials* 8 (2007): 381–399.

Hammer, S. M., D. A. Katzenstein, M. D. Hughes, H. Gundacker, R. T. Schooley, R. H. Haubrich, W. K. Henry, M. M. Lederman, J. P. Phair, M. Niu, M. S. Hirsch, and T. C. Merigan for the ACTG 175 study team. A trial comparing nucleoside monotherapy with combination therapy in HIV-infected adults with CD4 cell counts from 200 to 500 per cubic millimeter. *N Engl J Med* 335 (1996): 1081–1090.

Hammer, S. M., K. E. Squires, M. D. Hughes, J. M. Grimes, L. M. Demeter, J. S. Currier, J. J. Eron, J. E. Feinberg, H. H. Balfour, Jr., L. R. Deyton, J. A. Chadakewitz, and M. A. Fischl for the AIDS Clinical Trials Group 320 Study Team. A controlled trial of two nucleoside analogues plus indinavir in persons with human immunodeficiency virus infection and CD4 cell counts of 200 per cubic millimeter or less. *N Engl J Med* 337 (1997): 725–733.

Harden, V. A. *AIDS at 30: A history*. Washington, DC: Potomac Books, 2012.

Harden, V. A. Interview with James C. Hill. *In Their Own Words*, NIH Historical Office, October 4, 1988.

Hargrave, K. D., J. R. Proudfoot, J. Adams, K. G. Grozinger, G. Schmidt, G. Engel, W. Trummlitz, and W. Eberlein. 5,11-dihydro-6H-dipyrido(3,2-B:2',3'-E)(1,4)diazepines and their use in the prevention or treatment of HIV infection. U.S. Patent 5,366,972, issued November 22, 1994.

Harrington, M. The crisis in clinical AIDS research. *The Body*, December 1993.

Harrington, M. Once we were warriors: Activist corpses born in protest, furtive legislative coups, and the devastation that was Berlin. *The Body*, March 2002.

Harrington, M., and C. C. J. Carpenter. Hit HIV-1 hard, but only when necessary. *Lancet* 355, no. 9221 (2000): 2147–2152.

Hattox, S. E. Pharmacokinetics of nevirapine alone and in combination with zidovudine: The ACTG 164/168 Study Team. *Int Conf AIDS* 8: B185 (abstract no. PoB 3591), July 19–24, 1992.

Havlir, D., S. H. Cheeseman, M. McLaughlin, R. Murphy, A. Erice, S. A. Spector, T. C. Greenough, J. L. Sullivan, D. Hall, M. Myers, M. Lamson, and D. D. Richman. High-dose nevirapine: Safety, pharmacokinetics, and antiviral effect in patients with human immunodeficiency virus infection. *J Infect Dis* 171 (1995): 537–545.

Havlir, D., M. M. McLaughlin, and D. D. Richman. A pilot study to evaluate the development of resistance to nevirapine in asymptomatic human immunodeficiency virus-infected patients with CD4 cell counts of > 500/mm³: AIDS Clinical Trials Group Protocol 208. *J Infect Dis* 172 (1995): 1379–1383.

Havlir, D., R. Murphy, M. Saag, I. Kaul, V. Johnson, and D. D. Richman. Nevirapine: Further dose escalation of monotherapy (600 mg/daily) and combination therapy with zidovudine, *First Natl Conf Hum Retrovir Relat Infect* (abstract no. 1: 101), December 12–16, 1993.

Heldman, P. P. AIDS drug called promising. *Worcester Telegram & Gazette*, October 23, 1990.

Henry, K., A. Erice, C. Tierney, H. H. Balfour, M. A. Fischl, A. Kmack, S-H. Liou, A. Kenton, M. S. Hirsch, J. Phair, A. Martinez, and J. O. Kahn for the AIDS Clinical Trial Group 193A Study Team: A randomized, controlled, double-blind study comparing the survival benefit of four different reverse transcriptase inhibitor therapies (three-drug, two-drug, and alternating drug) for the treatment of advanced AIDS. *J Acquir Immune Defic Syndr and Human Retrovirology* 19 (1998): 339–349.

Heywood, M. Preventing mother-to-child HIV transmission in South Africa. *South African Journal on Human Rights* 19 (2003): 278–315.

Hilts, P. J. 82 held in protest on pace of AIDS research. *New York Times*, May 22, 1990.

HIV/AIDS Update—International conference paints bleak picture of pandemic with severe socioeconomic consequences. *MedPRO Month* 11 (1992): 116–119.

Ho, D. D. Dynamics of HIV-1 replication in vivo. *J Clin Invest* 99 (1997): 2565–2567.

Ho, D. D. Time to hit HIV, early and hard. *N Engl J Med* 333 (1995): 450–451.

Horwitz, J. P., J. Chua, and M. Noel. Nucleosides. V. The monomesylates of 1-(2'-Deoxy-β-D-Lysofuranosyl) thymine. *J Organic Chem* 29 (1964): 2076–2078.

The house that Harvey built. *Pharmaceutical Executive*, May 1983.

How to Survive a Plague. DVD, MPI Media Group, 2013.

Howse, J. Treatment Access March. *South African Medical Journal*, July 9, 2000.

Hoyle, P. C., and E. C. Cooper. Shortening the research and development time for new AIDS drugs: the pre-IND program and proactive clinical guidance at FDA's division of antiviral drugs. *Int Conf AIDS* 5: 552 (abstract no. M.C.P.61), June 4–9, 1989.

Huck, J. Breaking a silence: Starsky star, wife share their family's painful battle against AIDS. *Los Angeles Times*, August 25, 1989.

Huff, B. Let nevirapine do what it does best. *GMHC Treatment Issues*, March 2002.

Ismail, W. I. W., J. A. King, and T. S. Pillay. Insulin resistance induced by antiretroviral drugs: Current understanding of molecular mechanisms. *JEMDSA* 14 (2009): 129–132.

Jackson, J. B., R. W. Coombs, K. Sannerud, F. S. Rhame, and H. H. Balfour, Jr. Rapid and sensitive viral culture method for human immunodeficiency virus type 1. *J Clin Microbiol* 26 (1988): 1416–1418.

Jackson, J. B., G. Gecker-Pergola, L. A. Guay, P. Musoke, M. Mracna, M. G. Fowler, L. M. Mofenson, M. Mirochnick, F. Mmiro, and S. H. Eshleman. Identification of the K103N resistance mutation in Ugandan women receiving nevirapine to prevent HIV-1 vertical transmission. *AIDS* 14 (2000): F111–F115.

Jackson, J. B., P. Musoke, T. Fleming, L. A. Guay, D. Bagenda, M. Allen, C. Nakabiito, J. Sherman, P. Bakaki, M. Owor, C. Ducar, M. Deseyve, A. Mwatha, L. Emel, C. Duefield, M. Mirochnick, M. G. Fowler, L. Mofenson, P. Miotti, M. Gigliotti, D. Bray, and F. Mmiro. Intrapartum and neonatal single-dose nevirapine compared with zidovudine for prevention of mother-to-child transmission of HIV-1 in Kampala, Uganda: 18-month follow-up of the HIVNET 012 randomised trial. *Lancet* 362, no. 9387 (2003): 859–868.

James, J. S. Aerosol pentamidine, ganciclovir recommended for approval. *AIDS Treatment News* no. 78, May 5, 1989.

James, J. S. Convergent combination therapy. *AIDS Treatment News* no. 170, March 5, 1993.

James, J. S. ddC/ddI approval update. *AIDS Treatment News* no. 118, January 4, 1991.

James, J. S. ddI and ddC approval effort—interview with Martin Delaney. *AIDS Treatment News* no. 116, December 7, 1990.

James, J. S. Nevirapine triple combination: Preliminary results. *AIDS Treatment News* no. 211, November 18, 1994.

James, J. S. San Francisco AIDS Conference, related events: Issues and update. *AIDS Treatment News* no. 102, May 4, 1990.

Jerome P. Horwitz: AZT, the anticancer drug he developed 22 years ago, is now our best hope in the battle against AIDS. *People Magazine*, December 22, 1986.

Johnson, B. K., G. A. Stone, M S. Dogec, D. M. Asher, D. C. Cajdusek, and C. J. Gibbs, Jr. Long-term observations of human immunodeficiency virus-infected chimpanzees. *AIDS Res Hum Retroviruses* 9 (1993): 375–378.

Johnson, D. Ryan White dies of AIDS at 18: His struggle helped pierce myths. *New York Times*, April 9, 1990.

Johnson, N. Opening ceremony address, 13th International AIDS Conference, July 9, 2000.

Johnson, V. A., M. A. Barlow, D. P. Merrill, T-C. Chou, and M. S. Hirsch. Three-drug synergistic inhibition of HIV-1 replication in vitro by zidovudine, recombinant soluble CD4, and recombinant interferon-alpha A. *J Infect Dis* 161 (1990): 1059–1067.

Johnson/Johnson unit stays with AIDS drugs. Reuters News Service, November 27, 1991.

Johnston, M. I., and D. F. Hoth. Present status and future prospects for HIV therapies. *Science* 260 (1993): 1286–1293.

Jourdain, G., N. Ngo-Giang-Huong, S. LeCoeur, C. Bowonwatanuwong, P. Kantipong, P. Leechanachai, S. Ariyadej, P. Leenasirimakul, S. Hammer, and M. Lallemant for the Perinatal HIV Prevention Trial Group. Intrapartum exposure to nevirapine and subsequent maternal responses to nevirapine-based antiretroviral therapy. *N Engl J Med* 351 (2004): 229–240.

Kahn, J. O., S. W. Lagakos, D. D. Richman, A. Cross, C. Pettinelli, S-H. Liou, M. Brown, P. A. Volberding, C. S. Crumpacker, G. Beall, H. Sacks, T. C. Merigan, M. Beltangady, L. Smaldone, and R. A. Dolin. A controlled trial comparing continued zidovudine with didanosine in human immunodeficiency virus infection. *N Engl J Med* 327 (1992): 581–587.

Karim, S. A., Q. A. Karim, M. Adhikari, S. Cassol, M. Chersich, P. Cooper, A. Coovadia, H. Coovadia, M. Cotton, A. Coutsoudis, W. Hide, G. Hussey, G. Maartens, S. Madhi, D. Martin, J. M. Pettifor, N. Rollins, G. Sherman, S. Thula, M. Urban, S. Velaphi, and C. Williamson. Vertical HIV transmission in South Africa: translating research into policy and practice. *Lancet* 359, no. 9311 (2002): 992–993.

Karon, T. South African AIDS activist Zackie Achmat. *Time*, April 19, 2001.

Kasper, D. L., E. Braunwald, A. S. Fauci, S. S. Hauser, D. L. Longo, and J. L. Jameson, eds. *Harrison's Principles of Internal Medicine*, 16th ed. New York: McGraw-Hill, 2005.

Kelly, A. Background: HIV/AIDS in Uganda. *The Guardian*, December 1, 2008.

Kennedy, R. Elizabeth Glaser dies at 47: Crusader for pediatric AIDS. *New York Times*, December 4, 1994.

Kesho Bora Study Group. Triple antiretroviral compared with zidovudine and single-dose nevirapine prophylaxis during pregnancy and breastfeeding for prevention of mother-to-child transmission of HIV-1 (Kesho Bora study): A randomized controlled study. *Lancet Inf Dis* 11 (2011): 171–180.

Kessler, D. *A question of intent: A great American battle with a deadly industry*. New York: PublicAffairs, 2001.

Klunder, J. M., K. D. Hargrave, J. R. Proudfoot, K. G. Grozinger, E. Cullen, U. R. Patel, and S. R. Kapadia. Synthesis of a series of dipyrido[3,2-b:2',3'-e]diazepinones: Potent and selective non-nucleoside inhibitors of HIV-1 reverse transcriptase. *Int Conf AIDS* 7:109 (abstract no. W.A.1070), June 16–21, 1991.

Kohlsteadt, L. A., and T. A. Steitz. Reverse transcriptase of human immunodeficiency virus can use either human tRNA^{Lys3} or *Escherichia coli* tRNA^{Gln2} as a primer in an *in vitro* primer-utilization assay. *Proc Natl Acad Sci USA* 89 (1992): 9652–9656.

Kohlsteadt, L. A., J. Wang, J. M. Friedman, P. A. Rice, and T. A. Steitz. Crystal structure at 3.5 Å resolution of HIV-1 reverse transcriptase complexed with an inhibitor. *Science* 256 (1992): 1783–1790.

Kolata, G. AIDS researcher seeks wide access to drugs in tests. *New York Times*, June 26, 1989.

Kolata, G. Citing stress, FDA aide wants out. *New York Times*, December 22, 1990.

Kolata, G. FDA debate on speedy access to AIDS drugs is reopening. *New York Times*, September 12, 1994.

Kolata, G. FDA gives quick approval to two drugs to treat AIDS. *New York Times*, June 27, 1989.

Kolata, G. Innovative AIDS drug plan may be undermining testing. *New York Times*, November 21, 1989.

Kolata, G. Interest grows in licensing shortcut for 2 AIDS drugs. *New York Times*, September 25, 1990.

Kolata, G. Medical data: Who should hear it first? *New York Times*, May 22, 1990.

Kolberg, R. New AIDS drug may be less toxic, reach brain. United Press International, December 6, 1990.

Koop, C. E. Foreword. In *Pediatric AIDS: Challenge of HIV infection in infants, children and adolescents*, eds. P. A. Pizzo and C. M. Wilfert. Baltimore: Williams and Wilkins, 1991, vii–viii.

Kresge, K. J. Treatment is prevention. *IAVI Report* 15 (2011): 14–16.

Krogstad, P., S. Lee, G. Johnson, K. Stanley, J. McNamara, J. Moye, J. B. Jackson, R. Aguayo, A. Dieudonne, M. Khoury, H. Mendez, S. Nachman, A. Wiznia, and the Pediatric AIDS Clinical Trials Group 377 Study Team. Nucleoside-analogue reverse-transcriptase inhibitors plus nevirapine, nelfinavir, or ritonavir for pretreated children infected with human immunodeficiency virus type 1. *Clin Inf Dis* 34 (2002): 991–1001.

LaFraniere, S. South Africa rejects use of AIDS drug for women. *New York Times*, July 14, 2004.

Lagakos, S., J. Ware, R. Charo, E. Davidson, W. El-Sadr, M. Kline, J. Landis, G. Rutherford, and C. Van der Horst. *Review of the HIVNET 012 perinatal HIV prevention study*. Washington, DC: National Academies Press, April 7, 2005.

Lake, J. E., and J. S. Currier. Switching antiretroviral therapy to minimize metabolic complications. *HIV Ther* 4 (2010): 693–711.

Lallemant, M., G. Jourdain, S. LeCoeur, J. Y. Mary, N. Ngo-Giang-Huong, S. Koetsawang, S. Kanshana, K. McIntosh, and V. Thaineua for the Perinatal HIV

Prevention Trial (Thailand) Investigators. Single-dose perinatal nevirapine plus standard zidovudine to prevent mother-to-child transmission of HIV-1 in Thailand. *N Engl J Med* 351 (2004): 217–228.

Lambert, B. Jay C. Lipner, 46, a lawyer-lobbyist for victims of AIDS. *New York Times*, November 7, 1991.

Lamson, M. J., J. P. Sabo, T. R. MacGregor, J. W. Pav, L. Rowland, A., Hawi, M. Cappola, and P. Robinson. Single dose pharmacokinetics and bioavailability of nevirapine in healthy volunteers. *Biopharmaceutics & Drug Disposition* 20 (1999): 285–291.

Lange, J. M. A. Efficacy and durability of nevirapine in antiretroviral drug naïve patients. *J Acquir Immune Defic Syndr* 34, suppl. no. 1 (2003): S40-S52.

Larder, B. A., G. Darby, and D. D. Richman. HIV with reduced sensitivity to zidovudine (AZT) isolated during prolonged therapy. *Science* 243 (1989): 1731–1734.

Larder, B. A., P. Kellam, and S. Kemp. Convergent combination therapy can select viable multidrug-resistant HIV-1 in vitro. *Nature* 365 (1993): 451–453.

Lasagna, L., T. Cooper, G. Elon, E. Frei, S. Hellman, P. B. Hutt, C. Leighton, T. C. Merigan, Jr., and H. C. Pitot. *Final report of the national committee to review current procedures for approval of new drugs for cancer and AIDS.* National Cancer Institute, August 15, 1990.

Lauritsen, J. They left their HIV in San Francisco: A report on the sixth International Conference on AIDS. *New York Native*, June 24, 1990.

Lauritsen, J. Looking back on Berlin. *HEAL Newsletter*, Fall/Winter 1993.

Leary, W. E. Scientists optimistic on use of new therapies for AIDS. *New York Times*, June 15, 1996.

Leoung, G. S., D. W. Feigal, A. B. Montgomery, K. Corkery, L. Wardlaw, M. Adams, D. Busch, S. Corgon, M. A. Jacobson, P. A. Volberding, D. Abrams, and the San Francisco County Community Consortium. Aerosolized pentamidine for prophylaxis against *Pneumocystis carinii* pneumonia. *N Engl J Med* 323 (1990): 769–775.

Levi, J. Unproven AIDS therapies: The Food and Drug Administration and ddI. In *Biomedical Politics*, ed. K. E. Hanna, 9–42. Washington, DC: National Academy Press, 1991.

Lockman, S., R. L. Shapiro, L. M. Smeaton, C. Wester, I. Thior, L. Stevens, F. Chand, J. Makhema, C. Moffat, A. Asmelash, P. Ndase, P. Arimi, E. Van Widenfeit, L. Mazhani, V. Novitsky, S. Lagakos, and M. Essex. Response to antiviral therapy after a single, peripartum dose of nevirapine. *N Engl J Med* 356 (2007): 135–147.

Lodge, T. *Politics in South Africa.* Cape Town: David Philip, 2002.

Loecher, B. AIDS drug given another shot. *Danbury News-Times*, May 12, 1993.

Loubser, S., P. Balfe, G. Sherman, S. Hammer, L. Kuhn, and L. Morris. Decay of K103N mutants in cellular DNA and plasma RNA after single-dose nevirapine to reduce mother-to-child HIV transmission. *AIDS* 20 (2006): 995–1002.

Low, M., C. Tomlinson, M. Kardas-Nelson, K. Kim, and N. Geffen. *Fighting for our lives: The history of the Treatment Action Campaign 1998–2010.* Cape Town: Treatment Action Campaign, 2010.

Lublin, J. S. Scientists report discovering compounds that could lead to powerful AIDS drug. *Wall Street Journal*, February 1, 1990.

Luzuriaga, K., Y. Bryson, P. Krogstad, P., J. Robinson, B. Stechenberg, M. Lamson, S. Cort, and J. L. Sullivan. Combination treatment with zidovudine, didanosine, and nevirapine in infants with human immunodeficiency virus type 1 infection. *N Engl J Med* 336 (1997): 1343–1349.

Luzuriaga, K., Y. Bryson, G. McSherry, J. Robinson, B. Stechenberg, G. Scott, M. Lamson, S. Cort, and J. L. Sullivan. Pharmacokinetics, safety, and activity of nevirapine in human immunodeficiency virus type 1-infected children. *J Infect Dis* 174 (1996): 713–721.

Luzuriaga, K., Y. H. Chen, C. Ziemniak, G. Siberry, M. Strain, D. Richman, T-W. Chun, C. Cunningham, and D. Persaud. Absent HIV-specific immune responses and replication-competent HIV reservoirs in perinatally infected youth treated from infancy: Toward cure. *Conf Retrovir Oppor Infect* 20 (abstract no. 171LB), March 3–6, 2013.

Luzuriaga, K., M. McManus, L. Mofenson, P. Britto, B. Graham, and J. L. Sullivan for the PACTG 356 Investigators. A trial of three antiretroviral regimens in HIV-1-infected children. *N Engl J Med*, 350 (2004): 2471–2480.

Lyons, C., A. Mushavi, F. Ngobeni-Allen, and R. Yule. Ending pediatric AIDS and achieving a generation born HIV-free. *J Acquir Immune Defic Syndr* 60, suppl. 2 (2012): S35-S38.

MacDougall, D. S. The second conference on global strategies for the prevention of HIV transmission from mothers to infants. Global Strategies for HIV Prevention, September 2–5, 1999.

Marseille, E., J. G. Kahn, F. Mmiro, L. Guay, P. Musoke, M. G. Fowler, and J. B. Jackson. Cost effectiveness of single-dose nevirapine regimen for mothers and babies to decrease vertical HIV-1 transmission in sub–Saharan Africa. *Lancet* 354, no. 9181 (1999): 803–809.

Martinson, N. A., D. K. Ekouevi, F. Dabis, L. Morris, P. Lupodwana, B. Tonwe-Gold, P. Dhlamini, R. Becquet, J. G. Steyn, V. Leroy, I. Viho, G. E. Gray, and J. A. McIntyre. Transmission rates in consecutive pregnancies exposed to single-dose nevirapine in Soweto, South Africa and Abidjoan, Côte d'Ivoire. *J Acquir Immune Defic Syndr* 45 (2007): 206–209.

Marx, J. L. Drug-resistant strains of AIDS virus found. *Science* 243 (1989): 1551–1552.

Maugh, T. H. Studies of combined HIV drugs promising. *Los Angeles Times*, July 12, 1996.

Max Finland Award. Martin Hirsch biography. National Foundation for Infectious Diseases, 2008.

Mbeki, T. Health, human dignity and partners for poverty reduction. *ANC Today*, April 5, 2002.

McAlary, D. Study finds drug resistance fades quickly in key AIDS drug. *VOA News*, January 10, 2007.

McCaskell, T. Taking our place. *The Positive Side*, Summer 2011.

McConnell, M. S., P. Bakaki, C. Eure, M. Mubiru, D. Bagenda, R. Downing, F. Matovu, M. C. Thigpen, A. E. Greenberg, and M. G. Fowler. Effectiveness of repeat single-dose nevirapine for prevention of mother-to-child transmission of HIV-1 in repeat pregnancies in Uganda. *J Acquir Immune Defic Syndr* 46 (2007): 291–296.

McCullough, R., and L. Miller. Surveying the Global HIV/AIDS Landscape. In *From the ground up: Building comprehensive HIV/AIDS care programs in resource-limited settings*, eds. R. G. Marlink and S. T. Teitleman. Washington, DC: Elizabeth Glaser Pediatric AIDS Foundation, 2009.

McDonough, C. S. Africa court orders distribution of anti-AIDS drug. *VOA News*, March 25, 2002.

McDonough, C. S. Africa group says use of AIDS drug may harm pregnant women. *VOA News*, July 13, 2004.

McDonough, C. S. African group urges nationwide distribution of AIDS drug. *VOA News*, August 21, 2001.

McDonough, C. S. African activists sue for AIDS drug access. *VOA News*, November 26, 2001.

McDonough, C. S. Mbeki: Battle against AIDS "critically important." *World News Site*, April 24, 2002.

McGreal, C. Zackie Achmat: Profile. *The Guardian*, September 12, 2008.

McIntyre, J. A., M. Hopley, D. Moodley, M. Eklund, G. E. Gray, D. B. Hall, P. Robinson, D. Mayers, and N. A. Martinson. Efficacy of short-course AZT plus 3TC to reduce nevirapine resistance in the prevention of mother-to-child HIV transmission: A randomized clinical trial. *PLoS Medicine* 6 (2009): 1–9.

McKinney, R. E., Jr. Dr. Catherine Wilfert's indomitable will. In *Duke Magic: A History*, June 2009.

McKinney, R. E., P. A. Pizzo, G. V. Scott, W. P. Parks, M. A. Maha, S. N. Lehrman, M. Riggs, J. Eddy, B. A. Lane, S. C. Eppes, C. M. Wilfert, and Pediatric Zidovudine Phase I Study Group. Safety and tolerance of intermittent intravenous and oral zidovudine therapy in human immunodeficient virus-infected pediatric patients. *J Ped* 116 (1990): 640–647.

McMurran, K. After the tragedy, a call to arms. *People Magazine*, February 4, 1991.

Mellors, J. W., A. Muñoz, J. V. Giorgi, J. B. Margolick, C. J. Tassoni, P. Gupta, L. A. Kingsley, J. A. Todd, A. J. Saah, R. Detels, J. P. Phair, and C. R. Rinaldo, Jr. Plasma viral load and CD4+ lymphocytes as prognostic markers of HIV-1 infection. *Ann Intern Med* 126 (1997): 946–954.

Mellors, J. W., C. R. Rinaldo, Jr., P. Gupta, R. M. White, J. A. Todd, and L. A. Kingsley. Prognosis in HIV-1 infection predicted by the quantity of virus in plasma. *Science* 272 (1996): 1167–1170.

Merluzzi, V. J., K. Hargrave, K. Grozinger, M. Labadia, J. Adams, S. Hattox, K. Eckner, M. Skoog, R. Faanes, R. Koup, J. L. Sullivan, R. Eckner, and A. S. Rosenthal. Inhibition of HIV-1 reverse transcriptase by a non-nucleoside inhibitor, Abstract. *ICAAC*, October 1990.

Merluzzi, V. J., K. Hargrave, M. Labadia, K. Grozinger, M. Skoog, J. C. Wu, C-K. Shih, K. Eckner, S. Hattox, J. Adams, A. S. Rosenthal, R. Faanes, R. J. Eckner, R. A. Koup, and J. L. Sullivan. Inhibition of HIV-1 replication by a nonnucleoside reverse transcriptase inhibitor. *Science* 250 (1990): 1411–1413.

Merz, B. Aerosolized pentamidine promising in *Phenmocystis* therapy, prophylaxis. *JAMA* 259 (1988): 3223–3224.

Millenson, M. L. Cancer institute: AIDS drug unduly delayed. *Chicago Tribune*, January 5, 1998.

Miller, R. Boehringer HIV fighter drug looks promising. *Danbury News-Times*, December 16, 1994.

Mills, J. Ganciclovir for cytomegalovirus retinitis. *Western Journal of Medicine* 151 (1989): 543–544.

Mills, R. U.S. announces interim plan to help poor countries fight HIV/AIDS and other health crises. Office of the United States Trade Representative Press Release, December 20, 2002.

Mirochnick, M., T. Fenton, P. Gagnier, J. Pav, M. Gwynne, S. Siminski, R. S. Sperling, K. Beckerman, E. Jimenez, R. Yogev, S. A. Spector, and J. L. Sullivan for the Pediatric AIDS Clinical Trial Group Protocol 250 Team. Pharmacokinetics of nevirapine in human immunodeficiency virus type 1-infected pregnant women and their neonates. *J Infect Dis* 178 (1998): 368–374.

Mmiro, F. A., J. Aizire, A. K. Mwatha, S. H. Eshleman, D. Donnell, M. G. Fowler, C. Nakabiito, P. M. Musoke, J. B. Jackson, and L. A. Guay. Predictors of early and late mother-to-child transmission of HIV in a breastfeeding population: HIV network for prevention trials 012 experience, Kampala, Uganda. *J Acquir Immune Defic Syndr* 52 (2009): 32–39.

Mock, P. A., N. Shaffer, C. Bhadrakom, W. Siriwasin, T. Chotpitayasunondh, S. Chearskul, N. L. Young, A. Roongpisuthipong, R. Chinayon, M. L. Kalish, B. Parekh, and T. D. Mastro for the Bangkok, Collaborative Perinatal HIV Transmission Study Group. Maternal viral load and timing of mother-to-child HIV transmission, Bangkok, Thailand. *AIDS* 13 (1999): 407–414.

Mofenson, L. M. Protecting the next generation — Eliminating perinatal HIV-1 infection. *N Engl J Med* 362 (2010): 2316–2318.

Mofenson, L. M., J. Balsley, R. J. Simonds, M. F. Rogers, and R. R. Moseley. Recommendations of the U.S. Public Health Service Task Force on the use of zidovudine to reduce perinatal transmission of human immunodeficiency virus. *MMWR* 43, no. RR-11 (1994): 1–20.

Montaner, J. S. G., M. Harris, T. Mo, and P. R. Harrigan. Rebound of plasma HIV viral load following prolonged suppression with combination therapy. *AIDS* 12 (1998): 1398–1399.

Montaner, J. S. G., P. Reiss, C. Cooper, S. Vella, M. Harris, B. Conway, M. A. Wainberg, D. Smith, P. Robinson, D. Hall, M. Myers, and J. M. A. Lange for the INCAS Study Group. A randomized, double-blind trial comparing combinations of nevirapine, didanosine, and zidovudine for HIV-infected patients. *JAMA* 279 (1998): 930–937.

Moodley, D. The SAINT trial: Nevirapine (NVP) versus zidovudine (ZDV) + lamivudine (3TC) in prevention of peripartum HIV transmission. *Int Conf AIDS* 13: 16 (abstract no. LbOr2), July 9–14, 2000.

Moodley, D., J. Moodley, H. Coovadia, G. Gray, J. McIntyre, J. Hofmyer, C. Nikodem, D. Hall, M. Gigliotti, P. Robinson, L. Boshoff, and J. L. Sullivan for the SAINT investigators. A multicenter randomized controlled trial of nevirapine versus a combination of zidovudine and lamivudine to reduce intrapartum and early postpartum mother-to-child transmission of human immunodeficiency virus type 1. *J Infect Dis* 187 (2003): 725–735.

Moravick, A. M. Toward a common ground for activists and innovators. *Pharmaceutical Executive*, April 1991.

Morris, S. AIDS-related drug wins limited ok. *Chicago Tribune*, February 7, 1989.

Murphy, R. L. Defining the toxicity profile of nevirapine and other antiretroviral drugs. *J Acquir Immune Defic Syndr* 34 (2003): S15–S20.

Murphy, R. L., and J. Montaner. Drug evaluations antiinfectives: Nevirapine: A review of its development, pharmacological profile and potential for clinical use. *Expert Opinion on Investigational Drugs* 5 (1996): 1183–1199.

Musoke, P., L. A. Guay, D. Bagenda, M. Mirochnick, C. Nakabiito, T. Fleming, T. Elliot, S. Horton, K. Dransfield, J. W. Pav, A. Murarka, M. Allen, M. G. Fowler, L. Mofenson, D. Hom, F. Mmiro, and J. B. Jackson. A phase I/II study of the safety and pharmacokinetics of nevirapine in HIV-1-infected pregnant Ugandan women and their neonates (HIVNET 006). *AIDS* 13 (1999): 479–486.

Myburgh, J. Here is the evidence of Mbeki's denialism: A reply to the Minister in the Presidency, Essop Pahad. *Politicsweb*, July 12, 2007.

Myburgh, J. The Virodene affair (I): The secret history of the ANC's response to the HIV/AIDS epidemic. *Politicsweb*, September 17, 2007.

Myburgh, J. The Virodene affair (II): How Mbeki and Nkosazana Zuma allied with the Vissers against the MCC. *Politicsweb*, September 18, 2007.

Myburgh, J. The Virodene affair (III): How the MCC was eventually taken out, and why Virodene was nonetheless still banned in SA. *Politicsweb*, September 18, 2007.

Myburgh, J. The Virodene affair (IV): How the involvement in Virodene led to Thabo Mbeki's AIDS denialism. *Politicsweb*, September 20, 2007.

Myburgh, J. The Virodene affair (V): How the efficacy of Virodene was finally put to the test, and why the war on antiretrovirals ended. *Politicsweb*, September 21, 2007.

Myburgh, J. Virodene, transformation and the constitution. *Politicsweb*, March 19, 2012.

Myers, M. W., and J. G. Montaner. A randomized, double-blinded comparative trial of the effects of zidovudine, didanosine and nevirapine combinations in antiviral naïve, AIDS-free, HIV-infected patients with CD4 counts 200–600/mm^3. *Int Conf AIDS* 11: 22 (abstract no. Mo.B.294), July 7–12, 1996.

Ngobeni-Allen, F. AIDS@30. Harvard University address, December 2, 2011.

NIAID. HHS Secretary Louis W. Sullivan announces FDA's approval of ddI. Press Release, October 9, 1991.

NIAID. The HIVNET 012 study and the safety and effectiveness of nevirapine in preventing mother-to-infant transmission of HIV. Press Release, December 14, 2004.

NIAID. A Phase IIB randomized, controlled trial to evaluate the safety, tolerance, and HIV vertical transmission rates associated with short course nevirapine (NVP) vs. short course zidovudine (ZDV) in HIV infected pregnant women and their infants in Uganda. Press Release, July 12, 1999.

NIAID. Questions and answers: HIVNET 012. Press Release, July 14, 1999.

NIAID. Questions and answers: The HIVNET 012 study and the study safety and effectiveness of nevirapine in preventing mother-to-infant transmission of HIV. Press Release, April 7, 2005.

NIAID. Researchers identify a simple, affordable drug regimen that is highly effective in preventing HIV infection in infants of mothers with the disease. Press Release, July 14, 1999.

NIAID. Review of HIVNET 012 (A clinical trial to determine the efficacy of oral AZT and the efficacy of oral nevirapine for prevention of vertical transmission of HIV-1 infection in pregnant Ugandan women and their neonates). Press Release, March 22, 2002.

Nicholson, J., D. McCoy, M. Besser, R. Visser, and T. Doherty. Interim findings of the national PMTCT pilot sites: Summary of lessons and recommendations. *Health Systems Trust*, February 2002.

Novembre, F. J., M. Saucier, D. C. Anderson, S. A. Klumpp, S. P. O'Neil, C. R. Brown, II, C. E. Hart, P. C. Guenthner, R. B. Swenson, and H. M. McClure. Development of AIDS in a chimpanzee infected with human immunodeficiency virus type 1. *J Virol* 71 (1997): 4086–4091.

O'Brien, W. A., P. M. Hartigan, D. Martin, J. Esinhart, A. Hill, S. Benoit, M. Rubin, M. S. Simberkoff, J. D. Hamilton, and the Veterans Affairs Cooperative Study Group on AIDS. Changes in plasma HIV-1 RNA and CD4+ lymphocyte counts and the risk of progression to AIDS. *N Engl J Med* 334 (1996): 426–431.

O'Reilly, R., D. Kirkpatrick, C. B. Small, R. Klein, H. Keltz, G. Friedland, K. Bromberg, S. Fikrig, H. Mendez, A. Rubinstein, M. Hollander, F. Siegal, J. Greenspan, M. Lange, S. Friedman, R. Rothenberg, J. Oleske, C. Thomas, R. Cooper, A. de la Cruz, A. Minefore, I. Guerrero, B. Mojica, W. Parkin, M. Cowan, A. Ammann, D. Wara, S. Dritz, J. Chin, and M. Hammerschland. Unexplained immunodeficiency and opportunistic infections in infants — New York, New Jersey, California. *MMWR* 31 (1982): 665–667.

Orkin, A. Sixth international AIDS conference featured some notable absentees. *Can Med Assoc J* 143 (1990): 407–410.

Owor, M., M. Deseyve, C. Duefield, M. Musisi, T. Fleming, P. Musoke, L. Guay, F. Mmiro, and J. B. Jackson. The one year safety and efficacy data of the HIVNET 012 trial. *Int Conf AIDS* 13: 16 (abstract no. LbOr1), July 9–14, 2000.

Oxtoby, M. J. Perinatally acquired human immunodeficiency virus infection. *Pediatr Infect Dis J* 9 (1990): 609–619.

Pattishall, K. H. Discovery and development of zidovudine as the cornerstone of therapy to control human immunodeficiency virus infection. In *The search for antiviral drugs: Case histories from concept to clinic*, eds. J. Adams and V. J. Merluzzi, 23–43. Boston: Birkhäuser, 1993.

Pauweis, R. Discovery of TIBO, a new family of HIV-1 specific reverse transcriptase inhibitors. In *The search for antiviral drugs: Case histories from concept to clinic*, eds. J. Adams and V. J. Merluzzi, 71–104. Boston: Birkhäuser, 1993.

Pauweis, R., K. Andries, J. Desmyter, M. J. Kukla, J. Heykants, E. DeClercq, and P. A. J. Janssen. Potent and selective inhibition of HIV-1 replication in vitro by a novel series of tetrahydro-imidazo[4,5,1-JK][1,4]-benzodiazepin-2 (1H)-one and–thione

(TIBO) derivatives. In *Design of Anti-AIDS Drugs*, ed. E. DeClercq, New York: Elsevier, 1990, 103–122.

Pauweis, R., K. Andries, J. Desmyter, D. Schols, M. J. Kukla, H. J. Breslin, A. Raeymaeckers, J. Van Gelder, R. Woestenborghs, J. Heykants, K. Schellenkens, M. A. C. Janssen, E. De Clercq, and P. A. J. Janssen. Potent and selective inhibition of HIV-1 replication in vitro by a novel series of TIBO derivatives. *Nature* 343 (1990): 470–474.

Pear, R. Faster approval of AIDS drugs is urged. *New York Times*, August 15, 1990.

Pensi, T. Fixed-dose combination of lamivudine, stavudine and nevirapine in the treatment of pediatric HIV-infection: a preliminary report. *Indian Ped* 44 (2007): 519–521.

Persaud, D., H. Gay, C. Ziemniak, Y. H. Chen, M. Piatak, T-W. Chun, M. Strain, D. Richman, and K. Luzuriaga. Functional HIV cure after very early ART of an infected infant. *Conf Retrovir Oppor Infect* 20 (abstract no. 48LB), March 3–6, 2013.

Petra Study Team. Efficacy of three short-course regimens of zidovudine and lamivudine in preventing early and late transmission of HIV-1 from mother to child in Tanzania, South Africa, and Uganda (Petra study): A randomized, double-blind, placebo-controlled trial. *Lancet* 359, no. 9313 (2002): 1178–1186.

Pialoux, G., B. Dupont, M. Youle, B. Gazzard, S. Davies, G. F. M. J. Cauwenbergh, P. A. M. Stoffels, P. A. J. Janssen, and J. de Saint Martin. Pharmacokinetics of R 82913 in patients with AIDS or AIDS-related complex. *Lancet* 338, no. 8760 (1991): 140–143.

Pithouse, R. Report on global march for treatment access. *Treatment Action Campaign*, July 9, 2000.

Pitt researchers to investigate new drug combination for treatment of AIDS. Pittsburgh Press Release, PR Newswire February 24, 1993.

Pizzo, P. A., and C. Wilfert. Treatment considerations for children with HIV infection. In *Pediatric AIDS: Challenge of HIV infection in infants, children and adolescents*, eds. P. A. Pizzo and C. M. Wilfert. Baltimore: Williams and Wilkins, 1991, 478–494.

Positive Heroes. Vuyiseka Dubula. http://positiveheroes.org.za/vuyiseka-dubula/.

Power, S. The AIDS rebel. *The New Yorker*, May 19, 2003.

Prober, C. G., and A. A. Gershon. Medical management of newborns and infants born to seropositive mothers. In *Pediatric AIDS: Challenge of HIV infection in infants, children and adolescents*, eds. P. A. Pizzo and C. M. Wilfert. Baltimore: Williams and Wilkins, 1991, 516–530.

Project Inform. Project Inform statement regarding the use of single-dose nevirapine to prevent mother-to-child transmission of HIV. Press Release, December 15, 2004.

Raeymaekers, A., J. L. H. Van Gelder, M. J. Kukla, H. J. Breslin, and P. A. J. Janssen. Preparation and formulation of antiviral tetrahydroimidazo (1,4) benzodiazepine-2-ones. European Patent 336466, A1, issued October 11, 1989.

Rea, P. A., V. Zhang, and Y. S. Baras. Ivermectin and river blindness. *American Scientist*, July–August 2010.

Recent news about ddI. *The Body*, September 1999.

Recer, P. New compound blocks AIDS spread in test tube experiments, study says. Associated Press, December 6, 1990.

Rennie, J. Triple Whammy: Will an AIDS therapy live up to its advance billing? *Scientific American*, May 1993.

Rexroad, V. E., T. L. Parsons, F. M. Hamzeh, X. Li, M. L. Dreyfuss, P. D. Stamper, and R. H. Gray. Stability of nevirapine suspension in prefilled oral syringes used for reduction of mother-to-child HIV transmission. *J Acquir Immune Defic Syndr* 43 (2006): 373–375.

Richman, D. D. Loss of nevirapine activity associated with the emergence of resistance in clinical trials, The ACTG 164/168 Study Team. *Int Conf AIDS* 8: B183 (abstract no. PoB 3576), July 19–24, 1992.

Richman, D., D. Havlir, J. Corbeil, D. Looney, C. Ignacio, S. A. Spector, J. L. Sullivan, S. Cheeseman, K. Barringer, D. Pauletti, C-K. Shih, M. Myers, and J. Griffin. Nevirapine resistance mutations of human immunodeficiency virus type 1 selected during therapy. *J Virol* 68 (1994): 1660–1666.

Richman, D., A. S. Rosenthal, M. Skoog, R. J. Eckner, T-C. Chou, J. P. Sabo, and V. J. Merluzzi. BI-RG-587 is active against zidovudine-resistant human immunodeficiency virus type 1 and synergistic with zidovudine. *Antimicrob Agents Chemother* 35 (1991): 305–308.

Richman, D., C-K. Shih, I. Lowy, J. Rose, P. Prodanovich, S. Goff, and J. Griffin. Human immunodeficiency virus type 1 mutants resistant to nonnucleoside inhibitors of reverse transcriptase arise in tissue culture. *Proc Natl Acad Sci USA* 88 (1991): 11241–11245.

Rivers, B. KwaZulu-Natal — the saga continues. *Global Fund Observer Newsletter*, January 10, 2003.

Robertson, D. South Africa agency to appeal ruling on AIDS drug. *VOA News*, December 19, 2001.

Robertson, D. S. Africa court upholds decision on HIV drugs for pregnant women. *VOA News*, July 5, 2002.

Robertson, D. South African AIDS conference ends with renewed calls for government to provide HIV drugs. *VOA News*, August 6, 2003.

Robinson, P., D. Cotton, R. Curry, K. Henry, D. Hall, and M. Myers. Analysis of nevirapine (NVP) effect on clinical endpoints (CEs) of HIV progression or death in ACTG trial 193A, *Conf Retrovir Oppor Infect* 5: 210 (abstract no. 700), February 1–5, 1998.

Roehr, B. Articles criticising nevirapine trial may endanger babies' lives. *BMJ* 330 (2005): 61.

Roseberry, J. Catherine Wilfert Interview. *Women in Duke medicine: An oral history exhibit*, August 25, 2006.

Rossi, P. Maternal factors involved in mother-to-child transmission of HIV-1: Report of a consensus workshop, Siena, Italy, January 17–18, 1992. *J Acquir Immune Defic Syndr* 5 (1992): 1019–1029.

Saag, M. S., E. A. Emini, O. L. Laskin, J. Douglas, W. I. Lapidus, W. A. Schleif, R. J. Whitley, C. Hildebrand, V. W. Byrnes, J. C. Kappes, K. W. Anderson, F. E. Massari, and G. M. Shaw. A short-term clinical evaluation of L-679,661, a non-nucleoside inhibitor of HIV-1 reverse transcriptase. *N Engl J Med* 329 (1993): 1065–1072.

Saloojee, H. The real value of nevirapine. In *Nevirapine — godsend or drug from hell?* May 29, 2002. http://pmtct.org.za/docs/nevirapine.php.

Schneider, H., and D. Fassin. Denial and defiance: A socio-political analysis of AIDS in South Africa. *AIDS* 16, suppl. no. 4 (2002): S45–S51.

Schuler, J. Executive Profile: Digby Barrios. *Pharmaceutical Executive*, June 1985.

Schulman, S. David Z. Kirschenbaum Interview. *ACT UP oral history project*, no. 031, October 19, 2003.

Scott, E. Marinol: The little synthetic that couldn't. *High Times*, July 1994.

Sha, B. E., L. A. Proia, and H. A. Kessler. Adverse events associated with use of nevirapine in HIV postexposure for 2 health care workers. *JAMA* 284 (2000): 2722–2723.

Shaffer, N., R. Chauchoowong, P. A. Mock, C. Bhadrakom, W. Siriwasin, N. L. Young, T. Chotpitayasunondh, S. Chearskul, A., Roongpisuthipong, P., Chinayon, J., Karon, T. D. Mastro, and R. J. Simonds. Short-course zidovudine for perinatal HIV-1 transmission in Bangkok, Thailand: a randomized controlled trial. *Lancet* 353, no. 9155 (1999): 773–780.

Shapiro, R. L., M. D. Hughes, A. Ogwu, D. Kitch, S. Lockman, C. Moffat, J. Makhema, S. Moyo, I. Thior, K. McIntosh, E. Van Widenfelt, J. Leidener, K. Powis, A. Asmelash, E. Tumbara, S. Zwerski, U. Sharma, E. Handelsman, K. Mburu, O. Jayeoba, E. Moko, S. Souda, E. Lubega, M. Akhtar, C. Wester, R. Tuomola, W. Snoden, M. Martinez-Tristani, L. Mazhani, and M. Essex. Antiretroviral regimens in pregnancy and breast-feeding in Botswana. *N Engl J Med* 362 (2010): 2282–2294.

Shapiro, R. L., I. Thior, P. B. Gilbert, S. Lockman, C. Wester, L. M. Smeaton, L. Stevens, S. J. Heymann, T. Ndung'u, S. Gaseitsiwe, V. Novitsky, J. Makhema, S. Lagakos, and M. Essex. Maternal single-dose nevirapine versus placebo as part of an antiretroviral strategy to prevent mother-to-child HIV transmission in Botswana. *AIDS* 20 (2006): 1281–1288.

Sharpe, A. H., R. Jaenisch, and R. M. Ruprecht. Retroviruses and mouse embryos: A rapid model for neurovirulence and transplacental antiviral therapy. *Science* 236 (1987): 1671–1674.

Shih, C-K., J. Rose, G. L. Hansen, J. C. Wu, A. Bacolla, and J. Griffin. Chimeric human immunodeficiency virus type 1/type 2 reverse transcriptases display reversed sensitivity to non-nucleoside analog inhibitors. *Proc Natl Acad Sci USA* 88 (1991): 9878–9882.

Shilts, R. *And the band played on: Politics, people, and the AIDS epidemic*. New York: St. Martin's Griffin, 1987.

Sibert, L. Partnering with Community—Could the past hold more promise than the future? *Global Forum* 5 (2013): 31–40.

Siegel, J. E., and M. J. Roberts. Reforming FDA policy lessons from the AIDS experience. *Regulation* 14 (1991): 71–77.

Simonds, R. J., and L. Guay. Eliminating pediatric AIDS: What it will take and what it will bring. *AIDSTAR-One: Spotlight on Prevention*, April 2012.

Simonon, A., P. Lepage, E. Karita, D-G. Hitimana, R. Dabis, P. Msellati, C. Van Goethem, F. Nsengumuremyi, A. Bazubagira, and P. Van de Perre. An assessment of the timing of mother-to-child transmission of human immunodeficiency virus type 1 by means of polymerase chain reaction. *J Acquir Immune Defic Syndr* 7 (1994): 952–957.

Simpson, I., and S. Bolton. WHO publishes new guidelines on preventing mother to child transmission of HIV. WHO News Release, July 14, 2004.

Solomon, J. NIH dismissed concerns about AIDS treatment. Associated Press, December 14, 2004.

Solomon, J. NIH researcher seeks whistleblower protection. Associated Press, December 13, 2004.

Solomon, J. NIH review substantiates fired expert's concerns. Associated Press, July 4, 2005.

Solomon, J. Top U.S. officials warned of concerns before AIDS drug sent to Africa. Associated Press, December 13, 2004.

South Africa addresses AIDS. *New York Times*, August 18, 2003.

South Africa. *Global AIDS response progress report*. 2012. http://www.unaids.org/en/dataanalysis/knowyourresponse/countryprogressreports/2012countries/ce_ZA_Narrative_Report.pdf.

South Africa's Medicines Control Council may ban use of nevirapine only for prevention of vertical HIV transmission, official says. *The Body*, August 7, 2003.

Sperling, R. S., D. E. Shapiro, R. W. Coombs, J. A. Todd, S. A. Herman, G. D. McSherry, M. J. O'Sullivan, R. B. VanDyke, E. Jimenez, C. Rouzioux, P. M. Flynn, and J. L. Sullivan. 1996. Maternal viral load, zidovudine treatment, and the risk of transmission of human immunodeficiency virus type 1 from mother to infant. *N Engl J Med* 335 (1996): 1621–1629.

Stahl, J. W. A history of accelerated approval: Overcoming the FDA's bureaucratic barriers in order to expedite desperately needed drugs to critically ill patients. *Harvard Law School Third Year Paper*, March 31, 2005.

Steinbrook, R. FDA approves sale of AIDS pneumonia drug. *Los Angeles Times*, June 16, 1989.

Stern, J. O., P. A. Robinson, J. Love, S. Lanes, M. S. Imperiale, and D. L. Mayers. A comprehensive hepatic safety analysis of nevirapine in different populations of HIV infected patients. *J Acquir Immune Defic Syndr* 34 (2003): S21–S33.

Stringer, E. M., D. K. Ekouevi, D. Coetzee, P. M. Tih, T. L. Creek, K. Stinson, M. J. Giganti, T. K. Welty, N. Chintu, B. H. Chi, C. M. Wilfert, N. Shaffer, F. Dabis, and J. S. A. Stringer for the PEARL Study Team. Coverage of nevirapine-based services to prevent mother-to-child HIV transmission in 4 African countries. *JAMA* 304 (2010): 293–302.

Stringer, J. R., C. B. Beard, R. F. Miller, and A. E. Wakefield. A new name (*Pneumocystis jiroveci*) for Pneumocystis from humans. *Emerging Infectious Diseases* 8 (2002): 891–896.

Stringer, J. S. A., M. Sinkala, V. Chapman, E. P. Acosta, G. M. Aldrovandi, V. Mudenda, J. P. Stout, R. L. Goldenberg, R. Kumwenda, and S. H. Vermund. Timing of the maternal drug dose and risk of perinatal HIV transmission in the setting of intrapartum and neonatal single-dose nevirapine. *AIDS* 17 (2003): 1659–1665.

Sullivan, J. L. Prevention of mother-to-child transmission of HIV—What next? *J Acquir Immune Defic Syndr* 34 (2003): S67–S72.

Swarns, R. L. A bold move on AIDS in South Africa. *New York Times*, February 5, 2002.

Swarns, R. L. In a policy shift, South Africa will make AIDS drugs available to more pregnant women. *New York Times*, April 20, 2002.

Swarns, R. L. A move to force South Africa to give AIDS drug for newborns. *New York Times*, November 27, 2001.

Swarns, R. L. Safety of common AIDS drug questioned in South Africa. *New York Times*, November 25, 1999.

Swarns, R. L. South Africa may bar AIDS drug in childbirth. *New York Times*, August 7, 2002.

Swarns, R. L. South Africa to distribute $50 million in donated AIDS drugs. *New York Times*, December 2, 2000.

Taha, T. E., N. I. Kumwenda, D. R. Hoover, S. A. Fiscus, G. Kafulafula, C. Nkhoma, S. Nour, S. Chen, G. Liomba, P. G. Miotti, and R. L. Broadhead. Nevirapine and zidovudine at birth to reduce perinatal transmission of HIV in an African setting: A randomized controlled trial. *JAMA* 292 (2004): 202–209.

Thigpen, M. C., P. M. Kebaabetswe, L. A. Paxton, D. K. Smith, C. E. Rose, T. M. Segolodi, F. L. Henderson, S. R. Pathak, F. A. Soud, K. L. Chillag, R. Mutanhaurwa, L. I. Chirwa, R. J. Gvetadze, S. Johnson, T. Sukalac, V. T. Thomas, C. Hart, J. A. Johnson, C. K. Malotte, C. W. Hendrix, and J. T. Brooks for the TDF2 Study Group. Antiretroviral preexposure prophylaxis for heterosexual HIV transmission in Botswana. *N Engl J Med* 367 (2012): 423–434.

This week in science: Novel HIV-1 inhibitor. *Science* 250 (1990): 1315.

Thistle, P., R. F. Spitzer, R. H. Glazier, R. Pilon, G. Arbess, A. Simor, E. Boyle, I. Chisike, T. Chipato, M. Gottesman, and M. Silverman. A randomized, double-blind, placebo-controlled trial of combined nevirapine and zidovudine compared with nevirapine alone in the prevention of perinatal transmission of HIV in Zimbabwe. *Clin Inf Dis* 44 (2007): 111–119.

Thompson, M., M. Myers, M. Salgo, R. Rousseau, M. Odorisio, and M. Warburg. A master protocol to evaluate the safety and efficacy of multidrug combination antiretroviral therapy with zidovudine and zalcitabine with or without saquinavir or nevirapine for the treatment of HIV infection. *Conf Retrovir Oppor Infect* 4: 109 (abstract no. 242), January 22–26, 1997.

Top firms plan joint testing of AIDS drugs. *Wall Street Journal*, April 20, 1993.

UNAIDS. *AIDS epidemic update, December 2009.* Washington, DC: WHO Library, 2009.

UNAIDS. *Global plan towards the elimination of new HIV infections among children by 2015 and keeping their mothers alive.* Washington DC: WHO Library, 2011.

UNAIDS. *Global report: UNAIDS report on the global AIDS epidemic 2010.* Washington DC: WHO Library, 2010.

UNAIDS. *Report on the global AIDS epidemic 2008.* Washington, DC: WHO Library, 2008.

United Press International. Police arrest AIDS protesters blocking access to FDA offices. *Los Angeles Times*, October 11, 1988.

Van der Valk, M., J. J. Kastelein, R. L. Murphy, F. van Leth, C. Katlama, A. Horban, M. Glesby, G. Behrens, C. Bonaventura, R. K. Stellato, H. O. F. Molhuizen, and P. Reiss for the Atlantic Study Team. Nevirapine-containing antiretroviral therapy in HIV-1 infected patients results in an anti-atherogenic lipid profile. *AIDS* 15 (2001): 2407–2414.

Van Dyke, R. B., B. T. Korber, E. Popek, C. Macken, S. M. Widmayer, A. Bardeguez, I. C. Hanson, A. Wiznia, K. Luzuriaga, R. R. Viscarello, S. Wolinsky, and the Ariel Core Investigators. The Ariel Project: A prospective cohort study of maternal-child transmission of human immunodeficiency virus type 1 in the era of maternal antiretroviral therapy. *J Infect Dis* 179 (1999): 319–328.

Van Leth, F., P. Phanuphak, E., Stroes, B. Gazzard, P. Cahn, F. Raffi, R. Wood, M. Bloch, C. Katlama, J. J. P. Kastelein, M. Schechter, R. L. Murphy, A. Horban, D. B. Hall, J. M. A. Lange, and P. Reiss. Nevirapine and efavirenz elicit different changes in lipid profiles in antiretroviral-therapy-naïve patients infected with HIV-1. *PLoS Medicine* 1, no. 1 (2004): e19.

Van Wijk, J. P. H., and M. C. Cabezas. Review article: Hypertriglyceridemia, metabolic syndrome, and cardiovascular disease in HIV-infected patients: Effects of antiretroviral therapy and adipose tissue distribution. *Intl J Vascular Med* (2012) Article ID 201027, doi:10.1155/2012/201027.

Varmus, H., and D. Satcher. Ethical complexities of conducting research in developing countries. *N Engl J Med* 337 (1997): 1003–1005.

Vaughn, C. Diane Havlir: AIDS doctor. *UCSF Magazine*, June 2003.

Verweel, G., M. Sharland, H. Lyall, V. Novelli, D. M. Gibb, G. Dumont, C. Ball, E. Wilkins, S. Walters, and G. Tudor-Williams. Nevirapine use in HIV-1-infected children. *AIDS* 17 (2003): 1639–1647.

Vinikoor, M. Celebrating the end of the HIV/AIDS travel ban. *Health Affairs* blog, July 20, 2012.

Voice of America. S. Africa AIDS activists welcome spending increase. *VOA News*, October 31, 2001.

Voice of America. U.S. congressman slams South Africa's AIDS policies. *VOA News*, April 9, 2002.

Vyankandondera, J., S. Luchters, E. Hassink, N. Pakker, F. Mmiro, P. Okong, P. Kituuka, C. Ndugwa, N. Mukanka, A. Beretta, M. Imperiale, Jr., E. Loeliger, M. Giuliano, and J. Lange. Reducing risk of HIV-1 transmission from mother to infant through breastfeeding using antiretroviral prophylaxis in infants (SIMBA study), 2nd IAS Conference on HIV Pathogenesis and Treatment (abstract no. LB07), July 13–16, 2003.

Waldholz, M. Merck develops drug to combat virus causing AIDS: Human tests begun. *Wall Street Journal*, December 21, 1990.

Warren, K. J., D. E. Boxwell, N. Y. Kim, and B. A. Drolet. Nevirapine-associated Stevens-Johnson syndrome. *Lancet* 351, no. 9102 (1998): 567.

Watkins, J. D., C. Conway-Welch, J. J. Creedon, T. L. Crenshaw, R. M. Devos, K. M. Gebbie, B. J. Lee, III, F. Lilly, J. O'Connor, B. J. Primm, P. Pullen, C. Servaas, and W. B. Walsh. *The presidential commission on the human immunodeficiency virus epidemic report.* Washington, DC: NIH Library, June 24, 1988.

White, R., and A. M. Cunningham. *Ryan White: My own story.* New York: Signet, 1992.

Wines, M. Agreement expands generic drugs in South Africa to fight AIDS. *New York Times*, December 11, 2003.

Wockner, R. AIDS conference closes in chaos. *Outweek*, no. 54, July 11, 1990.

World Health Organization. *Antiretroviral drugs for treating pregnant women and preventing HIV infection in infants: Recommendations for a public health approach*. Geneva: WHO Library, 2010.

World Health Organization. *Antiretroviral therapy for HIV infection in infants and children: towards universal access: recommendations for a public health approach*. Geneva: WHO Library, 2010.

World Health Organization. *Global HIV/AIDS Response: Epidemic update and health sector progress towards universal access, Progress Report*. Geneva: WHO Library, 2011.

World Health Organization. WHO and UNAIDS continue to support use of nevirapine for prevention of mother-to-child HIV transmission. UNAIDS Media Center, March 22, 2002.

Wu, J. C., T. C. Warren, J. Adams, J. Proudfoot, J. Skiles, P. Raghavan, C. Perry, I. Potocki, P. R. Farina, and P. M. Grob. A novel, dipyridodiazepinone inhibitor of HIV-1 reverse transcriptase acts through a non-substrate binding site. *Int Conf AIDS* 7:108 (abstract no. M.A.1064), June 16–21, 1991.

Wu, J. C., T. C. Warren, J. Adams, J. Proudfoot, J. Skiles, P. Raghavan, C. Perry, I. Potocki, P. R. Farina, and P. M. Grob. A novel dipyridodiazepinone inhibitor of HIV-1 reverse transcriptase acts through a nonsubstrate binding site. *Biochem* 30 (1991): 2022–2026.

Yazdanian, M., S. Ratigan, S. Joseph, H. Silverstein, P. Riska, J. N. Johnstone, I. Richter, S. Norris, and S. Hattox. Nevirapine, a nonnucleoside RT inhibitor, readily permeates the blood brain barrier. *Conf Retrovir Oppor Infect* 4: 169 (abstract no. 567), January 22–26, 1997.

Zavis, A. U.S. accused of using Africans for tests. Associated Press, December 18, 2004.

Zonana, V. F. Top AIDS Drug regulator to step down: The FDA's Dr. Ellen Cooper asks for a job with less pressure. *Los Angeles Times*, December 22, 1990.

Zonana, V. F., and M. Cimons. Ease AIDS drug rules, health chief urges. *Los Angeles Times*, June 24, 1989.

Zuger, A. XI international AIDS conference: Two worlds, two hopes. *Journal Watch*, September 1, 1996.

Index

Page numbers in **_bold italics_** indicate pages with illustrations.

abacavir 250
Abbott Laboratories 182, 260, 289n65
accelerated approval of AIDS drugs 71, 90, 141–143, 155, 165, 168, 182, 211
Achmat, Zackie 216, 218, 220, 221, 232, 233, 236, 237, 240, 242, 262
acquired immune deficiency syndrome *see* AIDS
ACT UP 56, 59, 87, 92, 133, 262; Treatment and Data Committee of 92–95
ACTG 53, 54, 57, 60, 66, 69, 74, 75, 78, 81–83, 87, 88, 92, 95, 100, 113, 115–117, 119, 123–128, 131, 133, 137, 149, 151, 153–156, 158, 159, 161, 168, 174, 184, 207, 211; Community Constituency Group of 89, 90; Core Committee of 69; Executive Committee of 54, 90, 124; Master Protocol of 123–125; Pediatric Core Committee of 78, 115, 116, 118, 149, 185, 192, 253; Primary Infection Committee of 69; Working Group of 69
ACTG 076 clinical trial 119–121, 162, 191, 192, 194, 201, 253; treatment cost 197
ACTG 116A/B clinical trial 140–143, 277c14n18
ACTG 117 clinical trial 140–143, 277c14n18
ACTG 155 clinical trial *see* Concorde clinical trial
ACTG 164 clinical trial *see* Christmas tree clinical trial
ACTG 165 clinical trial 78, 79, 151–153, 246, 247, 270n31, 270n32
ACTG 168 clinical trial *see* Christmas tree clinical trial
ACTG 180 clinical trial 152–154, 206, 247, 278n34, 278n37, 278n39, 278n41, 278n45
ACTG 193a clinical trial 168, 210, 279c17n12, 280n14
ACTG 241 clinical trial *see* D'Aquila-Hirsch clinical trial
ACTG 245 clinical trial *see* pediatric salvage clinical trial
ACTG 250 clinical trial 185–186
acyclovir 9
Adams, Julian **_32_**, 32, 33, 35, 40, 42, 44, 48, 54, 57, 64–66, 80, 99, 102, 103, 112, 113, 116, 117, 121, 134–138, 260
advocacy groups 8–11, 52, 59, 63, 71, 83, 85, 86, 88, 89, 92, 95, 124, 127, 131–134, 140, 141, 152, 160, 165, 166, 178, 204, 214, 216, 224, 227, 233, 237, 239–242, 246, 255, 262; demonstration at FDA 85, 86; demonstration at International AIDS Conferences 87, 89, 90, 199, 216, 220; demonstration at NIH 89, 92; demonstration at pharmaceutical companies 91, 92
aerosolized pentamidine *see* pentamidine
African National Congress 216–220, 226, 229, 236, 242
African Renaissance 216, 219
AIDS 5–8, 13, 15, 16, 36, 91, 96, 139, 150, 178, 204, 222; barriers to treatment of 119, 204, 221, 222, 224, 226, 227, 229, 230, 232, 233, 236, 237, 240, 242, 252, 254, 255; death rate of 3, 4, 72, 108, 114, 243; epidemiology of 8, 36, 55, 72, 114, 118, 120, 156, 170, 182, 186–188, 199, 204, 214, 227, 243, 245, 247; functional cure of 247; victimization of patients 60, 61, 194, 204, 209, 238
AIDS Action Council 56
AIDS Action Now! 87
AIDS Clinical Trials Group *see* ACTG
AIDS Coalition to Unleash Power *see* ACT UP
AIDS Memorial Quilt 167
AIDS orphans 234, 254
AIDS Project Los Angeles 56
Ammann, Arthur 3, 4, **_110_**, 111, 112, 117, 147, 148, 191, 192, 198–203; first report of blood-borne HIV transmission 147–148; first report of mother-to-child-transmission 110–111
Amsterdam Cohort Study 113
Andrews, Laura 50–52, 56–58, 67–70, 75, 76, 167
antiretroviral therapy *see* HAART
Antiviral Drug Products Division of FDA 10, 57, 58, 71, 86–88, 90, 115, 140, 180–182, 207, 241, 265n39
Antiviral Drugs Advisory Committee of FDA 85, 86, 88, 115, 141–143, 146, 166, 168, 177–180, 182, 186
Ariel Glaser Pediatric AIDS Foundation 253, 291n48
Ariel Project 112, 118, 163, 200, 239
Ashe, Arthur 126
Aspen Pharmacare 239
Australian Drug Evaluation Committee 181
autoinduction 109
azidothymidine *see* AZT
AZT 8–10, 15–17, 24, 31, 34, 35, 38, 39, 45, 46, 55, 56, 64, 67, 68, 73, 74, 76, 77, 82, 85, 88, 90, 91, 97, 98, 102, 104–106, 108, 115, 123, 124, 126–131, 143, 146, 150, 153–155, 158–161, 163, 166, 168, 174–176, 197–199, 204, 206, 207, 213, 214, 218–221, 226, 238, 239, 247–249, 256, 267n8; approval of 9, 10, 14, 39, 71, 140, 141, 150, 155, 165, 219; first clinical trials of 9, 10, 15, 39, 83, 87, 118, 140; pediatric trials of 14, 15, 118, 149, 151, 157, 253; prevention of mother-to-child transmission 117–121, 162, 186, 191, 192, 194, 196, 200, 201, 212, 225, 240, 246, 253, 254; resistance to 34, 35, 39, 40, 45, 55, 67, 97, 100; side effects of 9, 30, 39, 73, 91, 118, 132, 183, 219; Thailand clinical trial of 121, 191, 194, 217, 275n62, 282n45; *see also* ACTG 076
AZT-like drugs *see* reverse transcriptase, nucleoside inhibitors of

Benkovic, Steven 62
BI Chemicals, Inc. 138, 180
BI development team 7–11, 28–36, 40–45, 47–52, 56–58, 62–64, 66–68, 97, 102; Merluzzi's leadership 28, 31, 47, 49, 50, 52, 69–71, 165
BI Pharmaceuticals, Inc. *see* Boehringer Ingelheim
BI project team 71, 76–82, 96–98, 100–103, 116, 117, 121, 124, 125, 129, 132–135, 137, 138, 140, 145, 146, 152–159, 163–165, 167–174, 177, 207, 224, 246; clinical planning 66–69, 74–76, 98, 104–109, 114, 135, 143, 185, 189, 190, 205, 212; discussions with patient advocates 95, 127, 160, 166, 177, 181; duck mascot *170*, 170, 171, 173, 178, 263; surrogate marker task force of 143–145
BI public relations task force 60, 62–65, 80, 83, 91–93, 127;
BI research team 27, 31, 32, *43*, 40–47, 50, 65, 98, 103, 124, 144, 145; Eckner's leadership 20, 47, 98; Grob's leadership 98, 99
BI 742 clinical trial (first nevirapine clinical trial) 66, 69, 72–74, 76, 77, 81, 96, 97, 100
BI 744 clinical trial *see* Christmas tree clinical trial
BI 834 clinical trial *see* Christmas tree clinical trial
BI 1011 clinical trial 279c16n8
BI 1037 clinical trial 278c14n37, 279c16n8
BI 1038 clinical trial 278c14n37, 279c16n8
BI 1046 clinical trial *see* INCAS clinical trial
BI 1090 clinical trial 168, 210, 211, 280n16
bioavailability 40–42, 44, 68, 74, 79, 100
biomarkers *see* surrogate markers
Bio-Méga 26, 28, 32, 33, 76,
Bio-Research Laboratories 268n15
BIRG-587 *see* nevirapine
BIRH-414 36, 42–47
blood bank 5, 139, 147, 148, 189; testing for HIV by 37, 91, 156, 189
Boehringer, Albert 24, *25*, 260
Boehringer Ingelheim 7, 11, 16, 60, 92, 128, 129, 205, 214, 238, 241, 260, 263; Administration Office Building of *101*, 101, 125, 159, 167, 171; Boehringer Ingelheim International GmbH 16, chemical archives of 18, 21–23, 27, 31; Manor House of 16, 17, 137; Nomenclature Committee of 63, 79; pilot plant of 29, 51, 52, 75, 101; Product Public Relations of 60, 62, 93; research and development laboratories of 16, 17, 20, 28, 29, 31, 33, 41, 49, 51, 52, 101; toxicology facilities 50, 52, 137

bootlegged drug supplies 93, 94
Bowen, John 87
breastfeeding 37, 111, 115, 121, 139, 186, 197, 198, 200, 212, 251, 252, 255
Brink, Anthony 219
Bristol-Myers Squibb 39, 40, 71, 86, 88, 91, 92, 95, 124, 126, 129, 132, 141–143, 165–167, 171, 250, 270c7n15, 275n12
Broder, Samuel 39, 40
broviac catheter 266c1n19
buffalo hump 183, 248
Burchett, Sandra 155, 157, 207
Burroughs Wellcome 9, 10, 14, 34, 39, 64, 85, 97, 126, 129, 130, 149, 267n12, 276n43
Bush, George H. W. 7, 86, 140, 141, 274n10
Bush, George W. 231, 234
butterfly effect 259
buyers clubs 94

Call to Action 200–202, 205, 213, 226, 231, 234, 235, 237, 253, 260
Cameron, Edwin *203*, 203–205, 221, 232, 262
CAPIC 134, 138, 277c13n17
Case Western Reserve University 103, 188, 189, 191
CCR5 gene 209
CDC *see* Centers for Disease Control and Prevention
CD4 cell counts 9, 13, 16, 37, 87, 91, 110, 140–145, 149, 159, 160, 162–164, 168, 175, 177, 181, 206, 211, 236, 238, 249, 271n67, 271n72, 277n4, 277c14n21, 277c14n27, 279c16n3, 279c16n4, 290n25
Centers for Disease Control and Prevention 14, 51, 72, 121, 122, 148, 249
cesarean section 37, 147, 251
Cheeseman, Sarah 66, 69, 70, 72–77, 79, 81, 82, 96–98
chickenpox 96, 156
Child Centered Family Care Clinic 252, 253
Chiron 140
Chow, Yung-Kang 123–131, 154, 155, 160, 182
Chris Hani Baragwanath Hospital 187, 222, 223, 243, 244
Christmas tree clinical trial 67–69, 75, 76, 82, 94–98, 100, 103–108, 123, 124, 134–136, 139, 140, 145, 146, 152–154, 174; split branches of 68, 69, 74, 102, 269c6n12, 270c7n11
clinical outcome trials 90, 141–143, 167, 168, 178, 180, 207, 210, 211
Clinton, Bill 234
Clinton Health Access Initiative 245
Clinton HIV/AIDS Initiative 234, 252
CMV *see* cytomegalovirus

CMV retinitis 85, 86, 90
Cohen, Ken 272n20
Colin (patient) 175, 179, 183, 280n50, 281n113
common cold 28, 60
Cooper, David 76, 160, 262
Cooper, Ellen 9, 10, 56–58, *57*, 71, 84, 86–88, 90, 115, 140, 219
community clinics 84, 86, 89, 92, 93, 133
Community Constituency Group *see* ACTG, Community Constituency Group of
compassionate use 85–87, 91, 128, 154
Concorde clinical trial 126, 130, 276n52
conditional approval of drugs 141–143, 221, 223; *see also* accelerated approval of AIDS drugs
Conference on Retroviruses and Opportunistic Infections 174, 176
Connor, Edward 119
Constitutional Court of South Africa 229, 230, 232, 233, 235, 238, 255, 262
convergent combination therapy 121–129, 154, 155, 160, 182; refuting and retraction of 130, 131
Coovadia, Hoosen "Jerry" 198, 220, 227, 236, 237, 242
CROI *see* Conference on Retroviruses and Opportunistic Infections
cryptococcal meningitis 221
cynomolgus monkeys 51
cytomegalovirus 85, 123

d4T 151, 165, 171, 284n14
D'Aquila, Richard 124, 126, 130, 131, 176
D'Aquila-Hirsch clinical trial 124, 126–129, 131, 137, 138, 143, 155, 158–165, 167, 174, 175, 177, 179, 276n25, 279c16n3, 279c16n4
darunavir 250
David (patient) 127, 128, 154, 155, 276n35
ddC 38, 40, 45, 46, 55, 58, 71, 77, 86, 94, 105, 123, 129–133, 146, 151, 259, 267n8; accelerated approval of 143, 164, 165, 278c14n35; clinical trials of 40, 86, 123, 132, 151, 275n11; side effects of 40, 133, 183
ddI 39, 40, 45, 46, 55, 58, 71, 77, 86, 88, 91, 94, 105, 108, 123–129, 146, 150, 154, 155, 158–161, 163, 171, 174, 175, 247, 267n17, 267n21, 270c7n15, 275n12, 281n113; advisory committee discussion of 142, 143; clinical trials of 39, 40, 86, 88, 123, 151, 270c7n15, 275n11, 277c14n18, 277c14n26, 277c14n27, 279n66, 279n15, 279c17n12, 284n9; expanded access to 88, 91, 92, 132, 133, 143, 276n3; New Drug

Application of 142; pediatric trials of 157, 206, 207; regulatory approval of 124, 133, 141–143, 164, 165; side effects of 39, 40, 183
Delaney, Martin 69, 87, 88, 141, 143, 178
DeLaurentis, Susan 56
Democratic National Convention 111
denialists of HIV/AIDS *see* dissidents of AIDS
DES *see* diethylstilbesterol
DHPG (dihydroxyphenylglycine) *see* ganciclovir
diabetes 44, 181, 248
dideoxycitidine *see* ddC
dideoxyinosine *see* ddI
diethylstilbesterol 118
dimethylformamide *see* Virodene
dissidents of AIDS 90, 219, 220, 230, 236, 242
Dlamini, Gugu 204
Doctors Without Borders 242
Dritz, Selma 148
Dubula, Vuyiseka 238, 255
duck *see* BI project team, duck mascot
Duke University 14, 15, 39, 118, 149, 200, 202, 253, 259
Durban Declaration 221

Eberlein, Wolfgang 267c3n38
Ebola virus 51
Eckner, Kristine 19–21, 27, 44, 65, **99**
Eckner, Robert **19**, 19–22, 24, 27, 31, 32, 34, 35, 40, 42, 44, 47, 65, 98, 259
efavirenz 250, 290n30
Eigo, Jim 87, 88
Elion, Gertrude 64, 271n60, 277n11
Elizabeth Glaser Pediatric AIDS Foundation 56, 61, 91, 111, 112, 150, 151, 163, 187, 191, 200–202, 205, 213, 226, 231, 234, 235, 237, 242, 251–254, 260
Elizabeth Glaser Scientist Awards 200
EMA *see* European Agency for the Evaluation of Medicinal Products
emtricitabine 247, 250
Engel, Wolfard 267c3n38
Epstein Barr virus 20, 148
Essack, Farid 220
etravirine 250
European Agency for the Evaluation of Medicinal Products 181; exceptional circumstances approval by 181, 207, 281n93
expanded access 40, 87, 88, 92, 94, 131–135, 137, 138, 141, 143, 165, 181, 267n21

Faanes, Ronald 269c5n27
Factor VIII 5, 6, 35
Faith Alive Foundation 3, **4**, 256
fast track drug development *see* accelerated approval of AIDS drugs
Fauci, Anthony 53, 86, 87, 88, 90, 94, 132, 250
FDA 9, 10, 50, 52, 54, 55, 60, 61, 71, 74–76, 82, 84–88, 119, 127, 132–134, 136, 140, 150, 162, 163, 166, 180, 191, 205, 206, 212, 219, 224, 228, 249; accelerated approval procedure of 71, 90, 141–143, 155, 165, 168, 182, 211; activist demonstrations at 85, 86; Investigational New Drug application to 56, 58, 69; New Drug Application to 167, 168, 210, 211; Parklawn Building of 57, 85, 86, 173; Pre-IND meetings of 57, 58; tentative approval procedure of 239; treatment IND procedure of 86, 88
Feigal, David 61, **84**, 83–86, 115, 180–182, 207, 241, 242
Fleishman Hillard 60, 62, 64
fluconazole 221
Food and Drug Administration *see* FDA

Gallo, Robert 174
gamma globulin 13, 15
ganciclovir 85, 86, 90, 270c8n15; Advisory Committee discussion on 85, 86; approval of 86; compassionate use of 85–87
Gastrozepin *see* pirenzepine
Gates Foundation 201
Gay Men's Health Crisis 56, 95
Gentille, Jamie 156, 157, **209**, 209, 210, **262**, 263, 279n64
Gerney, Brigitte 65
Gilead Sciences 250
Glaser, Ariel **14**, 13–16, 37, 55, 56, 60, 61, 91, 111, 112, 115, 127, 140, 149, 163, 209, 211
Glaser, Elizabeth 10, **37**, 37, 38, 42, 55, 56, 58, 60, 61, 90–92, 111, 112, 140, 149, 150, **150**, 151, 162, 163, 187, 200, 208–210, 234, 253, 254, 259, 260, 271n67, 271n70, 271n72, 271n74
Glaser, Jake **14**, 61, 112, 115, 149, 150, **150**, 152, 208, 209, 210, **261**, 263
Glaser, Paul Michael 16, 37, 61, 111, 208, 209
Glaxo Wellcome 176, 182, 218, 276n43
GlaxoSmithKline 238, 239, 250
Global Fund to Fight AIDS, Tuberculosis, and Malaria 231, 236
Global Strategies for HIV Prevention 191, 242; Montreal Conference of 199–202; Washington, D.C., Conference of 191–192
GM-CSF 16, 266n31
Goldrick, Sue **99**
Good Laboratory Practices 50
Gottlieb, Michael 37, 91, 111
Griffin, Johanna 99, 102, 103, 130, 144, 272n20

Grob, Peter 98, 99, 103, 124, 144, 167, 279c17n10
Grozinger, Karl **29**, 29, 30, 32, 33, 44–47, 51, 52, 56, 60, 65, 75, 78, 80, 94, 133–138, 261; kilo-laboratory of 30; pilot plant 29, 51, 52, 75, 101, 134
GSK· *see* GlaxoSmithKline
Guay, Laura 188, 189, 191, **193**, 193–198, 200–202, 213, 225, 228, 231, 232, 235, 240–242, 253–255
Gulf War 74
Guy's Drug Research Unit 218

HAART 182, 183, 210, 211, 213, 238, 243, 246–250, 256; treatment-as-prevention of 250; *see also* triple-drug regimen
half-life of a drug 41, 42, 44, 68, 74, 100
Hall, David 103, 115, 143, 160, 170, 171, 176, 177
Hargrave, Karl **19**, 20, 22–25, 27–33, 35, 41, 42, 44, 47, 63–65, 80, 98, **99**, 261
Harvard University 54, 98, 122, 123, 148, 149
Hattox, Susan 269c5n27
Hauwa 3, 4, 11, 256, 260
Havlir, Diane **104**, 103–108, 176, 261
Hawi, Amale 77, 78, 152, 153, 155, 156, 207
Health Protection Branch, Canada 76
Helms, Jesse 7
hematocrit 13
hemolytic uremic syndrome 13
hemophilia 5, 35, 36, 90, 111, 148, 152, 189, 215
hepatitis 5, 6, 7, 81, 97, 108, 109, 139, 147, 223, 248, 249, 263
herpes 6, 9, 20, 39, 51, 81, 106, 122; *see also* Epstein Barr virus
Highly Active Antiretroviral Therapy *see* HAART
Hill & Knowlton 95
Hirsch, Martin 54, 69, 98, 102, 112, **122**, 122–128, 130, 131, 154, 160, 176, 206, 246, 254, 275n5
HIV 5, 6, **43**, 123, 139, 266n39; accidental exposure to 117, 226, 248, 249; cell-based assays of 20, 21, **27**, 28, 32–36, 39, 44, 45, 52, 67, 68, 97, 102, 104, 113, 123, 151, 217, 267n41; eradication of 183, 209; HIV-1 35, 45, 46, 65, 98, 212; HIV-2 35, 45, 46, 98; integrase inhibitors of 250; mutations of 34, 35, 39, 40, 45, 97–100, 103–105, 123, 130, 144, 145, 212, 213, 272n22, 273n48; rates and infection with 3–7, 13, 15, 16, 37, 55, 112–115, 119–121, 163, 188, 197, 204, 208, 210, 211, 214, 239, 240, 251, 254, 255, 283n12; time to viral culture positivity assay of 174, 175; vac-

cines for 113, 126, 130, 246, 247, 249, 257, 262, 263; viral reservoirs of 183, 247
HIV Network for Prevention Trials *see* National Institute of Allergy and Infectious Diseases, HIVNET of
HIV protease 26
HIV protease inhibitors 26, 28, 32, 55, 76, 108, 162, 163, 165, 176, 178, 182, 206, 247, 250, 259, 260, 280n16, 290n8; side effects of 183, 184, 248
HIV reverse transcriptase *see* reverse transcriptase of HIV
HIV-RNA 140, 143–145, 159, 160, 168, 175, 177, 179, 181, 189, 197, 206, 211, 231, 273n63, 284n3
HIVNET *see* National Institute of Allergy and Infectious Diseases, HIVNET of
HIVNET 006 clinical trial 193
HIVNET 012 clinical trial 193–198, 200, 201, 205, 212, 213, 220, 224, 227–229, 232, 236, 241–243, 254, 282n44; BI audit of 225, 231, 235; complications of 194, 195, 196; data processing of 196, 197, 228, 282n61; Division of AIDS remonitoring of 228, 231, 235, 242; Institute of Medicine review of 241, 242, 289n84; open label protocol of 194; placebo controlled protocol of 191, 193, 228; Westat audit of 227, 228, 231, 232, 235, 241, 287n105; wire service criticism of 241, 242
Hlalele, Kgotso 223
Hlalele, Sarah 223, 225
Ho, David 112, 113, 182, 183, 192
Hoffmann-La Roche 40, 71, 86, 129, 132, 133, 143, 162, 176, 182, 259
Horwitz, Jerome *38*, 38–40
Hoth, Daniel 89
Hudson, Rock 204
human immunodeficiency virus *see* HIV
Hurley, Denis 220
Hussein, Saddam 74

ICAAC *see* Interscience Conference on Antimicrobial Agents and Chemotherapy
ICC 001 clinical trial 162, 279n14
ICC 002 clinical trial 162, 279n15
INCAS clinical trial 162, 174–177, 179, 180, 182, 183, 203, 206
IND *see* FDA, Investigational New Drug application to
indinavir 176, 182, 250, 281n104
INN *see* International Nonproprietary Name Expert Committee
Institute of Medicine 241, 242, 289n84
Inter-Company Collaboration for AIDS Drug Development 129, 130, 144, 162, 276n43

International AIDS Conference 7, 89, 199, 203, 212, 262; 5th in Montreal 87, 89, 123, 126, 199; 6th in San Francisco 7–9, 55, 58, 59, 63, 64, 80, 89, 90, 103; 7th in Florence 80, 81, 103; 8th in Amsterdam 103, 112, 114, 124; 9th in Berlin 126, 130, 175; 11th in Vancouver 176, 183, 186, 203, 204; 13th in Durban, South Africa 203–205, 212, 215, 216, 220, 221; 15th in Bangkok 240; 19th in Washington DC 261
International AIDS Society 191, 203, 212, 240, 262
International Nonproprietary Name Expert Committee 79
Interscience Conference on Antimicrobial Agents and Chemotherapy 62–64, 70, 80
Investigational New Drug application *see* FDA, Investigational New Drug application to
Irwin Memorial Blood Bank 148
ivermectin 116

Jackson, J. Brooks *188*, 188–191, 193, 194, 196–198, 201, 212, 213, 224, 225, 235, 240–242
Jaffe, Harold 148
Jane (patient) 120, 206, 207, 210, 211, 247, 275n55, 283c20n1, 284n14
Janssen Pharmaceuticals 59, 65, 81, 82, 100, 103, 124, 250; Research Foundation of 46
Jason (patient) 120, 206, 207, 210, 211, 247, 275n55, 283c20n1, 284n14
Johns Hopkins University 122, 191, 197, 212, 225
Johnson, Gail 215
Johnson, Magic 204
Johnson, Nkosi 215, 216, 222

Kamuzu Central Hospital 214
Kaposi's sarcoma 61, 96, 139, 248
Karl Thomae *see* Thomae
Keirns, James *41*, 41, 42, 44–46, 57, 58, 66, 68, 70, 73, 74, 107, 167
Kessler, David 88, 141, 142, 143
Kilimanjaro Christian Medical Center 251–253, 255
Kolbe, James 229
Koop, C. Everett 117, 118
Koup, Richard 65

"L" compounds of Merck 65, 81, 82, 93, 95, 99, 123, 124, 126, 127, 130, 250; resistance to 99, 100, 103, 127, 270n43
L-S 1170 24–36, 40, 45, 50, 60, 71, 267c2n28; bioavailability and half-life of 31, 40–42, 45; patent of 25, 26, 30, 31, 33; production of 28, 30, 32, 42, 44; *see also* BI development team; nevirapine
L-697,637 *see* "L" compounds of Merck

L-697,661 *see* "L" compounds of Merck
Labadia, Mark *18*, 18–28, 31, 33, 34, 36, 39–42, 47, 261, 267c3n28, 269c5n27
Lagakos, Steve 275n5
lamivudine *see* 3TC
LaMontagne, John 53, 54, 81
Lamson, Michael 107
Lange, Joep 69, 76, *113*, 113–117, 120, 121, 160, 186–188, 196, 198, 212, 213, 240, 252, 262
Large Simple Trial 133–135
Lasagna Committee 86, 90, 140, 141, 271n60, 274n10, 277c14n11
Leonard, Eileen 58
Leoung, Gifford 83
Lipner, Jay 90
lipodystrophy *see* buffalo hump
Luzuriaga, Katherine 79, 128, *151*, 151–155, 157, 206, 207, 246, 247, 261
LyphoMed 84–86

Mabale, Prudence 237
Maduna, Penuell 230
Makerere University 188, 189, 191, 193, 197, 212, 225
malaria 195, 200, 202, 221, 228, 253
Mandela, Nelson 216, 218, 219, 229, 232, 236
Mandela, Winnie 220
Maria (patient) 120, 206, 275n55, 283c20n1
Marinol 169
Massachusetts General Hospital 98, 122, 123, 126
Master Protocol 123–125, 162
Matebula, Vivienne 222, 223
Matsoso, Precious 232, 237
Mbeki, Thabo 214, 216–221, 224–227, 229, 230, 232, 236, 237, 240, 243, 245
Mbidde, Edward 192
McCaskell, Tim 87
McIntyre, James 237
Medicines Control Council of South Africa 217, 218, 220–222, 232, 233, 235–238, 240
Merck 16, 32, 33, 54, 65, 81, 82, 93, 95, 99, 100, 103, 123, 124, 126, 127, 129, 130, 176, 182, 250, 260; ivermectin clinical trials of 116
Merck 035 clinical trial 176, 182
Merigan, Tom 275n5
Merluzzi, Vincent "Jay" *17*, 17–22, 24, 27, 28, 31, 32, 34, 35, 45, 47–50, 52, 54, 56–58, 60, 62–66, 69–71, 76, 93, 95, 102, 165, 260
Mississippi baby 247, 290n8
Mmiro, Francis 188, 193–196, 201
Montaner, Julio 77, *161*, 160–162, 174–176, 179, 181, 183, 206, 207, 262
Montgomery, Bruce 83–86
Montreal Manifesto 87

Moodley, Dhayendre 187, 189, 190, 198
Moore, Malcolm 45
mother-to-child-transmission of HIV 3, 8, 35, 111, 112, 114–119, 162, 184, 186–189, 199, 200, 213, 239; first AZT clinical trial 118–121, 191, 253; prevention programs for 120, 201, 202, 205, 213, 216, 224, 226, 231–235, 237, 238, 245, 251–254, 256, 260; Thailand clinical trial with AZT 121, 191, 217, 275n62, 282n45; treatment regimens for 201, 254, 256, 291n62; *see also* HIVNET 012 clinical trial; nevirapine, prevention of mother-to-child transmission
MTCT *see* mother-to-child-transmission of HIV
Mtshali, Lionel 227
Mulago Hospital 193, 195, 196, 224, 225, 227, 228, 254
Mulroney, Brian 87
Musoke, Philippa 193
Mycobacterium avium-intracellulare 147
Myers, Maureen 53, 54, **81**, 81, 82, 93–95, 98, 100, 101, 103, 105–109, 113–117, 120, 121, 124, 127, 130, 133, 135, 137, 143, 144, 146, 153, 154, 157, 159, 160, 162, 165–168, 171, 173, 175–179, 181, 189, 191, 198, 205, 259, 260

National Cancer Institute 15, 39, 40, 53
National Education Association 6
National Institute of Allergy and Infectious Diseases 16, 53, 54, 81, 86, 94, 132; AIDS Division of 53, 54, 74, 81, 89, 124, 184, 190, 194, 196, 225, 228, 229, 231, 235, 241, 242; HIVNET of 190, 192, 194, 197, 235, 241
National Institutes of Health 20, 35, 39, 40, 53, 54, 56, 57, 60, 61, 74, 81, 85–87, 89, 94, 95, 111, 124, 142, 149, 151, 163, 174, 184, 188, 190, 192, 194, 196, 197, 212, 225, 228, 229, 231, 232, 235, 236, 241, 242, 259, 263; advisory committees of 35, 57; demonstration at 89, 92
National Minority AIDS Council 56
NDA *see* FDA, New Drug Application to
Ndungane, Njongonkulu 220
needle sticks 117, 226, 248, 249
nevirapine **27**, 36, 42, 47, 54, 74, 90, 119, 123–125, 127, 130, 163, 182, 204, 214, 221, 231, 236, 238, 250, 257, 263, 290n30; accelerated approval of 143, 156, 165, 168, 169, 177–181, 186, 206, 207, 223, 256, 280n87, 284n13, 284n15; ACT UP meeting about 92–95; ACTG presentations of 54, 55, 67, 69, 92; adult clinical trials of 10, 66, 69, 72, 73, 77, 93, 124, 126, 144–146, 154, 158, 160, 168, 174; Advisory Committee meetings of 168, 177, 178; bioavailability and half-life of 44–47, 66, 68, 74, 79, 100, 107, 125, 174, 185, 198, 211, 270c7n4, 273n11; blue specks in 136; bootlegged supplies of 93, 94; brand naming of 79, 129, 169; clinical investigator meetings of 74, 114; clinical outcome trials of 168, 178, 180, 207, 210, 211, 284n34; clinical supplies of 30, 49, 66, 75, 78, 94, 102, 103, 131–138, 152, 155–157, 165, 169, 190, 191, 205; commercial supplies of 138, 180; donation program of 205, 213, 221, 239, 285n62; expanded access of 93–95, 131–135, 137, 138, 181, 281n90; generic licenses of 239; generic naming of 62, 63, 79; hemihydrate of 78, 270n30; HIV prevention in chimpanzees 112, 113, 116, 117, 121; HIV protease inhibitor-sparing effect of 248; international clinical trials of 74–77, 102, 114, 133, 134, 160–162, 188, 212; Investigational New Drug application of 69–72, 269c6n19; liquid formulation of 77–79, 133, 152, 153, 155, 156, 165, 169, 190, 193, 207, **208**, 211; liquid placebo of 155, 190; liver toxicity of 108, 109, 146, 165, 178, 183, 179, 248, 249, 274c10n17, 274c10n18, 290n25; molecular mechanisms of 80, 103, 144, 145, 272n22, 273n48; New Drug Application of 165–167, 169–174, 176–180, 207, 224, 228, 236, 280n22; patent of 44, 113, 267c3n38; pediatric clinical trials of 10, 58, 68, 69, 74, 77–79, 94, 134, 151–158, 186, 206, 207, 211, 212, 246, 247, 270n31; pharmacologic properties of 45, 58; Pre-IND meeting of 57, 58, 67, 69; prevention of mother-to-child transmission 115, 116, 120, 165, 184–186, 189, 197, 201, 212, 213, 220, 224, 231, 237, 244, 254; public disclosure of 59, 62, 64, 65, 70, 82, 95, 100; public relations task force of 60, 62–65, 80, 83, 91–93, 127; regulatory interactions concerning 9, 10, 68–70, 75, 76, 82, 100, 128, 143, 166, 169–171, 173, 176, 177, 179–181, 207; resistance to 97–100, 102–105, 114, 134, 135, 144, 145, 152–154, 165, 176, 179, 212, 213, 224, 232, 233, 240, 256; scale up production of 44, 45, 51, 52, 94, 100, 102, 133–137, 155; selection for development 40, 42–47, 267n23; single-dose regimen of 3, 4, 185–190, 193, 194, 200– 202, 204, 205, 211, 213, 214, 222, 231, 232, 233, 235, 237, 240, 246, 251, 254–256; single-dose treatment cost 197; skin rash of 106–109, 135, 146, 153, 154, 165, 167, 169, 176, 178, 179, 183, 249, 274c10n13; stability testing of 78, 166, 167, 179, 198; surrogate marker analysis of 143–145, 168; tablet formulation of 48, 66, 73, 77–79, 100, 107, 128, 133, 135, 138, 166, 167, 169, 170, **180**, 181, 190, 206, 207, 211, 268n7; toxicology studies of 44, 45, 50–52, 56, 67, 68–70, 75, 76, 102, 103, 116, 133–138, 159, 169; traditional approval of 168, 210, 211, 223, 243; treatment during breastfeeding 186, 252; War Room for 167, 170, 172, 173; worker safety of 135
nevirapine development team *see* BI development team
nevirapine project team *see* BI project team
NIAID *see* National Institute of Allergy and Infectious Diseases
Nigeria 1, 3, 4, 239, 256, 285n62
NIH *see* National Institutes of Health
Ngobeni, Nomthunzi 186,
Ngobeni-Allen, Florence 186, 187, 243, **244**, 244, 245
Nkosi, Nonthlanthla Daphne 215
Nkosi, Xolani *see* Johnson, Nkosi
non-nucleoside reverse transcriptase inhibitors *see* reverse transcriptase, non-nucleoside inhibitors of
nucleoside reverse transcriptase inhibitors *see* reverse transcriptase, nucleoside inhibitors of
Nureyev, Rudolf 126

Obama, Barack 89, 261, 265n22
off-label prescription 8, 15, 85, 150,
opportunistic infection 6, 7, 10, 77, 83, 85, 87, 96, 108, 139, 140, 148, 186, 204, 221, 238, 247
Owor, Maxensia 212

p24 antigen 97, 100, 104, 105, 139, 140, 143, 154, 168, 272n3, 273n59
PACTG 316 clinical trial 190
parallel track 87, 88, 132; *see also* expanded access
Pascarelli, Terri 92, 93, 94, 95, 101
PCP *see* pneumocystis pneumonia
pediatric AIDS 5–8, 13, 15, 16, 35, 55, 111, 117, 147–150, 155, 186, 189, 200, 218, 222, 252; clinical trials of 10, 14, 15, 35, 58, 111, 149–151, 263
Pediatric AIDS Foundation *see* Elizabeth Glaser Pediatric AIDS Foundation
pediatric clinical research 8, 10, 14, 15, 56, 61, 69, 111, 112, 116, 149, 157, 163

Pediatric Core Committee *see* ACTG, Pediatric Core Committee of
pediatric salvage clinical trial 128, 155–157, 207, 279n48, 279n66, 284n9
pentamidine 83–85; aerosol of 73, 83–86, 91, 115, 199; approval of 86; community trial of 84, 86, 115
PEPFAR *see* President's Emergency Program for AIDS Relief
perinatal transmission of HIV *see* mother-to-child transmission of HIV
Perkins, Herbert 148
PETRA clinical trial 121, 191, 196, 198, 212, 252, 275n64
Pfizer 221
Pharma Research Ltd. 29
Phil (patient) 73, 74, 269c7n1
photoaffinity probe 80, 99, 272n22
PICNIC 134, 138
Piot, Peter 220
pirenzepine 24, 25, 30, 260, 266n57
placebo in controlled trials 14, 35, 85, 87, 121, 140, 155, 157, 191–194, 212, 228, 244, 277c14n26, 279n66
placenta previa 37
Pneumocystis carinii pneumonia *see* pneumocystis pneumonia
pneumocystis pneumonia 5, 6, 9, 61, 73, 77, 83, 86, 87, 91, 110, 111, 115, 139, 147, 148, 150, 199, 248, 265n9
Positive Women Network 237
President's Commission on AIDS 6
President's Emergency Program for AIDS Relief 234, 235, 239, 253, 288n27
Pretoria High Court 224, 226, 227, 229, 230
Project Inform 69, 87, 95, 141, 178, 262
Proudfoot, John 44, 80
Public Health Service, United States 120, 243, 249

raltegravir 250
Rega Institute 46
resistance, viral 34, 35, 39, 40, 45, 55, 67, 97–100, 102–107, 114, 117, 123, 124, 127, 130, 134, 135, 144, 145, 151–155, 161, 165, 174, 176, 179, 182, 209, 212, 213, 224, 232, 233, 240, 246, 256
retrovirus 19, 126, 182, 211, 212, 227, 238, 261, 266n39; *see also* HIV
reverse transcriptase of HIV 17, 18, 27, 35, 80, 123, 266n39, 266n46; HIV assays for 20–22, 24, 27, 33, 34, 39, 41, 42, 44, 45, 113, 267c3n28; molecular mechanisms of 80, 99, 103, 144, 145, 272n22, 273n48; mouse assays for 18–21, 39, 267n12; non-nucleoside inhibitors of 9, 35, 36, 46, 65, 80, 82, 98, 99, 100, 102, 103, 109, 113, 143, 162, 165, 182, 183, 248, 250, 268c3n46; nucleoside inhibitors of 17, 18, 22, 24, 30, 39, 47, 97, 109, 127, 151, 155, 161, 165, 182, 203, 248, 250; screening assays 18–22, 24, 25, 27, 31, 33, 36
reverse transcriptase research team *see* BI research team
Richman, Douglas *34*, 34, 35, 39, 44, 45, 52, 54, 58, 66, 67–69, 75, 82, 97–100, 102–104, 117, 176, 247, 261
rilpivirine 250
ritonavir 182, 206, 248, 260, 281n104
river blindness 116
Robbins, Frederick 188, 189
Roche Molecular Systems 140, 175, 181, 281n100, 284n3
Rose, Janice 272n20
Rosenthal, Alan 16–20, 22–33, 40, 41, 43, 50, 52, 54, 57, 58, 60, 62–66, 69, 70, 72, 79, 80, 102, 128, 135, 260
Roxane Laboratories 169, *180*, 181
Ruprecht, Ruth 118
Ryan White Care Act 262

SAINT clinical trial 190, 198, 220, 236, 237, 282n81, 286n40
Salk, Jonas 126
Samite 201
San Francisco General Hospital 61, 83, 103, 176, 261
San Francisco Health Department 148
saquinavir 162, 176, 182, 274c10n16, 281n104
Schmidt, Gunther 267c3n38
Schotze 16, 17
Schwartz, Racheline 272n20
Scolnick, Edward 129
Shih, Cheng-Kon *99*, 269c5n27, 272n20
shingles 6, 7
SIMBA clinical trial 252, *60 Minutes* 61, 111
skin rash 39, 106, 107–109, 117, 135, 146, 153, 154, 165, 167, 169, 176, 178, 179, 183, 185, 208, 249
Skoog, Mark *99*, 269c5n27, 272n20
Snow, William *93*, 92–95, 262
South Africa 1, 3, 121, 187, 189–191, 198, 204, 205, 212, 231, 235, 243; AIDS cases in 187, 188, 214, 243, 245, 254; apartheid in 187, 204, 216, 218, 236; AZT pilot program in 217–221, 226; Colleges of Medicine of 227; Competition Commission of 238, 239; Constitutional Court of 229, 230, 232, 233, 235, 238, 255, 262; Gauteng province of 222, 225–227, 233; Health Ministry of 218, 221, 224–227, 229, 237, 238, 245; KwaZulu-Natal province of 187, 189, 190, 198, 222, 227, 236; Mandela's Cabinet 216, 217; Mbeki's Cabinet 230, 237; Medicines Control Council of 217, 218, 220–222, 232, 233, 235–238, 240; national AIDS conference in 236, 237; nevirapine court case in 224–227, 229, 232, 240; nevirapine pilot program in 221–226, 229; Pretoria High Court of 224, 226, 227, 229, 230; Western Cape Province of 225, 227; *see also* SAINT clinical trial
South African Intrapartum Nevirapine Trial *see* SAINT clinical trial
Statistical Center for HIV/AIDS Research and Prevention (SCHARP) *see* HIVNET 012 clinical trial, data processing of
stavudine *see* d4T
Stefano (patient) 108, 109, 274c10n14
Steitz, Tom 99, 103, 272n22
Stevens-Johnson Syndrome 106, 183, 249, 274c10n13; *see also* skin rash
Strode, Pamela *172*, 165–174, 176–181, 211, 263, 279c17n8
Stuart (patient) 106, 273n1
Sullivan, John 20, 21, *21*, 24, 28, 32–36, 44, 45, 52, 54, 55, 57, 58, 64–67, 69, 78, 79, 103, 114–117, 120, 128, 148, 151–155, 185–190, 193, 198, 201, 206, 207, 236, 259, 260, 261
Sullivan, Louis 90
surrogate markers 139–143, 145, 161, 162, 164, 166, 168, 169; assays for 139, 140, 143–145, 174, 181
Swanstrom, Ronald 20, 21, 266n46
synergistic effect of antiviral drugs 67, 68, 98, 102
Syntex 85–87, 276n43

Tatu *251*, 251, 252, 255, 256
Tau, Hazel 238, 239
tenofovir 247, 250
tentative approval of generic AIDS drugs 239
tetrahydro-imidazo-benzodiazepinones *see* TIBO compounds
thalidomide 118
Thomae 24–26, 44, 260
Thomapyrin 24
Thompson, Conyers 87
3TC 121, 168, 176, 182, 191, 196, 198, 203, 204, 206, 212, 220, 238–240, 247–250, 252, 256, 275n64, 279n64, 279n15, 280n16, 281n104, 281n113, 282n81, 284n14, 286n40
thrush 6, 110, 147, 148, 204, 221, 238
Tiananmen Square 199
TIBO compounds 46, 47, 55, 59,

Index

64, 65, 81, 82, 103, 124, 250; patent of 46; resistance to 100, 103
Tiso, John 70–72, 98, 101, 165
Total Parenteral Nutrition 266c1n19
TPN *see* Total Parenteral Nutrition
Trade Office of the United States 234
traditional approval of drugs *see* FDA, New Drug Application to
travel ban on HIV-infected travelers 7, 89, 90, 261, 265n22, 271n52
Treatment Action Campaign 216, 218, 220, 221, 224–227, 229, 232, 235, 237–240, 242, 255, 262; Durban rally of 216, 220
Treatment and Data Committee *see* ACT UP, Treatment and Data Committee of
treatment-as-prevention 250
treatment experienced patients 161, 179
treatment IND 86, 88
treatment naïve patients 161, 162, 179
triple-drug regimen 122–131, 137, 138, 154, 155, 157–162, 168, 175, 176, 178, 179, 181–183, 186, 187, 190, 203, 204, 206, 207, 210–213, 217, 232, 233, 238–240, 243, 247, 248, 256; cost of 186, 204, 214, 217, 220, 239, 256; *see also* D'Aquila-Hirsch clinical trial; INCAS clinical trial; Merck 035 clinical trial
Trummlitz, Gunther 267c3n38
Tshabalala-Msimang, Manto 219–221, 224–227, 229, 230, 236, 237, 240, 245
Tsianco, Mike 171, 177, 178, 181
tuberculosis 77, 97, 98, 102, 123, 139, 161, 162, 195, 200, 221, 253
Tuskegee Study 192
Tutu, Desmond 229

UCLA 13, 15, 16, 150

UD-PM 0147BS 22, 266n57
Uganda 1, 121, 188–202, 212, 224–229, 231, 235, 241–243, 253; AIDS cases in 188, 214; Health Minister of 197; *see also* HIVNET 012 clinical trial
UNAIDS 121, 191, 205, 212, 220
Union Carbide corporate headquarters 28, 33, 101, 276n25
United States Adopted Name Council 63, 79
University of Alabama 124, 127
University of Amsterdam 113, 121
University of California Los Angeles *see* UCLA
University of California San Diego 34, 35, 44, 45, 66, 75, 76, 103, 108, 176, 261, 276n25
University of California San Francisco 110, 147, 148, 261
University of Massachusetts 19, 20, 24, 28, 35, 45, 57, 64–66, 70, 72, 73, 75, 76, 79, 98, 104, 120, 128, 148, 151–153, 155, 187, 206, 259, 261
University of Miami 15, 276n25
USAN *see* United States Adopted Name Council

vaccines *see* HIV, vaccines for
Vagelos, Roy 129
Vella, Stefano 76, 160, 262
vertical transmission *see* mother-to-child-transmission of HIV
viral load 82, 97, 100, 102, 103, 105, 107, 120, 125, 130, 139, 140, 143, 145, 146, 153, 159, 162, 164, 168, 174, 175, 176, 181, 183, 189, 190, 193, 197, 198, 206, 210, 211, 238, 239, 250, 251, 273n59, 273n63
viral resistance *see* resistance, viral
Viramune 79, 129, 169, 178, 180, **180**, 181, 190, 206, 207, **208**, 211, 239, 280n87, 290n25; *see also* nevirapine

Viramune donation program 205, 213, 221, 239, 285n62
Virodene 216–220, 226, 230
Visser, Olga 216–220, 226
Visser, Zigi 217–220, 226
Voltaire 256

Wainberg, Mark **175**, 174–176, 179, 203
Wanda (patient) 248, 249, 290n19
Warren, Tom 99, 272n22
Watkins Commission 274n10
Watson, Patricia 166, 279c17n8
Wellcome Research Laboratories *see* Burroughs Wellcome
Westat Corporation 225, 227, 228, 231, 232, 235, 241
White, Jeanne 5, 262
White, Ryan 5–11, 35, 58, 60, 140, 152, 211, 215, 216, 222, 262
white blood cells *see* CD4
Wilfert, Catherine 14, 15, **118**, 117–119, 149, 151, 192, 198, 200–202, 205, 213, **233**, **234**, 234, 235, 237, 253, 259, 260
World Bank 239
World Health Organization 2, 79, 114–116, 187, 205, 222, 229, 235, 240, 252, 255, 256; Clinical Research and Product Development branch of 114, 116; Global Program on AIDS of 114, 116; Model List of Essential Drugs of 222
Wright, James 48, **49**, 49, 66, 72, 77, 102, 107, 125, 133–138, 144, 166, 260
Wu, Joe 80, 81, 99, 103, 269c5n27, 272n22

Young, Frank 56

Zeegen, Susie 56
zidovudine *see* AZT
Zuma, Jacob 245
Zuma, Nkosazana 216–218

www.ingramcontent.com/pod-product-compliance
Ingram Content Group UK Ltd.
Pitfield, Milton Keynes, MK11 3LW, UK
UKHW050703160426
5217IPUK00038B/2043